LUMBAR SPINE SURGERY
TECHNIQUES & COMPLICATIONS

LUMBAR SPINE SURGERY

TECHNIQUES & COMPLICATIONS

Arthur H. White, M.D.
Director of St. Mary's Spine Center,
Senior Spine Consultant,
San Francisco Orthopaedic Residency Program,
San Francisco, California

Richard H. Rothman, M.D., Ph.D.
Professor of Orthopaedic Surgery,
University of Pennsylvania School of Medicine,
Chairman, Section of Orthopaedic Surgery,
Pennsylvania Hospital,
Philadelphia, Pennsylvania

Charles D. Ray, M.D.
Associate Director,
Institute of Low Back Care,
Minneapolis, Minnesota

With 406 illustrations and 14-color plate

The C. V. Mosby Company

St. Louis · Washington, D.C. · Toronto · 1987

A TRADITION OF PUBLISHING EXCELLENCE

Editor: Eugenia A. Klein
Assistant Editor: Lynn Gerdemann Hughes
Project Editor: Sylvia B. Kluth
Designer: Rey Umali
Production: Florence Achenbach

Copyright © 1987 by The C.V. Mosby Company

All rights reserved. No part of this publication may be reproduced, stored in a retrieval system, or transmitted, in any form or by any means, electronic, mechanical, photocopying, recording, or otherwise, without prior written permission from the publisher.

Printed in the United States of America

The C.V. Mosby Company
11830 Westline Industrial Drive, St. Louis, Missouri 63146

Library of Congress Cataloging-in-Publication Data

Lumbar spine surgery.

Includes index.
1. Vertebrae, Lumbar—Surgery. 2. Vertebrae, Lumbar—Surgery—Complications and sequelae. I. White, Arthur H., 1983-   . II. Rothman, Richard H., 1936-   .
III. Ray, Charles Dean. [DNLM: 1. Lumbar Vertebrae—surgery. 2. Postoperative Complications. WE 750 L9573]
RD768.L855   1987   617'.56   87-12402
ISBN 0-8016-5470-X

A/MV/MV 9 8 7 6 5 4 3 2 1   04/A/507

CONTRIBUTORS

Bryan Barber, M.D.
Orthopaedic Surgeon,
San Francisco, California

Sheldon Baumrind, D.D.S.
Professor, Department of Growth and
 Development,
University of California, San Francisco,
San Francisco, California

Bruce D. Beynnon
M.S. Research Engineer,
Department of Orthopaedics and Rehabilitation,
The University of Vermont,
Burlington, Vermont

Scott Blumenthal, M.D.
Division of Orthopaedics,
University of Texas Health Sciences Center,
Dallas, Texas

Neil Chafetz, M.D.
Associate Professor,
Department of Radiology,
University of California, San Francisco,
San Francisco, California

W. Bradford DeLong, M.D.
Assistant Clinical Professor,
Department of Neurosurgery,
University of California, San Francisco,
San Francisco, California

Richard Derby, M.D.
Department of Anesthesia,
Saint Mary's Hospital and Medicare Center,
San Francisco, California

Craig Derian, M.D.
Lumbar Spine Fellow,
University of Texas Health Sciences Center,
Division of Orthopaedic Surgery,
University of Texas Health Sciences Center,
Dallas, Texas

Drew Dossett, M.D.
Division of Orthopedics,
University of Texas Health Sciences Center,
Dallas, Texas

Stephen I. Esses, M.SC., M.D., F.R.C.S.C.
Assistant Professor,
Department of Orthopaedics,
University of Toronto,
Toronto, Ontario, Canada

John W. Frymoyer, M.D.
Professor and Chairman,
Department of Orthopaedics and Rehabilitation,
University of Vermont,
Burlington, Vermont

Noel Goldthwaite, M.D.
Staff Orthopaedic Surgeon,
St. Mary's Hospital,
San Francisco, California;
Research Director,
San Francisco Orthopaedic Residency Training
 Program;
Private Practice, Orthopaedic Surgery,
San Francisco, California

Robert J. Henderson, M.D
General and Vascular Surgeon,
Private Practice,
Dallas, Texas

Ken Hsu, M.D.
Attending Orthopaedic Surgeon,
San Francisco Orthopaedic Surgeon's Medical
 Group,
San Francisco, California

Hugo A. Keim, M.D., F.A.C.S.
Associate Professor of Clinical Orthopaedic
 Surgery,
Department of Orthopaedic Surgery,
Columbia University,
New York, New York

Felix O. Kolb, M.D.
Clinical Professor of Medicine,
University of California, San Francisco,
San Francisco, California

Martin H. Krag, M.D.
Assistant Professor,
Department of Orthopaedics and Rehabilitation,
University of Vermont,
Burlington, Vermont

Casey Lee, M.D.
Associate Professor,
Department of Orthopaedic Surgery,
UMDNJ—New Jersey Medical School,
Newark, New Jersey

Vert Mooney, M.D.
Professor and Chairman,
Divison of Orthopaedic Surgery,
University of Texas Health Sciences Center,
Dallas, Texas

James Morris, M.D.
Associate Professor, Orthopedic Surgery,
Department of Orthopaedic Surgery,
University of California, San Francisco,
San Francisco, California

Gary Onik, M.D.
Senior Scientist, Interventional Radiology,
Department of Neurosurgery,
Allegheny-Singer Research Institute,
Pittsburgh, Pennsylvania

Malcolm H. Pope, Ph.D.
Professor and Director of Research,
Department of Orthopaedics and Rehabilitation,
College of Medicine,
University of Vermont,
Burlington, Vermont

†Frank L. Raney, Jr., M.D.
Chief of Orthopedic Surgery,
Marshall Hale Memorial Hospital;
Associate Clinical Professor of Orthopedic Surgery,
University of California, San Francisco,
San Francisco, California

Wolfgang Rauschning, M.D.
Associate Professor,
Department of Ortopaetic Surgery,
University Hospital,
Uppsala, Sweden

Charles D. Ray, M.D., F.A.C.S.
Associate Medical Director and Chief,
Neuroaugmentive Surgery,
Institute for Low Back Care,
Minneapolis, Minnesota

R. Charles Ray, M.D.
Director, Scoliosis Program,
Mary Bridge Children's Hospital,
Tacoma, Washington

James Reynolds, M.D.
Instructor, San Francisco Orthopedic Residency Training Program;
Director, Low Back Clinic,
Permanente Medical Group,
Kaiser Foundation Hospital,
Oakland, California

Richard H. Rothman, M.D., Ph.D.
James Edwards Professor and Chairman,
Department of Orthopaedic Surgery,
Thomas Jefferson University,
Philadelphia, Pennsylvania

Jeffrey A. Saal, M.D.
Sports Orthopaedic and Rehabilitation Medicine Associates,
Portola Valley, California;
Associate Clinical Professor,
Department of Physical Medicine and Rehabilitation,
University of California, Irvine

Joel S. Saal, M.D.
Sports Orthopedic and Rehabilitation Medicine Associates,
Portola Valley, California

Jerome Schofferman
Assistant Clinical Professor of Medicine,
Department of Medicine,
University of California, San Francisco,
San Francisco, California

David Selby, M.D.
Associate Professor of Clinical Surgery,
Division of Orthopedics,
University of Texas Health Sciences Center,
Dallas, Texas

James Walter Simmons, M.D., F.A.C.S.
Orthopaedic Surgeon,
San Antonio, Texas

Robert Watkins, M.D.
Kerlan-Jobe Orthopedic Clinic,
Inglewood, California;
Clinical Associate Professor of Orthopaedics,
Department of Orthopedic Surgery,
University of Southern California School of Medicine,
Los Angeles, California

Arthur H. White, M.D.
Medical Director,
St. Mary's Spine Center,
San Francisco, California;
Senior Consultant, Spine Surgery,
San Francisco Combined Residency Program,
St. Mary's Hospital and Medical Center,
San Francisco, California

Augustus A. White III, M.D., Dr. Med. Sc.
Orthopaedic Surgeon-in-Chief,
Beth Israel Hospital;
Professor of Orthopaedic Surgery,
Department of Orthopaedic Surgery,
Harvard Medical School,
Boston, Massachusetts

---

†Deceased.

Leon L. Wiltse, M.D.
Honorary Clinical Professor of Surgery,
Department of Orthopaedics,
University of California, Irvine,
Long Beach, California

Ronald J. Wisneski, M.D.
Assistant Professor of Orthopaedic Surgery,
Hospital of the University of Pennsylvania;
Director, Department of Orthopedics,
Presbyterian-University of Pennsylvania Medical Center,
Philadelphia, Pennsylvania

Gar Wynne, M.D.
Director, San Francisco Orthopedic Training Program;
Attending Orthopedic Surgeon,
St. Mary's Hospital,
San Francisco, California

Michael R. Zindrick, M.D.
Assistant Clinical Professor,
Department of Orthopaedics, Surgery, and Rehabilitation,
Loyola University Medical Center,
Maywood, Illinois

James F. Zucherman, M.D.
Director of Orthopedics,
St. Mary's Spine Center;
Clinical Instructor,
Department of Orthopedics,
San Francisco Combined Orthopedic Residency Training,
San Francisco, California

This book is dedicated to Lloyd Taylor, Leon Wiltse, William Kirkaldy-Willis, Harry Farfan, and the other spinal surgery giants on whose shoulders we are standing as we reach for a better understanding of lumbar spinal problems.

PREFACE

This book is for you, the reader. Most books of this sort, which deal with procedures and techniques, are for the author who has mastered certain techniques and procedures and feels very strongly that those that he or she is advocating are the best.

This book is an attempt to do exactly the opposite. There is no single author. We have attempted to express every side of every issue. There is no "right" way to practice lumbar spine surgery. There are numerous techniques available and innumerable variations on those techniques.

Each of us has a different type of surgery practice and his or her own special set of talents. We must choose from our armamentarium that which will do our patients the most amount of good. A perfectly valuable surgical procedure done on the wrong patient or done ineptly may be of little or no value to the patient.

We therefore present each procedure in a variety of ways. Some procedures are presented by several authors in one section, and comments on a procedure have been made by other authors who have extensive experience with that procedure. The historical chapters further deal with each lumbar spine procedure through the perspective of time.

No one has the ultimate answer for the low back pain problem. There is no single surgical procedure that will work well for everyone. The ultimate solution to low back pain is not even surgical. It lies in prevention and conservative care. Changing the habits of our society to prevent low back pain will be a slow process. In the meantime, we have the stopgap measure of surgery. We need all the help we can get. There are a certain number of surgical tools available, and we should be familiar with each of those tools and use them as wisely as possible.

We have tried to present the surgical procedures and techniques available from a variety of standpoints. Our authors come from a broad geographical range with equally broad subspecialty training and experience in one or more of the surgical techniques. In addition, we have tried to select authors who have positive and negative experiences with a specific procedure. This might be confusing to casual reader; however, it is hoped that such an approach will provoke greater introspection before a spine surgeon "takes on" a procedure with which he or she is unfamiliar. Experienced surgeons who have mastered a specific procedure may not encounter complications that would be common for a novice.

Our desire to be successful as surgeons and our need to be right sometimes make it difficult for us to see, much less admit, our shortcomings. Great credit is due to the authors who have been able to break through the veil of optimism to help us avoid any disservice to our patients.

Arthur H. White, M.D.

CONTENTS

PART ONE: GENERAL PRINCIPLES

1. Introduction and purpose, 2
   Arthur H. White

2. History of lumbar spine surgery, 5
   Leon L. Wiltse

3. History: one neurosurgeon's viewpoint, 24
   Charles D. Ray

4. Some opinions of general orthopedists and superspecialists, 27
   Arthur H. White

5. Clinical biomechanics of lumbar spine surgery, 35
   Casey Lee

6. Normal biomechanics of the lumbar spine, 48
   Steven I. Esses, Augustus A. White

7. Surgical anatomy and nomenclature, 65
   Arthur H. White, Robert Watkins, Charles D. Ray

PART TWO: SURGICAL PROCEDURES

SECTION ONE—SURGICAL CONSIDERATIONS

8. Anatomic strategies of internal fixation, 74
   R. Charles Ray

9. Operative positioning for low back surgery, 86
   W. Bradford DeLong

10. Positioning the patient for lumbar decompressions or fusions, 95
    Charles D. Ray

SECTION TWO—LAMINECTOMY AND DISC EXCISION

11. Chemonucleolysis, 103
    James Walter Simmons

12. Microdiscectomy and percutaneous discectomy: indications, history and results, 115
    Ronald J. Wisneski, Richard H. Rothman

13. Microdiscectomy, 123
    W. Bradford DeLong

14. Exposures for lumbar decompressions and fusions, 134
    Charles D. Ray

15. Percutaneous nuclectomy, 141
    James Morris, Gary Onik

16. Laminectomy vs. laminotomy, 148
    Charles D. Ray

17. Extensive lumbar decompression: patient selection and results, 164
    Charles D. Ray

18. Far lateral decompressions for stenosis: the paralateral approach to the lumbar spine, 175
    Charles D. Ray

19. Failed posterior spine surgery, 187
    Arthur H. White, Ken Hsu

20. Disc herniations lateral to the intervertebral foramen, 195
    Michael R. Zindrick, Leon L. Wiltse, Wolfgang Rauschning

21. Methods of tissue dissection and resection in lumbar surgery, 208
    Charles D. Ray

22. Extensive lumbar decompression: autostabilization and other variations, 217
    Charles D. Ray

23. Lumbar decompression of osteophytes, spurs, and bony encroachment, 230
    Charles D. Ray

SECTION THREE—FUSION

24. History of spinal fusion, 237
    Hugo A. Keim

25. The effect of metabolic bone disease on spinal fusion, 246
    †Frank L. Raney, Jr., Felix O. Kolb

26. The technique of the bilateral-lateral lumbar spine fusion, 250
    Hugo A. Keim

27. Posterior intertransverse fusion: indications, pathomechanics, and results, 265
    Ronald J. Wisneski, Richard H. Rothman

†Deceased.

28. Spondylolisthesis, 279
    James Reynolds

29. Posterior lumbar interbody fusion, 286
    James Walter Simmons

30. Failed posterior lumbar interbody fusion, 296
    James F. Zucherman, David Selby, W. Bradford DeLong

31. Lumbar fusion with distraction rods, 306
    Arthur H. White

32. The Knodt rod: spare the rod and spoil the fusion, 315
    David Selby

33. Internal fixation with pedicle screws, 322
    Ken Hsu, James F. Zucherman, Arthur H. White, Gar Wynne

34. An internal fixator for posterior application to short segments of the thoracic, lumbar, or lumbosacral spine: design and testing, 339
    Martin H. Krag, John W. Frymoyer, Bruce D. Beynnon, Malcolm H. Pope

35. Anterior lumbar interbody fusion: step-by-step procedure and pitfalls, 368
    Bryan Barber

36. Anterior lumbar fusion, 383
    David K. Selby, Robert J. Henderson, Scott Blumenthal, Drew Dossett

37. The Raney technique of anterior interbody fusion, 403
    †Frank L. Raney, Jr.

38. Results of anterior interbody fusion, 408
    Robert G. Watkins

PART THREE—SPINE SURGERY: AN ANTHOLOGY

39. Bone grafts and implants in spine surgery, 434
    Ken Hsu, James F. Zucherman, Arthur H. White

40. Bone banking, 459
    James Walter Simmons

41. Synthetic bone graft, 471
    Vert Mooney, Craig Derian

42. Osteoporosis, 483
    Jerome Schofferman

†Deceased.

43. Computer assistance in spine surgery, 491
    Richard Derby, James F. Zucherman

44. Epidural fat grafts for the prevention of postoperative adhesions in the lumbar spine, 503
    Charles D. Ray

45. Toward percutaneous spine fusion, 512
    Noel Goldthwaite, Arthur H. White

46. Motion studies of the lumbar spine, 524
    Neil Chafetz, Sheldon Baumrind, James Morris

47. Electrophysiologic evaluation of lumbar pain: establishing the rationale for therapeutic management, 528
    Jeffrey A. Saal, Joel S. Saal

LUMBAR SPINE SURGERY

PART ONE

GENERAL PRINCIPLES

CHAPTER 1

INTRODUCTION AND PURPOSE

Arthur H. White

The study of low back pain and spinal surgery is the fastest growing subspecialty of medicine today. At least five new internal fixation devices for surgery of the lumbar spine have been developed recently. Ideas and techniques are changing so rapidly that it is difficult to stay abreast of them. The purpose of this book is to help spine surgeons understand the indications for specific types of spine surgery, the biomechanical advantages of each procedure, the technical means of performing the procedure, and the potential complications.

The lumbar spine subspecialty is bound inextricably with many other medical concerns, such as osteoporosis, metabolic bone disease, occupational medicine, pain clinics, rehabilitation medicine, spinal cord injury, spinal deformity, scoliosis, electrodiagnostics, bone banking, biomechanics, psychiatry, CT scanning, anesthesiology, and radiology. Not only are surgeons devoting their entire careers to low back pain, but now also are radiologists, anesthesiologists, physical therapists, psychiatrists, and neurologists.

Because of the rapid expansion of the spine specialties and the great diversity of the knowledge within the low back–pain field, it is impossible to keep up with all of the tools available in the successful treatment of patients with low back pain. Therefore groups of subspecialists with different interests in this field work together as units or in spine centers to more effectively diagnose and treat their patients. Each spine center has developed its own special approaches and algorithms, but no one algorithm or system has proved any better than another.

However, there are some common trends in most spine centers around the world.

The multidisciplinary trend achieves success by specialization of knowledge. Because many failures are caused by a lack of knowledge, specialization in such fields as metabolic bone disease, rehabilitation, electrodiagnostics, radiology, psychiatry, and surgical techniques can greatly raise the level of success in treating patients with low back pain.

The desire for the best "state-of-the-art" diagnostic tools has increased. Myelographic contrast materials have progressed from oil-based media to better and better water-soluble contrast media over the past 10 years. The CT scan has advanced to its third generation; now the multiplanar reformations are so good that many centers have virtually ceased using myelography. Electrodiagnostics has evolved from the use of simple EMGs and nerve conduction studies to the use of evoked potentials. Evoked responses are obtained not only from electrodes placed superficially over the spine but also from needle electrodes placed in the epidural space directly over suspected injury or disease. Diagnostic injection techniques have become progressively more popular. Discograms, rarely used 10 years ago, are now used almost universally in spine centers. Other diagnostic injection techniques, such as selective nerve root blocks, facet blocks, and indwelling epidural blocks, have become commonplace. Newer methods of placing needles, contrasting anesthetics, and placebos are being developed every day.

Another major trend in the low back-pain specialty is the search for the ultimate surgical procedure. The perfect spine surgery has not yet been developed, or we would all use only that procedure. Some surgeons are extremely competent in performing one technique, which has been perfected over many years. Since the procedure works well, they see no reason to change. Other surgeons, however, look for solutions to apparent inadequacies in old techniques. The basic laminectomy of 50 years ago has changed in many ways. For example, it has become smaller because surgeons are using microsurgical techniques and percutaneous microdiscectomy techniques. The ultimate in "small hole" surgery is chemonucleolysis. In the "bigger" direction the laminectomy has been expanded to the bilateral laminectomy, the facetectomy, and ultimately the removal of all posterior elements (the "Christmas tree" procedure).

Because of instability, fusions were added to laminectomies in various ways. At first a simple posterior fusion stabilized a segment but often "fused in" unsuspected underlying disease. The posterior interbody fusion allowed major decompression and stabilization. Others believed that more stability was required and therefore added wires and/or rods to the posterior fusion or interbody fusion. The Knodt rod and Harrington rod procedures were used to better hold stability and position while fusion took place. Greater amounts of stability then were offered by the Luque rods, intersegmental wiring, and pedicle screws. This book is intended to give the surgeon a broad look at techniques available and their variations, complications, and results. The spine surgeon should understand how to select one procedure from many so that the appropriate surgery for a specific patient will be chosen. We will not have a broad range of success in spine surgery if we keep trying to put a square peg in a round hole.

It has been demonstrated that time alone will "cure" the herniated disc 90% of the time. There are no reported surgical procedures with long range follow-up that have any better results. Perhaps surgery is indicated only in patients who are bedridden for months without improvement.

The time of 2 weeks of bed rest followed by a myelogram and laminectomy may be gone. Conservative measures can help an individual with a herniated lumbar disc to get out of bed and function somewhat normally while time is "curing the problem." We have epidural blocks and cortisone, flexion body jackets, manipulation-traction tables, gravity traction, and back schools. Bed rest can cause weakness, stiffness, and less physical and emotional ability to cope with a herniated disc. Although the occasional patient simply cannot get out of bed because of pain from a herniated disc, the vast majority can be reasonably active. If there is no improvement over many months, and if the patient finds the level of disability unacceptable, elective spinal surgery can be performed. Surgical intervention is mandatory only in the presence of progressive neurologic loss.

Lumbar spinal stenosis, spinal instability, and failed herniated disc surgery probably do not spontaneously improve with time. Conservative measures, such as exercise, injections, corsets and braces, traction, manipulation and medication, may all improve the pain and activity level of patients with these disorders. Again, if a specific patient finds that his or her life-style is too severely altered from normal despite good conservative measures, surgery may be chosen.

At this stage in our development of spine surgery education, there are not many broadly experienced spine surgeons who have crossed the multispecialty barrier. Most practicing spine surgeons who received their education more than 10 years ago learned basically one approach to the problem, which they continue to use. To learn other methods, the new surgeon must train with someone who looks at the problem in a different way. There are no good methods for accomplishing such training in our formal education system. There are some spinal fellowships available, but existing residency training programs and financial and malpractice restrictions make "itinerant training" difficult.

In this book we do not attempt to choose one surgical procedure as right or best. The choice of a particular procedure for a specific patient depends on the nature of the disease, the characteristics of the patient, the abilities of the surgeon, and other factors such as osteoporosis, blood transfusions, physical conditioning, pain behavior, job status, instruments and equipment, surgical assistants, and economic considerations. Each author presents a case for his favorite and most successful procedures and techniques. The reader then can compare the reasoning, biomechanics, success rates, and complications.

CHAPTER

2

HISTORY OF LUMBAR SPINE SURGERY

Leon L. Wiltse

This article is not intended to cover every aspect of the history of lumbar spine surgery. I do hope to touch on the early landmark advances and try to interpret the importance of these in light of subsequent developments.

In an article of this kind there are bound to be omissions of work that should be included. This is probably especially true of work done in countries with whose medical literature I am unfamiliar. For these I apologize at the outset.

While reviewing for this paper, I was again made exquisitely aware of how dependent we are for each new advance on the work of those who came before us. Many of the great advances seem to have been waiting to be made; the basic groundwork had all been done. When the discovery finally came, it often seemed to be accidental or, at least serendipitous. Even the remarkable discoveries of Conrad Roentgen[133] and Joseph Barr[11] came only after painfully slow lesser advances by other workers. Sir Isaac Newton[122] said it perfectly when he wrote in a letter to Robert Hooke, "If I have seen further [than others] it is by standing on the shoulders of giants."

Only rarely is a great leap forward precipitated by "a glimpse into infinity." I came across no such reports in this study of the history of lumbar spine surgery.

INTERVERTEBRAL DISC DISEASE AND DISC SURGERY

There is little doubt that low back pain and sciatica have been with us since antiquity. Skeletal remains contain an abundance of evidence of severe injury or disease that would surely have caused pain. Strangely, I found no mention of low back pain or sciatica in Nelson's concordance of the Bible. Perhaps in a day when terribly severe disease abounded, low back pain was not considered worthy of mention.

In Shakespeare's *Timon of Athens*,[143] when Timon is raging against his false and fickle erstwhile friends, we find the following: "Thou cold sciatica cripple our senators, that their limbs may halt as lamely as their manners." Thus the term *sciatica* appears to have been used for a long time.

An Italian physician, Domenico Cotugno,[33] gave the classic description of sciatica in 1764. He was the first to implicate the sciatic nerve as the cause. This line is taken from his article describing sciatica: "For it seems to be an acrid and irritating matter, which lying on the nerve, prays on the stamina, and gives rise to the pain." He did not incriminate the lumbar spine as the cause but believed that the pain arose from the nerve itself.

Valleix[158] in 1841 further defined the clinical picture of sciatica, describing tender spots along the course of the sciatic nerve. These became known as *Valleix's points*.

Virchow[162] in 1857 described what he called a fractured disc. This was an autopsy finding in a patient who died after a severe injury. He also described the gross and microscopic details of the intervertebral disc. In 1858 Von Luschka[164] described a posteriorly protruded disc, but he attached no clinical significance to it. Babinski[9] pointed out the frequent absence of the Achilles reflex on the painful involved side. Brissaud[20] described the inclination of the spine associated with sciatica and coined the term *sciatic scoliosis*. He recognized that at times the inclination was away from the side of the pain and at other times toward the painful side.

Toward the end of the nineteenth century a discovery was made of such magnitude that the practice of spine surgery was forever totally different. Conrad Roentgen,[133] a physicist of German ancestry who was born in Holland, discovered the x-ray while working at the University of Wurzberg. On Friday, November 8, 1895, he was experimenting with a Hittoff-Crookes tube. He had covered the tube with black paper, so no light could possibly get out, but he noticed that a fluorescent screen lying nearby glowed when the electric current was turned on. He became so fascinated with it that his wife barely got him to come to dinner that night. During the next few days he put wire and also his own thumb in the x-ray beam, making pictures of each one. He persuaded Frau Roentgen to hold her hand in the beam for 15 minutes, and a good reproduction of the bones of her hand was made on a photographic plate. Two rings on her fingers also show very clearly. This is probably the most famous roentgenogram in the world. It has been reproduced thousands of times and is remarkably good. Frau Roentgen was actually shocked and worried at seeing a picture of her bones. It seemed to her to portend death. Roentgen immediately recognized the implications of his discovery, and before the end of the next year x-ray machines could be found in physicians' offices in many places in the United States and Europe. Roentgen, true to the high scientific tradition of the day, refused to accept monetary gain from his momentous discovery. He did receive a Nobel prize and thus was compensated in the best way a true scientist could be.

To resume the saga of the disc, in 1896 Kocher,[90] a famous Swiss surgeon, reported a traumatic rupture of an intervertebral disc in a patient who had fallen 100 feet, landing in a standing position. The patient walked a few steps and then collapsed and died from visceral injuries. At autopsy Kocher found and described a posteriorly displaced disc between L1 and L2. He did not mention any possible connection between an extruded disc and sciatica.

In 1911 George Middleton,[113] a practicing physician, and John Teacher,[113] a pathologist at Glasgow University, described a case that was clearly a classical disc extrusion. A man had been lifting a very heavy plate on the deck of a ship and felt a "crack" in the small of his back. He had intense pain and was unable to straighten up. Paraplegia developed, and the patient died 16 days later from bedsores and septic cystitis.

At autopsy an extruded disc was found at about L1. Gross and microscopic studies confirmed that the extruded mass was nucleus pulposus that was pressing on the spinal cord. Middleton and Teacher described this extruded disc to perfection but, as did Kocher, failed to connect the ruptured disc to backache and sciatica.

It is easy to understand why these early physicians failed to connect the ruptured disc with the back pain and sciatica that were plaguing mankind then as now. We need only remember that these early observations were made from autopsy specimens.

Joel Goldthwait,[63] in an article published in 1911 on the lumbosacral articulation, showed how with loosening of the annulus fibrosus the pulpy nucleus could be projected backward to produce paralysis. He said that the time lapse for this displacement could be very short—weeks or even days. He included in this article a lateral drawing of a sagittal section showing a classical disc rupture at L5. He, as had others before him, failed to clearly associate disc rupture with sciatica, but he came very close because he did associate it with back pain.

In the 1920s Murray Danforth[43] and Phillip Wilson, Sr.[172] did quite a number of spine dissections. They recognized bulging discs, but, except for the hard bulging disc in the lateral canals, they did not connect them with sciatica. They also believed that a spinal nerve, especially the L5 spinal nerve, could be compressed in its lateral tunnel to produce sciatica. They even recognized that it could be compressed far laterally by ligaments, even beyond the pedicles. They described the lumbosacral ligament and called it the *sickle ligament,* which I think is a more appropriate name than the BNA name, the *lumbo-sacral ligament.* They were somewhat confused by the enlarged transverse processes noted in transitional vertebrae. They tended to believe these caused quite a bit of trouble. This is not surprising; in 1917 Bertolotti,[14] an Italian, had written about pressure on a spinal nerve due to enlarged transverse processes, which could cause sciatica. This belief was very popular for at least 20 years after Bertolotti published his paper.

Most of the surgeons of this era believed that a spinal nerve could be compressed in its lateral neurovascular canals by a buildup of osteophytes combined with narrowing of a foramen due to disc narrowing. In particular, Magnuson,[105] in addition to Danforth and Wilson, was a champion of this technique. Several surgeons even decompressed these nerves laterally by unroofing the lateral canals. A very modern concept, don't you think?

Walter Dandy,[42] professor of neurosurgery at Johns Hopkins, discovered in 1929 that nodules of discal origin could produce sciatica by compression and that their removal would cure the pain. In 1929 he reported two such cases in the *Archives of Surgery*. His drawings in this article are beautiful examples of herniated discs. He described them to perfection, along with his technique for removal, and he described how these masses produced sciatica. He even said he believed that in many cases they were produced by a series of small twisting injuries rather than by one major trauma. But he made the mistake of calling them "tumors" even though he was using the word in the generic sense since, strictly speaking, any abnormal mass in the body can be called a tumor. Because of this small mistake in semantics, little attention was paid to his article and the profession had to await the report by Mixter and Barr[114] for "the shot heard 'round the world."

Demonstrating how knowledge seems to advance in a parallel fashion in several of the countries of the civilized world, we read from an address given by Cauchoix[27] in 1978 that T.H. Alajouanine,[3] a Parisian neurologist in 1929, had a 20-year-old female patient with pain and sciatica plus a certain amount of motor paralysis. A Lipiodol myelogram showed an "impression" at the level of the third lumbar disc on the left. Surgery was performed through a transdural approach by D. Petit Dutaillis,[47] a general surgeon. A 7 to 8 mm projection was found, which was greater on the left side, and it was removed. Alajouanine and Dutaillis even said it came from the disc. They diagnosed the protrusion as a fibrocartilaginous lesion and called it a "disc tumor." The young woman recovered, but she continued to have weak ankle dorsiflexors. Again, the true nature of sciatica was not recognized, and again the relationship of ruptured discs to sciatica remained unclarified.

During the years before the publication of his classic work, George Schmorl,[141] at the Dresdon Institute of Pathology, is said to have studied 5000 to 10,000 human spines grossly, radiographically, and microscopically. In 1932 the classic book by Schmorl and Herbert Junghanns, entitled *The Human Spine In Health And Disease,* appeared. Dr. Joseph Barr,[11] a young orthopedic surgeon just out of his residency at the Massachusetts General Hospital, was assigned the job of writing a critique on Schmorl and Junghann's new book.

During June of that year Dr. Barr had a patient with what would be recognized now as an extruded lumbar disc. He kept the patient in bed, trying various types of conservative treatment, for about 2 weeks. Since the patient was not getting well, he called in Dr. Jason Mixter.[114] Dr. Kubick[11] did a Lipiodol myelogram and Dr. Mixter scheduled the patient for surgery on June 21, 1932. Dr. Barr was not present during the operation; however, on the following Sunday he stopped to see his patient, who was doing well. Dr. Barr went by the laboratory and asked to see the microscopic slides of the "tumor" that Dr. Mixter had removed. Dr. Mallory[11] had made some excellent slides that he showed to Dr. Barr.

It is essential to this story to mention again that Dr. Barr was at that moment reviewing Schmorl and Junghann's new book. The book was in German and it took him a very long time to "slog through it," as he later said. Incidentally, he memorized Schmorl's microscopic pictures of the disc. When Dr. Barr looked through the microscope that Sunday morning in June 1932, he recognized immediately that the "tumor" was actually nucleus pulposus, as Schmorl had so beautifully depicted in his photomicrographs. He and Dr. Mixter, along with Dr. Mallory, a pathologist at the Massachusetts General Hospital, studied the cases that had been done in the past few years that were called "chondromas," and related diagnoses. They decided that most of them were ruptured discs. On December 31, 1932, Dr. Barr and Dr. Phillip Wilson operated on the first patient for whom the preoperative diagnosis of "ruptured intervertebral disc" was made before surgery. A report of their observations was made on September 30, 1933, in an address by Drs. Mixter and Barr to the New England Surgical Society. Thus began the "Dynasty of the disc," as Farfan[54] has so eloquently stated.

Surgeons throughout the world quickly rushed to adopt disc removal. Workers with a bent toward basic science studied the structural characteristics of the intervertebral disc. Keyes and Compere[85] and Coventry[35] of the Mayo Clinic, in particular, conducted extensive studies of the microscopic characteristics of the disc. Arthur Naylor,[120] of Britain, and Carl Hirsch,[70,71] of Sweden, are also especially to be credited with contributing over the next 30 years to our basic knowledge of the intervertebral disc.

Love,[97] of the Mayo Clinic during the middle 1930s, developed a technique for extradural removal of the disc. It no longer was necessary to open the dura and go through both sides of the dural sheath to take out a disc.

Dr. Love[98] also presented a paper in

1939 showing how to remove the disc through a relatively small incision without removing any bone. This was a precursor of the microdiscectomy. The use of an actual microscope had not yet been described for back surgery.

In 1936 Shordania[144] introduced the concept of the "piriformis syndrome." The idea was that spasm of the piriformis muscle could cause compression of the sciatic nerve and thus cause sciatica.[13] Others followed with presentations of series of cases showing the value of piriformis section. The diagnosis of piriformis syndrome continues to be made occasionally. Treatment is now virtually always by injection rather than by surgical section. Whether piriformis spasm has anything to do with sciatica is in serious doubt today. An injection does seem to help in some cases.

In 1948 Lindbloom,[95] of Stockholm, introduced discography. This procedure has gradually gained in usage over the years but has never enjoyed really widespread popularity.[102]

Chemical dissolution of the disc was first introduced by Lyman Smith[148] in 1963. As with Dr. Barr's famous observation, which had been made possible by Schmorl's classic photomicrographs of the disc, Dr. Smith got the idea for chymopapain dissolution of the disc from an article by Thomas.[156] Thomas had injected papain into rabbits and noted that their ears drooped over. When he stopped giving the papain, their ears came upright again in a few days. Dr. Smith began his research in the late 1950s and published his first paper on chemonucleolysis in 1963. At present, chymopapain is being used fairly extensively throughout the world.[123]

Another enzyme, collagenase, was advocated by Bernard Sussman[155] in 1968. Collagenase is still in the experimental phase, but work on the enzyme is continuing.

The idea of using a microscope for microdiscectomy was introduced by Robert Williams[171] of Las Vegas, Nevada, in 1979. A very small skin incision is used, and no bone is removed. His operation differs from Grafton Love's[98] in that an even smaller approach is made, the ligamentum flavum and the annulus are split rather than partially removed, and only the protruding portion of the disc is removed. Others have modified the operation slightly. They still use a small incision, microdiscectomy instruments, and a microscope, but they decompress bone as necessary.[108]

Vascular studies of the spinal cord have contributed a great deal to our ability to operate around the spine with safety. The names of contributors that come to mind are Adamkiewecz,[2] Battson,[12] MacNab,[103] Dommisse,[45,46] and Crock.[37,38] The detailed and painstaking effort that went into their studies defies description.

It is my belief that the full import of the vascular supply to the spinal cord and the spinal nerves in their lateral canals has not been realized. Crock has repeatedly stated his belief that we are doing too much damage to the vessels that supply the spinal nerves when we do our decompressions and that this may be producing a claudicant type of pain. How to avoid this damage to the vessels and still decompress adequately remains to be learned.

The many years of painstaking research of Farfan[54,55] have been extremely important in explaining the biomechanics of the human spine. His concepts of rotary instability and the damage done by rotation were novel when first presented. They have proved to be correct and are of vital importance to our understanding of mechanical disorders of the spine.

There is little doubt that many others have contributed to the development of our surgical treatment of disc disease. Although most of the others did not describe actual surgical operations, their contributions have been vital. In particular, Roofe,[134] Inman[78] Hult,[75] Nachemson,[118,119] Graham,[64] Fraser,[56] Weber,[168] LaRocca,[94] Anderson,[5] and Spengler[151] should be mentioned. These are only a few. The literature on the intervertebral disc is mountainous.

DIAGNOSTIC TECHNIQUES

Air myelography was introduced by Dandy[41] in 1918. In 1921 Sicard and Forestier[146] published the first work using Lipiodol. In 1931 Arnell and Lidstrom,[6] of Sweden, recommended a water-soluble contrast, skiodan (Abradil). This was the first work with a water-soluble medium. This material was used for many years but never became popular because it could be used only in the lumbar spine area and required the use of anesthesia. There followed a succession of water-soluble materials advocated, including Thorotrast, Conray, Dimeray, Dimerex, and finally, in the 1970s, Metrizamide.

In 1941 Straen and coworkers[153] introduced Pantopaque, an oil-based material that remained the contrast of choice in the United States until Metrizamide was introduced. Metrizamide is still the water-soluble contrast most widely used; however, two new ones (Iohexol and Iopamidol) are being used extensively and have some advantages over Metrizamide.

The stories of the development of the CT scan and of the MRI are also interesting. In each case there was a step-by-step advance, and each forward step was totally dependent on a previous discovery that could not have been made without that discovery.

In the development of the CT scan Radon[131] in 1917 made a calculation that might have solved the problem of reconstruction. However, because the computer was not yet developed, nothing came of it. Then one evening in 1958 William Oldendorf,[124,125] a neurologist at UCLA, was at a cocktail party where some engineers were discussing an experimental x-ray machine that might be used by orange growers to detect dehydrated areas in oranges. Dr. Oldendorf believed that a similar system might show tumors in the brain and published his work in 1961,[125] which showed drawings of the basic apparatus for computerized tomography.

R.N. Bracewell,[17] an Australian radio astonomer between 1956 and 1979, made the necessary calculations for CT reconstruction, but he went no further.

In 1963 A.M. Cormak,[32] an American physicist, described the mathmatics related to Bracewell's lines but added one more critical ingredient, showing how such a reconstruction could be applied to tomography. During this time an English engineer and computer expert, G.N. Houndsfield,[74] began working in the central laboratories of E.M.I. Ltd. Beginning work in 1967, he was able to develop a functional scanner. He was exceedingly fortunate that computer technology had evolved to a level of sophistication necessary for his elaborate calculations.

The first good brain image was made in 1972. Houndsfield's breakthrough represents a fortunate confluence of engineering excellence, ingenuity, persistence, computer excellence, and the excellent facilities of the E.M.I. laboratory. In 1979 Houndsfield and Cormak shared the Nobel prize in medicine. Many believe that Oldendorf should have been included.

The history of the development of magnetic resonance imaging (MRI) is also fascinating,[147] again demonstrating that the development of most advanced techniques is a matter of inching forward, with many different scientists contributing vital fragments of knowledge. In 1869, Mendeleev,[112] a Russian, and

Meyer,[125] a German, within a few months of each other classified the 60 known elements into the periodic table. In about 1895 Rutherford,[137] a New Zealander working at Cambridge, discovered alpha, beta, and gamma radiation. He was the first to show that the atom had a nucleus that contained all of its positive charges. In 1913 Niels Bohr,[147] working at Cambridge, postulated that each atom had a number of electrons equal to the number of positive charges in the nucleus, which proved to be correct.

In 1952 Block,[15] at Stanford, and Purcell,[129] at Harvard, shared a Nobel prize for the discovery of the nuclear magnetic resonance (NMR) phenomenon.

In 1972 Damadian,[40] an American, patented an imaging device using the NMR principle. Others gradually pushed MRI to the point of medical usefulness. Moore and Hinshaw,[116] physicists at Nottingham, England, in particular are to be credited because they constructed a unit that produced the first head scan using MRI on May 18, 1979. A group at Aberdeen, Scotland, headed by Ried,[132] developed a unit that would give clearer and sharper images of the thorax and abdomen. They demonstrated this in the fall of 1980, 111 years after the publication of the periodic table by Mendeleev and Meyer.

Of course, our armamentarium is replete with other diagnostic techniques not available in 1932, when Joseph Barr made his epic observation. Among these are the electromyograph, conduction velocity studies, somatosensory evoked potentials, the various types of bone scan, and the ultrasonic,[22] which can be adapted for spine work. Mooney[115] has described a pain drawing that is very valuable in the diagnosis of the cause of low back symptoms. Wadell[165] has published a valuable study on the evaluation of spine pain by the nonorganic physical signs that the patient shows.

I believe our diagnostic abilities have reached a level of sophistication where to "explore" the back without knowing what is likely to be found before surgery is no longer acceptable.

LUMBAR SPINAL FUSION

The history of spinal fusion really begins in New York, with Fred Albee[4] and Russell Hibbs.[69] Each published the results of his spinal fusions in 1911. However, Albee probably antedated Hibbs by a short time. The fusion methods that they devised had been preceded by the attempts of several other surgeons to stabilize portions of the spine. In 1891, Berthold Hadra,[65] of Galveston, had successfully used wires wound around adjacent spinous processes in a case of fracture dislocation of the cervical spine. Hadra modestly gave credit to Dr. W. Wilkins,[65] who had performed a similar operation on the twelfth thoracic and first lumbar vertebrae previously with success. Fritz Lange,[93] of Munich, as early as 1909 tried to stabilize the spine by tying celluloid bars and later steel bars to the sides of the spinous processes, using silk and later steel wire. This was before the day of inert metals, and when metal was used for internal fixation, it was a race between the bony healing and liquification of the bone around the internal fixation device. Interestingly, Fritz Langes' idea[93] of using steel rods tied onto the spine with wire has a very modern ring, does it not?

Albee's method of fusion consisted of obtaining a strip of autogenous tibia, splitting the spinous processes, and laying the strip of tibia between the two halves of the spinous processes. He then sutured the soft tissues together very securely. Albee even designed a sterilizable motor saw to remove the strip of tibia. Hibbs's concept was in some ways more advanced. He denuded the laminae and feathered the bone, overlapping the bony strips. He did not get bone grafts from other sources, at least for the first several years.

Willis Campbell,[26] of Memphis, described his method of trisacral fusion in the mid-1920s. In this operation he tamped bone clear to the tips of the transverse processes of L5. He also used the principal of taking strips of iliac crest for graft. Later, it was natural to push bone out onto the transverse processes from L4 to S1 in doing lumbar spinal fusions. In a publication by Ghormley[60] in 1933, the use of iliac crest for graft was advocated and henceforth became the procedure of choice for most situations where autologous bone graft was needed. Strangely, it took 35 years after Campbell had described the placing of bone graft out to the tips of L5 before transverse process fusion became commonly used. Many older surgeons never stopped using simple posterior fusion as described by Hibbs, perhaps with some iliac crest graft added, even though including the transverse processes improved the fusion rate remarkably.

In 1948 Cleveland and Bosworth[28] recommended repairing pseudoarthrosis by going through the midline, exposing the transverse processes on only one side, and putting autologous iliac strips over this area. For some reason they did not place graft on both sides. Obviously, using both sides was a simple progression of the technique.[109] Reading their article emboldened me to start pushing bone graft out onto the transverse processes.

Melvin Watkins[167] in 1953 became the first to recommend approaching the transverse processes from far lateral. He approached the spine completely lateral to the sacrospinalis group of muscles. He recommended denuding the transverse processes and the lateral masses and laying a large slab of iliac crest along this area, fixing this slab of bone with screws. However, as early as 1936 Mathieu and Demirleau,[107] two French surgeons, had advocated far lateral grafting. They recommended driving a peg through a hole in the wing of the ilium and on over the transverse process. A small hole had to be made in the slab of graft to admit the transverse process. This procedure never gained popularity because it was technically difficult and fairly dangerous to the spinal nerve, which passes just anterior to the transverse process. The fact that such an operation could be done encouraged others to go out far laterally. Later, the sacrospinalis was split longitudinally in the cleft between the multifidous and the longisimus to reach the transverse processes and the lateral masses.[175]

Remarkable studies have been made in an effort to determine the effectiveness of spinal fusion in the relief of back pain. The work of DePalma and Rothman,[44] Rothman and Booth[135] in Philadelphia, Young[177] at the Mayo Clinic, and Frymoyer[58] at the University of Vermont should be mentioned.

METALLIC IMPLANTS

Up until the mid-1930s, surgeons had struggled with various materials for internal fixation. Gold did not produce electrolysis, but it was too soft and too expensive. Nothing worked well, and most devices had to be removed before they had really done their work.

In 1939 Venable and Stuck,[159] of San Antonio, Texas, published their brilliant work on the use of vitallium for internal fixation. They had studied this for several years before the book was published. Vitallium is a chrome-cobalt alloy that had been developed by dentists for mouth braces. Other metals used in the mouth had caused electrolysis, and fillings would loosen as a result. This was a remarkable step forward, because it made internal fixation really feasible.

Stainless steel was developed in the late 1930s, and of course other metals such as titanium and tantalum have evolved since. In addition, methylmethacrylate, other plastics, and ceramic have been introduced in the last 30 years.

INTERNAL FIXATION OF THE LUMBAR SPINE

As mentioned earlier, at the turn of the century, Hadra, Wilkins, and Lange had used internal fixation in the spine. Albee's graft was a form of internal fixation, but it was a slab of tibial bone. During the 1930s Phillip Wilson, Sr.[173] published his work describing the use of a plate that he bolted to the spinous processes, usually with a graft on one side and the plate on the other. However, this system was never very successful. The next step in the use of internal fixation of the lumbar spine was made by Don King,[86] of San Francisco, also during the late 1930s. He recommended using screws through the facets and first published his work in 1944. In 1959, Boucher,[16] of Vancouver, improved on the procedure by aiming the screws more medially so they went down into the pedicles; if driven further they would come out anterior to the base of the transverse processes. The plan, of course, was to keep them inside the bone.

The next great advance in spinal internal fixation was made by Harrington.[67,68] Although his rods are used much more extensively in scoliosis of the young, they may be used in the lumbar spine. Knodt[89] rods were developed in the 1950s and are used in the lumbar spine. The Luque[99,100] system, which consists of sublaminar wires and posterior rods, was developed during the 1970s. R. Judet,[82] since 1964, Roy-Camille,[136] since 1970, and Rene Louis,[96] since 1972, of France, have pursued the use of pedicle screws and plates. In the late 1970s Magerl[104] developed a system in which he inserted Schanz screws into the pedicles either percutaneously or by direct vision. These are held in place by an external fixator resembling a Hofmann apparatus. This system has been modified by Dyck[48] and others so that the fixator is internalized. Arthur Steffee,[152] of Cleveland, Ohio, since 1983 has also been working on a system of internal fixation by pedicle screws and plates. The Steffee system is being used experimentally now. Kraag,[91] working in Frymoyer's laboratory, has developed the Vermont System, which uses pedicle screws and connecting bars. The Edwards[49] system uses sacral screws fastened to Harrington-type rods. Marc Asher[8] has developed a plate that fastens to the sacrum by screws into the sacral pedicles. This plate serves as an anchor for Harrington-type rods. Zielke[178] has modified his screws slightly so they can be used in the pedicles and attached to his standard rods. Cotrel and Dubausset[34] have developed pedicle screws that can be attached to their posterior fixation rods. These are also valuable for reduction of scoliosis. At least two groups in Sweden[126] are working on the development of pedicle screw fixation. Kaneda,[83] of Japan, has developed pedicle screws that fasten to posterior rods.

Saillant,[139] Kraag,[91] and Zindrick[179,180] have studied pedicle anatomy extensively, especially as to size, shape, and direction of the pedicles at various levels. They have measured pull-out strength of various screw placements, including toggle strength and bone strength in various human age-groups.

Pedicle screws appear to have become safe enough for use by surgeons with special training in their insertion. Currently, there are at least 15 centers worldwide working on pedicle screws with either rods or plates. It is likely that the pedicle will be a most important area for attachment of screws to the vertebral body. With refinement and modification of existing systems, most of the necessary knowledge is now available for successful internal fixation of the lumbar spine by using the pedicles. Recognizing that the population is getting older and that older spines collapse, it is imperative that some method of internal fixation be found that will produce stability. If we are to decompress spinal stenosis adequately, we must find a method of internal fixation that will support the spine even though posterior bony stability has been lost. Until we find some chemical means of preventing osteoporosis, and perhaps even disc degeneration, internal support is the next best thing.

ANTERIOR INTERBODY FUSION

In 1933 Burns,[24] of Great Britain, performed a successful interbody fusion on a case of spondylolisthesis in a 14-year-old boy. He reported this in *Lancet* June 10 of that year. He drove an autogenous tibial peg from the abdominal aspect of the fifth lumbar vertebra into the sacrum. This is the first report of interbody fusion that I could find. There is a report of a Russian surgeon performing a similar procedure at about the same time, although I have been unable to find a reference. Jenkins,[81] of New Zealand, in 1935 reported a similar case to that of Burns, but he attempted to reduce the spondylolisthesis by extension, traction, and then fusion. Walter Mercer[111] of Edinburgh, reported his largely similar experiences in 1936.

In the years since, many modifications have been made. For instance, the retroperitoneal approach was described by Harman,[66] and of course it has its advantages. For the case of high grade spondylolisthesis, Freebody[57] reported the use of a large iliac graft, nearly filling the bodies of L5 and S1, instead of the tibial peg. In most surgeons' experience, the Freebody operation has worked very well. However, because the graft is soft the patient must be kept horizontal in plaster shells for 6 weeks. For cases of spondylolisthesis where there is virtually no slip, or for disc disease, the use of a hole saw and plugs have been reported. Paul Harmon,[66] in particular, has used this technique. More recently, Harry Crock,[37,38,39] of Australia, has developed a very elegant system for interbody fusion using a hole saw and perfectly fitted iliac grafts. His iliac grafts differ from others in that they are removed from the ilium from the crest downward.

Another surgeon who has been prominent in the development of the anterior interbody fusion of Hodgson,[72,73] of Hong Kong. He started his work with tuberculosis but extended it to intervertebral disc disease.

Even as early as the 1880s, anterior approaches to the vertebral column for the draining of tuberculous abcesses were fairly common, but it was a Japanese surgeon, Professor Ito,[77] who in 1934 refined the approach to the vertebral bodies to excise tuberculous tissue. His approach laid the groundwork for later surgeons' more complex procedures.

Horseshoe-shaped grafts from the iliac crest for use in the interbody area have been described by Goldner[61,62] and others. These grafts succeed well only if at least four or five grafts can be placed in the interbody space. They can be used best for disc disease or low grade spondylolisthesis since they need two large opposing vertebral surfaces.[166] Obviously, cases of high grade spondylolisthesis are not suitable. Fibular pegs are very successful when inserted in the vertical position under heavy pressure. If they tip over onto their sides, they will usually fail to fuse. Frank Raney,[130] of San Francisco, during the middle 1950s described his technique of using a large rectangular-shaped iliac graft in the posterior portion of the interbody space with three or four fibular struts anteriorly. These succeeded well.

Humphries,[76] of Cleveland, was the first to use a plate for anterior interbody fusion. During the 1950s he designed a compression plate that was fastened onto the anterior surfaces of the vertebra by screws. These were used especially at the lumbosacral joint. However, these plates have not been used to any great extent because of difficulty of application and possible danger to the great vessels.

Rene Louis[96] has recently described the use of a compression screw placed across the two vertebrae he is fusing from the anterior route.

POSTERIOR LUMBAR INTERBODY FUSION

The first published report I could find on the posterior lumbar interbody fusion (PLIF) was by Briggs and Milligan[19] in 1944. In the early 1940s these surgeons started packing bone between the vertebral bodies after discectomy. However, they believed the procedure did not work well because fusion failed. When they combined this procedure with a posterior fusion, they were then able to obtain solid fusion in most cases.

Cloward[29,30,31] reported that he had done a posterior lumbar interbody fusion in 1940, but he then did not do another until 1943. Irwin Jaslow,[80] an orthopaedic surgeon, in 1946 published his experiences with posterior lumbar interbody fusion. Thus began the PLIF. The Cloward operation is the classic. The problem with Jaslow's procedure, and others where fragments of local bone were tamped in, was that solid arthrodesis usually failed to result. This small amount of bone probably was no better regarding relief of pain than an ordinary discectomy and had the added disadvantage that these pieces of bone might migrate posteriorly.

There have been several other modifications of the PLIF since Briggs and Milligan made their report. These include the use of large autologous iliac crest grafts, large homologous iliac crest or tibial grafts and even small grape nut–like cancellous autologous or homologous grafts. Plug cutters were used posteriorly by Wiltberger[174] as early as 1957, and more recently Ma and Paulson[102] have advocated box chisels to place grafts in the interbody area from the posterior route. Recently, Selby[145] has adapted the Crock system for use from a posterior approach.

At present the PLIF is increasingly used in quite a number of centers throughout the world. It is another procedure that should be used only by those who have taken a special interest in its technical details.

FUSION OF THE SACROILIAC JOINT

There was a time in the 1920s when fusion of the sacroiliac joint was the surgical procedure of choice for low back pain and sciatica. Both Smith-Peterson[149] and Willis Campbell[26] wrote on the subject. Each described techniques of sacroiliac fusion. After surgery the patient was kept in bed, usually in a cast, for from 6 weeks to 3 months, and was then allowed up in a corset. Actually, the results were fairly good; at least two reports indicate that the good or excellent results were as high as 70%. It is very possible that if we were to put our present day disc patients to bed for 2 to 3 months, 70% would declare themselves well.

With the description of the herniated disc by Mixter and Barr in 1934, sacroiliac fusions for low back pain and sciatica stopped being done. Of course, sacroiliac fusion continued to be used for such things as fractured pelvis, tuberculosis of the sacroiliac joint, and a few other conditions.

REDUCTION OF SPONDYLOLISTHESIS

The idea of reducing the slip in spondylolisthesis has held a fascination for orthopedic surgeons since very early.[121] In 1936 Jenkins[81] tried to reduce by traction in extension and then fuse by an interbody graft. Recently Ascani and Monticelli[7] and others have improved on Jenkins's methods but still advocate reduction by extension associated with spinal fusion. Paul Harrington[67,68] was the first in America to reduce spondylolisthesis using rods. Mathias[106] has used a plate with sacral hooks and pedicle screws to reduce the condition. David Bradford,[18] McPhee, and John O'Brien[110] have been using combined posterior decompression with fusion then anterior fusion a few days later. Rene Louis plates and Steffee plates are being used to reduce the slip in a single operation.

Generally the Europeans have been more aggressive in reduction than have the Americans. Also, most Americans seem to believe that less than 50% olisthesis does not need reduction. Fusion in situ is still the most commonly used operation for spondylolisthesis.

Regarding fusion of the pars only for spondylolysis, Buck[23] was probably the first to attempt to internally fix the pars. He used a screw across the pars and bone-grafted the defect. Scott,[142] of Edinburgh, advocates a technique involving passing an 18-gauge wire around the base of the spinous process and the transverse process, bone grafting the pars, then twisting the wire tight.

Morscher[117] has recently designed a hook that attaches to the lamina with a screw attached that goes into the lateral mass. He bone-grafts the pars defect.

SPINAL STENOSIS

The condition that we now recognize as spinal stenosis has, of course, been with us since antiquity. Several Egyptian mummies have been found to have the condition, even though the ancient Egyptians generally did not live very long. Since spinal stenosis is usually a degenerative disease of the elderly, large numbers would not be expected to develop the condition.

Even some animals are afflicted with spinal stenosis. The dachshund and the Pekinese, in particular, frequently develop clinical symptoms due to spinal stenosis. German shepherds develop the disease in the lumbar area, and Wobbler's disease in horses is due to stenosis in the cervicothoracic area. However, for a surprisingly long time, in humans, it was not recognized as an entity that could be successfully treated by decompression.

In 1803 Portal,[128] of France, focused attention on changes in the size of the vertebral canal as a cause of spinal compression. He noted that abnormal curvature of the spine might produce deformity of the canal to the extent that severe cord compression, with paraplegia, might result.

In 1864 Jaccoud,[79] in a chapter on spinal cord compression due to spinal osseous processes, discussed Portal's report: "Before terminating the subject I must recall that singular form of paraplegia which [described by Portal] results from compression of the spinal cord by a spinal canal which is too narrow."

During the latter part of the nineteenth century a few authors wrote about this "strange condition" that seemed to respond simply to opening the back and exposing the dura. One of the very earliest examples of an operation to relieve spinal stenosis was reported by Arbuthnot Lane[92] in 1893. He had a patient with what was clearly degenerative spondylolisthesis producing cauda equina compression. He decompressed and relieved this patient. In 1893 Von Bechterew[163] proposed that there was an as yet undescribed disease of the spine that produced pain, weakness in the legs, parathesias, and the necessity of walking with the body bent forward. Another very early description of what was probably spinal stenosis was made in 1899 by Sachs and Fraenkel.[140] Their report came long before the introduction of myelography. Their patient had sacral and lumbar pain that caused him to walk bent far forward. This patient was eventually relieved by a two-level laminectomy. The surgeon, A. Gerster,[59] found neither tumor nor exudate but remarked upon the unusual heaviness of the laminae and the general thickness of the bone. After surgery the patient could straighten up and walk well. Sottac, in 1896, coined the term *intermittent claudication of the spinal cord* to describe the disease.[150]

In 1910 Sumita[154] described narrowing of the vertebral canal due to achondroplasia. He showed a schematic drawing of a cross-section of the narrowed vertebral canal in one of his cases.

In 1911 Bailey and Casamajor[10] described a patient with lower extremity pain and a weak left leg, who was obliged to walk with his body bent forward and who was unable to walk but for a short distance. He was cured after a laminectomy by Dr. Charles Elsberg[53] that revealed the laminae to be thicker than normal. No other explanation for the disorder could be found. Bailey and Casamajor stated that the spinal cord and the nerves of the cauda equina seemed susceptible to compression by arthritic abnormalities. They specifically emphasized the role of bony exostoses from articular processes and abnormalities of the ligamentum flavum that compressed the spinal roots from behind.

In 1913 Elsberg wrote of "a peculiar disease"[53] of the roots of the cauda equina with symptoms very much like those of tumor of the cauda equina, although no tumor was ever to be found at surgery. All of the patients improved very much after operation, and the good result was ascribed to the wide laminectomy. A year later, in 1914, Kennedy[84] gave further information about 22 patients with this disease. The roentgenograms of many of them showed arthritic changes, and most who had laminectomy were improved. In 1925 Parker and Adson[127] described spinal compression by hypertrophic arthritis, improved by laminectomy.

In 1931 Towne and Reichert[157] reported two cases of cauda equina compression improved by the removal of thickened, yellow ligaments at narrowed and hypertrophic interspaces.

In 1934 Cramer[36] described 26 patients, presumably those who had been operated upon by Elsberg and who had been regarded as examples of the "peculiar disease" that later was called "cauda equina radiculitis." Cramer suggested that this tumor-like syndrome was secondary to arthritic changes in the spine, since arthritic changes were well marked in two thirds of the cases. Most of these patients were improved after laminectomy. Many others contributed to the increasing knowledge of the disease.[141]

It was Henk Verbiest,[150,160,161] a neurosurgeon in Utrecht, Holland, who finally brought the condition into sharp focus. In 1949 he published his first article on the subject, and for the remaining 35 years of his professional life he probably did more than anyone else to delineate the condition and bring it to the attention of the medical profession.

Others who are prominent in the more recent development of our knowledge of spinal stenosis are Brodsky[21] and Ehni,[51] of Houston. Kirkaldy-Willis,[87,88] of Saskatoon, Saskatchewan, is credited with presenting the best classification and with bringing our attention to the lateral neurovascular canals as areas of compression. These appear to be even more important than the central canal.[25]

At present it appears likely that spinal stenosis is a much more common cause of back pain and sciatica than is the herniated disc. The major problem in the treatment of spinal stenosis is how to decompress adequately and still maintain stability. This is especially true of the lateral canals where, if we decompress to where the spinal nerve is unequivocally free, the spine may be unstable.

The advent of better methods of internal fixation may yet make it possible to take away the posterior bone and rigidly fix and fuse either in the same or an improved position.

In the last 3 or 4 years some authors have stated that a spinal nerve can be compressed even out beyond the lateral border of the pedicle.[176] In a way, we are coming full circle because, as mentioned earlier, in the 1920s and even up into the early 1940s authors such as Danforth and Wilson, Magnuson, Gormley, and the earliest of all, Bertolotti were suggesting that far lateral compression caused radiating pain into the leg. Abdullah,[1] in 1974, and very recently, Zindrick,[181] have reported on the finding of far lateral disc ruptures well out beyond the lateral border of the foramen. Because the spinal nerves are tightly bound in this far lateral area, an extruded disc lying underneath the nerve can cause identical symptoms to those of a ruptured disc in the central canal.

SUMMARY

The lumbosacral spine remains a most challenging area. Every new advance in surgical technique or diagnostic capability opens up new possibilities for treatment. I believe we are on the threshold of even greater moves forward.

However, many seemingly simple questions remain unanswered. For example, we don't know why some discs in the process of degeneration hurt while others do not. Why does the same degree of vertebral instability cause pain in some but not in others?[169] When should we fuse for instability?[170] When, if ever, should we fuse for disc disease?[134] Is the sacroiliac joint a frequent source of pain? (A significant number of health professionals believe that it is.) Why does spondylolisthesis slip farther in some children and not in others?

Probably the most pressing need of all is to develop better surgical treatment for degenerative scoliosis and degenerative spinal stenosis. Since our population is getting older, these conditions are on the increase. We must find better ways of stabilizing degenerative scoliosis, and we must learn to decompress spinal stenosis adequately and still maintain stability.

REFERENCES

1. Abdullah, A., et al.: Extreme lateral lumbar disc herniation, J. Neurosurg. **41:**229, 1974.
2. Adamkiewecz, A.A.: Ueber die Mikroskopischen Gefasse des Menschilichen Ruckeumarker, Transactions of the seventh session of the International Medical Congress, **1:** 155, 1881.
3. Alajouanine, T.H.: From the presidential address by Professor Jean Cauchoix before the annual meeting of the International Society for the Study of the Lumbar Spine, San Francisco, June 1978.
4. Albee, F.H.: Transplantation of a portion of the tibia into the spine for Pott's disease, JAMA **57:**885, 1911.
5. Anderson, G.B.J.: Epidemiological aspects of low backpain in industry, Spine **6:**53, 1981.
6. Arnell, S., and Lidstrom, F.: Mylography with skiodan (Abrodil), Acta Radiol. **12:**287, 1931.
7. Ascani, C., and Monticelli, G.: Reduction of spondylolisthesis, Paper presented at Sicot Congress, 1975.
8. Asher, M., et al.: Anthropometric studies of the human sacrum relating to dorsal transacral implant design, Manuscript submitted for publication, 1986.
9. Babinsky: Quoted from Reynolds, F., and Katz, S: Herniated lumbar intervertebral disc, American Academy of Orthopaedic Surgeons symposium on the spine, St. Louis, 1969, The C.V. Mosby Co.
10. Bailey, P., and Casamajor, C.: Osteoarthritis of the spine as a cause of compression of the spinal cord and its roots, J. Nerve Ment. Dis. **38:**588, 1911.
11. Barr, J.S.: Lumbar disc lesions in retrospect and prospect, Clin. Orthop. **129:**4, 1977.
12. Batson, O.V.: The function of the vertebral veins and their role in the spread of metastases, Ann. Surg. **1:**138, 1940.

13. Beaton, L.E., and Anson, B.J.: The relationship of the sciatic nerve and its subdivisions to the periformus muscle, Anat. Rec. **70:**1, 1937.
14. Bertolotti, La Radiologia Medica, 1917.
15. Bloch, F.: Nuclear induction, Physiol. Rev. **70:**460, 1946.
16. Boucher, H.H.: A method of spinal fusion, J. Bone Joint Surg. **41B:**248, 1959.
17. Bracewell, R.: Quoted by Oldendorf, W.H.: The quest for an image of the brain, New York, 1980, Raven Press.
18. Bradford, D.S.: Treatment of severe spondylolisthesis, Spine **4:**423, 1979.
19. Briggs, H., and Milligan, P.: Chip fusion of the low back following exploration of the spinal canal. J. Bone Joint Surg. **24:**125, 1944.
20. Brissaud: Quoted from Reynolds, F., and Katz, S.: Herniated lumbar intervertebral disc, American Academy of Orthopaedic Surgeons symposium on the spine, St. Louis, 1969, The C.V. Mosby Co.
21. Brodsky, A.E.: Low back pain syndrome due to spinal stenosis and posterior cauda equina compression, Paper presented to the Hospital Joint Diseases Annual Scientific Alumni Meeting, Houston, October 1969.
22. Brown, M.: Intraoperative ultrasonography, Personal communication, June 1984.
23. Buck, R.E.: Direct repair of the defect in spondylolisthesis, J. Bone Joint Surg. **52B:**432, 1952.
24. Burns, B.H.: An operation for spondylolisthesis, Lancet **1:**1233, 1933.
25. Burton, C., et al.: Causes of failure of surgery on the lumbar spine, Clin. Orthop. **157:**191, 1981.
26. Campbell, W.C.: An operation for extra articular arthodesis of the sacroiliac joint, Surg. Gynecol. Obstet. **45:**218, 1927.
27. Cauchoix, J.: Presidential address presented to the International Society for the Study of the Lumbar Spine, San Francisco, June 1978.
28. Cleveland, M., et al.: Pseudoarthrosis of the lumbosacral spine, J. Bone Joint Surg. **30A:**302, 1948.
29. Cloward, R.B.: History of posterior lumbar interbody fusion, Springfield, Ill., 1982, Charles C Thomas, Publisher.
30. Cloward, R.B.: New treatment of ruptured intervertebral discs, Paper presented to the annual meeting of the Hawaii Territorial Medical Association, May 1945.
31. Cloward, R.B.: The treatment of ruptured intervertebral discs by vertebral body fusion, Ann. Surg. **136:**987, 1952.
32. Cormack: Quoted by Oldendorf, W.H.: The quest for an image of the brain, New York, 1980, Raven Press.
33. Cortugno, D.: De Ischiade Nervosa Canmentarius, L. Naples, 1764, Simoncos Brothers.
34. Cotrel, Y., and Dubausset, J.: The use of pedicle screws and universal instrumentation for spinal fixation, Paper presented to the AO Trauma Course, Davos, Switzerland, December 1985.
35. Coventry, et al.: The intervertebral disc—its microscopic anatomy and pathology, J. Bone Joint Surg. **27:**105, 233, 460, 1945.
36. Cramer, F.: A note concerning the syndrome of cauda equina radiculitis, Bull. Neural. Inst. **3:**501, 1934.
37. Crock, H.: Isolated disc resorption as a cause of nerve root canal stenosis, Clin. Orthop. **191:**109, 1976.
38. Crock, H.: Isolated lumbar disc resorption as a cause of nerve root canal stenosis, Clin. Orthop. **115:**102, 1976.
39. Crock, H., et al.: Observations on the venous drainage of the human vertebral body, J. Bone Joint Surg. **55:**528, 1973.
40. Damadian, R.: Tumor detection by nuclear magnetic resonance, Science **171:**1151, 1971.
41. Dandy, W.E.: Ventriculography following the injection of air into the cerebral ventricles, Ann. Surg. **68:**5, 1918.
42. Dandy, W.E.: Loose cartilage from the intervertebral disc simulating tumor of the spinal cord, Arch. Surg. **19:**1660, 1929.
43. Danforth, M., and Wilson, P.: The anatomy of the lumbosacral region in relation to sciatic pain, J. Bone Joint Surg. **7:**109, 1925.
44. DePalma, A., and Rothman, R.: The nature of pseudoarthroses, Clin. Orthop. **59:**113, 1968.
45. Dommisse, G.F.: The blood supply of the spinal cord at birth, master's thesis, Cape Town, 1972, University of Cape Town, South Africa.
46. Dommisse, G.F.: The arteries and veins of the human spinal cord from birth, New York, 1975, Churchill Livingstone, Inc.
47. Dutaillis: Quoted from Reynolds, F., and Katz, S.: Herniated lumbar intervertebral disc, American Academy of Orthopaedic Surgeons symposium on the spine, St. Louis, 1969, The C.V. Mosby Co.

48. Dyck, W.: Fixator interne, Paper presented to the AO Trauma Course, Davos, Switzerland, December 1985.
49. Edwards, W.C.: The sacral fixation device: a new alternative for lumbosacral fixation, Paper presented to the meeting of the North American Spine Society, Laguna Niguel, Calif., July, 1985.
50. Ehni, G.: Seeking the hidden flaw, Presidential address, International Society for the Study of the Lumbar Spine, May 1980.
51. Ehni, G.: Significance of the small lumbar canal, I. J. Neurosurg. **31**:490, 1969.
52. Ehni, G.: Spondylolitic cauda equina radiculopathy, Tex. Med. **61**:746, 1965.
53. Elsberg, C.A.: Experiences in spinal surgery, Surg. Gynecol. Obstet. **16**:117, 1913.
54. Farfan, H.F.: Mechanical disorders of the low back, Philadelphia, 1973, Lea & Febiger.
55. Farfan, H.F.: The effects of torsion on the intervertebral joints canal, J. Bone Joint Surg. **12**:336, 1969.
56. Fraser, R.: Chymopapain in the treatment of intervertebral disc herniation—the final report of a double blind study, Spine **9**:815, 1984.
57. Freebody, D., et al.: Anterior transperitoneal lumbar fusion, J. Bone Joint Surg. **53B**:617, 1971.
58. Frymoyer, J.W., et al.: Disc disease and spine fusion in the management of low back disease: a minimum ten year follow-up, Spine **3**:1, 1978.
59. Gerster: Cited by Sachs, B., and Frankel, J.: Progressive ankylotic rigidity of the spine, J. Nerv. Ment. Dis. **27**:1, 1900.
60. Ghormley, R.K.: Low back pain with special reference to the articular facets with present attention of an operative procedure, JAMA **101**:1773, 1933.
61. Goldner, J.L., et al.: Anterior disc excision and interbody spine fusion for chronic low back pain, American Academy of Orthopaedic Surgery symposium on the spine, St. Louis, 1969, The C.V. Mosby Co.
62. Goldner, J.L.: Personal communication, February 1960.
63. Goldthwart, J.E.: The lumbosacral articulation, Boston Med. Surg. J. **164**:365, 1911.
64. Graham, C.E.: A preliminary report of a double blind study comparing chemonucleolysis and intradiscal cortisone in the treatment of backache and sciatica, Orthop. Clin. North Am. **6**:259, 1975.
65. Hadra, B.E.: Wiring of the spinous processes in Pott's disease, Transam. Orthop. Assoc. **4**:206, 1891.
66. Harmon, P.D.: Anterior extraperitoneal lumbar disc excision and vertebral body fusion, Clin. Orthop. **18**:169, 1960.
67. Harrington, P.R., and Dickson, J.H.: Spinal instrumentation in treatment of severe spondylolisthesis, Clin. Orthop. **117**:157, 1976.
68. Harrington, P.R., and Tullos, H.S.: Spondylolisthesis in children, Clin. Orthop. **79**:75, 1971.
69. Hibbs, R.H.: An operation for progressive spinal deformities, N.Y. J. Med. **93**:1013, 1911.
70. Hirsch, C.: An attempt to diagnose the level of disc lesion by disc puncture, Acta Orthop. Scand. **18**:132, 1948-1949.
71. Hirsch, C., and Schajowicz, F.: Studies on structural changes in the lumbar annulus fibrosis, Acta Orthop. Scand. **22**:184, 1953.
72. Hodgson, A.R., and Stock, F.E.: Anterior spine fusion for treatment of tuberculosis of the spine, J. Bone Joint Surg. **42A**:295, 1960.
73. Hodgson, A.R., and Wong, S.K.: A description of a technique and evaluation of anterior spinal fusion for deranged discs and spondylolisthesis, Clin. Orthop. **56**:133, 1968.
74. Houndsfield, G.: Quoted by Oldendorf, W.H.: The quest for an image of the brain, New York, 1980, Raven Press.
75. Hult, L.: The munk fors investigation, Acta Orthop. Scand. (suppl. 16), 1954.
76. Humphries, A.W., and Hawk, W.A.: Anterior spine fusion using an internal fixation device, J. Bone Joint Surg. **41A**:371, 1959.
77. Ito, H., et al.: A new radical operation for Pott's disease, J. Bone Joint Surg. **16**:499, 1934.
78. Inman, V.T., and Saunders, C.: Referred pain from skeletal structures, J. Nerve Ment. Dis. **99**:660, 1944.
79. Jaccoid, S.: Les Paraplegies et l'atorie du mouvement, Paris, 1864, Adriene Delahoye.
80. Jaslow, I.: Intercorporal bone graft in spinal fusion after disc removal, Surg. Gynecol. Obstet. **82**:215, 1946.
81. Jenkins, J.A.: Spondylolisthesis, Br. J. Surg. **24**:80, 1936.
82. Judet R., et al.: Osteosynthese: material, techniques complications, Actualities, De Chirurgie Orthopedique de L'Hopital, Raymond Pain Care, **7**:196, Paris, 1970, Masson & Cie, Editeurs.
83. Kaneda, K.: Personal communication, October 1985.
84. Kennedy, F., and Elsberg, C.A.: A peculiar and undescribed disease of the nerves of the cauda equina, Am. J. Med. Sci. **147**:645, 1914.

85. Keyes, D., and Compere, E.: The normal and pathological physiology of the nucleus pulposus and intervertebral disc, J. Bone Joint Surg. **14:**897, 1932.
86. King, D.: Internal fixation for lumbosacral fusion, Am. J. Surg. Arch. Surg. **66:**357, 1944.
87. Kirkaldy-Willis, W.H., et al.: Lumbar spinal stenosis, Clin. Orthop. **99:**30, 1974.
88. Kirkaldy-Willis, W.H., and McIvor, G.W.D.: Spinal stenosis, Clin. Orthop. **115:**1, 1976.
89. Knodt, T.H., and Larrick, R.: Distraction fusion of the lumbar spine, Ohio State Med. J. **12:**140, 1964.
90. Kocher, T.: Die Verlitzungen der Wirbelsaule Zurleich Als Beitrag zur Phyiologic des Menschlichen Ruchenmarks, Mitt Grenzgeb Med. Chir. **1:**415, 1896.
91. Kraag, M.H., et al.: An internal fixator for posterior application to short segments of the thoracic, lumbar or lumbosacral spine: design and testing, Manuscript submitted for publication.
92. Lane, W.A.: Spondylolisthesis associated with progressive paraplegia-laminectomy, Lancet **1:**991, 1893.
93. Lange, F.: Support of the spondylolitic spine by means of buried steel bars attached to the vertebrae, Am. J. Orthop. Surg. **8:**344, 1910.
94. LaRocca, H., and MacNab, I.: The value of pre-employment radiographic assessment of the lumbar spine, Can. Med. Assoc. J. **101**(7):49, 1969.
95. Lindbloom, K.: Diagnostic puncture of the intervertebral discs in sciatica, Acta Orthop. Scand. **17**(suppl. 4):231, 1948.
96. Louis, R.: Fusion of the lumbar and sacral spines by internal fixation with screw plates, Clin. Orthop. **203:**18, 1986.
97. Love, J.G.: Removal of intervertebral discs without laminectomy, Proc. Staff Meeting, Mayo Clinic **14:**800, 1939.
98. Love, J.G.: Removal of protruded intervertebral discs without laminectomy, Proc. Staff Meeting, Mayo Clinic **14:**800, 1939.
99. Luque, E.: Interpeduncular segmental screw fixation, Clin. Orthop. **203:**20, 1986.
100. Luque, E.: The anatomic basis and development of segmental spinal instrumentation, Spine, Vol. 7, Num. 3, 1982.
101. Ma, G., and Paulson: Interbody fusion of the lumbar spine with the use of box chisels, Paper presented at the meeting of the Western Orthopaedic Association, Oct. 1982.
102. MacNab, I.: Backache, Baltimore, 1977, Williams & Wilkins.
103. MacNab, I., and Doll, D.: The blood supply of the human spine, J. Bone Joint Surg. **53B:**628, 1971.
104. Magerl, F.: External skeletal fixation of the lower thoracic and lumbar spine: current concepts of external fixation of fractures, Berlin, 1982, Springer-Verlag.
105. Magnuson, P.B.: Differential diagnosis of causes of back pain accompanied by sciatica, Ann. Surg. **119:**878, 1944.
106. Mathias, H.H., and Heine, J.: The surgical reduction of spondylolisthesis, Clin. Orthop. **203:**34, 1986.
107. Mathieu, P., and Demerleau, J.: Surgical therapy of painful spondylolisthesis, Rev. Chir. Orthop. **23:**352, 1936.
108. McCullough, J.: Microdiscectomy, Paper presented at Surgery of the spine symposium, Melbourne, Australia, April 1985.
109. McElroy, K.D.: Lumbosacral fusion by bilateral lateral technique, Proc. Am. Acad. Orthop. Surg., J. Bone Joint Surg. **43A:**918, 1961.
110. McPhee, I.P., and O'Brien, J.P.: Reduction of severe spondylolisthesis, Spine **4**(5):430, 1979.
111. Mendeleev: Quoted by Oldendorf, W.H.: The quest for an image of the brain, New York, 1980, Raven Press.
112. Mercer, W.: Spondylolisthesis, Ed. Med. J. **43:**545, 1936.
113. Middleton, G.S., and Teacher, J.H.: Extruded disc at the T12-L1 level—microscopic exam showed it to be nucleus pulposus, Glasgow Med. J. I, A, VLXXVI.
114. Mixter, W.J., and Barr, J.S.: Rupture of the invertebral disc with involvement of the spinal canal, N. Engl. J. Med. **211:**210, 1934.
115. Mooney, V., et al.: A system for evaluating and treating chronic back disability, Western J. Med. **124:**370, 1976.
116. Moore and Henshaw: Quoted by Oldendorf, W.H.: The quest for an image of the brain, New York, 1980, Raven Press.
117. Morscher, E., and Gerber, B.: Surgical treatment of spondylolisis by bone grafting and direct stabilization of spondylolisis by means of a hook screw, Arch. Orthop. Traum. Surg. **103:**175, 1984.
118. Nachemson, A.: Lumbar intradiscal pressure, Acta Orthop. Scand. Suppl. **43:**104, 1960.
119. Nachemson, A.: The effect of forward leaning on lumbar intradiscal pressure, Acta Orthop. Scand. **35:**314, 1965.

120. Naylor, A.: The biophysical and biomechanical aspects of intervertebral disc herniation, Ann. R. Coll. Surg. Engl. **31**:91, 1962.
121. Newman, P.H.: A clincial syndrome associated with severe lumbosacral subluxation, J. Bone Joint Surg. **47B**:472, 1965.
122. Newton, Isaac: From a letter to Robert Hooke, February 7, 1695.
123. Nordby, E., and Lucas, G.: A comparative analysis of lumbar disc disease treated by laminectomy or chemonucleolysis, Clin. Orthop. **90**:110, 1973.
124. Oldendorf, W.H.: Displaying the internal structural pattern of a complex object, Ir. Trans. Bio-Med. Elect. BME. **8**:68, 1961.
125. Oldendorf, W.H.: The quest for an image of the brain, New York, 1980, Raven Press.
126. Olerud, S.: Stabilization of the spine with Schanz screws and an external fixator, Paper presented to the AO spine trauma course, Davos, Switzerland, December 1985.
127. Parker and Adson: Quoted from Reynolds, F., and Katz, S.: Herniated lumbar intervertebral disc, American Academy of Orthopaedic Surgeons symposium on the spine, St. Louis, 1969, The C.V. Mosby Co.
128. Portal, A.: Cours d'anatomie medicale ou elemens de l'anatemic de l'homme, Vol. 1, Paris, 1803, Baudouin.
129. Purcell, E.M., et al.: Resonance absorption by nuclear magnetic moments in a solid, Phys. Rev. **69**:37-38, 1946.
130. Radon: Quoted by Oldendorf, W.H.: The quest for an image of the brain, New York, 1980, Raven Press.
131. Raney, F.L. Jr., and Adams, J.E.: Anterior lumbar disc excision and interbody fusion used as a salvage procedure, J. Bone Joint Surg. **45A**:667, 1963.
132. Reid, A., et al.: Nuclear magnetic resonance imaging and its safety implications: follow-up of 181 patients, Br. J. Radiol. **55**:784-786, 1982.
133. Roentgen, C. In Talbott, J.: A biographical history of medicine, Orlando, Fl., 1970, Gurne & Stratton, Inc.
134. Roofe, P.G.: Innervation of the annulus fibrosis and posterior longitudinal ligament, Arch. Neurol. Psychol. (Suppl.) **46**:1, 1960.
135. Rothman, R., and Booth, R.: Failure of spinal fusion, Orthop. Clin. North Am. **6**:299, 1975.
136. Roy-Camille, R.: Internal fixation of the lumbar spine, Manuscript submitted for publication, 1986.
137. Rutherford: Quoted by Oldendorf, W.H.: The quest for an image of the brain, New York, 1980, Raven Press.
138. Sachs, B., and Frankel, J.: Progressive ankylotic rigidity of the spine, J. Nerv. Ment. Dis. **27**:1, 1900.
139. Saillant, G.: Etude anatomique der pedicles bertebraux application chiruguale, Rev. Chir. Orthop. **62**:151, 1976.
140. Sarpyener, M.A.: Congenital stricture of the spinal canal, J. Bone Joint Surg. **27**:70, 1945.
141. Schmorl G.: Die Pathologische Anatomie der Wirbelsaule, Verh. Deutsch. Ortho. Ges. **21**:3, 1926.
142. Scott, J.: Fixation of spondylolisis with circumferential wire around the transverse processes and spinous processes, Paper presented to the combined meeting of the English speaking orthopaedists of the world, Edinburgh, Great Britain, 1970.
143. Shakespeare, W.: Timon of Athens, Act 4, Scene 1, line 23.
144. Shordonia, J.F.: Die Chronische Entzundung des Piriformia Muscle, Med. Welt. **10**:999, 1936.
145. Selby, D.: A modification of the crock interbody fusion instruments for use in P.L.I.F., Personal communication, November 1985.
146. Sicard, J.A., and Forestier, J.: Methode radiographique d'exploration de la cavite epidurale par le Lipiodal, Rev. Neurol. **37**:1264, 1921.
147. Smith, F.W.: NMR historical aspects, Mod. Neuroradiol. **2**:7, 1983.
148. Smith, L.: Enzyme dissolution of the intervertebral disc, Nature **4887**:198, 1963.
149. Smith-Peterson, M.N., and Rogers, W.A.: End result study of arthrodesis of the sacroiliac joint for arthritis-traumatic and nontraumatic, J. Bone Joint Surg. **8**:118, 1926.
150. Sottac: Intermittent claudication of the spinal cord, 1896. Reported by Verbiest, H.: Neurogenic intermittent claudication, Amsterdam, 1976, North Holland Publishing Co.
151. Spengler, D.M., and Freeman, C.W.: Patient selection for lumbar discectomy, Spine **4**:129, 1979.
152. Steffee, A.: Segmental spine plates with pedicle screw fixation, Clin. Orthop. **203**:45, 1986.
153. Straen, W.H., et al.: Iodinated organic compounds as contrast media for radiographic diagnoses, iodinated aracyl esters, J. Am. Chem. Soc. **64**:1436, 1942.
154. Sumita, M.: Beitrage Zur Lehre von de Chronodystrophia Foetalis (Kaufmann) und Osteogenesis Imperfecta (Vrolik) mit Besonderer Berucksichtigung der Anatomishcen und Klinishcen differential Diagnose, Deutsch. Z. Chir. **107**:1-110, 1910.

155. Sussman, B.J.: Intervertebral discolysis with collagenase, J. Nat. Med. Assoc. **60**:184, 1968.
156. Thomas, L.: Reversible collapse of rabbit ears after intravenous papain, J. Exp. Med. **104**:245, 1956.
157. Towne, E.B., and Reichert, F.L.: Compression of the lumbosacral roots of the spinal cord by thickened ligamenta flava, Ann. Surg. **94**:327, 1931.
158. Valleix. Quoted from Reynolds, F., and Katz, S.: Herniated lumbar intervertebral disc, American Academy of Orthopaedic Surgeons symposium on the spine, St. Louis, 1969, The C.V. Mosby Co.
159. Venable, C.S., and Stuck, W.G.: Electrolysis controlling factor in the use of metals in treating fractures, JAMA **3**(1):349, 1939.
160. Verbiest, H.: Neurogenic intermittent claudication, Amsterdam, 1976, North Holland Publishing Co.
161. Verbiest, H.: Sur certaines former rares de compression de la queue de cheval hommage a clovis vincent, Paris, 1949, Malouie.
162. Virchow, R.: Untersuchunger über die enwickelung die Schadelgrunder, Berlin, 1857, G. Reimer.
163. Von Bechlerew, W.: Steifigheit der Wirbelsaule und ihre Verkrummung als Besondere Erkrankungsform, Neural Zentralb **12**:426-434, 1893.
164. Von Luschka, H.: Die Hagelenke des Menschlichen Korpers. IV. Berlin, 1858, G. Reimer.
165. Wadell, G., et al.: Non-organic physical signs in low back pain, Spine **5**:117, 1980.
166. Watkins, M.B.: Posterolateral fusion of the lumbar and lumbosacral spine. J. Bone Joint Surg. **35A**:1014, 1953.
167. Watkins, R., et al.: Anterior lumbar interbody fusion: a clinical review, Manuscript submitted for publication.
168. Weber, H.: Lumbar disc herniation: a controlled perspective study with ten years of observation, Spine **2**:131, 1983.
169. White, A.: Spondylolisthesis due to instability following massive posterior decompression, Paper presented to the meeting of the American Academy of Orthopaedic Surgeons, Las Vegas, Feb. 1975.
170. White, A.A., and Panjabi, M.: Clinical biomechanics of the spine, Philadelphia, 1978, J.B. Lippincott Co.
171. Williams, R.W.: Microsurgical lumbar discectomy, report to American Association of Neurology and Surgery, 1975, Neurosurgery **4**(2):140, 1979.
172. Wilson, P.: The anatomy of the lumbosacral region in relation to sciatic pain, J. Bone Joint Surg. **7**:109, 1925.
173. Wilson, P.D. and Straub, L.R.: American Academy of Orthopaedic Surgeons Institute course lecture, Ann Arbor, Mich. 1952.
174. Wiltberger, B.R.: The dowel intervertebral body fusion as used in lumbar disc surgery, J. Bone Joint Surg. **39A**:284, 1957.
175. Wiltse, L.L., et al.: The paraspinal sacrospinalis splitting approach to the lumbar spine, J. Bone Joint Surg. **50A**:919, 1968.
176. Wiltse, L., et al.: Alar transverse process impingement syndrome—the far out syndrome, Spine **9**:31, 1984.
177. Young, H., and Love, J.: End results of removal of protruded intervertebral discs with and without fusion, Instructional course lectures: The American Academy of Orthopaedic Surgeons, vol. 16, St. Louis, 1959, The C.V. Mosby Co.
178. Zielke, K., and Strempel, A.V.: Posterior lateral distraction spondylodesis using the twofold sacral bar, Manuscript submitted for publication, 1986.
179. Zindrick, M., et al.: A biomechanical study of intrapeduncular screw fixation in the lumbrosacral area, Clin. Orthop. **203**:99, 1986.
180. Zindrick, M., et al.: Analysis of the morphometric characteristics of the thoracic and lumbar pedicles, Manuscript submitted for publication, 1986.
181. Zindrick, M., et al.: Far lateral disc rupture—beyond the pedicle zone, Paper presented to the meeting of the Los Angeles chapter of the Western Orthopaedic Association, Arrowhead Springs, California, April 1985.

CHAPTER

3

HISTORY: ONE NEUROSURGEON'S VIEWPOINT

Charles D. Ray

Compared with the morbid seriousness of malignant gliomas, dysraphic states, or middle cerebral aneurysms, herniated discs have long seemed all too tame and unacademic for most neurosurgeons. They, then (and, alas, even now), have sometimes shown about as much excitement over "what's new" in lumbar spine surgery as general surgeons might show over hemorrhoidectomies. In a national survey Mendenhall and associates[2] found that "the greatest number of [patient] encounters and the greatest amount of the neurosurgeon's time [about 60%] involve disorders of the spine, with the single most common disease being displacement of an intervertebral disc." To me, it is a significant tragedy, in light of the above, that perhaps only 10% of the neurosurgical literature[1] and about 2% (by recent count) of the various clinical and scientific papers presented at national and international neurosurgical meetings relate to this area. Indeed, until the last few years, lumbar spine surgery had enjoyed relatively little enthusiasm in organized neurosurgery since the earlier work of Dandy, Mixter, Barr, Semmes, Murphey, Mayfield, and others.[3-5] Most recently, however, interest seems to be returning and becoming more visible. Early Age thinking about the lumbar spine is still very much in evidence, nonetheless, as reflected by persistent misconceptions or beliefs. For example, myelography is the "gold standard" of diagnosis (even as to lateral spinal stenosis!); a medical facetectomy is equated with foraminotomy; a total facetectomy in the presence of an open disc space (or a herniated disc) is an innocuous procedure; the mechanical low back syndrome is seldom a real clinical entity (of either facet or discogenic origin, or both) but is probably a "functional disorder"; fusion of one segment will cause the next one higher to subsequently break down, lateral stenosis is almost always a compression of an emerging "nerve root" caused by a hypertrophic facet joint; and there are few (if any) nerve-compressing lesions of importance (other than rare tumors) lateral to the pedicle.

Perhaps many practicing orthopaedists have similar misconceptions about these and other clinical details; fortunately most of these essentials are discussed and well rebutted in this book. I hope that the reader will find that many such myths are dissolving as a result of the growing, genuine, present revival of serious interest and creativity in this field. The lumbar spine is in a remarkable situation, being an area that has heretofore stimulated relatively limited basic scientific and clinical investigation yet being a topic of such widespread socioeconomic importance; it seems that almost everyone, sooner or later, has back trouble, much of which is serious enough to alter their lifestyle. On the other hand, virtually no one ever dies of these diseases or disorders, although they may effectively cause "premature aging" of one's life-style.

Personally, I feel like a "direct descendent" of original lumbar spine surgeons when I review the fascinating article by my old chief, Francis Murphey, relating to the early days of neurosurgery.[3] He writes that in 1934, "during the month of elective neurosurgery (at the Harvard Service of the Massachusetts General Hospital) under Dr. Jason Mixter, I had an old Italian come in who had severe sciatica screaming 'dolor, dolor' which he traced down the back of his leg . . . . I assisted Dr. Mixter because the resident was sick. Dr. Tracy Mallory, pathologist at the Mass General, reported the specimen to be nucleus pulposus, which was the first to be identified as such and led to the recognition of the ruptured disc by Dr. Mixter."

Dr. Murphey continued, "in 1937 I did the first disc operation to be done in Memphis. After this Dr. R.E. Semmes and I had a long discussion with Dr. Willis Campbell, head of the famous Campbell Orthopedic Clinic. He said that he didn't want anything to do with intraspinal surgery and this is the reason that to this very day no one but neurosurgeons have done discs in Memphis" (and in many other locations). "After two years of routine [Lipiodol] myelograms, I analyzed the accuracy of this procedure . . . and found that there was a 25% false-negative . . . and a 15% false-positive. This was presented . . . in 1939."[4] Semmes and Murphey never liked myelography; they believed that it was all too often used as a substitute for a careful physical examination.[5] Further, nearly all of their intraspinal surgeries were performed with the patient under local anesthesia (Semmes had learned this from its pioneer, Halstead, while training under him at Johns Hopkins), so that the patient could help guide the surgeon to the exact part of the root or spinal nerve that was entrapped, whether caused by disc, bone (stenosis), or whatever. He clearly admonished that, "You should follow the tender root involved around the pedicle below—even out into the retroperitoneal space if necessary."[3]

"I will never forget the day Dr. John Shea, Sr., after watching us struggle with the usual neurosurgical rongeurs to expose a ruptured disc . . . introduced us to the Kerrison rongeur. . . . Glen Spurling and Frank Mayfield introduced us to the pituitary rongeur to pull out the extruded fragment and to clean out the disc space. Dr. Semmes initially presented these two contributions of our to the Cushing Society (which Semmes helped found) on . . . Dr. Cushing's 70th birthday party."[4] "In those days, lumbar fusions were tried and then abandoned, to be revived by Dr. Ralph Cloward, on the neurosurgical side."[3]

Although a large number of things in lumbar spinal surgery have undergone major changes since 1940, much that is old continues to be interwoven with the newer methods and thinking. Certainly there is a place for local anesthesia, exactly as Semmes and Murphey described it, in selected cases and also combined with light epidural anesthesia by indwelling microcatheter placed at about L2 and above (which they didn't use). On the other hand, these pioneers did not understand the "sore disc disease" as they called it; that is, the cases having segmental instability with discogenic (and often facetogenic) pain. They noted these problems when the patient, under local anesthesia, complained of severe, deep-seated back ache as the disc space was being curetted or mechanically shifted. We know now that many of these instability cases will have persistent, even disabling, mechanical low back pain and perhaps repetitive re-herniations of a given disc until the segment becomes autostabilized or is fused.

REFERENCES

1. Burton, C.V.: Full-thickness autogenous fat grafts in the prevention of epidural fibrosis, Contemp. Neurosurg. **5:**1, 1982.
2. Mendenhall, R.C., et al.: Neurosurgery in the United States: a log-diary study, Neurosurgery **8:**267, 1981.
3. Murphey, F.: The early days of neurosurgery as I remember them, with emphasis on disc surgery, Neurosurgery **17:**370, 1985.
4. Semmes, R.E.: Diagnosis of ruptured intervertebral disc without contrast myelography and comments upon recent experience with modified hemilaminectomy for their removal, Yale J. Biol. Med. **11:**433, 1939.
5. Semmes, R.E.: Ruptures of the lumbar intervertebral disc, Springfield, Ill., 1964, Charles C Thomas, Publisher.

CHAPTER

4

SOME OPINIONS OF GENERAL ORTHOPEDISTS AND SUPERSPECIALISTS

Arthur H. White

The general orthopedist does not have the opportunity to express ideas adequately in literature and at meetings. Frequently the general orthopedist believes that those who are writing and talking are "ivory tower specialists" without an understanding of what is going on "in the trenches."

Sometimes superspecialists think that they have all the answers, and that general orthopedists do not appreciate the nuances of the superspecialty field.

I was recently given some letters and papers written by Dr. William Knapp in the 1960s that clearly show that general orthopedists of the Tri-State Orthopaedic Society were quite aware of what was going on in the spinal world and knew almost as much as we know now. They were asking themselves the same questions and coming up with some of the same answers that we do today. Since they believed instability played some part in the postoperative patient's pain, they looked for better ways of stabilization. They knew that myelograms could not adequately predict surgical pathologic findings, and they thought that facet joints had a part in chronic low back pain.

In the following 1967 survey of the members of the Tri-State Orthopaedic Society, we discovered that opinions varied greatly. Of the 114 members 77 responded, and the surgeons were often almost equally divided in their answers. There was quite a variation of opinions concerning questions that generally require yes or no answers. It is surprising that surgeons with good training and experience could answer so dividedly. Dr. Knapp concludes that answers to the problems in spine surgery are not as clear-cut as the "ivory tower" specialist thinks they are.

There is every reason to believe that the questionnaire was answered sincerely,

28 *General Principles*

	% Yes	% No
1. Do you think disc instability is a factor in low backache preoperatively?	88	12
2. Do you think disc instability is a factor in low back pain after simple discectomy or laminectomy?	78	22
3. Do you think one has to have anterior nerve root irritation to have backache and leg pain in disc disease?	41	59
4. Do you think the catch in the low back, which often comes on while bending over, is a shift in the nuclear material inside the disc, causing stretch on the annulus and pain?	42	58
5. Do you believe that the relief of back and leg pain one sometimes sees with traction and/or with manipulation is due to a shift of nuclear material within the disc?	38	62
6. Do you think this catch is a simple muscular strain or tear in the ligaments of the low back?	59	41
7. Do you think scleratome distribution of pain to the hip or leg from irritation of the posterior division of the nerve root, which comes from the facets, ligaments, etc. is a reality?	87	13
8. Do you think a chronic low back pain can come from irritation, sprain, or arthritic manifestations in the facets?	94	6
9. Do you think one can get chronic low back symptoms of pain from poor postural strains of the facets, ligaments, and annulus fibrosa?	97	3
10. Do you think one can get mechanical foraminal compression phenomenon of the spinal nerve roots from narrowing of the disc space before or without surgery of any type?	84	16
11. Do you think one can get mechanical foraminal compression phenomenon of the spinal nerve roots from narrowing of the disc space after simple laminectomy-discectomy type surgery?	78	22
12. Do you think assymetric facets are a factor in chronic low backache?	69	31
13. Do you think rudimentary development of facets is a factor in low backache?	69	31
14. Do you think unequal leg length of ¼ to ½ inch can be a factor in producing shearing force with disc and facet stress and low back pain?	57	43
15. Do you think the low backache in spondylolisthesis is due to shearing stress on the disc (annulus fibrosa or ligaments)?	54	46
16. Do you think the low backache in spondylolisthesis is due to stress on the fibrous tissue at the arch defect areas?	51	49
17. Do you think the leg pain in spondylolisthesis may be due to nerve root irritation as it is stretched over or around the fibrocartilaginous mass, which is built up at the posterior arch defect?	95	5
18. Do you believe that disc instability and bulging is the great factor in backache and leg pain in spondylolisthesis?	33	67
19. Do you think that, with surgery for spondylolisthesis, the area should be stabilized with spinal fusion?	92	8

	% Yes	% No
20. In cases of disc disruption, with surgery, would you fuse all cases if you were sure there would be an uneventful fusion?	27	73
21. Do you think much of the postoperative back stiffness and disability after spinal surgery is due to prolonged splinting of flexible structures from wearing of a brace, etc., rather than the bony instability of the fused segment?	54	46
22. Do you think the decreased back bending, with postoperative bracing, may let the neural elements adhere down more firmly than if free excursion were allowed during the back healing period?	46	54
23. Once a disc herniates, do you think this weakened area can heal and prevent recurrences?	65	35
24. Do you think the prolonged wearing of a corset or brace has any curative effect?	41	59
25. Do you think the prolonged wearing of a corset or brace has a weakening effect on the trunk muscles?	86	14
26. Do you think repeated episodes of nerve root trauma by a herniating disc can cause adhesive scarring down of the nerve root?	93	7
27. Given a case of undoubted ruptured disc with sciatica, do you advise surgery on the first episode?	18	82
28. Do you do myelograms if you don't intend to operate?	18	82
29. Given a case with clinical symptoms of a herniated disc, do you only operate if the myelogram is positive?	15	85
30. Do you believe there are false negative myelograms?	95	5

31. Do you think that all motion can be effectively eliminated at the lumbosacral or L4-L5 level by
   a. Camp type lumbosacral support?
   b. Jewett type hyperextension brace?
   c. flexion type brace?
   d. chair back brace?
   e. Taylor brace?
   f. body cast?
   g. one-legged spica?
   h. two-legged spica?
	almost 100% no	

32. Do you think that all motion can be effectively eliminated at the lubosacral or L4-L5 levels (or both), at the time of surgery by
   a. facet props?
   b. facet screws?
   c. H-graft?
   d. Wilson plate?
   e. Knodt bars?
   f. posterior interbody dowels or "chunk" grafts?
   g. anterior interbody dowels or "chunk" grafts?
   h. anterior plates or staples?
	almost 100% no	

33. Do you do laminectomies and fusions
   a. yourself?
   b. with a neurosurgeon?
   c. fusions at the request of a neurosurgeon?
   d. refer operative back cases to a neurosurgeon?
	83
	38
	59
	25
		17
		62
		41
		75

	% Yes	% No
34. If answer to Question 33 is (a), do you		
a. routinely do laminectomy and discectomy only, without fusion?	39	61
b. routinely do both discectomy and fusion?	22	78
c. decide to do a fusion at the time of operation by manual testing of vertebral motion, etc.?	45	55
35. Do you tell patients that have had only a discectomy that a fusion may be necessary in the future if they continue to have, or if they develop, back pain?	70	30
36. Do you do discograms?	7	93
37. How long do you keep patients recumbent following		
a. discectomy alone?	3 days	
b. laminectomy and fusion? *average*	20 days	
c. fusion only?	20 days	
38. Do you have your postoperative back cases wear a brace? If so, for how long? *average 5 months*	73	27
39. Do you prescribe braces as a nonoperative method of treating low back pain?	96	4
40. Do you prescribe exercise as nonoperative treatment of low back pain?	93	7
41. Do you prescribe exercise as postoperative treatment?	82	18
42. Do you ever do spinal fusions alone without exploration of the disc space?	70	30
43. Do you use autogenous or homogenous bone, or both, when doing spinal fusions?	97	
44. How long does it usually take you to do a laminectomy (one interspace) and fusion? *45 minutes to 3½ hours—average 2 hours*		
45. If disc pathology exists at L4–L5 only and you elect to do a fusion, do you include L5–S1?	77	23
46. If disc pathology exists at L5–S1 only, do you extend a fusion to include L4–L5?	17	83
47. How many years, after your training, have you been in orthopedic practice? *average 18 years*		
Comments:		

and Dr. Knapp was at a loss to understand the rationale of some of the treatment in view of the stated beliefs.

Despite the fact that Dr. Knapp was sold on complete immobility for the developing bony union, he was convinced that methods of immobilizing the back in the past had been not only inefficient but, in many respects, deleterious. Dr. Knapp was looking for a logical explanation of why a large percentage of the orthopedists did a simple discectomy, relieving the nerve root irritation, and yet did not do a stabilizing procedure in this defective area. It seemed, in fact, that the surgeons should do just exactly the opposite of what the majority are doing. Dr. Knapp was certain that to the run-of-the-mill orthopedist in practice, the solution to the back problem is not as cut and dried as the authorities would lead them to believe.

In the same vein as the 1967 questionnaire, I asked 12 contributors to this book to fill out questionnaires and rate the frequency with which they use many of the specific surgical procedures discussed in this book. We also asked them to evaluate the complication rate associated with each procedure.

A summary of these questionnaires points out that the laminectomy is the most common surgical procedure these physicians use. Posterior intertransverse fusions are the second most common. Internal fixation is then most frequently used, followed by anterior interbody fusion. The least used surgical procedures are about equally the posterior interbody fusion and microdiscectomy. Chemonucleolysis is used least of any of the surgical procedures.

The questionnaire asked for those who have "experienced significant complications with this procedure." The significant complications have been extensively explained in the chapters on the specific procedures. As with all procedures, the complications include infection and damage to neurologic structures attributable to a specific procedure, which may not have been experienced with a simpler or more standard procedure.

Complications unique to the anterior and posterior interbody fusions are the displacement of the bone graft from the interbody position.

A complication unique to the internal fixation procedures is displacement of the internal fixation devices, requiring replacement or creating neurologic damage.

Chemonucleolysis carries with it the well-known complication of anaphylaxis and the other major neurologic injuries, such as transverse myelitis. It is also well known that postchemonucleolysis instability and stenosis can occur.

Epidural fat grafts have some unique complications to the area from which the fat was obtained, such as hematoma or cosmetic deformity. Some individuals have experienced the fat graft to create neurologic pressure over the epidural space and become responsible for further symptoms.

The failure of a particular procedure to "cure the patient" is not truly a complication. There is a known and published success and failure rate for each of these procedures. At times, however, many of the authors have used a procedure on a specific patient and then experienced failure to obtain an acceptable result. When such a failure is attributable to inherent problems with that specific type of surgery, the author considers it a complication. For example, immediate breakdown at the level above a solidly fixed fusion may be considered a complication. Laminectomy, discectomy, or chemonucleolysis, which results in the immediate need for a second surgery, might be considered a complication.

The complications as discussed in this section are not the minor complications anticipated with any surgery, such as urinary tract infection, pneumonia and complications associated with a general anesthetic, or the underlying diseased process that led to the surgery, that is, continued neurologic deficits that were present before the procedure.

Clearly, 20 years later there is no unanimity of opinion. We are still asking the same questions, trying to be scientific in our approaches, and hoping that in another 10 years we can answer these same questions.

QUESTIONNAIRE

1. I find this procedure to be of what value?
2. I have experienced significant complications with this procedure.
3. What percentage of the surgery that you do involves this procedure?

John W. Frymoyer

Procedure	Question 1			Question 2		Question 3
	No value	Some value	Great value	Yes	No	%
Anterior interbody fusion		X		X		5
Posterior interbody fusion		?			X	0
Posterior intertransverse fusion			X		X	40
Laminectomy			X	X		40
Internal fixation		X			X	10
Use of bank bone		?			X	0
Microdiscectomy		X			X	5
Chemonucleolysis		X			X	5
Epidural fat grafts		X			X	50

Hugo Keim

Procedure	Question 1			Question 2		Question 3
	No value	Some value	Great value	Yes	No	%
Anterior interbody fusion		X		X		1
Posterior interbody fusion		X		X		1
Posterior intertransverse fusion			X		X	95
Laminectomy			X		X	80
Internal fixation		X		X		40
Use of bank bone	X			X		2
Microdiscectomy		X			X	1
Chemonucleolysis		X			X	5
Epidural fat grafts		X			X	30

Vert Mooney

Procedure	Question 1			Question 2		Question 3
	No value	Some value	Great value	Yes	No	%
Anterior interbody fusion			X	X		40
Posterior interbody fusion		X		X		5
Posterior intertransverse fusion			X		X	15
Laminectomy			X		X	40
Internal fixation			X	X		10
Use of bank bone		X			X	40
Microdiscectomy	X				X	0
Chemonucleolysis		X		X		0
Epidural fat grafts		X		X		90

Charles D. Ray*

Procedure	Question 1			Question 2		Question 3
	No value	Some value	Great value	Yes	No	%
Anterior interbody fusion			X	X		0
Posterior interbody fusion			X	X		0
Posterior intertransverse fusion			X	X		30
Laminectomy (laminotomy)			X	X		70
Internal fixation			X	X		0
Use of bank bone			X	X		30
Microdiscectomy			X	X		50
Chemonucleolysis			X		X	2
Epidural fat grafts			X	X		90

*Dr. Ray wrote "Most Usual Reason for 'Complication': It didn't work in about one fifth to one third of all cases (that is, technique inadequate to fully address problem or failure to 'take')."

David Selby

Procedure	Question 1			Question 2		Question 3
	No value	Some value	Great value	Yes	No	%
Anterior interbody fusion			X		X	40
Posterior interbody fusion		X		X		10
Posterior intertransverse fusion			X		X	20
Laminectomy			X		X	30
Internal fixation			X		X	50
Use of bank bone			X		X	50
Microdiscectomy	X				X	0
Chemonucleolysis	X				X	0
Epidural fat grafts	X			X		0

Leon L. Wiltse

Procedure	Question 1			Question 2		Question 3
	No value	Some value	Great value	Yes	No	%
Anterior interbody fusion		X	X		X	10
Posterior interbody fusion				X		1
Posterior intertransverse fusion			X		X	70
Laminectomy			X	X		70
Internal fixation			X		X	10
Use of bank bone		X		X		1
Microdiscectomy			X		X	1
Chemonucleolysis			X		X	10
Epidural fat grafts	X			X		0

Robert Watkins

Procedure	Question 1			Question 2		Question 3
	No value	Some value	Great value	Yes	No	%
Anterior interbody fusion			X	X		20
Posterior interbody fusion			X	X		10
Posterior intertransverse fusion		X			X	30
Laminectomy (stenosis)			X	X	X	30
Internal fixation			X		X	20
Use of bank bone	X			X		
Microdiscectomy			X		X	30
Chemonucleolysis			X		X	0
Epidural fat grafts		?			X	30

Arthur H. White

Procedure	Question 1			Question 2		Question 3
	No value	Some value	Great value	Yes	No	%
Anterior interbody fusion		X				1
Posterior interbody fusion		X		X		5
Posterior intertransverse fusion			X			80
Laminectomy			X			95
Internal fusion			X	X		80
Use of bank bone		X				2
Microdiscectomy	X					0
Chemonucleolysis		X				5
Epidural fat grafts	X					5

Richard H. Rothman

Procedure	Question 1			Question 2		Question 3
	No value	Some value	Great value	Yes	No	%
Anterior interbody fusion		X			X	5
Posterior interbody fusion	X					0
Posterior intertransverse fusion			X		X	10
Laminectomy			X		X	80
Internal fixation		X			X	5
Use of bank bone		X			X	5
Microdiscectomy		X			X	10
Chemonucleolysis	X				X	0
Epidural fat grafts		X			X	80

CHAPTER 5

CLINICAL BIOMECHANICS OF LUMBAR SPINE SURGERY

Casey Lee

HISTORICAL REVIEW

Clinical biomechanics for lumbosacral spine surgery has evolved around the following:

1. To fuse or not to fuse the lumbosacral spine for idiopathic low back pain
2. Iatrogenic instability after disc excision
3. Determination of degenerative instability of a spinal motion segment

These questions emerged many decades ago and have remained unanswered.

Before the report of successful treatment of low back pain and sciatica by surgical excision of the herniated disc by Mixter and Barr,[40] spinal fusion was a commonly accepted procedure for patients with low back pain caused by structural anomalies or facet trophysm of the lumbrosacral spine.* Until recently, enthusiasm for spinal fusion has diminished as the disc excision procedure became popular. The herniated disc problem was known to be a manifestation of a degenerative process of the disc, and the disc excision for herniated disc was generally thought to cause further mechanical instability of the spine. Although the combined procedure of disc excision and spinal fusion was advocated by many surgeons[3,4,21,59,60] but its efficacy for pain relief was questioned by some.[8,16,52] Is mechanical instability of a spinal motion segment caused by degenerative processes of the disc, by the surgical procedure of partial excision of the disc, or by the combination of both?

A biomechanical study of a partial excision of the disc demonstrated no significant alterations of biomechanical behavior of the disc.[27,28,39,55] This study suggests that the disc excision procedure does not contribute to the instability of the motion segment.

Others[15,25,41] observed that instability of the lumbosacral spine was occasionally associated with degenerative changes of the disc and was a common cause for chronic low back pain. In these patients satisfactory relief of low back pain was obtained by spinal fusion.[41,53,54]

In recent years spinal surgeons, not having answers to these fundamental questions, are confronted with further

---

*References 2, 5, 9, 10, 14, 24, 29, 30, 47, 56.

problems as we are performing more complicated surgical procedures such as extensive decompression for spinal stenosis, use of various internal fixation devices, and choices of different type of fusion procedures.

PHYSIOLOGIC PAIN MECHANISM

Three common causes for idiopathic low back pain are ligamentous sprain causing nociceptive irritation, neural compression as in disc herniation or spinal stenosis, and biochemical irritation of nociceptive endings by inflammation-provoking degenerative byproducts. These three pain mechanisms are all closely related to the structural integrity, external loads, structural response to the applied loads, and kinematics of spinal motion segment. Further explanations of this relationship between pain mechanisms and biomechanics of a spinal motion segment are made in the subsequent paragraphs.

The annulus fibrosus, various ligamentous structures of the spinal motion segments, and joint capsules of the facet joint are richly innervated by nociceptive endings and are common sources for idiopathic low back pain. The physical deformations of these structures (strain) beyond their physiologic limit is defined as sprain (excessive strain)* in clinical practice. Therefore sprain of various structures, including the annulus fibrosus, depends largely on two factors—applied load and structural response to the applied load. The applied load to a specific ligamentous structure about a joint causes two significant biomechanical changes—forces acting on the structure (stress) and deformation of the structure (strain). These two biomechanical factors caused by external loads are closely related to the movement patterns of the joint (kinesiology).

Normal structures of the annulus fibrosus, joint capsules of the facet joint, and various ligaments of a spinal motion segment require greater amounts of force (stress) to make these structures deform beyond the physiologic limit (sprain). Degenerated and attenuated structures of annulus, ligaments, or capsules have altered biomechanical response to the applied forces. In this circumstance a physiologic loading condition can become an abnormal loading condition to these structures, causing abnormal excessive strain (sprain). Abnormal motion pattern (hypermobility or irrational motion) can also alter the stress and strain responses of these structures to external loads.

Clinical biomechanics for diagnosis and treatment of idiopathic low back pain encompasses studies on loads to the spine, stress/strain characteristics of normal and degenerated structures of annulus, ligamentous structures and joint capsule, and motion studies.

A spinal motion segment is a compound joint that is made of a three joint complex. The posterior two joints are the facet joints, which are true synovial joints. The anterior joint is the intervertebral disc. The disc has many similarities, as well as dissimilarities, with a synovial joint; it is a highly specialized joint to accommodate specific physiologic requirements—movements, stability, load bearing capacity, and protective mechanism to the neural contents.

The structural specifications of the disc are designed to provide maximum stability with a relatively small but important amount of motion and load transmission. In a typical large weight bearing synovial joint such as the knee joint, the movement is primarily guided by geometric configuration of the articulating surfaces, joint capsule, and surrounding ligaments

---

*The biomechanical term *strain* refers to the deformation of structures caused by forces applied on them (stress). The clinical term *strain* refers to the excessive deformation of the muscle-tendon unit (sprain of ligaments vs. strain of muscle).

(probably in the order of significance). In the disc the articulating surface of the joints, the "vertebral end-plates," are simple and made of two relatively fat and parallel surfaces. The guidance of motion of the disc is therefore heavily dependent on the annulus fibrosus (capsular component of a synovial joint) and the adjacent facet joints. The anterior and posterior longitudinal ligaments are important for flexion and extension of a motion segment in the saggital plane but do not significantly contribute to guidance and stabilization for torsion, side bending, and horizontal translation. In a large weight bearing synovial joint, most of the weight bearing function is provided by the articular cartilage. This function of a synovial joint is transformed into a very special design arrangement in the disc as a form of annulus fibrosus and nucleus pulposus.

The spinal motion segment is a functional unit of the spinal column that is made of a three joint complex—one disc and two facet joints. The concept of a three joint complex is not new but is very important to understanding low back pain problems. Historically, we have been conditioned to think only of the disc problems whenever we are faced with patients with low back pain and sciatica, and we have neglected problems arising from the other two joints—facet joints.

THE DISC

The disc is a nonsynovial joint and the largest avascular structure in the human body. A disc is made of three component structures: the vertebral end-plates, the annulus fibrosus, and the nucleus pulposus.

The vertebral end-plate provides a comparable function to the subchondral bone plate in a synovial joint to disperse the load to the adjacent nucleus pulposus and annulus fibrosus. However, the vertebral end-plate, unlike the subchondral bony plate in which no fluid exchanges between the joint cavity and subchondral bony sinusoid, permits fluid diffusion between vertebral sinusoids and the nucleus pulposus and annulus fibrosus.[42] This fluid exchange through the vertebral end-plates plays a major role in the nourishment of the largest avascular structure of the disc. When the disc is loaded on axial compression, the vertebral end-plate is the weakest structure among the three component structures of the disc.[7,42]

The nucleus pulposus, which has no cells, consists of a three-dimensional network of collagen fibers (mainly type II) embedded in a mucoprotein gel.[27] It is located near but slightly posterior to the geometric center of the disc. Acid mucopolysaccharide is the main component of the ground substance. Water content of the nucleus pulposus is about 80% in a young adult and decreases with age.[48] The nucleus pulposus is incompressible material, and it bulges out when the disc is cut through the nucleus pulposus. In physiologic status in vivo, the nucleus pulposus is compressed by the elastic properties of the ligamentum flavum, maintaining the disc height. It also acts like a ball bearing when the vertebral bodies roll in flexion and extension. The center of rotation within the disc changes instantaneously, depending on the position of the spine during flexion and extension.[28,50] In the degenerated disc the instant center of rotation tends to move posteriorly,[11] and an increased stress is applied to the facet joints. The nucleus pulposus transforms the vertebral compression forces into tangential stresses (Hoop stress) in the annulus fibrosus.[43]

The nucleus pulposus has no nociceptive endings. Therefore any biochemical or morphologic change of the nucleus pulposus does not set up direct nociceptive stimulation. However, these changes can produce secondary changes of the biomechanical behaviors of the motion segments and can set up nociceptive stimulation. Degeneration of the nucleus pulposus may lead to loss of disc height and altered load transmission across the disc and the facet joints.

The annulus fibrosus is made of concentric lamellae of collagen fibers (type II and I), which expand obliquely across the disc space between vertebral end-plates. The fibers in each lamella run obliquely 30 degrees to the end-plate. Thus two adjoining lamellae run in the opposite direction and fibers cross each other at 120 degrees. The annulus is stiffest and has lowest deformation and energy dissipation in this arrangement.[18,19]

The interlamellar spaces are filled with abundant amounts of proteoglycan. The mechanical properties of the annulus for these physiologic functions are from mechanical behavior of the composite material (collagen fibers and proteoglycan). The proteoglycan component of the composite material binds collagen fibers and lamellae and provides water-binding capacity. Abnormal biomechanical behaviors of degenerated discs are commonly associated with changes in composition of proteoglycan, which cause changes in collagen-binding capacity and water-binding capacity of the disc. Whether these changes are secondary to repetitive trauma to the disc or are the primary cause for disc disruption is not clear. Nevertheless, changes in biochemical composition caused by aging produces susceptibility of the disc to trauma by delamination of the annulus fibrosus and abnormal strain to the collagen fibers.

The annulus fibrosus is the most important component structure in a spinal motion segment for biomechanical stability and for transmitting vertical weight bearing forces.[50] The visocoelastic behavior of the annulus fibrosus in relation to the load bearing ability and stability of a spinal motion segment in normal and abnormally degenerated discs has been extensively studied with static or dynamic compression tests.*

Under the axial compressive load the disc fails at the vertebral end-plate. The normal annulus fibrosus can withstand much greater stress than the failure stress of the vertical end-plate, and it does not fail first under the axial load. The vertical compressive load applied on the vertebral body is transmitted to the annulus fibrosus as the tangential hoop stress through the end-plate and the nucleus pulposus.

Studies on the disc bulge and intradiscal pressure have been frequently quoted subjects in the literature in attempts to correlate back pain to pathologic conditions of the disc degeneration and to various physiologic postures and activities. The amount of disc bulge under controlled axial loads was higher in the degenerated disc.[26] In the degenerated disc the amount of disc bulge under controlled axial loads was much higher (30%), and the annulus was subjected to higher vertical stress and lower tangential forces because of loss of hydrostatic behavior of the degenerated nucleus pulposus. However, it is not clear that the lateral bulge of the annulus fibrosus under the axial load produces abnormal strain on the annulus fibers and causes pain by stimulation to the nociceptive endings within the outer layers of the annulus. An abnormal amount of bulge beyond a certain critical level may exert direct pressure on the nerve root, causing radiculopathy.

Bulging of a disc under a given amount of axial compressive load can be manifested as two very different phenomena, depending on the status of component structures of composite material of the annulus fibrosus—proteoglycan and collagen framework.

When the disc is loaded externally, the

---

*References 7, 39, 43, 50, 59, 62.

external load is counterbalanced by an internal resistive force of the disc (joint reaction force). Two main components of the internal resistive force of the disc are osmotic pressure and solid structural stiffness (networks of the annulus fibrosus). The osmotic pressure is provided by the proteoglycan component of the annulus fibrosus and nucleus pulposus.

When the applied axial compressive load causes disc space narrowing by less internal resistive pressure of the disc caused by changes in proteoglycan components with low osmotic pressure, the outer layer of the annulus will bulge out by the buckling phenomenon. In this case the bulged annulus does not have any significantly increased stress or strain. This situation is similar to a deflated balloon between the two solid objects. When two solid objects are squeezed together, the balloon will bulge out but the balloon's wall will not be stretched much.

When external compressive load is applied to the disc with a good osmotic pressure mechanism but weaker solid structural frame, the disc wall (annulus) will bulge out with increased stress and strain (stretched out wall). When the same load is applied to a disc with normal osmotic pressure mechanism and intact solid structure force, the disc bulge and increased stress and strain of the wall will be minimal, but the intradiscal pressure will become very high. The intradiscal pressure in the disc with normal osmotic pressure mechanism but weak solid structure frame will have only a moderate level. The intradiscal pressure in the disc with low osmotic pressure but normal solid structural frameworks will be lower than the above cases, and the intradiscal pressure in the disc with low osmotic pressure and weak solid structure frame will be the lowest among all.

Therefore abnormal bulge of the annulus fibrosus does not necessarily mean increased stress and strain on the fibers of the annulus or the overlying posterior longitudinal ligament, and it does not necessarily cause stimulation to nociceptive endings contained in these structures. This may be a reason why some patients with bulging disc are asymptomatic as long as the disc bulge is not causing direct radicular compression.

Intradiscal pressure may not necessarily represent the stress or strain status of the fibers of the annulus fibrosus. The relationship between the factors (intradiscal pressure and stretch of outer layer of the annulus) is also greatly influenced by the integrity of the solid structures. The results of measurements of intradiscal pressure have been applied to clinical care for patients with low back pain to guide postures and activities for less pain. The relationship between the intradiscal pressure and pain in various stages of disc degeneration and in various postures and activities is not completely understood.

The annulus fibrosus provides maximal stability against horizontal displacement.[19] It also provides a very significant amount of torsional stability of a motion segment (40% to 50%), and an approximately equal amount of torsional stability is provided by the posterior lumbar facet joints.[11] The annulus fibrosus provides minimal resistance in tension to angular motion of the motion segment.

The posteriorly located two facet joints are the other part of the three joint complex of a motion segment. The facet joint is a true synovial joint and is richly innervated by nociceptive endings. The primary function of the lumbar facet joint is to provide torsional stability of a motion segment.[11] The facet joints have very small amounts (less than 20%) of the weight bearing capacity in normal physiologic conditions. The resection of the facet joints (partial or complete) as a part of posterior spinal decompression for spinal stenosis can compromise the torsional stability of the whole motion segment and probably place extra burdens to the annulus fibrosus.

SURGICAL PROCEDURES, DISC DEGENERATION, STABILITY, AND LOW BACK PAIN

Low back pain in degenerative disc disease is commonly caused either by abnormal strain (sprain of ligaments and capsules) of the annulus fibrosus and the posterior longitudinal ligament or by mechanical or chemical irritation of the degenerative facet joints. The abnormal strain on the annulus fibrosus, posterior longitudinal ligament, and facet joints capsule is produced either by nonphysiologic external overloading to the normal structures (common cause of injury to normal healthy structures) or by physiologic loading to the degenerated abnormal structures.

In biologic systems the degenerative process is almost always accompanied by the biologic reparative system. The identifiable evidences of reparative processes in the degenerated spinal motion segments are increased surface area of the vertebral end-plates by local or circumferential ridging or osteophyte formation, increased surface areas of the facet joints with change of geometric joint configuration, and scarring or thickening of the outer layer of the annulus fibrosus, ligamentum flavum, and facet joint capsule. Accurate measurements of the degree of the negative effect (structural weakness, destabilization) of degenerative processes and of the degree of the positive effect (structural enhancement, self-stabilization) of the reparative processes have not been obtained.

The three most common pathologic conditions for treatment by spinal surgeons are disc herniation, spinal instability, and spinal stenosis.

Disc herniation is a manifestation of a spectrum of degenerative processes of the disc. The successful choice of surgical procedures for a herniated disc depends on the proper evaluation of biomechanical function of the whole motion segment. Partial excision of a herniated disc (degenerated nucleus pulposus and inner layers of the annulus) through a laminotomy does not appear to cause serious biomechanical derangement of the motion segment, if the herniated disc is a relatively isolated pathologic condition. A biomechanical study on fresh human cadaver lumbar spine demonstrated a self-sealing effect of the disc after a simulated procedure of disc excision on the motion segment.[39] The mechanism of pain relief of sciatica after disc excision is probably due to removal of mechanical pressure and the source of chemical irritation to the nerve root. The relief of back pain in disc herniation is not often predictable either by surgical excision or discolysis. A possible mechanism for back pain relief by discolysis is decreased intradiscal osmotic pressure and decreased strain on the outer layer of the annulus fibrosus.

Spinal Instability and Mechanical Low Back Pain

Clinical stability is defined as "the ability of the spine under physiologic loads to limit patterns of displacement so as not to damage or irritate the spinal cord or nerve root and, in addition, to prevent incapacitating deformity or pain due to structural changes."[58] Clincial instability for low back pain can be caused by abnormal displacement under physiologic loading (hypermobility) and also by structural changes without evidence of hypermobility.

Clinicians in practice use the term *spinal instability* to designate the condition of painful hypermobility and the term *mechanical low back pain* to designate the condition of low back pain caused by abnormal structural behavior under physiologic loading without evidences of hypermobility.

Spinal hypermobility caused by degenerative processes (degenerative spondylolisthesis) has long been recognized as an important cause of low back pain. The hypermobility of the motion segment can be manifested in any plane of motion. The most commonly observed type is translation on the horizontal plane. In a normal spinal motion segment there is no translation of one vertebral body on the other in the horizontal plane throughout the physiologic ranges of motion of the lumbosacral spine. Translation in excess of 2 to 3 mm in either extension or flexion is considered to be clinically significant for instability.[41,46]

The most common type of hypermobility observed in practice is excessive angular displacement in the saggital plane. Excessive disc space angle, greater than 9 degrees above the normal (1 degree for L5-S1) is considered to be significant for clinical instability.[46] Farfan and associates[12] reported that the principal pathomechanics of degenerative spondylolisthesis is the torsional translation of a vertebra to the adjacent vertebra. Pearcy and his associate[45] performed an in vivo motion study of degenerative spondylolisthesis and reported that there is no detectable movement across the segment of the degenerative spondylolisthesis. It is quite common in clinical practice, however, for definitive hypermobility to be detected on flexion and extension roentgenograms of the lumbosacral spine of patients with degenerative spondylolisthesis, especially during the early stage.

It is probable that the end stage of many hypermobile segments reaches static equilibrium between the degenerative and reparative processes. Any disturbances in this equilibrium will result in a dynamic instability with hypermobility. Such unstable hypermobility is frequently observed after decompressive surgery for spinal stenosis caused by degenerative spondylolisthesis.

The term *mechanical low back pain* was discarded either because it lacks precision in meaning or because it does not describe a verifiable condition. Can any abnormal pattern (erratic motion but within the magnitude of movements that can be detected by conventional evaluation techniques of the lateral flexion-extension roentgenogram) be the cause of pain from the degenerated motion segment? An erratic motion pattern within a motion segment may produce abnormal strain in certain parts of the motion segment without producing hypermobility that can be detected by conventional techniques of lateral flexion-extension roentgenogram. Clinicians have occasionally observed patients with chronic low back pain whose symptoms were thought to be due to abnormal movements, although there are no signs of hypermobility and their symptoms are relieved successfully by a spinal fusion procedure alone.

Unfortunately, no reliable technique to diagnose this condition exists. Some clinicians use a conventional trial method of external immobilization of the lumbrosacral spine by applying a pantaloon-type cast. This technique is useful but lacks specificity for establishment of non-hypermobile instability. The presence of traction osteophytes was thought to be indicative of segmental instability,[37] but when it becomes significant for production of pain symptoms is not known. I could establish no significant relationship between the size of the traction spur and biomechanical characteristics of the motion segment (kinematic and load bearing capacity) in a preliminary study on fresh human cadaveric spine. The presence of traction spurs indicates the past biomechanical history of the motion segments, but it does not tell us the current status regarding load bearing capacity of the motion segment.

Nonhypermobile abnormal motion patterns may be detected by special techniques. A very minute degree of abnormal motion patterns may be detectable by stereophoto-roentgenography, and an erratic motion pattern may be detected by determination of a locus of instantaneous centers of rotation of a motion segment.[20] However, the clinical relevance of these new techniques of detecting fine movement patterns is not established.

Discometric evaluation of the disc can provide useful information concerning the clinical relevance of disc degeneration. The acceptance capacity of volume and pressure increase within a disc, its pain production, and morphologic grading of the disc degeneration can provide us physiologic responses of the disc and their pain production mechanism. Pain from the outer layers of the annulus fibrosus caused by abnormal strain (stretching) due to increased disc volume and/or pressure is probably a good indicator of the structural integrity of the disc, providing that there is a constant relationship between the disc pressure and volume and the annulus strain. As mentioned in the discussion of disc pressure, the responses of the annulus to these tests are probably variable depending on the types of degeneration (solid framework vs. ground substance), leakage of the annulus, and the biomechanical property of scarred outer layers of the annulus fibrosus.

The diagnosis of clinical instability of a spinal motion segment can be established when pain is caused by demonstrable hypermobility. The diagnosis of clinical instability is very difficult to establish when pain is caused by nonhypermobile abnormal motion and/or abnormal biomechanical response of structures to a physiologic loading situation. In this case, the physician may use other criteria based on empirical experiences, traction spur and other roentgenographic findings,[18] discogram, and trial immobilization.

Posterior Spinal Decompression and Spinal Instability

How much of posterior spinal structures can the surgeon remove and yet maintain stability of the motion segment? The question has been asked frequently since the extensive posterior decompressive procedure became popular for the treatment of spinal stenosis.

Posner and associates[46] found that a functional spinal motion segment failed under simulated flexion loading conditions when all the posterior components plus one anterior component had been destroyed during laboratory testing on fresh human cadaveric spines. This suggests that no immediate disastrous instability of a motion segment will result when all posterior structures are surgically removed as long as the anterior structures have normal biomechanical load bearing functions. Two unknown factors for the postdecompression instability in clinical practice are structural integrity of the anterior structures (amounts of degenerative and reparative processes) and fatigue behavior of the anterior structures with increased stress by removal of posterior structures.

The incidence of postdecompression spondylolisthesis is reported to be 2% among 182 patients reviewed by White and Wiltse[57] and 10% among 59 patients reviewed by Shenkin and Hash.[51] In a study group of patients with no preoperative evidence of olisthesis, the postdecompression incidence of olisthesis was 3.7%.[32] Progressive spondylolisthesis after decompressive laminectomy in those patients with preoperative degenerative spondylolisthesis was observed in all cases. The two most important factors for stability after posterior decompression are the extent of decompression in width and the functional integrity of the other remaining structures.

Incremental loss of functional stability of a spinal motion segment can be expected when more posterior spinal structures are surgically removed. Clinical experience[12,32] suggests that no gross instability is expected when a less than bilateral one half facetectomy is performed on a motion segment provided that the anterior spinal structures are able to provide a relatively normal load bearing function. However, it is not known if the increased stress on the annulus fibrosus and posterior longitudinal ligament by loss of posterior supporting structures can produce nociceptive irritation without detectable gross instability. Fractures of pars interarticularis or the inferior articular process have been observed[12] in those patients who were treated with bilateral medial one half process fracture, indicating stress concentration of the remaining structures. Multilevel decompression was reported to have higher incidence of postcompression olisthesis,[50] but the true incidence rate per level is not clearly known. Four levels of decompression will have approximately a four times higher incidence rate of postdecompression olisthesis, but the per level incidence rate will be constant. There is no clear biomechanical understanding how multiple levels of decompression will affect one level within the multiply decompressed levels, in comparison to one level of decompression alone.

The determination of functional integrity of the anterior structure is very difficult (see the discussion on segmental instability). The normal disc height of the motion segment to be decompressed was considered to be a contributing factor for postdecompression olisthesis.[57] The normal height of the disc space does not always mean that the disc has normal load bearing capacity. I have found no consistent relationship between the disc height and the incidence of postdecompression olisthesis. Narrow disc space with exuberant osteophyte formation may be indicative of reparative effects. The literature indicates that these patients with sufficient preoperative amounts of reparative processes with self-stabilizing segmental instability will most probably have further instability after a posterior decompressive procedure. Spinal fusion with internal stabilization may be necessary in these cases.

Postdecompression spinal instability can be expected in the following circumstances: (1) the presence of preoperative segmental instability (either static or dynamic hypermobility, and pain by abnormal biomechanics of the motion segment even in the absence of gross hypermobility) and (2) posterior decompression involving more than bilateral one half facetectomies and disc excision combined with extensive posterior decompression.

BIOMECHANICS OF SPINAL FUSION

The rationale for spinal fusion procedures for treatment of low back pain was based on the thought that painful symptoms can be relieved by elimination of the degenerated or unstable spinal motion segment by fusion. Some authors[8,16] reported that spinal fusion offered few benefits in the management of lumbar disc disease. Spinal fusion, however, has become important for the treatment of low back pain. The effectiveness of spinal fusion for low back pain can be measured on the parameters of relief of the pain symptoms, achievement of stabilization of the fused segments, and the incidence of adverse effects. Failure of pain relief by spinal fusion may be from several sources: (1) poor indication, (2) failure of stabilization of the fused segments, and (3) complications of fusion.

A poor indication for spinal fusion is probably the most common cause for poor results. The best indication for spinal fusion is clinical spinal instability due to degeneration, trauma, or surgical decompression. In all of these cases the achievement of successful spinal fusion is usually difficult because of the presence of inherent instability and abnormal shear stress across the segment to be fused. Other indications of spinal fusion for idiopathic low back pain are poor, such as for herniated disc or chronic low back pain without localizing signs and recurrent disc herniation without signs of clinical instability. Spinal fusion is occasionally well indicated even with no definitive hypermobility on flexion-extension lateral roentgenogram of the lumbosacral spine, when there is sufficient indirect evidence of spinal instability identified by physical examination, plain x-ray films, and discographic examination.[13]

Failure to achieve adequate stabilization of the segments to be fused is another important source for poor results. The inadequate stabilization may be due to failure of fusion (pseudoarthrosis) or inadequate mechanical support by the fusion mass. Pseudoarthrosis has been considered generally to be a leading cause for poor results, although its significance for persistent symptoms after spinal fusion has been questioned.[49] The two most common causes for pseudoarthrosis are (1) the presence of preexisting instability with a significant amount of shear stress across the segment to be fused and (2) inadequate technique. The successful achievement of spinal fusion in cases with grossly hypermobile degenerative spondylolisthesis is often very difficult, unless the abnormal shear stress of the segment is neutralized with either an internal or external immobilization or fixation system. The common technical errors responsible for pseudoarthrosis are inadequate preparation of the graft bed (insufficient amount of graft bed or inadequate decortication) and poor availability of the graft material (inadequate amount, poor osteogenic or osteoconductive graft).

Inadequate mechanical support by the fusion mass may result in continuous motion of the diseased parts within the fused segments and may produce persistent symptoms. The posterior spinal fusion is observed to allow a significant amount of detectable motion across the disc of the same segment under compression and torsional loadings.[34,39] Both the anterior fusion and bilateral lateral intertransverse processes fusion provide adequate stabilizing efforts on the segment to be fused.[34,50]

Complications of the lumbosacral spinal fusion are spondylolysis acquisita and spinal stenosis. The incidence of postfusion spinal stenosis has ranged from 11% to 41%.[6,38] The most common type of postfusion spinal stenosis is associated with posterior spinal fusion and is usually found within the fused segment. However, I find that posterior fusion also causes a high incidence of spinal stenosis at the adjacent free level. Postfusion stenosis and spondylolysis acquisita at the level above the fusion segments (juxta-fused) are indicative of clinical manifestations of abnormal stress increase at the juxta-fused level. Biomechanical fusion studies on fresh human cadaveric spines and mathematical analysis of the stress redistribution due to various types of spinal fusion procedures revealed abnormal stress concentration at the juxta-fused segment after all types of fusion procedures.[34] Posterior fusion gave highest abnormal stress at the juxta-free segment, especially about the facet joints.

INTERNAL FIXATION OF THE LUMBOSACRAL SPINE

The internal fixation system is used during the surgical treatment of low back pain to prevent or correct deformity such as spondylolisthetic slip and to neutralize normal shear stress across the segment to fuse and to achieve solid fusion.

Because of the anatomic arrangement of the greater vessels anterior to the lumbosacral spine, most of internal fixation systems are designed for posterior spinal fixation. The use of the internal fixation system for the lumbosacral spine has not been popular until recently, because the lumbosacral joints are highly mobile joints with high stress and also because of short segments fixation, problems of secure fixation of the device to the sacrum, and the lumbosacral angle.

Various types of internal fixation systems have been used for lumbosacral spinal fusion: Harrington rods, Knodt rods, Luque rods, Luque rectangular rods, Harrington rods with sublaminar wiring, and a few systems using pedicular screws with plates, rods, or cables.

Harrington rods are biomechanically unstable systems in flexion and torsion, and they cannot be readily contoured for the lumbrosacral angle.[23] The sacral hooks for Harrington rods or Knodt rods are not well tolerated and often cause painful symptoms under high stress. The Knodt rods system provides very poor stabilization in flexion and poor torsion.[1,23,35] Although the posterior Harrington distraction rods and Knodt rods can provide flexion posture of the lumbosacral spine, clinical evidence of benefit is doubtful.[36] For a short segment fusion at the lumbosacral junction, it is very important to maintain the proper lumbosacral angle to minimize untoward effects on the juxta-fused free segments. The Luque rectangular system with sublaminar wiring or wiring around transverse processes or with pedicular screws provides much more stable fixation and provides better clinical results.[23,33] Other systems using pedicular screws with plates or rods (Zielke, Steffee, and Wiltse) can also provide more rigid internal fixation.

The use of rigid fixation systems for spinal fusion is best indicated when any significant amount of posterior decompression is contemplated on the segment with preoperative gross instability. In such case, successful achievement of solid fusion becomes very difficult because of increased instability and reduced graft bed size due to decompression. Failure to obtain solid fusion after repeated bone grafting for pseudoarthrosis is an additional indication for the use of internal fixation devices. Another indication is correction (reduction) of deformities caused by trauma or degeneration. Although the rigid fixation of a short segment can provide good stabilization of the segment to be fused, it can also produce increased untoward effects on the juxta-fused segment. Only prudent indications of various internal fixation systems can provide the maximal benefit of stabilization and minimal adverse effects.

REFERENCES

1. August, A.C., et al.: A bimechanical comparison of methods of posterior fixation in lumbosacral spine fusion, Transactions of the thirty-first annual meeting, Orthop. Res. Soc. **10:** 333, 1985.
2. Ayers, C.E.: Further case studies of lumbosacral pathology with considerations of the involvement of the intervertebral discs and facets, New England J. Med. **213:**713, 1935.
3. Barr, J.S.: Ruptured intervertebral disc and sciatic pain, J. Bone Joint Surg. **29:**429, 1947.
4. Barr, J.S.: Low back and sciatic pain: results and treatment, J. Bone Joint Surg. **33A:**633, 1951.
5. Brailsford, J.F.: Deformities of the lumbosacral region of the spine, Brit. J. Surg. **16:**562, 1928-1929.
6. Brodsky, A.E.: Post-laminectomy and post-laminectomy and post-fusion stenosis of the lumbar spine, Clin. Orthop. **115:**130, 1970.
7. Brown, T., et al.: Some mechanical tests on the lumbosacral spine with particular reference to the intervertebral disc, J. Bone Joint Surg. **39A:**1135, 1957.
8. Caldwell, G.A., and Sheppard, W.B.: Criteria for spinal fusion following removal of protruded nuclear pulposus, J. Bone Joint Surg. **39A:**1971, 1948.
9. Chandler, F.A.: Spinal fusion operations in the treatment of low back and sciatic pain, JAMA **93:**1447, 1929.

10. Danforth, M.S., and Wilson, P.D.: The anatomy of lumbosacral region in relation to sciatic pain, J. Bone Joint Surg. **6**:109, 1925.
11. Farfan, H.F., et al.: The effects of torsion on the lumbar intervertebral joints: the role of torsion in the production of disc degeneration, J. Bone Joint Surg. **52A**:468, 1970.
12. Farfan, H.: The pathological anatomy of degenerative spondylolisthesis: a cadaver study, Spine **5**:412, 1980.
13. Farfan, H.: The use of mechanical etiology to determine the efficacy of active intervention in single joint lumbar intervertebral joint problems: surgery and chemonucleolysis compared, Unpublished manuscript, 1986.
14. Ferguson, A.: The clinical and roentgenographic interpretation of lumbosacral anomalies, Radiology **22**:548, 1934.
15. Friberg, S., and Hirsch, C.: Anatomical and clinical studies on lumbar disc degeneration, Acta Orthop. Scand. **19**:222, 1950.
16. Frymoyer, J.W.: The role of spine fusion: question 3, Spine **6**:248, 1981.
17. Frymoyer, J.W., et al.: Disc excision and spine fusion in the management of lumbar disc disease: a minimum ten-year follow-up, Spine **3**:1, 1978.
18. Fung, Y.B.: Biomechanics: its scope, history and some problems of centenuum mechanics in physiology, Appl. Mech. Rev. **21**:1, 1968.
19. Galante, J.L.: Tensile properties of the human lumbar annulus fibrosus, Acta Orthop. Scand. Suppl. **100**, 1967.
20. Gertzbein, S.D., et al.: Determination of a locus of instantaneous center of rotation of rotation of the lumbar disc by Moire fringes: a new technique, Spine **9**:409, 1984.
21. Ghormley, R.K., et al.: The combined operation in low back and sciatic pain, JAMA **120**:1171, 1942.
22. Goldworth, J.E.: The lumbosacral articulation: an explanation of many cases of lumbago, ischias and paraplegia, Boston Med. Surg. J. **164**:365, 1911.
23. Guyer, D., et al.: Biomechanical comparison of seven internal fixation devices for the lumbosacral junction, Paper presented to the second NASA meeting, Laguna Niguel, Calif., July 25-27, 1985.
24. Hibbs, R., and Swift, W.: Development abnormalities at the lumbosacral juncture causing pain and disability (a report of 147 patients treated by the spine fusion operation), Surg. Gynecol. Obstet. **48**:604, 1929.
25. Hirsch, C.: Studies on the mechanism of low back pain, Acta Orthop. Scand. **20**:261, 1951.
26. Hirsch, C., and Nachemson, A.: New observations on the mechanical behavior of lumbar discs, Acta Orthop. Scand. **23**:254, 1954.
27. Hirsch, C., et al.: Biophysical and physiological investigation on cartilage and other mesenchymal tissues. VI. Characteristics of human nuclei pulposi during aging, Acta Orthop. Scand. **22**:179, 1952.
28. Hoag, J.M., et al.: Kinematic analysis and classification of vertebral motion, J. Am. Osteopath. Assoc. **59**:899, 982, 1960.
29. Key, A.J., and Ford, L.T.: Experimental intervertebral disc lesion, J. Bone Joint Surg. **30A**:621, 1948.
30. Kimberly, A.G.: Low back pain and sciatica, Surg. Gynecol. Obstet. **65**:195, 1937.
31. Knutsson, F.: The instability associated with disc degeneration in the lumbar spine, Acta Radiologica **25**:593, 1944.
32. Lee, C.K.: Lumbar spinal instability (olisthesis) after extensive posterior spinal decompression, Spine **8**:429, 1983.
33. Lee, C.K.: A clinical comparison study for internal fixation systems for lumbosacral spinal stenosis, paper presented at the annual meeting of the International Society for the Study of the Lumbar Spine, Dallas, May 29-June 1, 1985.
34. Lee, C.K., and Langrana, N.A.: Lumbosacral spinal fusion: a biomechanical study, Spine **9**:574, 1984.
35. Lee, C.K., and Langrana, N.A.: Biomechanical study of the Knodt rods in fresh human cadaveric lumbosacral spines, Unpublished manuscript.
36. Lee, C.K., and DeBari, A.: Lumbosacral spinal fusion with Knodt distraction rods, Spine **11**:373, 1986.
37. MacNab, I.: The traction spur: an indicator of segmental instability, J. Bone Joint Surg. **53**:663, 1971.
38. MacNab, I., and Dall, D.: The blood supply of the lumbar spine and its application to the technique of intertransverse lumbar fusion, J. Bone Joint Surg. **53B**:130, 1970.
39. Markoff, K.L., and Morris, J.M.: Structural component of the intervertebral disc, J. Bone Joint Surg. **56A**:675, 1974.
40. Mixter, W.J., and Barr, J.S.: Rupture of the intervertebral disc with involvement of the spinal canal, New England J. Med. **211**:210, 1934.
41. Morgan, F.P., and King, T.: Primary instability of lumbar vertebrae as a common cause of low back pain, J. Bone Joint Surg. **39B**:6, 1957.

42. Nachemson, A., et al.: In-vitro diffusion of dye through the end plate and the annulus of human lumbar intervertebral disc, Acta Orthop. Scand. **41:**589, 1970.
43. Nachemson, A.: Lumbar intradiscal pressure: experimental studies on postmortem material, Acta Orthop. Scand. Suppl. **43,** 1960.
44. Overton, L.J.: Arthrodesis of the lumbosacral spine (a study of end results), Clin. Orthop. **5:**97, 1955.
45. Pearcy, M., and Sheperd, J.: Is there instability in spondylolisthesis? Spine **10:**175, 1985.
46. Posner, I., et al.: A biomechanical analysis of the clinical stability of the lumbar and lumbosacral spine, Spine **7:**374, 1982.
47. Putli, V.: New conceptions in the pathogenesis of sciatic pain, Lancet **2:**53, 1927.
48. Puschel, J.: Der wssergehald normalerr und degenerieter zweischenwirbel scheiben. Bietr. Path. Anat. **84:**123, 1930 (quoted by Galante).
49. Rothman, R.H., and Booth, R.: Failure of spinal fusion, Orthop. Clin. North. Am. **6:** 299, 1975.
50. Rollander, S.D.: Motion of the spine with special reference to stabilizing effect of posterior fusion, Acta Orthop. Scand. Suppl. **90,** 1966.
51. Shenkin, H.A., and Hash, C.J.: Spondylolisthesis after multiple bilateral laminectomies and facetectomies for lumbar spondylosis: follow-up review, J. Neurosurg. **50:**45, 1979.
52. Spurling, R.G., and Grantham, E.G.: Ruptured lumbar discs in lower lumbar region, Am. J. Surg. **75:**140, 1948.
53. Unander-Scharin, L.: Spinal fusion in low back pain, Acta Orthop. Scand. **20:**335, 1951.
54. Unander-Scharin, L.: On low back pain with special reference to the value of operative treatment with fusion, Acta Orthop. Scand. Suppl. **5,** 1950.
55. Virgin, W.: Experimental investigation into the physical properties of the intervertebral disc, J. Bone Joint Surg. **33B:**607, 1951.
56. Wagner, L.C.: Congenital defects of the lumbosacral joints with associated nerve symptoms, Am. J. Surg. **27:**311, 1935.
57. White, A.H., and Wiltse, L.L.: Spondylolisthesis after extensive lumbar laminectomy, Paper presented at the forty-third annual meeting of the American Academy of Orthopaedic Surgeons, New Orleans, February 1976.
58. White, A.A., and Panjabi, M.M.: Clinical biomechanics of the spine, Philadelphia, 1978, J.B. Lippincott Co.
59. Wu, H.C., and Yao, R.F.: Mechanical behavior of the human annulus fibrosus, J. Biomech. **9:**127, 1976.
60. Young, H.H., and Walsh, A.C.: Combined operation for low back and sciatic pain: follow-up study, Collected papers of the Mayo Clinic and Mayo Foundation, **39:**475, 1948.
61. Young, H.H., et al.: Low back and sciatic pain: long term results after removal of protruded intervertebral disc with or without fusion, Clin. Orthop. **5:**128, 1955.
62. Zie, N.: Load capacity of the low back, J. Oslo City Hosp. **16:**75, 1966.

CHAPTER

6

NORMAL BIOMECHANICS OF THE LUMBAR SPINE

Stephen I. Esses   Augustus A. White

With the ever-increasing knowledge in science and medicine, there are numerous opportunities for progress at the crossroads of a variety of disciplines. A prototypical example of this has been in the fields of orthopedic surgery and mechanical engineering. More specifically, advances in the clinical understanding, evaluation, and treatment of problems of the lumbar spine have occurred as the result of the collaborative research endeavors of clinical scientists and bioengineers. This chapter is a review of the cogent clinical biomechanics of the normal lumbar spine. The synopsis includes the basic engineering principles and data necessary to identify the motion, stresses, and stability in the normal lumbar spine. We know that by delineating and understanding the normal biomechanics of the vertebral column, we will be better prepared to recognize and correct the abnormal.

BIOMECHANICS OF THE LUMBAR SPINE
Intervertebral Disc

The intervertebral disc has been implicated in many of the numerous causes of low back pain. It consists of three parts, each of which seems ideally suited, in structure and composition, to withstand large forces and moments.

The nucleus pulposus is a semiliquid with a water content of 70% to 90%. Collagen fibrils, mainly type II, are not arranged in any particular pattern and make up 15% to 20% of the nucleus. In cross-section the nucleus pulposus of the lumbar intervertebral disc comprises 30% to 50% of the total disc area.

The annulus fibrosus consists of fibrocartilaginous fibers that are arranged in a concentric and lamellar fashion enveloping the nucleus. The fibers of each layer run parallel to each other and are arranged with a 30-degree orientation to the plane of the disc. Horton[37] has demonstrated that the fibers of adjacent lamellae run in opposite directions and thus have an interception angle of 120 degrees. The inner one third of fibers attach to the endplates, and the outer two thirds attach to the intervertebral body. This latter attachment is extremely strong, as there is an attachment into the bone through Sharpey's fibers. It is of interest to note that there are nerve endings present in the outer portion of the annulus. The endplate is simply hyaline cartilage resting on a subchondral bone plate.

Studies have been conducted to determine the loads on a normal lumbar intervertebral disc. This has required the in vivo measurement of intradiscal pressures using a needle with a pressure-sensitive polytheylene membrane at its tip.[52] After needle introduction a discogram is performed to confirm placement of the needle tip in the nucleus pulposus and to ensure a relatively normal disc. It has been shown in normal discs obtained at autopsy that the pressure in the nucleus pulposus is one-and-one-half times the externally applied loads per unit of area.[49] By using this relationship and the pressure data obtained in vivo, the load per unit of area can be calculated. Furthermore, by estimating the surface area of the interspace, the total load at that level can be approximated. A correlation exists between the total load on the disc (T.L.) and the body weight above the disc (B.W.), which can be expressed as:

T.L. = 2.8 B.W. + 30

In the sitting position the range of pressures in the nucleus pulposus of 15 patients measured 1013 to 1496 kilopascals (kPa). In the standing position there was an average decrease in pressure of 30%. These figures are higher than those reported by Andersson, Ortengren, and Nachemson,[5] as well as those measured by Quinnell, Stockdale, and Willis.[67] However, all investigations have confirmed the relative changes that occur with different positions: an increase in pressure in the nucleus pulposus with sitting and a decrease with standing and recumbency.

In the standing position the intradiscal pressures reported by Nachemson and Elfstrom[51] ranged from 600 to 900 kPa, whereas in the studies of Quinnell, Stockdale, and Willis the pressures ranged from 400 to 750 kPa.

Spinal loads in vivo can be evaluated not only by intradiscal pressure measurements, but also with electromyography of trunk muscles or by measuring intraabdominal pressures. These latter techniques were employed by Marras, King, and Joynt[46] during controlled isometric and isokinetic conditions. Subjects were able to produce the greatest torque with the back under isometric conditions, and this torque potential increased as the trunk flexion angles were increased. By measuring intradiscal pressures, myoelectric signals, and intraabdominal pressures, Schultz and associates[73] validated their biomechanical analysis of loads on the lumbar spine. Another innovative technique for evaluating spinal load has been developed by Eklund and Corlett.[22] They propose using changes in body height as a measure of disc compression caused by creep. They have shown that both shrinkage and recovery follow a pattern similar to exponential curves.

Hirsch[32] has examined the manner in which intervertebral discs react to loading. With statically applied loads the disc compresses and bulges circumferentially. The deformation, however, is small. With 100 kg loading, the compression is less than 2 mm and the deformation anteriorly is less than 1 mm. Most of this deformation in the disc occurs in the initial 30 seconds, although absolute equilibrium is never attained. Lin and associates[41] demonstrated that the anterior bulge is usually greater than the lateral bulge during axial loading. They also confirmed that most of the disc bulging occurs at the onset of loading. The way in which dog and rabbit discs bulge has been studied by Klein, Hickey, and Hukins.[38] They have noted that, during compression of a disc, the shape of the bulge viewed in profile approximates the arc of a circle. Markolf[45] has noted that, after the load is removed, the load deformation curve is different from the loading curve, presumably as a result of hysteresis.

The effect of a long-term axial compressive loading on human intervertebral joints has been examined recently by Burns, Kaleps, and Kazarian.[14] They have shown that under static compressive loading the strain-time data exhibits creep. The parameters of this creep phenomenon appear to be a function of the morphologic condition of the disc. If nuclear herniation is present then the ability of the disc to accommodate axial compressive loads is compromised. Koreska and colleagues[39] from Toronto have studied the effect of pure axial compression on the composite behavior of the intervertebral disc. They have demonstrated an exponential relationship between axial compressive load and axial deformation. With eccentric compression the relationship between the applied moment and lateral displacement is linear in the range of normal static physiologic loads. However, the behavior is nonlinear for the lower lumbar spine when the posterior elements are removed.

Axial compressive forces result in bulging of the disc and, thus, results in circumferential tensile stresses. Galante[27] has investigated the tensile properties of the human lumbar annulus fibrosus. As previously noted, the fibers in each lamella run in an opposite direction to the previous one and form an angle of 30 degrees with the horizontal. Because of this orientation, the annulus fibrosus is stiffer between the horizontal and the two fiber direction axes. It is most extensible along the vertical direction. Galante also showed that the anterior annulus is stiffer than the posterior annulus and that stiffness increases toward the periphery.

The Vertebrae

Mechanical studies on human vertebrae have been performed by Bell and associates.[10] They showed that the stress-strain curve of a vertebra subjected to compression approximates a straight line. Interestingly, the strain of the elastic limit appears to be independent of the breaking stresses. Put another way, the deformation required to produce failure of a vertebral body is independent of its strength. Olof Perey[62] has shown that vertebral bodies are compressed about 16% on average before their breaking point is reached. This means that the elasticity of the disc and the vertebral body is similar. In considering the mechanical properties of the vertebra, it is worth using a model consisting of two end-plates, vertical trabeculae or "struts" that are loaded in compression, and transverse trabeculae or "ties" that act to reinforce the struts. Review of Euler's formula serves to emphasize the importance of the lateral supports. We recognize that in osteoporosis it is the transverse trabeculae that are initially predominantly lost. This, according to Euler's theorem, will result in a greater reduction in vertebral strength than would otherwise have been expected on the basis of simple loss of bone content. This has been found indeed to be the case, as evidenced by the experimental work of Bell and associates.[10] The application of the Euler's theorem to the human spine is limited, however. This is due to the fact that the spine is curved before loading, whereas the Euler equation applies only to straight columns. A critique of application of Eulerian theory to the human spine has been published by Owens and colleagues.[55]

It has already been stated that the trabeculae within the vertebral body constitute a three-dimensional grid. The outer cortical shell is thin and, according to Bell and associates,[10] plays very little role in vertebral strength. However, in their work there was no isolated measurement of cortical strength, and their conclusion was arrived at indirectly. Bartley and coworkers[7] investigated the differences between crushing a whole vertebral body and crushing a vertebra trimmed of its cortical bone by using a band saw. In this study there was no statistically significant difference between the crushing strengths of entire vertebral bodies and those of the trabecular bone samples. Rockoff and associates[71] measured the peak nondestructive compression strength of intact vertebral bodies, as well as the compression strength of the same bodies either after cortical removal or after division of the central trabeculae. Their results suggest that the loss of strength resulting from removal of the cortex is greater than 40%, and that relatively little force is transmitted by way of the central trabeculae, especially in subjects over 40 years of age. Perhaps the reason for the apparent discrepancy in these studies is that power tools were used to remove the cortex; this probably destroys some of the trabecular bone, creating localized stress concentrations. To obviate this problem, McBroom and associates[47] tested intact vertebral bodies, as well as those from which the cortex had been removed by manual sanding. The results of this study demonstrated only a 10% reduction in strength of vertebral bodies after cortical sanding. Their work shows that axial compressive stresses in the interior trabecular bone are the most important feature of vertebral loading in compression.

Review of the raw data from the previously mentioned articles seems to indicate that the failure strength of the intervertebral disc and vertebral body is higher than that of the vertebral end-plate. Indeed, work by Hirsch[33] demonstrates that, when large static or dynamic loads are applied to the spine, fracture of the vertebral end-plate with leakage of disc contents into the centrum occurs. In testing to failure of numerous specimens, Lin and colleagues[41] found no evidence of failure of the annulus. The extensive investigation by Perey[2] supports this view that under normal circumstances end-plate fracture will occur before failure of the rest of the vertebral body or disc. This has recently been confirmed by McBroom and associates.[47] Of 16 vertebrae tested to maximum compressive load, all failed by end-plate fracture. Horst and Brinckmann[36] have measured the distribution of axial stress on the end-plate of the vertebral body. They have shown that the stress distribution depends on the state of degeneration of the intervertebral disc and the relative position of adjacent end-plates.

Load Sharing

In many studies of spinal biomechanics the posterior elements are removed from the specimens prior to testing, because it was thought that a vertical load is transmitted from one vertebral body to the next via the intervening disc. Hirsch and Nachemson[34] were unable to show any change in the amount of disc compression after removal of the pedicles and facets on one or both sides of postmortem specimens. Nachemson[49] demonstrated an increase in the pressure of the nucleus pulposus after removal of the arches and articular facets. The average increase was 18%, although the differences between specimens were large. He felt that this data implied that in vertical loading the facets take up about 20% of the load.

Adams and Hutton[1] have examined the effect of posture on the role of the apophyseal joints in resisting intervertebral compressive forces. With the spine 2 degrees extended, a position simulating erect standing posture, the facet joints carry 16% of the compressive force. In a slightly flexed posture, similar to unsupported sitting, the apophyseal joints take no part in resisting the intervertebral compressive force.

The effect of the posterior structure on

stiffness has been shown by Markolf.[45] It was noted that in the lumbar spine the posterior structures contribute substantially to stiffness both in extension and in torsion. Lin and colleagues[41] placed strain gauges near the articular processes on laminae to study the strain in the posterior elements with loading. During anterior compression there was very little load bearing in the posterior elements. With posterior compression, however, large strains were recorded that indicate the activation of a second major load path through the articular processes. Prasad, King, and Ewing[66] have investigated the role of the articular facets during caudocephalad acceleration of the spine, using both strain gauges and intervertebral load cells to obtain data. Their work demonstrates that the facets are, indeed, capable of bearing compressive and tensile loads, the proportion varying inversely with decreasing levels of acceleration. Furthermore, hyperextension of the spine transfers more load to the facets. With respect to intradiscal pressures, Berkson and associates[12] demonstrated little effect with pure compression after posterior element excision. Recently, Young and King[87] have performed a series of elegant experiments that better establish the mechanism for transmission of axial load across a facet joint. Their work suggests that there is bony interaction between the tip of the inferior facet and the pars interarticularis of the vertebra below. They believe that the transmission of compressive facet load occurs through this bony contact.

Mathematic Modeling

As a result of problems with the availability of specimens, materials, and funding, experimental data concerning the biomechanics of the lumbar spine is limited. One method of overcoming these limitations is to use finite element analyses. A finite element analysis generates a mathematic model that can be used to predict the mechanical behavior of a system.

Sonnerup[75] developed a semi-experimental stress analysis of the human intervertebral disc in compression. Using theoretic analysis, he was able to determine the tangential and radial stress distributions of the annulus fibrosus. The results show that inhomogeneity considerably influences the distribution of tangential stress, even when only pure compression of the disc is considered. With refinements in technique and greater familiarity with the use of finite element analysis in dealing with orthopedic problems, a more sophisticated model was developed by Belytschko and associates.[11] By employing an axisymmetric linear model, they demonstrated that an adequate representation of intervertebral disc behavior requires the inclusion of material anisotropy. The same group[40] went on to develop a nonlinear analysis, which is an important step, because the collagenous fibers of the annulus cause it to demonstrate nonlinear behavior. Their studies showed that hoop stresses play an important role in lumbar discs. Thus the fiber stress in the annulus of a lumbar disc is tensile throughout, increasing toward the outer boundary.

A hybrid-stress, finite element model of the intervertebral disc was developed by Spilker.[76] Using this contrast, he was able to assess effects of disc geometry and material properties on predicted radial disc bulge, vertebral deflection, and intradiscal pressure increases under compressive loading. Broberg and von Essen[13] have proposed a model with rotational symmetry of the intervertebral disc. The nucleus is assumed to be an incompressible fluid while the annulus is modeled by multiple fiber layers with alternating fiber inclination. Using this model, the authors have shown that small changes in fiber geometry yield dramatic changes in fiber strains and pressures in the nucleus pulposus.

A three-dimensional finite element analysis of a vertebra has been formulated by Hakim and King.[31] The model predicts large areas of strain in the anterior aspect of the vertebra, as well as at the junction of the pedicles and vertebral body. These investigators also carried out controlled static and dynamic loading experiments. They were able to show good correlation between observed and predicted values. Gracovetsky, Farfan, and Lamy,[29] from Montreal, have attempted to express in mathematic terms what happens when a subject lifts an object. They have hypothesized that the particular way in which someone lifts a weight is determined by minimizing a function of the shear at all intervertebral joints. In spite of the increasing sophistication of these mathematic models, it is important to remember that their relevance to clinical orthopedics ultimately depends on accurate experimental data and clear validation.

Clinical Relevance

The term *low back pain* refers to a wide variety of conditions, all of which result in the perception of pain in the region of the lumbosacral spine. Clearly, not all these entities have a mechanical basis, though mechanical factors probably do play an etiologic role in some low back pain. From the preceding discussion we can hypothesize that under some circumstances axial loading results in disc bulges large enough to trigger the nerve endings of the annulus fibrosis and provide a nociceptive stimulus. It is interesting to note that in clinical practice there are a group of patients in whom low back pain is exacerbated by prolonged sitting. The increase in intradiscal pressures that occur in the sitting position may well account for this phenomenon. As the load-bearing role of the articular facets is being better documented, it is worth speculating on the relationship of facet load to low back pain. Mathematic modeling has shown an increase in facet load with disc degeneration. This increased facet load tends to deform the joint capsule and may well stimulate the receptor nerve endings to fire.

KINEMATICS OF THE LUMBAR SPINE
Coordinate System

In initiating a discussion of kinematics, it is wise to define a system whereby position and motion can be described. An orthogonal or Cartesian system has many advantages and is widely used; White, Panjabi and Brand[83] have demonstrated its clinical value. This central coordinate system has its origin between the cornua of the sacrum. The negative-Y axis is described by a plumb line dropped from the origin with the subject standing in the anatomic position. The positive-X axis points to the left at a 90-degree angle to the Y axis, and the positive-Z axis points forward at a 90-degree angle to both the X and Y axis.

Motion can be described as either rotation, translation, or a combination of the two. Rotation occurs when there is a spinning or angular displacement of a body about an axis. Put another way, a body is in rotation when movement is such that all particles along some straight line in the body or a hypothetical extension of it have zero velocity relative to a fixed point. Translation, on the other hand, occurs when all particles in the body have the same direction of motion relative to a fixed point. A vertebra can either translate along or rotate about any of the three axes in the central coordinate system and thus is said to have 6 degrees of freedom. In general, motion of the spine is a combination of rotation and translation. We can simplify the clinical nomenclature of spine movement to the coordinate system designation as follows.

Flexion	+X
Extension	−X
Left axial rotation	+Y
Right axial rotation	−Y
Right lateral bending	+Z
Left lateral bending	−Z

When one component of motion is always associated with another component, the two or more components are referred to as coupled. The extent to which coupling occurs in the spine is very large. The facet joints in the lumbar spine are arranged at a 45-degree tilt to the X,Y plane and at 90 degrees to the X,Z plane. Because of this orientation, there is well-defined coupling between each of the three components of motion in both the sagittal and frontal planes.

Range of Motion: Clinical Studies

Many attempts have been made to document the range of motion of the lumbar spine. Accurate clinical assessment is fraught with problems and has led investigators to devise a variety of techniques. Some of these and their associated difficulties have been reviewed by Troup, Hood, and Chapman.[79] This group measured the maximal range of lumbar sagittal mobility by using a modification of the method described by Lindahl.[42] Calculations of lumbar movement were made by subtracting the range of flexion and extension at the hip joints from the range of motion of the hips and lumbar spine combined. This latter measurement was made by estimating the angle between the femora and a tangent to the contour of the spine at the lowest thoracic level in both the fully flexed and extended positions. Their study of 230 young, healthy adults demonstrated a mean lumbar flexion and extension of about 80 degrees. This figure is approximately 10 degrees less than that found by Clayson and coworkers[15] and by Lindahl.[42] This discrepancy may be due to the fact that in the former study all subjects were slender young women. The greater range of motion found by Lindahl is probably due to the difference in the method of determining the inclination of the upper limit of the lumbar region. Unfortunately, the techniques used by both Lindahl and by Troup, Hood, and Chapman are unsuitable for clinical practice. They require awkward posturing by patients and involve some discomfort. It is also important to note that these techniques are limited to spinal measurement in the sagittal plane.

Moll and Wright[48] measured spinal mobility in three planes by means of objective clinical methods. To determine anterior spinal flexion, they inked the skin overlying the lumbosacral spine in three spots and then measured the distances between the marks with the subject bending forward. The amount of distraction between the marks had previously been reported to correlate with anterior flexion measured radiographically by Macrae and Wright.[44] Similar methods were used in this study to measure lateral spine flexion and spine extension. Moll and Wright had shown that these clinical determinations correlate with measurements made radiographically. In reviewing the motions of 237 normal subjects, they concluded that the distribution of measurements in each plane of spinal movement followed a Gaussian pattern. Spinal mobility was found diminished by almost 50% between youth and old age. Interestingly, these investigators also found that male mobility exceeded female mobility in the sagittal plane but not in the coronal plane.

Van Adrichem and van der Korst[80] used a similar technique to assess the flexibility of the lumbar spine in children and adolescents. They noted that there is a gradual decrease in flexion of the lumbar spine as one moves cranially from the fifth lumbar vertebra. Some caution is needed, however, in evaluating these articles. Portek and associates[64] have compared clinical and radiologic techniques of measuring lumbar spine movement and found very little correlation. Indeed, their work suggests that the use of skin marks is prone to large errors. This is probably due to the mobility of skin over bony landmarks and the extensibility of the skin.

Clinical quantification of axial rotation of the lumbosacral spine is difficult. Detailed measurements of axial rotation in living subjects were made by Gregersen and Lucas.[30] Steinmann pins were placed in the spinous processes of subjects, and angular displacement of the pins was recorded. With the patients standing, rotation in the lumbar spine ranged from 13 to 18 degrees at each level. In two instances axial rotation at the lumbosacral joint was measured while the subjects were seated. It was found to be significantly less than that observed in the same subjects while they were standing. Further work in this area was carried out by Lumsden and Morris.[43] They measured axial rotation of the lumbosacral joint during various activities, with and without restraints. The average total rotation was found to be 5.9 degrees while the subjects were standing, and lumbrosacral axial rotation was noted to be less than 2 degrees while the subjects were walking.

Range of Motion: Radiographic Studies

It would seem that radiographic assessment of motion of the lumbar spine would be superior to the clinical techniques previously discussed. Tanz[77] obtained x-ray films of 55 subjects in maximum flexion, extension, and right and left lateral bending. The amount of movement taking place at each interspace was calculated by superimposing the films such that the vertebrae caudad to the level being assessed coincided in both films. Tanz found very large differences in normal spinal motion between individuals. He noted a smaller range of lateral bending of the lumbosacral joint than at other levels. In addition, there appears to be a significant decrease in motion range by age 35 years.

A radiographic investigation of lumbar spine movement was also undertaken by Allbrook.[4] He obtained lateral x-ray films of 32 subjects in full flexion, erect, and in full extension. The radiographs were superimposed such that the shadows of the sacra coincided, and the total amount of motion of the lumbar column was measured. Individual vertebral movement was calculated by subtraction. The data show that the lower vertebrae have the most movement and that the range gradually decreases in the upper lumbar spine. In a study of fresh cadaveric lumbar motion segments it was noted by Nachemson and associates[53] that age does not seem to affect their mechanical behavior.

RANGE OF MOTION: SUMMARY

Table 6-1 summarizes the current information regarding ranges and representative figures for the lumbar spine. These figures are taken from the work of White and Panjabi[82] and represent both a review of the literature and their own analysis.

Instantaneous Axis of Rotation

The instantaneous axis of rotation (IAR) is a line that is perpendicular to the plane of motion of a rigid body. The position of the IAR and the magnitude of the rotation about it define plane motion. It is important to note that a given IAR depends on the structure and the type of loading. Motion segments consist of two adjacent vertebrae and all intervening soft

56 *General Principles*

Table 6-1 *Estimated range and representative degree of rotation*

Area of spine	Flexion-extension, X-axis rotation		Lateral bending, Z-axis rotation		Axial rotation, Y-axis rotation	
	Compiled rotary range (degrees)	Representative angle (degrees)	Compiled rotary change (degrees)	Representative range (degrees)	Compiled rotary change (degrees)	Representative angle (degrees)
L1-L2	9-16	12	3-8	6	<3	2
L2-L3	11-18	14	3-9	6	<3	2
L3-L4	12-18	15	5-10	8	<3	2
L4-L5	14-21	17	5-7	6	<3	2
L5-S1	18-22	20	2-3	3	<3	5

*Adapted from White, A.A. and Panjabi, M.M.: Spine **3**:12, 1978.

tissues. Also known as functional spinal units, these segments represent the smallest mechanical unit of the spine involving kinetics, as well as kinematics. Many investigators have attempted to document the IAR of lumbar motion segments. Since these studies have often used different loading techniques, the results are understandably disparate. Pennal and associates,[61] from Toronto, attempted to find this "point of zero instant velocity" by superimposing lateral radiographs taken in flexion and extension. They then determined the point about which motion occurs for each intervertebral level. The normal subjects were found to have a "point of motion" clustered within a specific zone approximately 2.5 cm square. In 65% of subjects that had confirmed spine pathology, the point of motion fell outside this zone.

Rolander[72] noted that healthy discs show a concentration of instantaneous centers of ventroflexion in the dorsal part of the disc, and vice versa. Furthermore, with rotation in the frontal plane there is a tendency for the instantaneous centers to be concentrated to the left median for flexion to the right, and vice versa. In the work of Tanz[77] superimposed films demonstrated that the IAR in flexion and extension is anterior to the articular facets. In lateral bending the center of motion is medial to these joints. Dimnet and associates[21] further investigated lateral flexion of the lumbar spine. They studied a series of seven radiographs obtained during lateral flexion of each subject to define the curve of change in angle and the paths of the IAR. Among other conclusions, they were able to show that the vertebrae from T11 and L5 participate in a comparable fashion in the movement of the column as a whole. Cossette and colleagues[16] addressed themselves to determining the IAR of the third lumbar intervertebral joint during torsion. The angle of rotation was restricted to 6 degrees or less, as this is believed to be the physiologic range (vide supra). The centers of rotation were found to lie anterior to the facet joints in the region of the posterior nucleus and annulus. There also appears to be a correlation between the location of the center of rotation and the direction of rotation, with the IAR lying toward the side to which rotation is forced. Seligman and associates,[74] have developed an accurate method for determining the IAR by using a computer and digitizer. The angle of rotation for the L4-L5 motion segment was measured at 3-degree levels from maximum extension to flexion. The loci were located in the posterior one half of the disc. These investigators noted a difference between the normal loci and the loci of motion segments affected by degenerative disc disease.

An innovative technique involving moire fringes has been used by Gertzbein and coworkers.[28] Two moire screens with engraved reference lines were superimposed on two positive prints of radiographs of a motion segment rotated through 3 degrees. The primary fringes were then identified and the IAR was recorded as the intersection of both primary fringes that intersect at 90 degrees to each other. A locus of centers of rotation of the L4-L5 spinal segment was found to lie in the posterior half of the disc, in agreement with other studies.

Coupling, Preload, and Helical Axis of Motion

The concept of coupling has already been introduced, and the reader will appreciate that, in the studies previously reviewed, only planar motion has been investigated. To examine three-dimensional movement, Rab and Chao[68] have used biplane radiographs. Pope and associates[63] have employed this technique in conjunction with an apparatus that permits the study of segmental vertebral motion under conditions of loading, both in living human subjects and in fresh cadaveric specimens. They have documented the coupling motion of the lumbar spine and have shown that axial rotation is uniformly associated with lateral bend. Indeed, with more complex movements, they have demonstrated a summation effect. Thus there is an increase in lateral translation when both axial rotation and lateral bend are introduced, as compared to when only the latter is affected. Frymoyer and associates[26] have further investigated this phenomenon of coupling in living subjects. The complex coupling that occurs in vivo is similar to that which has been reported by Panjabi[56] in studies of vertebral motion segments.

In most of the studies of mechanical behavior and lumbar spine motion performed in vivo, physiologic loads are applied to the specimens. However, in vivo preloads are present and can be very large, as shown by Nachemson.[50] These preloads are due to body posture and superimposed body weight. Panjabi and coworkers[58] have studied the effects of preload on load displacement curves of the lumbar spine. They showed that, when the preload is present and directed laterally or anteriorly, the spine becomes more flexible; whereas the spine becomes less flexible in the presence of preload when it is subjected to axial tension or torsion. Furthermore, the main motion curve, as well as the coupled motion curve, is affected by the inclusion of preloads. The preload is, in large part, the result of muscle forces. Unfortunately, there is a paucity of information concerning their structured orientation, and it is difficult to quantify their contributions. Rab and associates[69] have performed a mathematic analysis of the musculature about the lumbar spine. They approximated the potential forces and direction of action that the muscles could generate by using cross-sectional and three-dimensional centroid lines of the muscles. Their calculations suggest that the maximum total extensor moment is 2860 kg cm. This value is comparable to that estimated by Troup and Chapman.[78]

As further descriptions of the coupling patterns of the lumbar spine become available, it is increasingly evident that pure planar motion rarely occurs. Thus in the strict sense it is inaccurate to try and identify instantaneous axes of rotation. The helical axis of motion (HAM) is the three-dimensional equivalent of the IAR. A rigid body moving in three-dimensional space can be said to rotate and translate about a certain axis. The location and orientation of this HAM along with information about its rotation and translation constitute a complete three-dimensional description of the motion. White,[81] in collaboration with Panjabi, applied these concepts to an analysis of the mechanics of the thoracic spine in 1969. A technique for measuring three-dimensional, six degrees-of-freedom motion of a body joint has been developed by Panjabi, Krag, and Goel.[60] The great advantage of their methodology is that the six-dimensional motion vector, so determined, can be transformed into six parameters that describe the instantaneous HAM of the joint. The technique uses three spheres that are rigidly attached to the moving body, and six linear variable differential transformers. This represents a considerable improvement over the experimental technique previously employed by Panjabi and White[57] in an attempt to analyze three-dimensional mechanics of the spine.

Facet Orientation

Before concluding our discussion of kinematics, it is worthwhile discussing the spatial orientation of facet joints and its relation to intervertebral disc failure. In theoretic modeling of the spine we usually assume that there is symmetry about the midsagittal plane. There is, however, a high incidence of asymmetry of the posterior facets referred to as "articular tropism." Studies by Badgley,[6] Willis,[86] and Farfan[23] have measured the orientation and tropism of the articular facets. In the Farfan study it was noted that there is a 23% incidence of joint asymmetry in patients without complaints of back pain. The normal functions of the facet joints include the control of spine motion. By restricting certain patterns of movement, it is thought that the facet joints act to protect the discs and ligaments. The clinical study of Farfan and Sullivan[24] suggests that there is a high correlation between asymmetric facet orientation and the level of disc pathology in patients with low back pain. They have hypothesized that intervertebral joint instability is related to facet orientation. Farfan and associates [25] have further investigated this and have calculated that 35% of the resistance to torque of an intact intervertebral joint is supplied by the disc, with the remaining resistance supplied by the facet joints. They have postulated that in vivo disc degeneration is due to torsional strains. Therefore, if there is articular facet joint dysfunction, there would be a greater risk of disc injury. Indeed, in the study of Cyron and Hutton[17] lumbar intervertebral joints were subjected to compressive and shear forces. It was found that joints with articular tropism rotated to the side of the more oblique facet. This may cause additional stress on the annulus fibrosus on the side of the less oblique facet. The importance of torsion to disc degeneration is still unclear, however. Adams and Hutton[2] have shown that torsion of the lumbar spine is predominantly resisted by the apophyseal joint that is in compression and that this facet is the first structure to yield at the torsional limit. They found that this occurs at about 2 degrees of joint rotation and that much greater angles are required to injure the intervertebral disc. In a more recent publication by these authors[3] experiments were performed that suggest the facet joints do, indeed, prevent excessive motion from damaging the intervertebral discs.

Clinical Relevance

The purpose of studying spine kinematics is, in part, to better identify the abnormal. In the preceding discussion it is clear that there is evidence to suggest that many patients with spine pathology have different IARs from the rest of the population. Whether this is cause or effect has yet to be established. With refinements in our understanding and techniques it may well be possible to obtain kinematic profiles of patients and use this information to identify different etiologic entities. Although much work remains to be done in detailing the kinematics of the lumbar spine column, it is clear that great strides have been made in this area over the past 3 decades. With additional research and improved methodologies, the validity of our data and models will allow us to better understand spine kinematics, both in normal and in pathologic situations.

STABILITY OF THE LUMBAR SPINE

Over the past few decades the term *stability* has crept into the orthopedic and bioengineering vocabulary. Its use has increased to the point that the term now is often bandied about without adequately defining it. We have decided with some recalcitrance to use this word, but to emphasize two caveats: first, stability is relative, and second, its measure depends on the observer's vantage (for example, the surgeon, engineer, or anatomist). We will discuss lumbar spine instability from several perspectives.

Stability of Fractures

In 1949 Nicoll[54] published a review of thoracolumbar fractures and noted that they could be classified as either stable or unstable. In the former the intraspinous ligaments remain intact, and in the unstable types these ligaments are ruptured. Holdsworth[35] elaborated on this classification and proposed that it form a rational basis for treatment. He also emphasized the dependence of stability on the status of the posterior ligament complex. However, Bedbrook[8] showed that, even if the entire posterior ligamentous complex is disrupted, the spinal column remains stable. He demonstrated that for instability to occur the disc must be disrupted and the anterior longitudinal ligament stripped, in addition to the posterior ligamentous injury. After careful review of these articles, the clinical criteria the authors used to define stability are still unclear. Holdsworth[35] alluded to the presence of pain and neurologic deficit. However, he realized that, because the posterior ligaments are not damaged in burst fractures, they would be classified as stable by his definition, in spite of the fact that they are extremely painful and often associated with neurologic deficit. Bedbrook[8,9] addressed the issue of mechanical instability with deformity, but he stressed that stability is often not easy to assess in the initial stages after a fracture.

Any classification of stability that has relevance to the spine surgeon must include assessment both of deformity and of neurologic deficit, as well as the potential for both to occur. Indeed, Whitesides[85] has defined a stable spine as one that can withstand stress without progressive deformity or further neurologic damage. This concept has been further refined by the introduction of the concept of the three-column spine. Denis and Armstrong[20] and Denis[18] have described the third or middle column as the posterior longitudinal ligament, the posterior annulus fibrosus, and the posterior wall of the vertebral body. The posterior column is formed by the posterior bony arch and posterior ligamentous complex. The anterior column is composed of the anterior longitudinal ligament, the anterior annulus fibrosus, and the anterior part of the vertebral body. By assessing the mode of failure of the three columns, a fracture can be categorized as to its degree of stability.

Denis[18,19] has classified instability into three grades. Instability of the first degree occurs when the spinal column can angulate or buckle, as in severe compression or seat-belt fractures. Instability of the second degree applies to fractures that can result in neurologic deficit. Burst fractures provide a good example. Third degree instability refers to mechanical and neurologic instability, as in fracture dislocations. Although this classification is a significant advance in relating fracture type to stability, it is important to remember that neurologic damage to the cord can occur without concomitant overt trauma to the spine. Riggens and Kraus,[70] in relating neurologic deficit to type of vertebral spinal cord injuries, have noted a 17% incidence of traumatic spinal cord injuries in which there was no radiographic evidence of vertebral injury. Although this circumstance is more common in the cervical and thoracic spine, Riggins and Kraus have documented posttraumatic paraplegia and paraparesis in the absence of vertebral injury.

Evaluation of Stability

We feel that it is unreasonable to try to equate fracture type with stability, because many other factors are crucial to that assessment. Furthermore, guidelines for lumbar spine instability should apply not only to posttraumatic situations but also to cases of disease, tumor, and surgery. In an attempt to develop more global guidelines for assessing spinal instability, investigators have performed biomechanical analysis of functional spinal units. This work has been reported for the cervical spine by White and associates[84] and Panjabi and others.[59]

More recently, Posner and coworkers[65] have studied the mechanics of the lumbar spine as a function of the transection of its components, by using flexion, extension, and preload forces alone and in combination. In flexion testing all specimens were stable if the anterior components plus two additional components were intact; whereas in extension testing all specimens were stable if the posterior components plus one additional component were intact. Using the results of this study, the authors refined a checklist for

Table 6-2 *Checklist for the diagnosis of clinical instability in the lumbar (L1-L5) spine*

Element	Point value*
Cauda equina damage	3
Relative flexion sagittal plane translation >10% or extension sagittal plane translation >10%	2
Relative flexion sagittal plane rotation >10°	2
Anterior elements destroyed	2
Posterior elements destroyed	2
Dangerous loading anticipated	1

Modified from White, A.A., and Panjabi, M.M.: Clinical instability of the spine. In Evarts, C.M., editor: Surgery of the musculoskeletal system, New York, 1983, Churchill Livingston, Inc.
*Total of 5 or more, Clinically unstable.

Table 6-3 *Checklist for the diagnosis of clinical instability in the lumbosacral (L5-S1) spine*

Element	Point value*
Cauda equina damage	3
Relative flexion sagittal plane translation >5% or extension sagittal plane translation >10%	2
Relative flexion sagittal plane rotation >0 degrees	2
Anterior elements destroyed	2
Posterior elements destroyed	2
Dangerous loading anticipated	

Modified from White, A.A., and Panjabi, M.M.: Clinical instability of the spine. In Evarts, C.M., editor: Surgery of the musculoskeletal system, New York, 1983, Churchill Livingston, Inc.
*Total of 5 or more, Clinically unstable.

assessing clinical instability of the lumbar and lumbosacral spine. The rationale of using a checklist with numeric values is that relevant anatomic, biomechanical, and clinical factors can be individually weighed. Clearly, each of these areas is crucial in the total evaluation of the patient. There is a great deal of difference between two patients with similar fracture patterns if one is elderly and neurologically intact and the other is a football player with a neurologic deficit. Tables 6-2 and 6-3 are checklists that provide a systematic approach to patient assessment for the diagnosis of clinical instability in the lumbar and lumbosacral spine, respectively.

SUMMARY

The spinal surgeon is being confronted with more and more biomechanically related data. To critically evaluate this material, we must understand basic engineering principles. This chapter has reviewed the recent literature dealing with biomechanics, kinematics, and stability of the lumbar spine. The reader will appreciate that many of the articles cited have not only increased our basic science knowledge, but have also provided us with information leading to significant advances in patient care. Although significant strides have been made in spine biomechanics, much remains to be done. By meticulously investigating the mechanical design of the normal spine, our understanding of pathologic situations will improve. In this way our ultimate goal of accurate diagnosis and successful treatment of patients may well be achieved.

REFERENCES

1. Adams, M.A., and Hutton, W.C.: The effect of posture on the role of the apophyseal joints in resisting intervertebral compressive factors, J. Bone Joint Surg. **62B:**358, 1980.
2. Adams, M.A., and Hutton, W.C.: The relevance of torsion to the mechanical derangement of the lumbar spine, Spine **6:**241, 1981.
3. Adams, M.A., and Hutton, W.C.: The mechanical function of the lumbar apophyseal joints, Spine **8:**327, 1983.
4. Allbrook, D.: Movements of the lumbar spinal column, J. Bone Joint Surg. **39B:**339, 1957.
5. Andersson, G.B.J., et al.: Intradiskal pressure, intra-abdominal pressure and myoelectric back muscle activity related to posture and loading, Clin. Orthop. **129:**156, 1977.
6. Badgley, C.E.: The articular facets in relations to low back pain and sciatic radiation, J. Bone Joint Surg. **23:**481, 1941.
7. Bartley, M.H., Jr., et al.: The relationship of bone strength and bone quantity in health, disease, and aging, J. Gerontol. **21:**517, 1966.
8. Bedbrook, G.M.: Stability of spinal fractures and fracture dislocations, Paraplegia **9:**23, 1971.
9. Bedbrook, G.M.: Treatment of thoracolumbar dislocation and fractures with paraplegia, Clin. Orthop. **112:**27, 1975.
10. Bell, G.H., et al.: Variations in strength of vertebrae with age and their relation to osteoporosis, Calc. Tiss. Res. **1:**75, 1967.
11. Belytschko, T., et al.: Finite element stress analysis of an intervertebral disc, J. Biomech. **7:**277, 1974.
12. Berkson, M.H., et al.: Mechanical properties of human lumbar spine motion segments, J. Biomech. Eng. **101:**53, 1979.
13. Broberg, H.G., and von Essen, H.O.: Modeling of intervertebral discs, Spine **5:**155, 1980.
14. Burns, M.L., et al.: Analysis of compressive creep behavior of the vertebral unit subjected to a uniform axial loading using exact parametric soluion equations of Kelvin-solid models, J. Biomech. **17:**113, 1984.
15. Clayson, S.J., et al.: Evaluation of mobility of hip and lumbar vertebrae of normal young women, Arch. Phys. Med. **43:**1, 1962.
16. Cossette, J.W., et al.: The instantaneous center of rotation of the third lumbar intervertebral joint, J. Biomech. **4:**149, 1971.
17. Cyron, B.M., and Hutton, W.C.: Articular tropism and stability of the lumbar spine, Spine **5:**168, 1980.
18. Denis, F.: The three-column spine and its significance in the classification of acute thoracolumbar spine injuries, Spine **8:**817, 1983.
19. Denis, F.: Spinal instability as defined by the three-column spine concept in acute spinal trauma, Clin. Orthop. **189:**65, 1984.

20. Denis, F., and Armstrong, G.W.D.: Compression fractures versus burst fractures in the lumbar and thoracic spine, J. Bone Joint Surg. **63B:**462, 1981.
21. Dimnet, J., et al.: Radiographic studies of lateral flexion in the lumbar spine, J. Biomech. **11:**143, 1978.
22. Eklund, J.A.E., and Corlett, E.N.: Shrinkage as a measure of the effect of load on the spine, Spine **9:**189, 1984.
23. Farfan, H.F.: Referred to in Farfan, H.F. and Sullivan, J.D.: The relation of facet orientation to intervertebral disc failure, Can. J. Surg. **10:**179, 1967.
24. Farfan, H.F., and Sullivan, J.D.: The relation of facet orientation to intervertebral disc failure, Can. J. Surg. **10:**179, 1967.
25. Farfan, H.F., et al.: The effects of torsion on the lumbar intervertebral joints: the role of torsion in the production of disc degeneration, J. Bone Joint Surg. **52A:**458, 1970.
26. Frymoyer, J.W., et al.: The mechanical and kinetic analysis of the lumbar spine in normal living human subjects in vivo, J. Biomech. **12:**165, 1979.
27. Galante, J.O.: Tensile properties of the human lumbar annulus fibrosis, Acta Orthop. Scand. Suppl. 100, 1967.
28. Gertzbein, S.D., et al.: Determination of a locus of instantaneous centers of rotation of the lumbar disc by moire fringes, Spine **9:**409, 1984.
29. Gracovetsky, S., et al.: A mathematical model of the lumbar spine using an optimized system to control muscles and ligaments, Orthop. Clin. North Am. **8:**135, 1977.
30. Gregersen, G.G., and Lucas, D.B.: An in vivo study of the axial rotation of the human thoracolumbar spine, J. Bone Joint Surg. **49A:**247, 1967.
31. Hakim, N.S., and King, A.I.: A three-dimensional finite element dynamic response analysis of a vertebra with experimental verification, J. Biomech. **12:**272, 1979.
32. Hirsch, C.: The reaction of intervertebral discs to compression forces, J. Bone Joint Surg. **37A:**1188, 1955.
33. Hirsch, C.: The mechanical response in normal and degenerated lumbar discs, J. Bone Joint Surg. **38A:**242, 1956.
34. Hirsch, C., and Nachemson, A.: New observations on the mechanical behavior of lumbar discs, Acta Orthop. Scand. **23:**254, 1954.
35. Holdsworth, F.W.: Fractures, dislocations, and fracture-dislocations of the spine, J. Bone Joint Surg. **45B:**6, 1963.
36. Horst, M., and Brinckmann, P.: Measurement of the distribution of axial stress on the end-plate of the vertebral body, Spine **6:**217, 1981.
37. Horton, G.W.: Further observations on the elastic mechanism of the intervertebral disc, J. Bone Joint Surg. **40B:**552, 1958.
38. Klein, J.A., et al.: Radial bulging of the annulus fibrosus during compression of the intervertebral disc, J. Biomech. **16:**211, 1983.
39. Koreska, J., et al.: Biomechanics of the lumbar spine and its clinical significance, Orthop. Clin. North Am. **8:**121, 1977.
40. Kulak, R.F., et al.: Nonlinear behavior of the human intervertebral disc under axial load, J. Biomech. **9:**377, 1976.
41. Lin, H.S., et al.: Mechanical response of the lumbar intervertebral joint under physiological (complex) loading, J. Bone Joint Surg. **60A:**41, 1978.
42. Lindahl, O.: Determination of the sagittal mobility of the lumbar spine, Acta Orthop. Scand. **37:**41, 1966.
43. Lumsden, R.M., and Morris, J.M.: An in vivo study of axial rotation and immobilization at the lumbosacral joint, J. Bone Joint Surg. **50A:**1591, 1968.
44. Macrae, I.F., and Wright, V.: Measurement of back movement, Ann. Rheum. Dis. **28:**584, 1969.
45. Markolf, K.L.: Deformation of the thoracolumbar intervertebral joints in response to external loads, J. Bone Joint Surg. **54A:**511, 1972.
46. Marras, W.S., et al.: Measurements of loads on the lumbar spine under isometric and isokinetic conditions, Spine **9:**176, 1984.
47. McBroom, R.J., et al.: Prediction of vertebral body compressive fracture using quantitative computed tomography, J. Bone Joint Surg. **67A:**1206, 1985.
48. Moll, J.M.H., and Wright, V.: Normal range of spinal mobility, Ann. Rheum. Dis. **30:**381, 1971.
49. Nachemson, A.: Lumbar intradiscal pressure, Acta Orthop. Scand. Supp. 43, 1960.
50. Nachemson, A.: The load of lumbar discs in different positions of the body, Clin. Orthop. **45:**107, 1966.
51. Nachemson, A., and Elfstrom, G.: Intravital dynamic pressures in lumbar discs, Scan. J. Rehab. Med. Supp. **1:**1, 1970.
52. Nachemson, A., and Morris, J.M.: In vivo measurements of intradiscal pressure, J. Bone Joint Surg. **46A:**1077, 1964.
53. Nachemson, A.L., et al.: Mechanical properties of human lumbar spine motion segments, Spine **4:**1, 1979.

54. Nicoll, E.A.: Fractures of the dorso-lumbar spine, J. Bone Joint Surg. **31B:**376, 1949.
55. Owens, E.F., et al.: A critique of applications of the Euler equation to the human spine, J. Manipulative Physiol. Ther. **6:**67, 1953.
56. Panjabi, M.M.: Experimental determinations of spinal motion segment behavior, Orthop. Clin. North Am. **8:**169, 1977.
57. Panjabi, M., and White, A.A.: A mathematical approach for three-dimensional analysis of the mechanics of the spine, J. Biomech. **4:**203, 1971.
58. Panjabi, M.M., et al.: Effects of preload on load displacement curves of the lumbar spine, Orthop. Clin. North Am. **8:**181, 1977.
59. Panjabi, M.M., et al.: Stability of the cervical spine under tension, J. Biomech. **2:**189, 1978.
60. Panjabi, M.M., et al.: A technique for measurement and description of three-dimensional six degree-of-freedom motion of a body joint with an application to the human spine, J. Biomech. **14:**447, 1981.
61. Pennal, G.F., et al.: Motion studies of the lumbar spine, J. Bone Joint Surg. **54B:**442, 1972.
62. Perey, O.: Fracture of the vertebral end-plate in the lumbar spine, Acta Orthop. Scand. Supp. 25, 1957.
63. Pope, M.H., et al.: Experimental measurements of vertebral motion under loads, Orthop. Clin. North Am. **8:**155, 1977.
64. Portek, I., et al.: Correlation between radiographic and clinical measurement of lumbar spine movement, Br. J. Rheum. **22:**197, 1983.
65. Posner, I., et al.: A biomechanical analysis of the clinical stability of the lumbar and lumbosacral spine, Spine **7:**374, 1982.
66. Prasad, P., et al.: The role of articular facets during +G2 acceleration, J. App. Mech. **41:**321,1974.
67. Quinnell, R.C., et al.: Observations of pressures within normal discs in the lumbar spine, Spine **5:**166, 1983.
68. Rab, G.T., and Chao, E.Y.: Three-dimensional roentgenographic analysis of the lumbar spine. Paper presented to Twenty-Seventh Annual Conference on Engineering in Medicine and Biology, October 10, 1974.
69. Rab, G.T., et al.: Muscle force analysis of the lumbar spine, Orthop. Clin. North Am. **8:**193, 1977.
70. Riggins, R.S., and Kraus, J.F.: The risk of neurologic damage with fractures of the vertebrae, J. Trauma **17:**126, 1977.
71. Rockoff, S.D., et al.: The relative contribution of trabecular and cortical bone to the strength of human lumbar vertebrae, Calc. Tiss. Res. **3:**163, 1969.
72. Rolander, S.D.: Motion of the lumbar spine with special reference to the stabilizing effect of posterior fusion, Acta Orthop. Scand. Supp. **90:** 1966.
73. Schultz, A., et al.: Loads on the lumbar spine, J. Bone Joint Surg. **64A:**713, 1982.
74. Seligman, J.V., et al.: Computer analysis of spinal segment motion in degenerative disc disease with and without axial loading, Spine **2:**566, 1984.
75. Sonnerup, L.: A semi-experimental stress analysis of the human intervertebral disc in compression, Exp. Mech. **12:**142, 1972.
76. Spilker, R.L.: A simplified hybrid-stress finite element model of the intervertebral disc. In Gallagher, R.H., et al., editors: Finite elements in biomechanics, New York, 1982, John Wiley & Sons, Inc.
77. Tanz, S.S.: Motion of the lumbar spine, Am. J. Roent. **69:**399, 1953.
78. Troup, J.D.G., and Chapman, A.E.: The strength of the flexor and extensor muscles of the trunk, J. Biomech. **2:**49, 1969.
79. Troup, J.D.G., et al.: Measurements of the sagittal mobility of the lumbar spine and hips, Ann. Phys. Med. **9:**308, 1968.
80. Van Adrichem, J.A.M., and van de Korst, J.K.: Assessment of the flexibility of the lumbar spine, Scand. J. Rheum. **2:**87, 1973.
81. White, A.A.: Analysis of the mechanics of the thoracic spine in man. Acta Orthop. Scand. Supp. 127, 1969.
82. White, A.A., and Panjabi, M.M.: The basic kinematics of the human spine, Spine **3:**12, 1978.
83. White, A.A., et al.: A system for defining position and motion of the human body parts, Med. Biol. Eng. **13:**261, 1975.
84. White, A.A., et al.: Biomechanical analysis of clinical stability in the spine, Clin. Orthop. **109:**85, 1975.
85. Whitesides, T.E.: Traumatic kyphosis of the thoracolumbar spine, Clin. Orthop. **128:**78, 1977.
86. Willis, T.A.: Lumbosacral anomalies, J. Bone Joint Surg. **41A:**935, 1959.
87. Yang, K.H., and King, A.I.: Mechanism of facet load transmission as a kyphosis for low back pain, Spine **9:**557, 1984.

ADDITIONAL READINGS

Farfan, H.F.: Mechanical disorders of the low back, Philadelphia, 1973, Lea & Febiger.

Morris, H.M., and Markolf, K.L.: Biomechanics of the lumbosacral spine, Atlas of orthotics: The American Academy of Orthopaedic Surgeons, St. Louis, 1975, The C.V. Mosby Co.

Schultz, A.B.: Mechanics of the human spine, Appl. Mech. Rev. **27:**1487, 1974.

White, A.A.: Analysis of the mechanics of the thoracic spine in man, Acta Orthop. Scand. Supp. 127, 1969.

White, A.A., and Panjabi, M.M.: Clinical biomecanics of the spine, Philadelphia, 1978, J.B. Lippincott Co.

White, A.A., et al.: Biomechanics of lumbar spine and sacroiliac articulation: relevance to idiopathic low back pain. In White, A.A., and Gordon, S.L., editors: Symposium of idiopathic low back pain, St. Louis, 1982, The C.V. Mosby Co.

White, A.A., et al.: Spinal stability: evaluation and treatment. In Murray, D.G., editor: Instructional course lectures: The American Academy of Orthopaedic Surgeons, St. Louis, 1982, The C.V. Mosby Co.

CHAPTER

7

SURGICAL ANATOMY AND NOMENCLATURE

Arthur H. White   Robert Watkins   Charles D. Ray

One can never emphasize enough the importance of knowing the exact location of the lesion that causes a clinical syndrome and how to reach it surgically without creating new problems. The experienced surgeon knows this almost reflexively, but the less-traveled neuro-orthopedist faces difficult trials. One should carefully study a skeletal model side by side with plain films and CT scan images to create a three-dimensional mental image of the structures to be operated on, those to be removed or altered, and those to be left alone. It seems almost sophomoric to suggest that one review and recite the anatomy in question, but these are indeed serious elements of our business, almost identical with skills and details of navigation required of the long-distance pilot or captain. In general, the most important parameters of exposure are: restraints placed by the anatomy, knowledge of permissible technique (that is, what one can get away with), visibility (the factor largely related to size of the incision, retraction, illumination and visual contact, and maneuverability of instruments and tissues), subsequent closure of the wound, and patient positioning and comfort. It is certainly not enough to speak of exposure solely in terms of how to get to the target by the shortest and safest route.

Several anatomic landmarks are important in the approach to the lumbar spine. The first is the relationship of the disc to the interlaminar area. One must realize that the disc space progresses cephalad faster than the interlaminar area (Fig. 7-1). That is, the fifth lumbar disc is approximately at the L5-S1 interlaminar area, while the second disc is under the lamina of L2, cephalad to the interlaminar area of L2-L3. The importance of the disc level is immediate, in that it determines the skin incision. If the majority of the intracanal work is to be done on the disc, the skin incision should be centered over the disc. The radiographic marker for the skin incision is inserted just lateral to the spinous process at the disc level. After performing the skin incision, incise the subcutaneous fat.

THE ANATOMY OF THE LIGAMENTUM FLAVUM

It must be understood that the ligamentum flavum inserts approximately

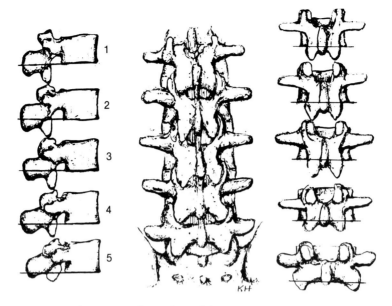

Fig. 7-1 Relationship of disc space to lamina.

under 50% of the cephalad lamina into the edge of the caudad lamina. Laterally, it bends with the facet joint capsule and forms a more vertical portion of the ligamentum flavum in the lateral recess. The ligamentum flavum likewise has a superficial portion and a deep portion. The undersurface of the ligamentum flavum is nature's dural protectant, and postoperative fat or Gelfoam should be considered a second-best substitute to the undersurface of the ligamentum flavum.

The next concept is that of the transversing and exiting nerve root. At each disc space and interlaminar area there will be a transversing dural sac, nerve root, and exiting nerve root. Identify each of these structures as separate entities, and orient the pathology according to these structures. Lateral recess stenosis and a central-to-medial disc herniation should predominantly affect the transversing nerve root, whereas foraminal stenosis at the same level of the operation should affect the exiting nerve root.

The key landmark for intracanal pathology is the pedicle. Identify the pedicle as the hallmark of safe exploration inside the spinal canal. The pedicle is identified usually at the base of the superior facet. With the identification of the pedicle, usually with a nerve hook just under the edge of the facet joint, several structures then become known in relation to the pedicle. Sometimes the medial portion of the facet joint must be removed to reach the pedicle. The pedicle, likewise, will be more cephalad as you progress cephalad in the spine. The pedicle vascular supply at the base of the pedicle can be quite profuse. The vascular leash exits above and below the pedicle, but more prominantly above it. Also, the disc space is less than 1 cm cephalad to the pedicle. The transversing nerve root is medial to the pedicle and exits around the caudal portion. Of course, there is an intervertebral foramen above and below the pedicle, but if the operation is done for disease or injury of the transversing nerve root, then the intervertebral foramen with which you are interested is caudad to the pedicle.

THE FACET JOINT

The facet joint consists of a more dorsal, inferior facet, sweeping down off the cephalad lamina and a more volar, superior facet coming off the pedicle and the inferior lamina. Dissection should not remove the external facet joint capsule for an interlaminar operation, and great care must be taken to preserve the fat pad inside the facet joint when performing an operation for intradiscal pathology. The superior facet and facet joint often can protrude quite far into the spinal canal, such as in a trefoil canal shape. Both articulations of the facet must be identified to proceed to the next step of identification of the pedicle, which should be at the base of the superior facet.

In the coming months and years interest in lumbar spine surgical anatomy will become even more focused on structures adjacent to and lateral to the pedicle. Tethering of the nerve structures by several small perineural ligaments and the neurovascular bundle comprising the Von Luschka nerve all probably act to prevent the root, ganglion or spinal nerve from being able to move about. Thus, the laterally passing root cannot "escape" the onslaught of a rapidly compressing disc herniation, hematoma, or facet capsular hydrops. Likewise, it may be unable to evade the slowly evolving disc bar, uncinate spur, hypertrophic facet, or spondylolisthesis.

Further lateral to the "far out" syndrome (compression of the spinal nerve by a stenosis between the sacral ala and the transverse process of L5) is the probably more common entrapment of the nerve between a lateral disc bar of S1 and its adjacent ala. Of course, there has been much controversy as to how a nerve structure may be entrapped within a nonmoving, tight passage or between prominent, opposing surface structures (that is, dorsal and ventral walls of the lateral recess, between pedicle and spur, spur and ala, or superior lamina and posterior vertebral body) where the structures arise from one and the same segment. This relative entrapment in a previously adequate passage must be related to nerve swelling. Nerves may enlarge rapidly as a result of interstitial edema or perineural vascular engorgement; they may also enlarge slowly, on both sides of a stenotic area due to a buildup of axonally transported materials, or as a result of a progressive development of perineural fibrosis. The latter two phenomena may require weeks or months to develop, but the first two may occur in minutes, hours, or days after minor trauma, traction injury, or local inflammation; these first two are also more likely to be reversible by the systemic or epidural administration of a glucocorticoid.

There are far out ligaments of importance in lumbar nerve entrapment. For example, the intertransverse ligament (a rather thin, broad, sheetlike band extending between the transverse processes all along the lumbar spine; below L5 this ligament merges onto the presacral fascia) may lie ventral or dorsal to iliolumbar ligaments. The nerve passes immediately ventral to this confluence of structures. A posterolateral disc osteophyte lying ventral to the nerve will press it dorsally against these ligaments, causing an entrapment syndrome; this may be the source of neurogenic claudications often seen in osteophytosis. This lateral anatomy is becoming clearer with the increased use of a paralateral approach to decompression, as described in Chapter 18.

Another lateral structure, as yet not clearly appreciated, is the complex nerve sheath. This is a rather loose envelope that begins as a poorly organized tissue layer surrounding the dural sac and is contiguous with the loose sheath to accompany the root sleeve, to pass around the ganglion, down the presacral space beneath the inferior extension of the L5-sacral intertransverse ligament, around the confluence of the sciatic nerve elements, out the sciatic notch and down the leg. This sheath can be demonstrated by injection of contrast, using digital x-ray

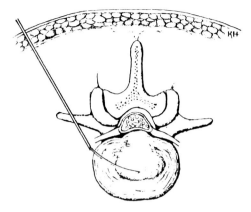

Fig. 7-2 Chemonucleolysis, double needle technique.

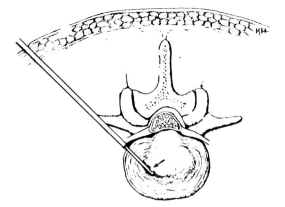

Fig. 7-3 Percutaneous nuclectomy with suction-cutting apparatus.

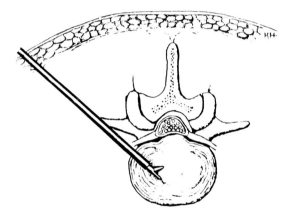

Fig. 7-4 Percutaneous nuclectomy done with rongeurs.

subtraction, or with subsequent CT scanning. The clinical importance of this sheath is not yet clear; however, there may be a rather lymphatic function with a fluid passage in which the nerve is able to slide about freely. This sheath probably should be preserved during surgery in order to maintain normal nerve mobility on traction. Sheath injections with contrast medium may prove important for study of far out nerve entrapment.

The nomenclature of lumbar spine surgical procedures has become confusing as new procedures have been added by specialists from various disciplines in different countries. It is hard to define where a laminotomy ends, a laminectomy begins, and where a laminectomy becomes a wide decompression.

The smallest hole that we can make to do a surgical procedure in the lumbar spine is with a needle. A 25- or 22-gauge needle is sufficient to do chemonucleolysis with chymopapain or collagenase (Fig. 7-2).

The second smallest hole for doing spinal surgery is probably in percutaneous nuclectomy with the use of a scope (Fig. 7-3). A scope can be passed posterolaterally in the same direction that a needle is passed for chemonucleolysis and instruments then used through the scope to remove disc material (Fig. 7-4).

Microdiscectomy is another very small incision (approximately 1 inch) through the midline at one of the lumbar disc levels. The dissection can be carried down to the ligamentum flavum with or without a microscope. The ligamentum flavum can be partially or totally excised. The vertebral canal can then be entered and the disc and nerve roots evaluated. It is difficult through this incision to do much bone removal or exploration of the lateral recess and intervertebral foramen. Various probes and instruments have been developed for such evaluation. The disc can be "trimmed." Some entry into the intradiscal space can be obtained but thorough removal of the interstasies of a disc is not

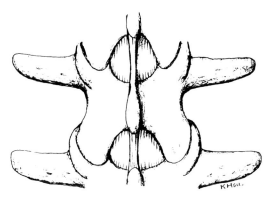
Fig. 7-5 Normal anatomy.

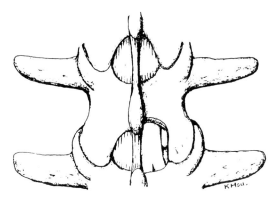
Fig. 7-6 Laminotomy.

possible through this small incision. With a slightly larger incision, a lamina distractor can be used to give more working room. As we require greater amounts of disc removal, nerve passageway exploration and decompression, we need to have larger incisions, more muscular retraction, and more bone excised from the lamina.

When we begin removing bone from the lamina of one of the lumbar vertebra, we are doing a laminotomy (Figs. 7-5 to 7-7). Since the lamina extends from the base of the spinous process to the pars interarticularis, a laminectomy is a complete removal of this structure (Fig. 7-8). When the entire lamina is removed from both sides of a single vertebra, we have done a bilateral laminectomy (Fig. 7-9). Since the spinous process is supported by the lamina on both sides, a bilateral laminectomy necessitates that the spinous process is also removed.

Is a bilateral laminectomy a wide decompressive laminectomy? How much more bone can we remove laterally before we have sacrificed the pars interarticularis or one of the articular processes? The latter would certainly be called a broad or wide decompressive laminectomy and would probably have added to the definition a facetectomy if the entire facet joint was removed. If only part of the facet joint was removed it

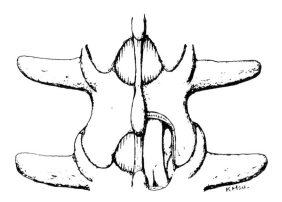
Fig. 7-7 Laminotomy with partial facetectomy.

could be called a hemifacetectomy. The hemifacetectomy allows us to decompress the lateral recess or spinal nerve channel before it exits the intervertebral foramen. To enlarge the intervertebral foramen, we can remove increasing amounts of articular process, vertebral body, or pedicle. A total facetectomy would, by definition, be also a foramentomy.

Far lateral herniated discs and nerve root entrapments imply that the diseased process and procedure necessitated is outside the intervertebral foramen. The intervertebral foramen probably can be considered to end at the lateral border of the pedicle.

Other terms such as hemilaminectom, autostabilization, "Christmas tree" procedure, and partial laminectomy are not broadly accepted terms with well-

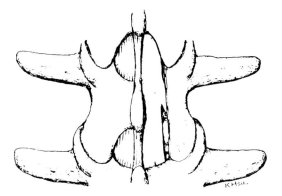

Fig. 7-8 Total unilateral laminectomy.

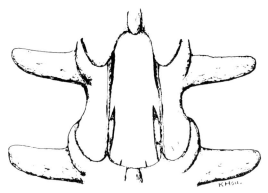

Fig. 7-9 Bilateral laminectomy.

accepted definitions.

The nomenclature for surgical procedures on a disc is even less standardized and more confusing. We speak of discectomy, which might imply the complete removal of a disc. The closest thing we can come to a total disc removal is during an anterior interbody fusion, at which time we do remove nearly the complete disc. From a posterior approach, however, the typical laminectomy removes only approximately one fourth to one third of a disc. With a posterior interbody fusion we may remove as much as three fourths of a disc substance. There are terms such as to "trim" a disc, which I assume means simply the removal of the extruded portion of the disc. There are not any good or standard names for these partial disc excision procedures. One might use the term sequestrectomy for removing a sequestered disc or extruded disc removal for an extruded disc. When the disc is entered bilaterally we may use the term bilateral disc excision or discectomy. When the end-plates of the disc are curetted, the name and description of the procedure could so state.

There is less confusion about lumbar fusions. Although an anterior fusion can be done in several different fashions, there is really only one term for all the different styles of the anterior interbody fusion. Similarly, the posterior interbody fusion has only one name despite the various techniques. There should be a specific name for a posterior interbody fusion that is done unilaterally and for one that is done with small fragments of bone vs. large "bone plugs." A posterior intertransverse fusion implies that the bone is placed over the transverse processes and along the lateral faces of the superior facets. Many people assume that an intertransverse fusion also includes placing bone within the facet joint. A facet joint fusion implies only the placement of bone within the facet joint.

When the posterior elements are left intact and a fusion placed over the lamina and spinous processes, the term used is a *posterior fusion*. This does not usually include an intertransverse fusion. It may well include the facet joints. Specific names have been given to these posterior fusions, such as those of Hibbs and Albee.

The nomenclature for internal fixation with fusions is burgeoning. In the 1960s we had only the Knodt and Harrington rods from which to choose. In the 1970s the Luque rods developed with intersegmental wiring with combinations of Harrington rods and Luque rods. Facet screws have been used for over 20 years. Techniques for placing screws in the pedicle have developed in Europe over the past 10 years and now in the United States many variations have developed that are included in chapters in this book. The pedicle screws have attachments for plates, dual rods, threaded rods, Harrington rods, and Luque rods. The fusions that can be used in addition to these internal fixations are usually posterior. These can be posterior interbody fusions or posterior intertransverse fusions. There is internal fixation for anterior fusions also in the form of screws, which have various forms of cables and rods attached.

In the following chapters you will see descriptions of all of these procedures and why they may be selected by the surgeon as the procedure of choice in a particular circumstance. It may be confusing when you read that one qualified surgeon finds a procedure extremely valuable while another finds it useless. There are many reasons for this variation in opinion. One reason is the selection of patients. A surgeon may be working with a population of patients who are very hardy with high pain tolerances and high frustration tolerances. His patients may put up with spinal instability or backache, whereas another surgeon may be dealing with demanding patients with low pain tolerance who do not cope well with backache. The latter group of patients may do better with some form of internal fixation or fusion, whereas the former may be totally successful with laminectomy alone. It is well known that patients with classical herniated discs experience a high success rate with laminectomy and disc excision alone. Patients with degenerative disc disease, spinal stenosis, and instability do not do well with laminectomy. Some surgeons believe that surgery is totally unwarranted in patients with various forms of degenerative disc disease unless there is a frank herniated disc with nerve root involvement. Other surgeons believe that they have the tools to help patients deal with backache and forms of degenerative disc disease.

PART TWO

SURGICAL PROCEDURES

SECTION ONE

SURGICAL CONSIDERATIONS

CHAPTER

8

ANATOMIC STRATEGIES OF INTERNAL FIXATION

R. Charles Ray

Why should the use of internal fixation in the lumbar spine fusion be controversial? Few present-day orthopedic surgeons question the use of internal fixation in other parts of the body. Intramedullary femoral rods hold shattered femurs in proper alignment, resisting great stresses, yet allow early ambulation without external casts or braces. Healing rates with "rigid" internal fixation are at least as good, and probably better, than with nonfixation methods. In addition, the A/O group has shown a basic microscopic difference in bone healing with "rigid" internal fixation. Shenk and Willenegger[8] have shown that with the absence of motion primary vascular bone healing can occur. In the presence of motion without sufficient internal fixation bony healing occurs by calcification of fibrocartilaginous tissue matrix. There are other advantages as well. Much has been written in this area about early mobilization of nonoperated parts to prevent disuse atrophy, soft tissue scarring, and other attributes of "fracture disease."

The principle of rigid internal fixation that enables patients to be quickly mobilized without external supports and promotes rapid and secure bony healing has great appeal to the spine surgeon. Significant advances have been made with spinal instrumentation in the last 20 years. With internal fixation scoliosis surgeons have made dramatic progress in the decrease of nonunion rates and rapid patient mobilization with maintenance of spinal alignment. Routine reoperation with fusion mass exploration, which was once advised, no longer is routinely performed.

Why, then, the controversy when the same principles are applied to the lumbar spine? It is because there are so many conflicting reports in the literature as to success rates in lumbar fusion operations, both with and without internal fixation.

Fusion rates without internal fixation have been quoted anywhere from 56% to 96%,[9] whereas fusion rates with internal fixation have shown a similar spread. What then is wrong with the methods of fixation and how can they be improved?

Perhaps the forces of the lumbar spine, with the weight of the trunk meeting the fixed segment of the pelvis, is too much for the puny forces of our present-day fixation methods. One should remember that these alignments must be maintained not only when the patient is recumbent but also when the patient is ambulating, which tends to put a spiraling force couple across the lumbosacral junction with each step. Perhaps we should be comparing our present methods of spine fixation not with modern intramedullary rods but with Parnam bands and four-hole plate methods of treating femoral fractures of the last century. We need to reexamine the anatomy of the lumbar spine and seek an anatomic strategy of fixation.

There are several problems with current fixation methods. As already stated, there is no clear-cut evidence that they work. They often distort anatomy, creating loss of the normal lumbar lordosis and altering spine mechanics. They often encroach on the canal size, which is sometimes a negligible problem and sometimes the cause for their emergent removal. They often require excessive dissection above and below the level of interest.

Metallic implants, which include most of the fixation methods, interfere with further workup procedures, especially CT scans. Some improvement in technology has enabled this to be less of a problem than it was previously, but even more problems will be encountered with nuclear magnetic resonant (NMR) scanning. The implants may fail and cause direct neurologic damage, increased irritation, and the need for repeat surgery.

There is still the unanswered question of remote scarring or mutagenic potential with the current stainless steel implants over an extended period of time.

The ideal fixation for the lumbar spine has seven basic attributes. First, it restores the relationship between the disc, pedicle, nerve root, and facet joint to a more normal alignment. Second, the fixation should be rigid enough to obviate the need for external immobilization and allow for mobilization of adjacent nonfixed structures. Third, it should not interfere with further workup such as NMR scanning or CT scans. It also should block all planes of motion, including sagittal, coronal, and translational, as well as rotational planes. It should not excessively stress-shield the spine fusion mass, ideally tapering its strength over time to allow gradual transfer of stress to the fusion mass. In addition, it should restore and maintain sagittal plane curvatures normally found in the spine. Finally, it should be relatively simple, easy, and safe to perform.

A detailed consideration of the biomechanics of the spine is not appropriate for this section, but it is important to remember that the forces acting on the implant causing it to fail are, in large part, a result of the distance from the center of instant axis of rotation of the motion segment. The greater the distance from that axis, the greater is the implant's lever arm in restricting forces close to the axis rotation and the greater the forces acting on the implant as well. The exact type and amount of motion varies from level to level and patient to patient. The lumbar facets have different orientations at each level and occasionally even at the same level on different sides. Disc height, capsular laxity, and ligamentous structures greatly influence potential amounts of range of motion. The forces on a hypermobile L4-L5 level with a tall disc space and partially removed facets and ligaments are different from the end stage–narrowed L5-S1 disc with hypertrophic facet joints. The type of fusion and fixation may need to be varied from patient to patient and possibly level to level.

Certain basic anatomic considerations should be remembered. The lumbar spine is comprised of interconnected segments joined in three places at each level by two different types of articulations. The disc anteriorly is somewhat constrained by the superficial thickening of the annulus that compromises the anterior and posterior longitudinal ligaments. In general the disc allows the two adjacent segments to move in nearly any direction: in sagittal or coronal planes, in rotation, or in distraction and compression. Most restriction of range of motion occurs by the facet joints, which, by their relative oblique orientations to the sagittal plane, allow little rotation while minimally restricting flexion and extension. This is an important point since one can direct the internal fixation to further limit this naturally restricted range of motion unless the facet joints are nonfunctional secondary to degeneration or surgical removal. This latter case greatly increases the rotational stresses on the implant.

The anatomy of the sacrum differs from the lumbar segments in terms of fixation potential in three important areas. The thickness of the sacral lamina usually is much thinner and sometimes nonexistent. The spinous process often is small, if present at all. The relative size of the spinal canal is small in relationship to adjacent structures so that any encroachment by wires or hooks may have significant neurologic impingement effects that would not be found at other levels.

The various anatomic structures for fixation and their relative merits will now be considered.

SPINOUS PROCESS

The spinous process was the first structure used for internal fixation in the spine. Hadra of Galveston used a figure of eight silver wire in 1891 in the treatment of a cervical fracture. Albee popularized the interspinous process fusion originally described in 1911. Since he used a tibial graft held in place by sutures, this construct was of questionable significance as far as internal fixation is concerned. In 1931 Gibson used a tibial graft that blocked extension by fitting snugly between the bases of the spinous processes. The "clothespin" graft, as it has been called, was recognized to restore facet alignments, reduce lumbar lordosis, and open intervertebral foramina. It has the added advantage of not using metal. The Wilson plate described in 1952 used metal on one side of the spinous process for stability and bone graft bolted to the other side for the fusion mass.

The simplest construct for spinous process fixation remains the tension band wire, either in the form of a simple loop placed through holes or around the ends of the spinous process as a whole. Converting this to a figure of eight changes little in the properties of the fixation. This construct, which restricts flexion only, tends to cut through bone with the same principle used to make cheese cutters. With the current emphasis on adequate decompression, the spinous process seldom is left totally intact. The bone quality is mostly cancellous with a very thin cortical shell and hence is a poor choice in terms of relative strength for a fixation device. Although the spinous process is easy to approach, its distance from the instant axis of rotation and great subsequent forces imposed on it greatly limits its use.

The area of the junction of the spinous process with the lamina has received increased attention recently as an alternative to sublaminar wiring. Drummond and Keene from Wisconsin have developed a fixation technique using the relatively strong bone in the junctional area of the spinous process and the lamina (Fig.

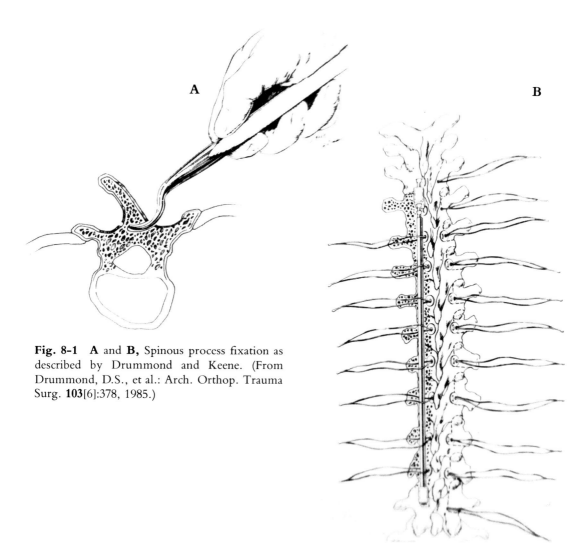

Fig. 8-1 **A** and **B,** Spinous process fixation as described by Drummond and Keene. (From Drummond, D.S., et al.: Arch. Orthop. Trauma Surg. **103**[6]:378, 1985.)

8-1). The forces on the cortex are dissipated by using a washer buttress for the wire. This increases pull-out strength by 40% over the wire alone. The use of this technique with double Harrington or Luque rods shows promise for multiple-level fixation as a safer alternative than sublaminar wiring.

LAMINA

The lamina is, by far, the most commonly used area of lumbar fixation. It can be thinned and partially resected for decompression while still maintaining adequate strength for fixation. Laminar fixation usually takes the form of Knodt, Harrington, or Luque rods. The difference between the Knodt and Harrington rod is primarily one of size. Both systems attach at the two end segments by a hook that intrudes to a greater or lesser extent into the canal space. Both Harrington and Knodt systems can be applied either in distraction, as most commonly used, or in compression, but usually not both simultaneously. In pseudarthrosis repair with minimal motion, excellent fixation can be obtained by using two, or even three, Knodt rods in compression across the fusion mass. A tension band wire around the spinous process can be used in most cases as an adjunct to a distraction system (Fig. 8-2). If applied first, it can prevent overdistraction and loss of lumbar lordosis, which are common problems with too zealous tightening of the

78 Surgical Procedures

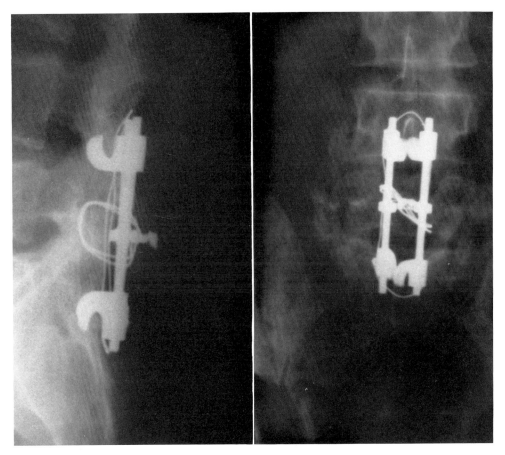

Fig. 8-2 Distraction force via Knodt rods with compression and limitation of distraction via spinous process tension band. Supplemented with sublaminar wires at L4.

distraction rods. The Knodt rods, because of the nut-thread configuration, cannot be contoured to match or maintain lordosis. However, Harrington systems can be contoured to maintain the lordosis by using square-ended rods to prevent rod rotation (Fig. 8-3). Edward sleeves also can be used to exert pressure against the lamina to achieve the same results.

One must also be careful with any compression system not to create foraminal stenosis by overzealous tightening or inadequate bony resection. Weiss springs now modified with an internal rod splint are undergoing some resurgence of popularity because of their ability to maintain constant corrective forces. Fixed systems such as Harrington rods, in contrast, have been shown by Nachemson to lose significant amounts of distraction forces over time.

Because of the presence of lumbar lordosis and the relative tilt of the L5 and sometimes L4 and S1 lamina, standard hooks often do not fit the superior aspect of the lamina in the proper manner. This sometimes causes an occult compromise of the neural canal as the tip of the hook protrudes farther into the canal than would be anticipated. This problem has been somewhat alleviated by changing the rod-lamina axis in such hooks as designed by Andre.

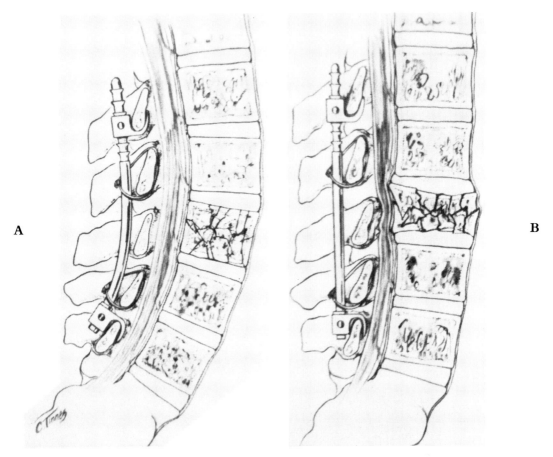

Fig. 8-3 Contouring of Harrington rods to preserve lordosis combined with sublaminar wires. **A,** Proper alignment with rod contouring. **B,** Poor alignment without contouring rod. (From Dewald, R.: Clin. Orthop. **189**:150, 1984.)

PEDICLE FIXATION

Pedicular fixation has a varied history of contributors. Louis[5] of Marseilles, France, described a plate-screw fixation for one or two levels at the lumbosacral junction. (Fig. 8-4.) Professor Arthur Yau of Hong Kong used Dwyer screw fixation of the pedicles for posterior fixation for kyphosis. The concept of pedicular fixation is an attractive one. The pedicles are seldom involved in decompressive resection until the end stage of compressive disease is seen. Quality of bone varies from nearly all cortical in the young patient, to a thin cortical tube in the elderly. Most of the fixation is above the floor of the canal, so a great depth of penetration to the vertebral body is not necessary. The angles of the pedicle-body alignment and the cross-sectional sizes of the pedicles can all be determined by preoperative CT scans.

Pedicular fixation is achieving renewed interest in the form of an external fixation system designed by Friedrich Magerl[6] and in the form of an extended plate and screw fixation system designed by Arthur Steffee (Fig. 8-5). Several different pedicle screw-rod constructs have emerged in 1985. Some of these allow translational sagittal plane realignment, such as spondylolisthesis reduction, never before possible. Just as long bones undergo certain changes with age, the

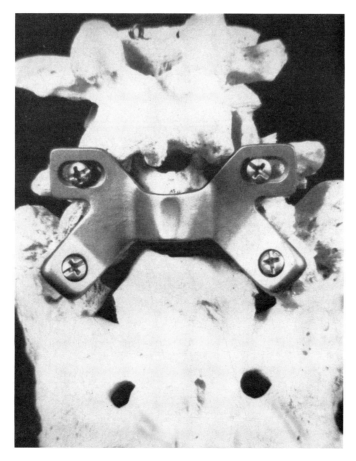

Fig. 8-4 Louis plate and pedicle screw fixation. (From Louis, R.: Clin. Orthop. **203**:18, 1986.)

pedicle undergoes similar changes. There is a gradual enlargement resulting from periosteal new bone formation with thinning of the cortex and enlargement of the medullary canal accompanied by loss of trabecular bone centrally. This accounts for the cephalad-craniad foraminal stenosis seen in the elderly, along with disc space narrowing and other factors.

Pedicular fixation usually takes the form of screws attached to some other fixation device. These include flexible Dwyer cables, solid rods, and rigid plates. The pedicle screws can also serve directly as attachment points for Knodt rods or indirectly via wires for Harrington or Luque rods. The increased rigidity afforded by segmental fixation at every level is attractive. How rigid the fixation becomes depends in large measure on the degree with which the pedicular screws are fixed to each other. Dwyer cables provide tension forces but little else. Substituting a rod for the cable provides resistance to both flexion and extension, but this is not useful for segmental stepoff such as with spondylolisthesis. More rigid plate attachment, such as the plate and screw devices of Louis and Steffee, provides not only resistance to flexion and extension but also some resistance to torsional forces, as well. Due to the cantilever of the screw off the plates, how much distraction across the disc space they can maintain is unclear. This is an area of active research and interest.

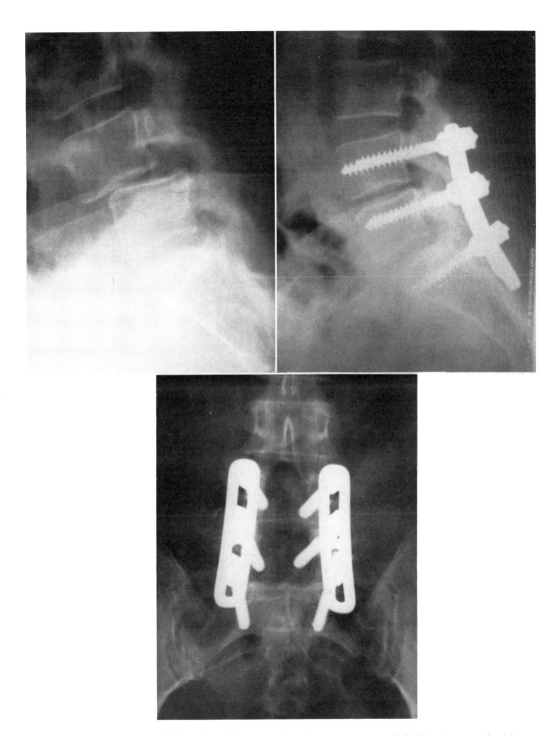

Fig. 8-5 A 56-year-old female with progressive degenerative spondylolisthesis treated with Steffee instrumentation.

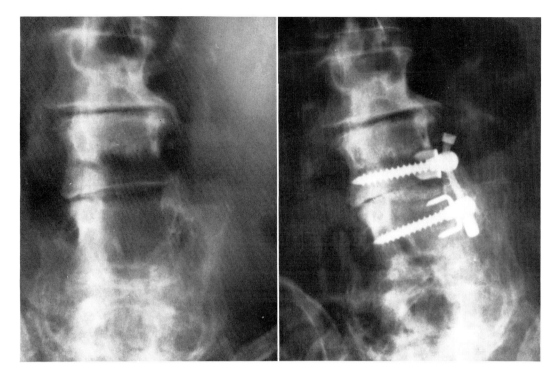

Fig. 8-6 A 51-year-old female with multiple posterior surgeries with L3-L4 nonunion and instability secondary to total facet removal treated with anterior Dwyer instrumentation and fusion.

VERTEBRAL BODIES

In 1969 Dwyer[4] introduced the concept of a tension band fixation applied to the vertebral body on the convexity of the scoliotic curve (Fig. 8-6). This used a flexible cable attached to a staple-screw device at each level. The success of his device has received variable reports with different spine centers. Its use, in conjunction with posterior instrumentation for severe paralytic or neuromuscular curves, is well established. The use of this device alone has not been as well received.

An advance on the Dwyer apparatus was made by Zilke by modifying the screw-staple arrangement and substituting a threaded rod and nuts for the flexible cable. This allowed for a more controlled determination of the loss of lordosis seen with the Dwyer apparatus and allowed a greater correction of rotational deformity. Both types of fixation suffer from two basic flaws. First, instrumentation to L5 can be difficult, and to the sacrum essentially impossible. Second, the risk, however low, of retrograde ejaculation in males exists. Certain other risks with this approach to the spine include renal failure secondary to retroperitoneal fibrosis, direct trauma to the iliac veins, spleen or ureters, and late arterial damage caused by erosive pressure of the metal on iliac vessels.

The vertebral body, featuring a cortical shell and cancellous bony core, requires a fairly large screw thread for fixation. Forces on the cortical shell need to be distributed by a washer or staple device. The best fixation is achieved by engaging the far cortex with the screw. Because of the short distance to the axis of rotation, fairly large forces have to be generated to achieve correction of the curve. A similar device featuring more rigid fixation for the treatment of spine fractures through an anterior approach has been devised by Dunn[3] (Fig. 8-7). This device uses a com-

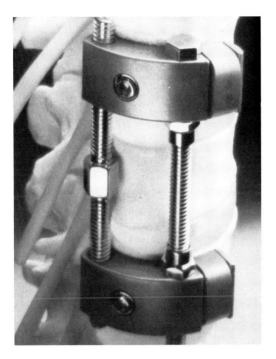

Fig. 8-7 Dunn device for anterior instrumentation. (Zimmer Spinal Product Systems, Zimmer USA, Inc., Warsaw, Ind.)

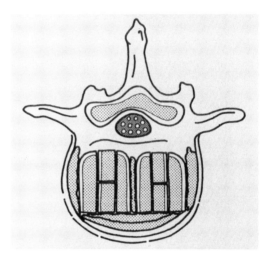

Fig. 8-8 Lin's interbody fusion technique. (From Lin, P.M., editor: Posterior lumbar interbody fusion, Springfield, Ill., 1982, courtesy of Charles C Thomas, Publisher.)

bination of plate, staple, and screw at the level above and below the unstable segment. These two plates are connected by two threaded rods and nuts. Although not a biomechanically perfect device, it is the most rigid to be devised so far. It is really only applicable at levels above L5.

DISC SPACE

Blocking motion by fixation of the area where motion occurs around the axis of rotation has long been attractive. The disc is the site primarily of compressive loading, which should stimulate bony healing. The vertebral end-plates form a large area for graft incorporation. The materials used for fixation of this area have included bone, coral plugs, and cintered metal plugs. The treatment of discogenic pain by attempting to stop disc motion at sites other than the disc has always seemed peculiar to me. Rolander[7] has shown how some disc motion occurs even with rigid fixation of all the posterior elements as a result of the viscoelastic behavior of bone.

Spine surgeons contemplating fixation across the disc space, especially with rigid structures such as an iliac bone plug, have found similar problems encountered by their colleagues doing total knee replacements at the tibial plateau. Resection of the cortical end-plate, although sometimes desirable, weakens the supporting structure for the implant. Substituting a cancellous bone bed for the original cortical plate greatly enhances the bony incorporation of the fusion, but the strength of the bone in resisting impaction of the grafts diminishes rapidly with the distance from the end-plate.

This has led numerous authors to suggest distributing the forces as widely as possible by "filling up the interspace" with graft material[2] (Fig. 8-8). When an interbody fusion is done through a posterior approach, fixation achieved anteriorly by the bone plugs is well supplemented by some sort of posterior compressive fixation across either the lamina or spinous process to help prevent posterior dislocation of the bone plugs. This compression fixation may take the form of either a single tension band wire around the spinous processes or Weiss springs attached to the lamina. Interbody fusions done from a posterior approach are probably the most technically demanding of the fixation techniques and are associated with some of the potentially greatest risks, including cauda equina syndrome, nerve root impingement by displaced plugs, and possibly excessive scar formation. Many authors believe this scar formation is due to excessive motion during the incorporation phase of the bone plugs. Supplemental posterior fixation and careful attention to technical details ensuring good plug interbody fit will probably reduce this problem.

FACET JOINTS

Since the spine moves at the disc and facet joints and since facet joint degeneration is a common cause of back pain, it seems reasonable to approach back pain by fixating and fusing the painful facet joints themselves. Screw fixation was described in 1959 by Boucher.[1] Unfortunately, more and more emphasis is being placed on resecting various aspects of the facet joints to accomplish spinal decompression. The remaining portion of the facet joints allows fairly little area for screw fixation. The proximity of the nerve root, running adjacent and beneath the joints, has lead to reports of direct injury to the roots by the screws themselves. The quality of bone is variable and often less suitable for fixation than the ajdacent pedicle or lamina. A variation on this technique described by Magerl[6] increases the fixation by incorporating part of a lamina and pedicle in the facet fixation (Fig. 8-9).

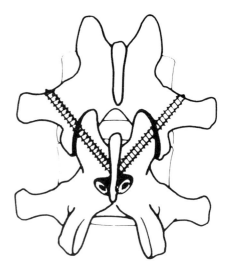

Fig. 8-9 Mangerl's facet joint fixation. (From Mangerl, F.: Clin. Orthop. **189**:125, 1984.)

SACRAL FIXATION

The sacrum presents unique problems and challenges with regard to spinal fixation. The body area anteriorly is difficult to reach. Work in this area is associated with its own unique potential hazards. The lamina posteriorly is sometimes absent and is often thin when compared to the lamina of the ajdacent segments. The relative canal size at the sacrum is often small, allowing less degree of safety for hooks that protrude into the canal itself.

The alar-pedicle area, representing enlargement of the transverse processes, however, presents a large, strong area for fixation not found in the lumbar spine. The pedicles of S1 are fairly large and largely cortical in most patients. The position of this area for fixation, however, is fairly far lateral to the midline, making midline insertion of distraction forces over short segments more difficult. Harrington rods attached to alar hooks can be contoured into the midline if at least three levels are instrumented.

Some of these problems have been avoided with bypassing the sacrum and fixating to the ilium. The Alan-Ferguson

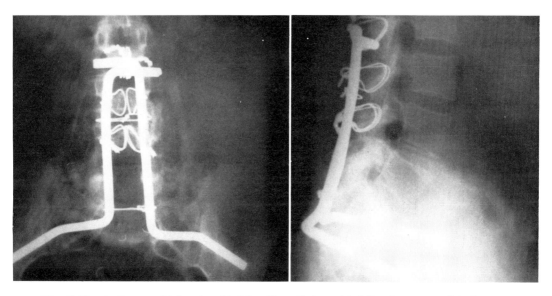

Fig. 8-10 A 42-year-old female with L2 to ilium fusion with Allen-Ferguson pelvic fixation for Luque rods for sacral neurolemmoma.

method of attaching Luque rods to the pelvis is, by far, the strongest pelvic fixation available (Fig. 8-10). This, however, poses the additional problem of the fixation crossing the unfused segment sacroiliac joint, which has led to some cases of symptomatic sacroilitis.

Sacral fixation poses the greatest unsolved problems in lumbosacral fixation. It is an area of active research and development.

SUMMARY

There are many unsolved problems in the field of spinal instrumentation in the lumbar spine. The spinal surgeon should be able to tailor the fixation method used to the individual patient's needs and unique anatomy.

Rigid fixation is not available in the lumbar spine. Future developments will need to be based on a sound knowledge of anatomic structure, relative mechanical strengths, and physiologic loads.

The ideal implant would provide immediate, secure fixation, allow additional investigative studies to be performed, and not stress-shield the spine by being bioincorporable.

REFERENCES

1. Boucher, H.: A method of spinal fusion, J. Bone Joint Surg. **41B:**248, 1959.
2. Cloward, Ralph B.: Posterior lumbar interbody fusion, Springfield, Illinois, 1982, Charles C Thomas, Publishers.
3. Dunn, K.: Anterior stabilization of thoracolumbar injuries, Clin. Orthop. **189:**116, 1984.
4. Dwyer, A.F., et al.: An anterior approach to scoliosis: a preliminary report, Clin. Orthop. **62:**192, 1969.
5. Louis, R.: Fusion of the lumbal and sacral spine by internal fixation with screw plates, Clin. Orthop. **203:**18, 1986.
6. Magerl, F.: Stabilization of the lower thoracic and lumbar spine with external skeletal fixation, Clin. Orthop. **189:**125, 1984.
7. Rolander, S.D.: Motion of the lumbar spine with special reference to the stabilizing effect of posterior fusion, Doctoral thesis, University of Gothenburg, Sweden, 1966.
8. Schenk, R.H., and Willenegger, H. Zum Histologischen Bild Der Sogenannten. Primarheilung der Knochenkomdak ta Nach Experimentellen Osteotomien Am Hund. Experientia (Basel) **19:**593, 1963.
9. Stauffer, R., and Coventry, M.: Anterior interbody lumbar spine fusion, J. Bone Joint Surg. **54A**(4):756, 1972.

CHAPTER 9

OPERATIVE POSITIONING FOR LOW BACK SURGERY

W. Bradford DeLong

If ideal operative positioning for low back surgery were possible, it would achieve the following benefits.

1. It would provide expandable access to the operative field.
2. It would decrease blood loss.
3. It would provide the anesthesiologist with unrestricted access to the patient's airway and would support the patient's respirations.
4. It would allow unrestricted use of x-rays or the C-arm fluoroscope during the operative procedure.
5. It would avoid pressure or traction on peripheral nerves or other susceptible areas.
6. It would be easy to achieve without requiring expensive paraphernalia.

Let's examine these considerations in more detail, since in practice there is no ideal method of operative positioning. Trade-offs exist, and choices must be made.

ACCESS TO THE OPERATIVE FIELD

The operative position must not restrict the surgeon if he or she decides that the surgical exposure must be developed further as the case proceeds. The incision may have to be extended superiorly or inferiorly, or a unilateral procedure may have to be expanded into a bilateral approach. If an unanticipated spinal fusion becomes necessary, the surgeon will need access to a bone graft donor site.

The position of the patient should not interfere with the surgeon's use of the operating microscope. Some positions place the surface of the patient's back high off the floor. Use of the microscope is then awkward, since most microscope stands will not lift the microscope high enough.

The ideal operative position would facilitate interlaminar access during the decompressive portion of the procedure by initially placing the curve of the lumbosacral spine in a neutral position, but it would allow the surgeon to restore some degree of lordosis before performing a fusion.

Some operative positions place the lumbosacral spine in a considerable amount of lumbosacral flexion, which can lead to such problems as allowing a periosteal elevator to slip into the spinal canal unexpectedly. This mishap can result in a dural tear at best and neural damage at worst. Excessive flexion can also tighten the paravertebral muscles against the spinous processes, making satisfactory retraction difficult. If the patient's spine is fused in pelvic flexion, the procedure can lead to severe lumbosacral mechanical problems postoperatively.

If an orthopedic team is to perform a fusion after a neurosurgical team performs the spinal decompression, it is important for the neurosurgeons to anticipate the needs of the orthopedists. If a bilateral posterolateral fusion is planned, for example, then the initial operative positioning should provide for the wide exposure that will be required later for the fusion. The position chosen should also allow the orthopedists to fuse the spine in an anatomic degree of lumbosacral lordosis.

DECREASED BLOOD LOSS

If a patient requires a blood transfusion because of surgical blood loss, he or she is exposed to the risks of transfusion reaction, coagulation problems, hepatitis, or acquired immune deficiency syndrome. The autodonation of blood or the use of designated donors can lessen these risks, but it is safest and easiest to use optimal operative positioning to minimize blood loss in the first place.

The key to minimizing intraoperative blood loss is abdominal decompression. If the patient's position puts pressure on the abdomen, the vena cava will be compressed. This, in turn, increases the pressure in the spinal venous complex, particularly the epidural veins, making intraspinal operative exposure difficult and bloody. On the other hand, if the patient's abdomen is hanging freely, then the epidural veins will contain blood under relatively low pressure. Under these circumstances, hemostasis is rarely a problem. Any bleeding that occurs stops promptly with the temporary application of Gelfoam soaked in thrombin or with bipolar coagulation.

Abdominal compression can lead to problems other than increased intraoperative blood loss. If the vena cava is compressed, cardiac return can be severely compromised and hypotension can occur. This situation can lead the anesthesiologist to think that blood loss has been greater than it actually has been. The patient might then be overtransfused in a futile attempt to correct the hypotension.

A theoretic advantage of optimal abdominal decompression is the lessening of the risk of an intraabdominal vascular catastrophe. It is well known that if an instrument accidently penetrates the anterior boundary of the disc space, then the aorta, vena cava, or iliac vessels can be lacerated, resulting in an extreme emergency. If the abdomen is well decompressed, then the vena cava and iliac veins will be relatively flaccid and the aorta and iliac arteries will not be pushed back against the spinal column. Under these conditions, the vessels stand a better chance of remaining unscathed should they be approached by a disc rongeur, curette, or some other instrument.

ANESTHESIA ACCESS

The operative postion should support respiration by allowing free excursion of the patient's chest and by permitting free diaphragmatic excursion through satisfactory abdominal decompression.

The anesthesiologist must have unrestricted access to the patient's head to deal with any problems that arise from the endotracheal tube and to protect the patient's eyes from pressure.

The anesthesiologist must also have access to intravenous and intraarterial lines. This is best accomplished by abducting the patient's upper extremities on arm boards, allowing the hands to rest beside the head.

If a Foley catheter is used, the operative

position should allow the nursing staff access to the catheter if any drainage problems arise.

The patient's lower extremities should be gently compressed by elastic stockings or wraps to encourage efficient venous return.

X-RAY ACCESS

X-rays are often needed during spinal surgery. This need cannot always be anticipated, and it is important that the operative position not restrict the placement of the x-ray film cassette or the alignment of the x-ray beam itself.

If lateral x-rays are required, a cassette holder can usually be positioned with relative ease. However, various pieces of the frame or holding device can obstruct the x-ray beam if the possible need for x-rays is not kept in mind during positioning of the patient.

Posteroanterior x-ray films can be difficult or impossible to obtain if the patient is positioned in one of the various frames available, because the acute angle of the patient's hips causes the thighs to block placement of the film cassette.

Satisfactory use of C-arm biplane fluoroscopy usually requires the use of a "diving board" extension on the operating table, although some of the frames might allow placement of the C-arm tube beneath the prone or kneeling patient for anteroposterior views.

PROTECTION OF PERIPHERAL NERVES

The brachial plexus must be protected from traction injuries by avoiding excessive anterior sagging of the shoulders and upper extremities. Similarly, the shoulders should not be forced posteriorly during the procedure. Pads should not press against the axilla during the procedure.

Postoperative ulnar neuropathy can be avoided by paying attention to two points. First, the ulnar nerve should be protected against direct pressure in the ulnar groove at the elbow. This can be done by proper padding and positioning. Second, the ulnar nerve should be protected against a traction injury by avoiding acute flexion of the elbow during surgery.[3] Ulnar neuropathy arising from elbow flexion is less well recognized than neuropathy arising from direct pressure, but both etiologies are important and care should be taken to avoid them.

The common peroneal nerve at the fibular head must be protected from direct pressure, which can occur if the patient's knee migrates laterally against the frame after the operation is under way.

The sciatic nerve must be protected from pressure at the gluteal fold. Such pressure can occur if the patient is sitting back against a frame that allows the lower edge of the gluteal support to cut in at the gluteal fold.

The lateral femoral cutaneous nerve can sustain a pressure injury if a pad, sandbag, or frame presses against it during the case. This obviously should be avoided, since it can lead to prolonged or permanent dysesthesia of the lateral thigh.

PROTECTION OF MISCELLANEOUS PRESSURE POINTS

The patient's head must be well supported to avoid accidental pressure over the eyes. Even a few minutes of direct pressure over an eye can cause permanent loss of vision.

If the patient is in a lateral or semiprone position, the neurovascular structures of the axilla must be protected by a roll supporting the upper chest.

If the patient is in a kneeling position, extreme flexion of the hip should be avoided to maintain femoral arterial and venous circulation.

Pressure over the anterior superior iliac spines, the knees, the ankles, and the toes should be avoided. If the patient is kneeling, the knees must rest on padding.

When the patient is turned supine to prone and back again, the downward upper extremity should be placed along the patient's side to avoid levering the shoulder into a sprain or even a dislocation.

POSITIONING TECHNIQUES

The operative position should be safely attainable with a minimum of operating room personnel required for turning and positioning. The necessary positioning equipment should be readily available for a reasonable cost.

A number of positioning techniques are available. Many attain the ideal in some respects but fall short in others. Let us examine the advantages and disadvantages of the most common positions.

Lateral or Semilateral

This positioning technique places the patient either on his or her side in a full lateral position or on the side rolled toward a prone position, in which case the position is called "semilateral" or "semiprone."

The use of either variation—full lateral or semilateral—is generally limited to unilateral discectomy. The pathologic side is placed uppermost. The axillary structures are protected with a roll supporting the chest, and a pillow is placed between the knees. If the patient is in a semilateral position, the uppermost hip and knee are flexed and the uppermost knee brought anterior to the lower knee, providing stability. A wide strap or strip of tape can be placed across the chest to provide further stability, although it should not be severely tightened or respiration will be restricted.

A suction-activated "bean bag" can be used to help stabilize the patient, although x-ray films will be degraded somewhat if the x-ray beam passes through this device.

Advantages of this position include ease of positioning, excellent access to the airway and intravenous lines, and good support of respiration by providing free excursion of the chest and abdomen. Excellent abdominal decompression is provided, minimizing blood loss. In addition, it is relatively easy to use the operating microscope in this position.

Disadvantages of this position include the lack of flexibility of the surgical exposure. If the exposure must be extended to the opposite side, it is difficult to visualize the downward side of the operative field. Other problems include difficulties in surgical orientation, especially in the semilateral variation. Since the patient is neither fully prone nor fully lateral, he or she is not "square" to the floor of the operating room, and the surgeon can become disoriented in regard to the location of the lateral and/or anterior aspect of the vertebral body.

Another disadvantage is the restriction of the assistant's ability to see and help with the procedure. It is also difficult or impossible to obtain truly lateral or posteroanterior x-ray films if the patient is not truly lateral or prone.

Prone on Bolsters

If the patient is placed prone, he or she must be supported on bolsters of some sort. Chest rolls are important to maintain adequate chest excursion, but it is unwise to use chest bolsters alone. The abdomen must also be decompressed for the reasons mentioned previously.

Prone on chest rolls and separate iliac crest supports

The patient is placed prone with short chest rolls supporting the chest. The anterior iliac crests are supported separately by padded sandbags or some other firm support. The abdomen is left free between the chest rolls and the iliac crest supports. The operating table can be "broken" (flexed) to bring the lumbosacral spine to a more nearly neutral position. The patient is stabilized by a wide strap secured around the thighs. A footboard can also be used for additional stabilization.

Advantages of this position include some measure of abdominal decompression, which enhances respiratory support. Satisfactory lateral x-ray films can be obtained easily.

Disadvantages include less-than-optimal abdominal decompression, which contributes in some instances to greater blood loss than necessary. Satisfactory posteroanterior x-ray films are difficult to obtain if the operating table is flexed, since the film cassette cannot be positioned for optimal visualization of the entire lumbosacral spine. In this position the lumbosacral lordosis is not neutralized. This may inhibit access to the spinal canal.

Prone on bolsters extending from the chest to the iliac crests

This is a variation of the immediately previous technique. Long bolsters are used that support the chest, then they are brought around the lateral aspect of the abdomen and are curved back in to support the iliac crests.

The single advantage of this technique over the previous technique is the somewhat increased ease of positioning the patient.

Disadvantages are the same as those of the previous technique, with the added problem of poorer abdominal decompression. It is difficult to position the middle of the long bolsters far enough laterally to avoid abdominal compression.

Prone on the Hall Frame

Several frames place the patient in a prone position by supporting the chest and the anterior iliac crests on pads. These include the Hall, Relton, Basildon (Gardner), and Norfolk frames. The basic frame in this category is the Hall spinal frame. The supporting pads are adjustable for width but not for height. The pads of the Relton frame adjust for height as well as width. The Basildon (Gardner) frame is similar to the Hall frame, but it provides a horseshoe headrest as part of the device. The Norfolk frame is similar to a Relton frame with a horseshoe headrest.

These frames provide the abdominal decompression necessary to support respiration and minimize blood loss. X-ray access is satisfactory for both lateral and posteroanterior x-ray films.

Disadvantages include the pressure placed on the anterior iliac crests by the pads, which can lead to skin problems and/or compromise of the lateral femoral cutaneous nerves. This position does not neutralize lumbosacral lordosis, and access to the spinal canal can be less than satisfactory, although the maintenance of lordosis is desirable if a fusion is being performed.

These frames provide a convenient method of positioning children or small adults and are especially suited for the surgery of scoliosis, where extensive access to the lumbosacral spinal canal is not necessary.

Knee-Chest Position Without a Frame

This technique places the patient in a kneeling position on the surface of the operating table. The patient is secured with wide tape or straps. The position provides good abdominal decompression.

However, serious disadvantages exist. The position is difficult to achieve and maintain. Considerable flexion of the hips and knees is necessary to provide stability, and this degree of flexion can lead to compromise of the femoral arterial and/or venous circulation. This degree of flexion can also widen the interlaminar space to a surprising extent, a situation that can lead to accidental interlaminar penetration by a periosteal elevator. This position also tenses the paravertebral muscles against the spinous processes, making retraction of the muscles difficult at times.

In addition to these disadvantages, posteroanterior x-ray films cannot be obtained because there is no room to position the film cassette anterior to the patient's abdomen. The patient's back is high, and use of the operating microscope is difficult.

Kneeling on the Operating Table, Supported by a Frame

Several frames are available that support the patient in a kneeling position on the surface of the operating table. These include the Hastings frame, the Hicks frame, and the Tarlov seat. The use of these frames has a clear advantage over the simple knee-chest position without a frame. A frame can support the patient in a less extreme kneeling position, protecting circulation to the lower extremities.

Advantages include excellent abdominal decompression, which enhances respiration and minimizes blood loss. The lumbosacral lordotic curve can be neutralized, providing better access to the spinal canal. Frames of this type are relatively simple in design and can be purchased or constructed relatively inexpensively.

Disadvantages include the difficulty of obtaining satisfactory posteroanterior x-ray films and the difficulty of using the operating microscope when the patient's back is high above the surface of the operating table. If care is not taken, the patient can be positioned in the frame in rather extreme flexion of the hips and knees, leading to circulatory problems in the lower extremities and to the potential for accidental interlaminar penetration when the paravertebral muscles are being stripped from the spinous processes and laminae.

It may be difficult to position and stabilize a particularly tall or obese patient in any of these frames.

Kneeling on the Andrews Frame

The Andrews frame uses an assembly that bolts onto the foot section of the operating table. When the foot section is cranked down to a vertical position, the assembly supports a horizontal padded plate on which the patient kneels (Fig. 9-1). The patient's feet are fastened to the horizontal plate by straps attached to padded boots. The patient's chest rests on pillows or pads placed on the surface of the operating table, and his or her hips are supported by a gluteal plate. Stabilization is completed by using lateral thigh supports and/or a strap around the thighs (Fig. 9-2).

The operative position achieved by the Andrews frame is similar to the Troncelliliti position used at Pennsylvania Hospital in Philadelphia by Doctors Richard H. Rothman and Frederick A. Simeone.[1,2]

Advantages of the Andrews frame include the ease of positioning the patient, even one who is obese or tall. Excellent abdominal decompression is achieved, which enhances respiration and minimizes intraoperative blood loss. It is easy to protect pressure points. The lumbosacral lordotic curve can be partially neutralized by allowing the patient to sit back against the gluteal support with the hips and knees in mild flexion, but lordosis can be restored if a lumbosacral fusion is to be done. The patient's back is at a normal level, enhancing use of the operating microscope.

Disadvantages include the difficulty of obtaining posteroanterior x-ray films, because the flexion of the thighs blocks optimal positioning of the film cassette. The frame is more complex than some of the other frames available and is therefore more expensive.

92 *Surgical Procedures*

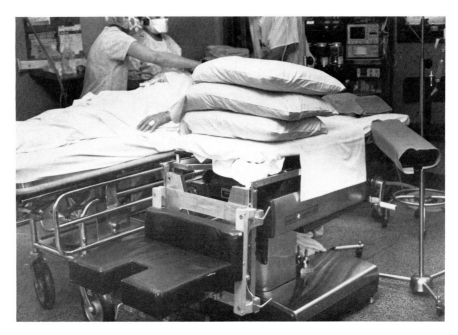

Fig. 9-1 Andrews frame assembly, ready for patient positioning.

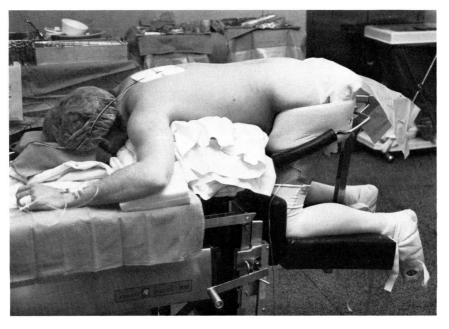

Fig. 9-2 Patient positioned on the Andrews frame. Feet are secured with padded boots that attach to buckles on undersurface of the horizontal plate. Gluteal plate is adjusted so that patient sits back slightly against the plate, placing lumbosacral curve in a neutral position. Upper thighs are stabilized by lateral thigh supports and/or wide strap. Three or four pillows support the chest. Elbows are not flexed past 90 degrees, and ulnar grooves are protected from pressure.

Technique of positioning in the Andrews frame

The use of any specific positioning technique becomes easier as an operating team gains experience with the technique. The following are details of the Andrews frame technique I have developed after using the device in several hundred cases of low back surgery.

1. The kneeling plate is attached to the Andrews frame assembly, and the foot of the operating table is cranked down to a 90-degree vertical position, so that the kneeling plate is horizontal.

2. Three or four pillows are placed on the operating table to support the patient's chest.

3. The patient is placed under anesthesia, and intubation is performed while the patient is supine on the gurney.

4. The patient's legs are wrapped. The foot boots are placed on the patient before turning.

5. The gurney is moved down so that the lower margin of the patient's rib cage is adjacent to the vertical foot section of the operating table. This step requires moving the gurney considerably more than the anesthesiologist would generally anticipate, and care must be taken that the breathing circuit tubing has sufficient slack to allow movement of the gurney to this extent.

6. The patient's hips and knees are flexed to 90 degrees before turning.

7. At least four people turn the patient. If the patient is exceptionally tall or obese, more than four people should be used. One person (usually the anesthesiologist) supports the patient's head; one person turns the patient's torso; another person catches the torso; and the fourth person turns the pelvis and flexed lower extremities, easing the knees down onto the horizontal kneeling plate. The foot boots are strapped into the buckles on the kneeling plate.

8. The kneeling plate then is elevated to adjust the height of the patient's pelvis. The gluteal support is put into place, and the patient is moved toward the foot of the operating table so that his or her hips and knees are flexed slightly past 90 degrees. The head of the operating table is elevated slightly so that the patient is sitting back against the gluteal support. The lower edge of the gluteal support must not press into the sciatic nerves at the gluteal folds. The chest pillows are adjusted to achieve maximal abdominal decompression.

9. Arm boards are attached to the center section of the operating table, and the patient's upper extremities are adjusted so the forearms and hands rest beside the head. The shoulders should neither sag too far anteriorly nor be pushed too far posteriorly. The ulnar nerves should be free of pressure at the ulnar grooves. To avoid stretching the ulnar nerves the elbows should not be acutely flexed.

10. If lateral thigh supports are used, they should angle downward toward the floor so they will not impair visualization of the spine on lateral x-ray views (Fig. 9-3). A wide strap is placed around the patient's upper thighs to secure him or her against the gluteal support and prevent forward sliding during the procedure (see Fig. 9-3).

Variations of the Andrews frame technique include the following:

1. Intubation can be performed while the patient is awake. The patient can then assist in turning himself or herself into a kneeling position on the frame. This may be a useful technique for a particularly obese patient.

2. The foot section of the operating table can be left flat until after the patient is turned. Then the patient's knees can be flexed to 90 degrees and the kneeling plate attached. The foot section is then cranked down 90 degrees to a vertical position, as the patient is gradually moved caudally to the proper position.

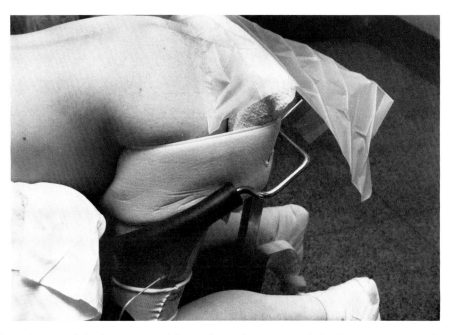

Fig. 9-3 Lateral thigh supports of the Andrews frame are angled inferiorly so they will not interfere with localizing roentgenograms. Note optimal degree of abdominal decompression achieved.

The technique of moving the patient from the Andrews frame back onto the gurney includes the following:

1. After the dressing is applied and the drapes are removed, the patient is supported manually while the upper thigh supports and gluteal support are removed.
2. The foot boots are removed. One strap of each boot is unbuckled, and the boot is taken off the patient's foot. The boot then dangles from the kneeling piece by the remaining strap. This minimizes the risk that the boot will be discarded with the disposable operating room debris.
3. The operating table is raised above the level of the gurney.
4. The patient's knees and hips are both maintained in 90 degrees of flexion, and the patient is rolled onto the gurney with the knees and hips maintained in flexion. This allows easy turning with minimal lifting by the operating room personnel. Before turning, the downward arm is moved from the abducted position to a position alongside the patient's torso.

SUMMARY

Each operative position presents advantages and disadvantages. At the very least, the positioning technique chosen should allow the surgeon to extend the operative exposure if necessary, and it should provide maximal abdominal decompression to enhance respiration and minimize blood loss.

REFERENCES

1. Finneson, B.E.: Low back pain, ed. 2, Philadelphia, 1980, J.B. Lippincott Co.
2. Rothman, R.H., and Simeone, F.A.: The spine, ed. 2, Philadelphia, 1982, W.B. Saunders Co.
3. St. John, J.N.: The elbow flexion test in ulnar entrapment neuropathy, Paper presented to the annual meeting of the Western Neurosurgical Society, Jackson Hole, Wyo., September 1982.

CHAPTER

10

POSITIONING THE PATIENT FOR LUMBAR DECOMPRESSIONS OR FUSIONS

Charles D. Ray

CUSHIONS, ROLLS AND FRAMES

Nearly all cases of lumbar spinal surgery are performed with the patient in the prone position. A number of authors have described the lateral recumbent position for lumbar discectomies, but this is an uncommon choice.[2] Since the patient is to be face down when operated on, particular problems arise regarding the application of pressure against the thorax, abdomen, brachial plexus, neck, and face or head. Additional considerations may be made as to whether the lumbar spine should be positioned in flexion or extension. Further, as the neck is generally rotated to one side, preexisting cervical spine problems may be aggravated.

A number of frames, platforms, and cushions have been devised and are available commercially to address some or several of these problems; none of the currently available systems appears to address them all.[3,5,10,11] Therefore in each case the surgeon, anesthesiologist, and operating room team must improvise, for example, with additional cushions, towel rolls, tape, and pads. Fortunately this combination usually suffices except in unusual cases, with very obese patients, or with those whose procedure requires many hours on the operating table. Such latter patients should be warned in advance that there may be a problem with pressure points, skin "burns" or stiffness of joints that may well arise in the postoperative period.

In general, there should be a distribution of the pressure so that at no place on the skin does the pressure exceed the capillary perfusion pressure, otherwise burns or necrosis of the skin may likely occur. Occasional patients will have a short-lived numbness of the forehead, the chin, or at scattered areas around the chest or arms or legs. There is considerable misunderstanding about the simple physics of cushions and padding. One must remember that the weight applied against the supporting surface (for example, the operating table, platform, and frame) resulting from gravity, remains the same with or without cushions or foam rubber padding. These latter aids simply help to distribute the pressure more evenly around the dependent tissues, and in doing so they prevent pressure points, especially over bony prominences or susceptible structures.

A major additional purpose for a variety of surgical frames, lateral cushions, or attachments is to permit the abdomen to remain pendulous thus reducing intraabdominal and intrathoracic pressures, lowering venous back-pressure. These effects result in a significant reduction in blood loss from epidural and other extradural venous sources compared to a flat-abdomen position of the patient, particularly an obese one.[1,3,5,10,11] In fact, the blood loss difference may be as much as 300% to 400% between the flat abdomen and the free-hanging one.

The kneeling, "tuck," knee-chest, or prone-sitting positions have been preferred techniques in lumbar surgery for some years.[1,5,10,11] There are advantages and disadvantages to the use of each of them. A considerable amount of lumbar spine, hip, and knee flexion is obtained in the extreme "tuck" position, for example, and it has been shown that this may produce vascular and nerve compression particularly in the posterior compartment of the knees. In addition, with prolonged spinal surgical procedures this position has been found to produce permanent changes, albeit rarely, in some of the nerves, for example, the sciatic and peroneal; there may also occur a subsequent massive release of myoglobin (from hypoxic, ischemic damage to the muscles of the lower leg) resulting in acute renal failure.[4] This extreme flexed position may so tighten the posterior paraspinal erector muscles that lateral retraction, may be quite difficult.[6,7,8] Additionally, extreme flexion is not tolerable to patients with hip or knee joint disorders, joint destruction, or prosthetic replacements.

EXTENSION VS. FLEXION OF THE LUMBAR SPINE

In general, there are reasonable arguments in favor of positions that promote hyperextension, as well as for those that result in hyperflexion. Hyperextension or hyperlordosis (downward swaying of the low back and a free abdomen) is particularly helpful where the posterior musculature must be relaxed, as in cases where a posterolateral fusion is being performed. Proponents of the hyperflexion concept argue that this position promotes an increased opening of the posterior bony structures to facilitate surgical decompressions. Indeed, when dealing with ordinary discectomy or the decompression of stenoses, hyperextension may so closely approximate the posterior structures that access through the interlaminar spaced may be somewhat more difficult. On balance and in practice, however, the relaxation of musculature provided by extension of the lower back is more important than would be a mild, additional opening of the posterior bony interspaces achieved through hyperflexion positions. If one does require an increase in the distance between posterior elements (laminas or dorsal spinous processes) at a given lumbar level, then a simple lamina spreader provides excellent localized posterior distraction (effectively a hyperextension of that particular segment).

One should be careful that prolonged forceful retraction of tight paraspinal muscles does not result in a postoperative compartment syndrome. This painful complication probably occurs with some frequency and is usually unrecognized.

CUSHIONING AND THE PRONE-SITTING (KNEELING) FRAME

In all of the surgical frames, rolls, and cushions indicated previously, the patient's body weight is in various ways

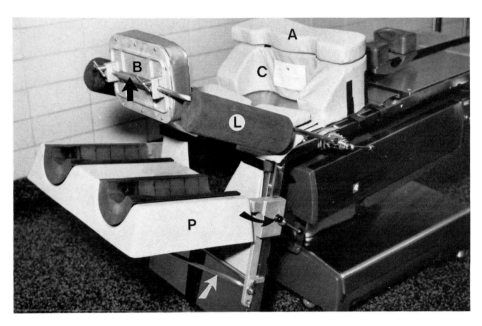

Fig. 10-1 Prone-sitting platform *(P)* is attached to foot piece of standard operating table. Chest cushion *(C)* lies against table. An auxillary cushion *(A)* is removable to accommodate patients of varying neck length. Yoke to hold buttocks cushion *(B)* attaches to lateral mounting sockets of operating table side rails, secures lateral cushions *(L)*, and passes behind *(short black arrow)* buttock cushion mount *(B)*. Long, **V**-shaped stabilizer rod *(white arrow)* is folded beneath the platform. Slide locks *(curved black arrow)* hold the platform on the side rails of the foot piece of the operating table.

distributed among pressure areas on the upper chest, the knees, buttocks, and possibly the anterior iliac spine. For a kneeling or prone-sitting frame most important is the distribution of weight between the upper chest and knees. Iliac spine elevation by lateral padding has been used (not very successfully) to reduce hyperlordosis which occurs in most of the dependent abdomen frame systems. Chest cushions should distribute the weight principally along the upper clavicular and manubrial areas; there should be little pressure against the breasts and certainly not on the superior axillary (or lateral subclavicular) areas, which might promote compression of the brachial circulation or nerve plexus. If the arms are brought overhead or laterally, one must be careful about brachial plexus stretch or compression and shoulder capsule stretch. Alternatively, the arms and hands may be brought downward to pass beneath then anterior to the abdomen. If needed, an additional cushion(s) may be placed on top of the chest cushion to raise the chest farther above the level of the operating table surface, increasing the chest-to-table distance and increasing the angle to which the head and neck will fall forward.

The new knee cushions and lower leg cushions are shaped with a rounded cavity configuration, like troughs, made into the platform of the frame to more evenly distribute the weight applied to the upper tibias, as shown in Fig. 10-1. In addition, there is a gap between the upper portion of these rounded cushions and the operating table; the patellas lie in this gap so that no weight is directly borne by them. The majority of the weight is therefore dis-

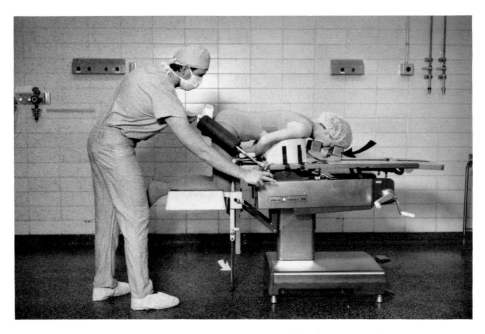

Fig. 10-2 Patient is placed on frame and face rest *(curved black arrow)*, and position of yoke is set by tightening side rail mounting sockets as shown. Stabilizer rod *(short white arrow)* is positioned against floor. Face rest unit has a rocker bottom that can be positioned to permit neutral positioning of neck.

tributed along the two tibial plateaus. Further, the lower leg cushion is shaped so that the ankle portion is elevated relative to the knee, as is the normal kneeling position.

With this attachment frame it is almost impossible to flex the thighs more than 90 degrees relative to the trunk or flex the lower leg less than 90 degrees relative to the thighs. In this way the position of the hip joints and knees are quite neutral and optimal; in addition, the stretch on the sciatic nerve is reduced by the bent-knee position.

Additional cushions are positioned along the break in the operating table where there is a rather prominent edge. Buttock and thigh cushions are mounted on a large yoke that is attached to the lateral rails of the operating table (Fig. 10-2). Relatively little pressure is applied to the buttocks; this has helped reduce some of the postoperative sciatic complaints that occur with some of the hyper-flexion frames. With the latter there may also be significant pressure against the sciatic notches. Incidentally, leaning against one of the lateral thigh cushions is comfortable for the surgeon while operating. The cushioning was developed to optimally accommodate the patient, anesthesia team, and surgeon.[9]

ATTACHING AND ADJUSTING THE PLATFORM AND CUSHIONS

The foot portion of the standard operating table remains in the horizontal position as the present kneeling platform is slid into place on the side rails and locked in location at the anticipated correct height for the particular patient's knees (tibial length) (see Figs. 10-1 and 10-2). The foot and platform are then positioned perpendicular to the floor.

The chest cushion is laid on the table and bound in place with Velcro tabs. The surfaces of the platform and chest cushion are covered with a cotton sheet, smooth-

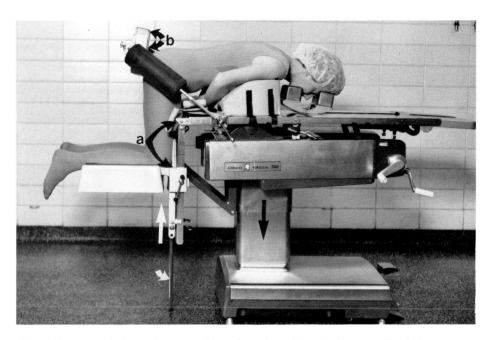

Fig. 10-3 Patient's buttocks are positioned too low *(short dual arrows, b)* relative to upper back. Platform is therefore also too low *(long dual arrows, a)*. With stabilizer *(short white arrow)* against floor, platform is unlocked and table hydraulic piston lowered *(large straight arrow)*. Platform "rises" *(large white arrow)* as will buttocks, until desired position is reached and platform is then locked. Stabilizer is retracted and table lowered to suit the surgeon. Note also that the forearms lie against removable cushions so that they need not be wrapped. In regular surgical use all body cushions are covered with thin cloths.

ly applied without wrinkles. The anesthetized, intubated or awake (locally anesthetized) patient is placed on the kneeling platform by simple bent-knee transfer from the litter. The yoke is now attached and adjusted to accommodate the size of the patient. The lateral thigh cushions are mounted eccentric as to their long axes and may be rotated about that axis (the rod of the yoke) to position them closer or farther apart; this accomodates all patients with various widths of hips and buttocks. Thigh and buttocks cushions are covered with cotton pillow cases. If the knee cushions become soiled beyond easy cleaning they may be replaced easily.

For many patients it may be necessary to raise or lower the position of the buttocks relative to the chest, thus bringing the dorsal surface of the lumbar spine into a parallel position with the floor. To change the height of the kneeling platform and thereby the buttocks, the table is pumped up with its hydraulic piston and with the sequential use of the stabilizer legs and rail locks, as shown in Fig. 10-3, the vertical position of the platform may be raised or lowered along the side rails of the operating table as needed. Moving the platform correspondingly changes the buttock elevation relative to that of the chest (which does not change its distance to the operating table surface). The entire table and patient may be lowered to suit the surgeon's own height and the degree of leaning he or she will assume over the patient's body. Safety pawls prevent the platform from slipping off the side rails, should the side locks be forgotten.

Some patients will tend to drift upward

100 *Surgical Procedures*

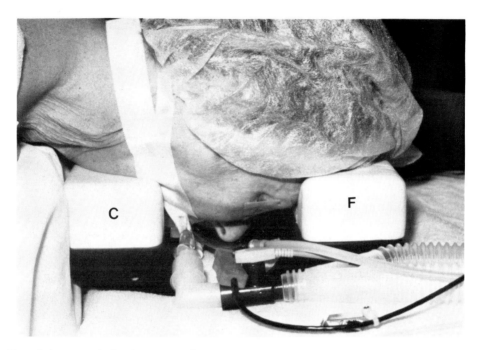

Fig. 10-4 Patient's face lies against face rest, which has forehead *(F)* and chin *(C)* cushions; distance between them can be adjusted to suit face size and rocker positioned to permit normal cervical lordosis. Washable replaceable face cushions are not covered. Note the emergence of tubes, cables, wires, and the free access to facial structures.

on the operating table, especially those who are under local (deep paraspinal infiltration) anesthesia or those having fusions where considerable motion is employed by the surgeon. In such cases shoulder braces (not illustrated) may be positioned above (cephalad to) the chest cushion to prevent upward drifting of the torso.

THE CUSHIONED FACE REST

Many patients who have disorders of their lumbar spine also have cervical spine problems. When using an ordinary laminectomy frame in the prone position, the head and neck are rather sharply rotated to one side or the other. For the intubated patient, such a rotation may present undue lateral pressure against the vocal cords and glottis, as well as an undesirable posture of the neck. If simple forehead cushioning is used, the neck may be hyperextended, as well as rotated. It is thereby not uncommon for some patients to complain of neck or throat difficulties for days or even weeks after procedures performed on a standard laminectomy frame. The cushioned face rest described here, for use with the prone-sitting frame, obviates abnormal positioning of the head and neck.[9] (Figs. 10-3, 10-4, and 10-5.)

After the patient is brought into the operating room on the stretcher, endotracheal intubation is performed and the face rest is positioned over the patient's face. The distance between the forehead and chin cushions is adjusted and locked. The patient is then turned over onto the operating table and positioned on and in the present prone-sitting frame; the face rest is adjusted for elevation of the chin to neutralize almost any curvature of the neck. The face rest cushions are carefully

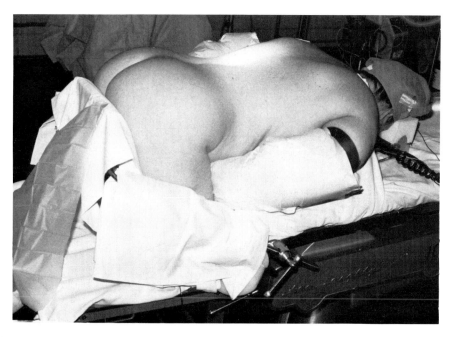

Fig. 10-5 View of patient's right side as she lies against chest cushions and on face rest. Note full extent of cushioning and its draping. Lower arms have been padded with foam cushion and tucked in beneath abdomen. There is a lumbar hyperlordosis produced by the positioning.

checked so that supraorbital ridges, eyes, and the lower lip are free from contact or pressure points.

SUMMARY

The anesthesia team and the surgeon should strive to develop or use patient positions that are comfortable and safe, reliable, and relatively simple. Clearly, the positioning must permit the surgeon to visualize, approach, and perform the procedure with relative comfort, especially when the operating time is very long. In today's litigious world, a skin slough, weakened facial muscle, or nerve loss traceable to patient positioning (regardless of the length of the surgical procedure), brings with it the specter of potential legal action if any of these or other effects persist and produce patient discomfort or discontent. With the use of the present platform and its ergonomically-oriented cushions, there has been a definite reduction in postoperative knee, hip, leg, and sciatic complaints, as well as those involving the neck, scalp and face. Lumbar hyperextension produced by this frame has been a distinct advantage in the reduction of paraspinal muscle and tendon tightness, particularly valuable during posterolateral fusions.

An important, unexpected effect of the use of this system is the reduction in arterial pressure. When using a modified Tarlov frame, it was usually important to perform fusions under hypotensive anesthesia; for this procedure an arterial catheter was routinely placed. With the use of the new prone-sitting frame, on the other hand, arterial pressure remains slightly low; thus hypotensive agents have seldom been required. Nonetheless, true hypotension as a surgical complication is not seen. Some patients, on the other hand, have significant fluid loading during the surgery, perhaps related to the dependency of the abdomen and legs. They require subsequent diuresis.

A few other benefits have been seen. For example, for most patients the frame brings the patient sufficiently close to the operating room floor so that the usual stack of platforms is not required. Furthermore, I have noted less hyperextension of my own knees and my associates have experienced less low backache compared with the use of some of the other surgical frames, since we now can stand somewhat closer to the patient and lean against the lateral cushions.

ACKNOWLEDGMENTS

I wish to express my appreciation for the assistance and diligence shown this project by Richard Steller. Helpful suggestions were made by my associates at the Institute for Low Back Care, especially Dr. Richard Salib and Mr. Kevin Gracie. Drs. Stuart Weatherhead and Russell Bagley, Department of Anesthesiology, Abbott-Northwestern Hospital, also contributed valuable criticism. Patents have been applied for on all major elements of these systems. The platform, cushions, and face rest units are manufactured by CeDaR Surgical, Inc., 15265 Minnetonka Blvd., Minnetonka, MN, 55345.

REFERENCES

1. Eckert, A.: Kneeling position for operations on the lumbar spine, especially for protruded intervertebral discs, Surgery **25:**112, 1949.
2. Cannon, B.W., and Ray, C.D.: The lateral position for lumbar disc surgery. University of Tennessee and Baptist Memorial Hospital, Memphis, Tenn. Annual meeting of the Southern Neurosurgical Society, Miami, 1959. (Film.)
3. Cloward, R.B.: Cloward surgical saddle, Honolulu, 1984 Surgical Equipment International.
4. Keim, H.A., and Weinstein, J.D.: Acute renal failure—a complication of spine fusion in the tuck position, J. Bone Joint Surg. **52A:**1248-1250, 1970.
5. Orthopedic Systems, Inc.: Andrews spinal surgery frame (monograph), Hayward, Calif., 1983.
6. Ray, C.D.: New techniques for decompression of lumbar spinal stenosis, Neurosurgery **10:**587-592, 1982.
7. Ray, C.D.: The paralateral approach to lumbar decompressions, Proceedings of the annual meeting of the American Association of Neurological Surgery, April 1983.
8. Ray, C.D.: Lateral spinal decompression using the paralateral approach. In Watkins, R.G., editor: Principles and techniques of spine surgery, Rockville, Md., 1987, Aspen Press.
9. Ray, C.D.: Head and chin cushioned face-rest for surgery in the prone position, Anesthesiology **64:**301, 1986.
10. Tarlov, I.M.: The knee-chest position for lower spinal operations, J. Bone Joint Surg. **49A:**1193-1194, 1967.
11. Wayne, S.J.: The tuck position for lumbar-disc surgery, J. Bone Joint Surg. **49A:**1195-1198, 1967.

SECTION TWO

LAMINECTOMY AND DISC EXCISION

CHAPTER

11

CHEMONUCLEOLYSIS

James Walter Simmons

"If the science of medicine is not to be lowered to the rank of a mere technical profession, it must preoccupy itself with its history."
Emile Littre (1801-1881)

The procedure of chemically dissolving herniated nucleus material by injection with the enzyme chymopapain has developed over 40 years since the isolation and naming of chymopapain in 1941 by Jansen and Balls.[12] Lewis Thomas[24] in 1956 was the first to demonstrate the enzymatic properties that crude papain exhibits on the mucoid portion of the cartilage. He observed that, within 18 hours after rabbits were injected with a solution of crude papain, the structural integrity of the ear cartilage was disrupted. Larger injection doses of papain involved the joint cartilage, epiphyseal growth plate, tracheal cartilage, and bronchial cartilage. It was noted that "apart from the unusual cosmetic effect, the animals exhibited no evidence of systemic illness or discomfiture." With time, the ears replenished the basophilic chondroid matrix and regained their original shape. Subsequent research has proved that inactivated forms of the enzyme bypass serum protein and selectively bind to cartilage matrix, enabling it to effectively lyse the proteoglycans of the cartilage.

In 1959 Carl Hirsch[11] indicated that he believed an enzyme would be discovered that would dissolve the collagen of the disc and be used as treatment for low back pain secondary to disc problems. He believed this enzyme would probably come from bacteria. Joe Barr[1] in 1961 stated that it might be possible to shrink the lesion and stabilize the spine by biochemical methods.

Lyman Smith[20] first injected chymopapain into the lumbar intervertebral discs of 22 dogs previously paralyzed because of herniation of the discs; 14 demonstrated a reversal of their paralysis. A postmortem analysis failed to demonstrate any adverse effect attributable to the enzyme. This study laid the foundation for the clinical use of chymopapain. In 1964 10 patients were injected with chymopapain intradiscally; seven experienced immediate relief from leg and back pain. Smith was extremely encouraged by this study and went on to treat 30 more patients with favorable results. The initial surgical technique used by Smith in these experiments was the posterolateral approach, where the needle passes laterally to the dura but within the bony canal and into the center of the disc.

Extensive pharmacologic and toxicologic studies were performed in 1965 by Garvin and associates[7] to assess the effectiveness and safety of chymopapain in removing the nucleus pulposus. Five conclusions were drawn from this study. (1) Low doses of approximately 0.01 mg per disc in rabbits and dogs effectively dissolved the nucleus pulposus; however, doses of 5 to 20 mg per disc affected the annulus fibrosis. (2) Doses of chymopapain up to 100 times the optimum effective dose were tolerated well when injected intravenously, intradiscally, and epidurally. (3) Chymopapain injected intrathecally was highly toxic. (4) Lethal doses of chymopapain ruptured fine blood vessels of the microcirculation. (5) Nerve tissue was not affected.

In 1967 Smith and Brown[20] injected 75 patients intradiscally, achieving 76% overall success. However, 86% of patients without previous spinal surgery experienced favorable results. During this series of studies the lateral approach for injecting the lumbar discs came into use. This method was rapid and offered less resistance, compared to the resistance of bone, because the needle passed through soft tissue. This study also confirmed that the use of sodium diatrizoate in discography should be avoided because of its allergenic quality.

In 1971 MacNab and coworkers[14] discovered several factors that influenced the use of intradiscal injection. Of 100 patients injected, the best results were seen in patients with severe sciatica of short duration associated with marked root tension. The worst results were demonstrated in those patients displaying obesity, diabetes, or emotional breakdown.

Before 1975, 19 open-label uncontrolled clinical trials were published that involved 3845 patients with a reported success rate of 75.6%.[21] A controversial study done at Walter Reed Army Medical Center[17] in 1975 triggered the withdrawal of the New Drug Application that had been filed with the U.S. Food and Drug Administration (FDA) for use in the treatment of intervertebral disc disease with Discase (chymopapain). This study reported no statistical difference in instance or quality of improvement between the placebo group (49% success rate) and the group tested with Discase (58% success rate). Brown and Daroff[2] criticized the Walter Reed study because of (1) the early code break, (2) the lack of the inert placebo, (3) the insufficient dose of Discase, and (4) the lack of technical expertise.

Physicians in the United States who had been using the drug with excellent results were disheartened when no progress had been made toward an FDA approval. Subsequently, in 1977 a group was formed and chartered for the sole purpose of making chymopapain available in the United States for commercial use. The group was named CADUCEUS (Committee Advocating the Development and Use of Chymopapain to Eliminate Unnecessary Surgery). When no significant progress was made in gaining federal approval for chymopapain, efforts were initiated to seek approval for its production and use through state legislatures. Three states—Illinois, Indiana, and Texas—had the necessary vehicles established to allow the intrastate use. However, only Texas had an environment that would support the growing of the papaya fruit, which provides the crude latex required for the manufacture of the finished drug product. Chemolase became legal to use in the state of Texas in September 1979. A review of 21 physicians' records of 919 patients who underwent chemonucleolysis with Chemolase in Texas between 1981 and 1982 demonstrated a 93% success rate with no deaths.[19]

Chymodiactin, the chymopapain produced by Smith Laboratories, Inc., received FDA approval in November 1982, after nationwide clinical studies between 1980 and 1982.[19] Preceding the 1982 FDA approval of Chymodiactin was a multicentered double-blind study of 108 patients, showing 80% good results at 6 weeks, with 73% good results at 6 months. This was followed by a multicenter open-label study of 420 patients, which was reported 90.5% successful, with 1.42% incidence of anaphylaxis and two deaths. Robert Fraser[4] of Adelaide, Australia, did a double-blind study of 60 patients that indicated an 80% success rate with no anaphylaxis, a 57% placebo effect, and no deaths.

Because of the reports revealing instances of ascending transverse myelitis associated with the injection of chymopapain, the FDA drug bulletin of August 1984[3] recommended modification of chymopapain administration procedures. These recommendations were based on the Smith Laboratories, Inc., report of 30 serious neurologic events in 72,000 patients and on the Baxter-Travenol Laboratory report of 16 serious neurologic complications in 50,000 patients. These complications included paraplegia and/or paresis, cerebral hemorrhage, and transverse myelitis.

The labeling was changed to reflect these findings. Modifications in the administration of the procedure were recommended that consisted of avoiding multiple level injections, using supplemental local anesthesia, and training physicians adequately. The labeling further stated that 27 of 29 serious neurologic complications occurred when general anesthesia was used.

Until further improvements are made on the compound to eliminate the problems of anaphylaxis and ascending transverse myelitis, the most important controllable factors are adequate physician training and technique.

PHARMACOLOGY AND TOXICOLOGY
Source and Description

Chymopapain is a proteolytic enzyme derived from papaya latex. The latex is obtained by cutting vertical slits in the skin of the papaya fruit and collecting the exuded latex. This crude latex then is processed, and the purified chymopapain is isolated. The enzyme chymopapain has a molecular weight of 34,000 and contains 275 amino acids.[22]

Chymopapain hydrolyzes the noncollagenous protein that interconnects long-chain mucopolysaccharides. When injected into the nucleus pulposus of the lumbar intervertebral disc, it tightly binds to the mucopolysaccharide protein complex and rapidly hydrolyzes the noncollagenous polypeptides.[6,23] These compounds are responsible for the strong water-binding capacity of the nucleus pulposus.[10,15,16] The depolymerization of the nucleus pulposus lowers the intradiscal pressure and frequently provides relief from the pain.

Assay

The analysis of the activity of chymopapain was first done by using casein as the substrate. The nonlinearity and lack of reproducibility of this method caused Pharmotex* researchers to develop an assay utilizing the synthetic substrate DL-benzoyl arginine-p-nitroanilide (BAPNA). Such a method has been developed (U.S. patent pending) with activity being reported in International Enzyme Units (IEU). This assay, done under optimal conditions for catalytic activity, is reproducible, linear, and capable of continuous monitoring of the reaction velocity. Each vial of Chemolase contains 6 IEU of chymopapain. An IEU is the amount of enzyme that produces 1 μM of p-nitroaniline per minute from a 5 mM solution of BAPNA at 37° C and at a pH of 6.4.

Metabolism

The pharmacologic use of chymopapain is contingent on its specific localization; thus absorption, distribution, and excretion are reduced in practical importance. After intradiscal injection, chymopapain or its immunologically reactive fragments diffuse rapidly into the plasma.[13] Chymopapain is absorbed into the blood and is inhibited by the alpha-2-macroglobulins, which occur naturally in plasma. After use of chymopapain in humans, a moderate increase in urinary acid mucopolysaccharides occurs.

Margin of Safety

Rabbits will tolerate an intradiscal or epidural dose 1000 to 3000 times the minimum effective dose.[9] Watts[25] has demonstrated that in humans the minimum effective dose for dissolving the nucleus pulposus was approximately 2 to 4 mg per disc, whereas the maximum tolerated dose was about 600 mg per disc.

---

*Pharmotex, Inc.: Texas-based company organized to obtain U.S. Food and Drug Administration approval of the drug Chemolase (chymopapain).

Therefore the tolerated dose is 150 to 300 times greater than the effective dose.

Effect on Surrounding Tissue

The annulus fibrosus has a high collagen content and is resistant to damage from chymopapain. Doses of enzyme beyond the therapeutic range have no deleterious effect on ligaments, bone, or dura.[8] The margin of safety is reduced should the enzyme enter the subarachnoid space through improper injection, although doses several times the therapeutic dose would still be safe in humans. An intrathecal injection can cause subarachnoid hemorrhage.[18] Studies in dogs have indicated that intrathecal chymopapain can be tolerated at doses much higher than the therapeutic range.

Effect on Blood Vessels

Large doses in animals produce capillary hemorrhages by destroying the endothelial cell cement. This reaction may be localized or systemic, depending on the distribution of the injected enzyme. Massive intravenous doses, such as 15 mg per kg of body weight in rabbits, cause acute hemorrhaging in the lung, pericardium, liver, and peritoneum. The small vessels are particularly susceptible.[14]

Effect on Nerve Tissue

The spinal nerves are protected by a thick protective dura that is unaffected by chymopapain. Garvin and associates[7] showed that the epidural injection of chymopapain in dogs, even up to a lethal dose, did not penetrate the intact dura. The concentration of chymopapain that might leak into the epidural space would be much less than that injected into the nucleus pulposus as a result of binding at the site and inactivation by plasma alpha-2-macroglobulins, giving a further margin of safety.

Antigenicity

As a foreign protein chymopapain can induce antibody production. In one study chymopapain did not produce anaphylaxis in sensitized rabbits after injection into the nucleus pulposus of normal discs.[8] However, Kapsalis and coworkers,[13] using radioimmunoassay techniques, showed that in humans immunoreactive proteins of the enzyme did appear in the circulation within 30 minutes. Garvin and associates[7] found the minimum anaphylactic dose of chymopapain to be 0.24 mg per kg in guinea pigs. It was 20 times less likely to cause anaphylaxis than ovalbumin and 40 times less likely to produce anaphylaxis than horse serum.

A review of 28 studies involving 4897 patients revealed an approximate anaphylaxis rate of 0.8% after the injection of chymopapain. All patients experiencing anaphylaxis had uneventful recoveries after resuscitation.[19]

Localization

Two major factors are responsible for the localization of injected chymopapain.
1. Chymopapain binds to the mucopolysaccharides of the nucleus pulposus.
2. The surrounding annulus fibrosis has a high collagen content that is not affected by chymopapain in therapeutic doses.

PATIENT SELECTION

Proper assessment of the patient is vital to the success of chemonucleolysis. Approximately 80% of all patients experiencing leg pain from disc displacement will respond favorably to conservative measures, such as bed rest, exercise, anti-inflammatory drugs, body corset, epidural blocks, physical therapy, and traction. Only after all conservative resources have failed should the more aggressive management be considered.

A physician then is faced with two options: surgery or chemonucleolysis. A small percentage of patients who fail to respond to the conservative management require immediate surgical intervention to offer relief of nerve compression that causes a rapidly progressing neurologic deficit.

The ideal candidate for disc surgery is the ideal candidate for chemonucleolysis. A series of diagnostic steps will aid the judgment of the surgeon. A complete medical patient history that includes the following should be taken.
1. Allergies
2. History of symptoms
    a. Total duration of back pain
    b. total duration of sciatica
    c. Location of sciatica
3. Other significant medical history
4. List of medications
5. Neurologic and muscle testing
    a. Muscle strength testing
    b. Deep tendon reflexes
    c. Sensation
    d. Mechanical tests
    e. Sciatic stretch
    f. Sitting straight leg raising
    g. Supine straight leg raising

Neurologic and musculoskeletal assessment, including the evaluation of sensation, muscle strength, and deep tendon reflexes, should be well recorded. The mechanical and sciatic stretch tests, including sitting and supine straight leg raising, weakness, muscle wasting, and dermatomal dysesthesia all contribute to the clinical diagnosis of radiculopathy, secondary to herniated nucleus pulposus, which might be responsive to chemonucleolysis.

In addition, laboratory studies include:
1. Routine lumbosacral roentgenographic studies
2. CT scan
3. Myelogram
4. Enhanced CT scan
5. Discography
6. Electromyogram

A positive myelogram, CT scan, or enhanced CT scan should be required before chemonucleolysis unless clinical evidence of discogenic disease has been proved by discography. Electromyography is used frequently to confirm the extent of the radiculopathy and to help locate the position of the lesion. Other studies considered to be of value include epidural venography and epidurography. These studies should be used within the scope of the expertise of the physician performing and using the studies.

Additional valuable studies and information that might be taken into consideration are the Minnesota Multiphasic Personality Inventory, pain drawing, previous surgery, and litigations. These particular studies should not be used to determine whether the patient should receive the chemonucleolysis; however, if these factors are positive and there is other confirming evidence, they may indicate a decreased chance of the patient's responding to chemonucleolysis.

The following list of criteria for chemonucleolysis can be consulted when receiving all the data collected from the patient assessments.

CRITERIA FOR CHEMONUCLEOLYSIS

1. The patient must not have a known allergy to meat tenderizer or papaya. If such exists, an allergy consultation should be obtained for clearance.
2. The patient must not have a previous chymopapain injection history.
3. Leg pain is the dominant symptom when compared with back pain. Ideally, it should affect one leg and follow a typical sciatic or femoral nerve distribution.
4. Straight leg raising is usually reduced to 50% of the normal. The pain crosses over to the symptomatic leg when the unaffected leg is elevated, or pain radiates proximally or distally with digital pressure on the tibial nerve in the popliteal fossa (or a combination of these signs).
5. Motor weakness and/or reflex abnormality is present.
6. The myelogram, CT scan, or enhanced CT scan should be abnormal, corresponding to the level of herniation determined clinically.
7. A focal or localized posterolateral bulge or prolapse is displayed as determined by computerized tomography or myelography.
8. Leg and back pain must be refractory to conservative therapy (bed rest, activity modification, brace support, and/or analgesics).
9. The safety and effectiveness of chymopapain has not been studied in pregnant animals or in pregnant patients. It is also not known whether chymopapain can cause fetal harm. Therefore chymopapain should not be used in pregnant women.
10. The safety and efficacy of chymopapain has not been studied in children. Therefore chymopapain should not be used in children.
11. The differential diagnosis must not indicate the possibility of:
    a. Spinal cord tumor
    b. Metastatic cancer
    c. Vertebral osteomyelitis
    d. Disc space infection
12. X-ray findings should not indicate:
    a. Mechanical insufficiency
    b. Spinal stenosis
    c. Spondylolisthesis
    d. Blockage by cervical or thoracic disc as demonstrated by myelogram
    e. An inability to reach disc space via a lateral route

f. An intrathecal or intravascular flow of contrast dye with discography

PREOPERATIVE EVALUATION AND PREPARATION

Chemonucleolysis is not a cure for all low back pain. Careful preoperative screening should be done in all cases, although no hard criteria exist.

Certain materials should be available for each candidate before chemonucleolysis. An adequate lumbar spine x-ray series is necessary to assess the various physical properties of the lumbar spine segment(s) to be injected. These x-ray films permit an evaluation of the L5-S1 angle; the location, shape, and size of anticular processes; the presence of osteophytes or lumbar spine anomalies, and spinal disc width. This evaluation can help safely expedite the needle placement.

Chemonucleolysis is a safe and effective procedure for treatment of discogenic disease, low back pain, and sciatica. Although its safety and effectiveness have been established, the procedure still must be viewed as an elective invasive treatment. The patient who chooses to undergo chemonucleolysis must be completely informed of the procedure. Standard informed consent procedures, acceptable to local institutions, should be executed in accordance with state and federal laws.

TECHNIQUE FOR INJECTION

The technique for chemonucleolysis is the intradiscal injection of chymopapain for appropriately diagnosed patients. Before injection, all patients are required to have myelographic and/or CT scan confirmation of discogenic disease unless clinical evidence has been proved by discography.

Injection of chymopapain is restricted to the operating suite or x-ray department and is administered using a local, supplemental local, or general anesthetic as deemed appropriate by the attending physician. Chemonucleolysis is done under strict aseptic conditions. Preoperative sedation is given as indicated.

The patient is placed on a radiolucent table, usually in the left-lateral position. A portable image intensifier or biplane fluoroscopy is used to provide both lateral and anteroposterior views of the spine. The image intensifier is maneuvered to adequately demonstrate the disc. The patient's back is prepared for surgery and draped in the usual surgical manner. The free-hand technique is most commonly used.

The L4 intervertebral disc space is approached using the lateral technique from a point at the level of the iliac crest and 8 to 10 cm lateral to the midline (according to the body structure of the patient). A 7-inch, 18-gauge needle is inserted at an angle of 45 degrees to the sagittal plane in the direction of the intervertebral disc space. The lateral image confirms the direction and positioning of the needle.

Several technical considerations must be noted. First, when the tip of the advancing needle reaches a line adjoining the posterior borders of the vertebral bodies, one should obtain a firm, gritty sensation from the annulus. If the tip of the needle passes anterior to this line before the sensation is obtained, the needle will not enter the nucleus of the disc but will pass anterior and lateral to it. If this occurs, the needle should be inserted at a more acute angle to the sagittal plane. If the angle is to be changed, the needle should first be withdrawn close to the skin surface.

The second consideration is related to the bony obstructions found in the transverse process, the pars interarticularis, or the facet joint. The structures causing bony obstruction can be determined on lateral roentgenographic projection. Obstruction at the level of the upper half of the vertebral body is probably due to the transverse process. Obstruction at the level of the lower half of the vertebral body is probably due to the pars interarticularis. Opposite the disc space, obstruction is probably due to the facet joint. If the transverse process causes obstruction, the site of the needle insertion is moved in a cephalad direction for the L4 intervertebral disc space. If the pars interarticularis or facet joint causes obstruction, the angle of the needle insertion needs to be reduced.

For the L5 intervertebral disc space the image intensifier is repositioned laterally. The L4 needle serves as a landmark and guide to the position of the L5 disc space. The L5 needle is inserted at the same angle to the sagittal plane, that is, 45 degrees, and is directed approximately 45 degrees caudally. This angle is adjusted until the tip of the needle is level and adjacent to the posterior aspect of the vertebral bodies (the L5 disc space). This is of great importance in assessing bony obstruction. Obstruction by the transverse process necessitates complete repositioning of the needle. Obstruction by the pars interarticularis or facet joint necessitates reducing the angle of the needle relative to the sagittal plane.

Sometimes a broad transverse process of L5 obstructs this approach. If this occurs, the double-needle technique is necessary: a 22-gauge needle is placed through the 18-gauge needle with the tip of the 18-gauge needle lying just at the level of the inferior of the L5 vertebral body. By curving the distal one half inch of the 22-gauge needle with the bevel up, the needle will curve downward and into the L5 intervertebral disc space as it passes out of the tip of the 18-gauge needle. It is imperative that the surgeon has visually verified the correct needle tip placement by using image intensification. Discography with metrizamide is done to confirm needle placement and evaluate the continuity and pathology of the disc. (Resistance to flow will give some indication of the integrity of the disc.)

Problems arise if too much attention is paid to the angle of the needle insertion and too little attention is paid to the overall size and shape of the patient. A clear, three-dimensional mental image of the lower lumbar region is essential. An articulated specimen of the spine in the operating room is helpful.

Next, 0.5 ml of chymopapain solution is injected into the involved disc space, and a period of 10 minutes—by the clock—is allowed to pass before the injection of the remainder of the solution. This is based on the possibility that there may be an autoimmune reaction to the nuclear protein, or a reaction to the enzyme, the extent of which may be dose related. Drapes are removed to observe the patient for early systemic reactions. The patient is observed for 20 minutes—by the clock—before returning the patient to recovery.

"A Sterotaxic System for Chemonucleolysis at L5" has been described by Froning.[5] Surgical preparation, image intensification, and technical considerations are the same as for the free-hand technique.

Actual disc center depths must be used with the stereotaxic device. Magnified radiographic film distances can be easily converted to actual distances by a simple x-ray pelvimetry-like technique. A preprocedure lateral film is exposed with a skin-adherent, lead vinyl strip placed over the spinous processes, and a radiographic centimeter ruler is positioned opposite this strip (Fig. 11-1). Magnified film distances are corrected to actual distances by placing a protractor from disc center to the lead vinyl strip and then over the ruler image in the film. Thus individual disc center depths are premeasured in each patient. This film may be made by

Chemonucleolysis 111

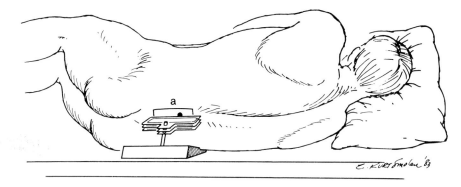

Fig. 11-1 Actual disc center depth determination using simple x-ray pelvimetry-like technique.

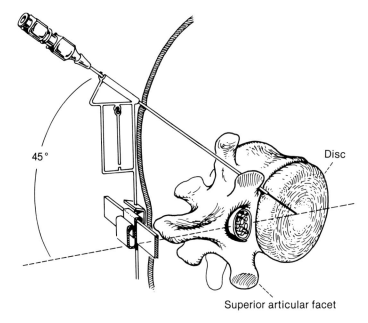

Fig. 11-2 Visual parallels for steriotaxic passage of needle, 45-degree angle guide, and disc parallel guide.

the technician the day before the chymopapain procedure is scheduled, so that disc center depths may be measured in conjunction with other preprocedure plain film planning.

The accuracy requirements of a sterotaxic system prohibit the unreliability of estimating disc depths. Disc center depths are measured from the skin surface at the midsagittal plane. Skin entry is measured as an offset from the midsagittal plane. A 45-degree angle guide contains a plumb chain to help orient it to the vertical. The midsagittal plane is oriented to the horizontal by positioning the patient in true lateral. The vertical and horizontal form the right angle of this 45-degree right triangle (Fig. 11-2).

The two visual parallels for stereotaxic passage of the needle are the 45-degree angle guide and the disc parallel guide (see Fig. 11-2). The parallel guide is maneuvered on magnetic bridges until its image bisects the disc end-plates (Fig. 11-3). Ideal skin entry is prelocated as a combination of sagittal offset equal to indi-

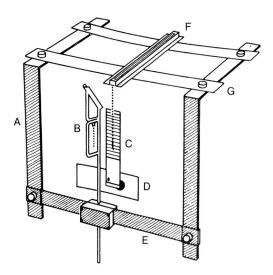

Fig. 11-3 Prelocation of ideal skin entry using stereotaxic guidance frame. *A*, Guidance frame (2); *B*, angle guide; *C*, offset ruler; *D*, radiopaque skin tab, two shapes (4); *E*, malleable bridge (and angle guide holder); *F*, parallel guide; *G*, magnetic bridge (2).

vidual premeasured disc center depths and a plumb chain from the parallel guide (see Fig. 11-3).

Blunt dissection is provided by use of a double needle, in which the outer needle consists of a 17-gauge flat-ended cannula fitted with a round-ended obturator. The surgeon maneuvers the cannula into the nerve axilla to dock directly on the disc surface. The outer needle, with its flat end resting on the disc surface, protects the spinal nerve from the sharp dissection of the inner tapering 22-gauge needle (see Fig. 11-2).

SUMMARY

When injected into the intervertebral disc, chymopapain binds and hydrolyzes the nucleus pulposus, reduces the intradiscal pressure, and relieves pain. Intrathecal injection is the most toxic route, and anaphylaxis is the most dangerous side effect.

REFERENCES

1. Barr, J.S.: Lumbar disk lesions in retrospect and prospect, Clin. Orthop. **129**:4, 1977.
2. Brown, M., and Daroff, R.B.: The double blind study comparing discase to placebo: an editorial comment, Spine **2**:33, 1977.
3. Food and Drug Administration: FDA drug bulletin, vol. 14, No. 2, August 1984.
4. Fraser, R.D.: Chymopapain for treatment of intervertebral disc herniation: a preliminary report of double blind study, Spine **7**(6):608, 1982.
5. Froning, E.C.: Individual orthopaedic instruction (IOI), Paper presented to the annual meeting of the American Academy of Orthopaedic Surgeons, Atlanta, Feb. 1984.
6. Garvin, P.J., and Jennings, R.B.: Long-term effects of chymopapain on intervertebral discs of dogs, Clin. Orthop. **9**(2):281, 1973.
7. Garvin, P.J., et al.: Chymopapain: a pharmacologic and toxicologic evaluation in experimental animals, Clin. Orthop. **41**:204, 1965.
8. Garvin, P.J., et al.: Enzymatic digestion of the nucleus pulposus: a review of experimental studies with chymopapain, Orthop. Clin. North Am. **8**(1):27, 1977.
9. Gesler, R.M.: Pharmacology properties of chymopapain, Clin. Orthop. **67**:47, 1969.
10. Hendry, N.G.C.: The hydration of the nucleus pulposus and its relation to intervertebral disc degeneration, J. Bone Joint Surg. **40B**:132, 1958.
11. Hirsch, C.: Studies on the pathology of low back pain, J. Bone Joint Surg. **41B**(2):237, 1959.
12. Jansen, E.F., and Balls, A.K.: Chymopapain: a new crystalline proteinase from papaya latex, J. Biol. Chem. **137**:459, 1941.
13. Kapsalis, A.A., et al.: The fate of chymopapain injected the therapy of intervertebral disc disease, J. Lab. Clin. Med. **83**:532, 1974.
14. MacNab, I., et al.: Chemonucleolysis, Can. J. Surg. **14**:280, 1971.
15. Naylor, A.: The biophysical and biochemical aspects of intervertebral disc herniation and degeneration, Ann. R. Coll. Surg. Engl. **31**:91, 1962.
16. Naylor, A., and Smare, D.L.: Fluid content of the nucleus pulposus as a factor in the disc syndrome, Br. Med. **2**:975, 1953.
17. Schwetschwenau, P.R., et al.: Double-blind evaluation of intradiscal chymopapain for herniated lumbar discs, J. Neurosurg. **45**:622, 1976.
18. Shealy, C.N.: Tissue reactions to chymopapain in cats, J. Neurosurg. **26**:327, 1967.

19. Simmons, J.W., et al.: Update and review of chemonucleolysis, Clin. Orthop. **183:**51, March 1984.
20. Smith, L.: Enzyme dissolution of the nucleus pulposus in humans, JAMA **18:**177, 1964.
21. Smith, L., and Brown, J.: Treatment of lumbar intervertebral disc lesions by direct injection of chymopapain, J. Bone Joint Surg. **498:**502, 1967.
22. Stern, I.J.: Biochemistry of chymopapain, Clin. Orthop. **67:**42, 1969.
23. Stern, I.J., and Smith, L.: Dissolution of chymopapain in vitro of tissue from normal or prolapsed intervertebral discs, Clin. Orthop. **50:**269, 1967.
24. Thomas, L.: Reversible collapse of rabbit ears after intravenous papain, and prevention of recovery by cortisone, J. Exp. Med. **104:**245, 1956.
25. Watts, C., et al.: Chymopapain treatment of intervertebral disc disease, J. Neurosurg. **42:**374, 1975.

EDITORIAL COMMENTARY

Few of the authors are using chemonucleolysis to any significant degree at this time. Richard Rothman finds chemonucleolysis of no value and does not use the procedure at all. As Vert Mooney states, "I think chymopapain eventually will be relegated to a historic procedure. Its unpredictability and its lack of equal efficiency, when compared to surgery, eventually will lead to its demise." He believes that percutaneous discectomy will supplant chymopapain in an ideally suited candidate.

William Kirkaldy-Willis states that in his community the patients "are usually prepared to wait for 3 months. During this time 75% of them become almost symptom-free." He still finds chemonucleolysis successful 70% of the time, but only one third of his good candidates are willing to accept the procedure.

Leon Wiltse, of course, has been one of the prime advocates of chemonucleolysis for the past 20 years. He still uses the procedure when patients are willing to accept it after informed consent, which is becoming less and less frequent.

C.D. Ray has some poignant remarks regarding chemonucleolysis. He states that "chemonucleolysis stands as a monument to medical herd instinct behavior. Like the annual suicidal migration of the wildebeest of Africa, at one time it seemed that everybody needed chymo. Now it seems that nobody needs chymo. Neither extreme has proved correct. Chemonucleolysis has been far more carefully studied than operative discectomy (including microdiscectomy). The effects, failures, and the terrible neurologic lesions of the central nervous system have been well documented and widely publicized. The overall morbidity and mortality now that the dust begins to actually settle are better with chemonucleolysis than with discectomy, albeit by a small margin. Certain post-procedural complications, for example, severe low backache and segmental instability, may be more common after chymopapain, but the frightening sequela of paresis, plegias, or bleeds are too rare to deserve the attention given them. Studies in the baboon, showing that simultaneous arachnoidal injections of contrast agent and enzyme proved to be far more damaging to the spinal cord and other CNS structures led to the recommendation that either saline acceptance discography alone be performed, or no discography at all immediately prior to interdiscal enzyme injection." Dr. Ray has published in the *Journal of Neurosurgery* in 1984 the "Danger of Intravenous Injection During Chemonucleolysis." He found that with moderate injection pressures the discographic dye not infrequently gained direct or indirect access to venous drainage and the vena cava. Therefore he strongly recommends that contrast discography be performed immediately before the injection of the enzyme. If vascular access is seen, chymopapain should not be injected.

In San Francisco, Bradford DeLong, Jim Morris, and the other authors have almost ceased doing chemonucleolysis because of adverse publicity and patient and physician fears. Our success rate during our active use of the drug was only about 50%. We find chemonucleolysis to be less reliable, less successful, and less predictable than surgery. It is extremely frustrating and time consuming for a patient to undergo chemonucleolysis, wait for 3 to 5 months to see if there is going to be a success, and then have to undergo surgery that had a 90% probability of success to begin with.

We are seeing the long-range development of spinal stenosis after chemonucleolysis as we have seen with discectomy.

At this time, it looks as though chemonucleolysis has not stood up to the test of time.

Only one of our authors found chemonucleolysis of no value. Most felt that it was of some value, and a few felt that it was of great value. Only one of our authors has experienced significant complications with the procedure. However, it is the least used procedure of any of the seven major surgical procedures reviewed in this book.

Arthur H. White

CHAPTER

12

MICRODISCECTOMY AND PERCUTANEOUS DISCECTOMY: INDICATIONS, HISTORY, AND RESULTS

Ronald J. Wisneski   Richard H. Rothman

MICRODISCECTOMY TECHNIQUES

The year 1984 marks the fiftieth anniversary of Mixter's and Barr's[10] classic address at the Massachusetts General Hospital, illustrating for the first time the surgical cure of sciatica by excision of a herniated lumbar disc. It is therefore appropriate that we consider how our surgical armamentarium has evolved in dealing with neural compression from a herniated nucleus pulposus.

Throughout these past 5 decades we have come to understand the precision, beauty, and ability to promptly and dependably eradicate the pain of a compressed nerve by using discectomy procedures, but we have also come to understand the misery and suffering that can be wrought by the misapplication of the surgical techniques. To emphasize this point, one need only look at the review published by Aitken and Bradford in 1947.[1] They investigated 170 surgical cases from the files of a large national compensation carrier between 1940 and 1944; only 17% of the patients had good results, and 45% were judged poor or "bad." The review showed that discs were removed at levels that did not correlate with the neurologic examination or the myelogram. Extensive laminectomies were performed for single-level disc disease. Postoperative x-ray films demonstrated laminectomies performed at the wrong levels. Within 2 months of the first episode of lumbar pain one seventh of the patients were operated on. In another one seventh of the cases there was ample preoperative evidence of a psychoneurotic disorder. The mortality rate in the 170 cases was 3%. Complications such as postoperative foot drop developed in six cases, and paralysis of the quadriceps muscles developed in three cases. A major review summarizing the experience in over 13,000 operations performed in 35 investigations for lumbar disc degeneration was published in 1961.[7] Unfortunately it is often difficult to compare findings from one investigation to the next, but two factors are unequivocal. The first is complete relief of pain, which was achieved in only 46% of the cases, a mark quite short of an ideal goal. The second factor, complete failure of pain relief, is constant at 10%.

We have found that the three factors that have the greatest predictive value in determining disc herniation are the presence of a positive myelogram, a positive tension sign, and a neurologic deficit. If all three factors are present, one is almost assured of uncovering mechanical nerve root compression at surgery. There remains a guiding principal, and this cannot be stressed too strongly, that the degree of herniation noted at surgery is the most important factor in determining the quality of surgical result. If one correlates the degree of herniation with complete relief of sciatica, one sees an almost linear relationship between these two factors. With complete herniations, there is at least a 90% complete relief of sciatica, falling to a 40% placebo effect with a negative exploration.

An equally significant criterion is an initial lack of psychosocial complications in the patient's history. Psychosocial problems clearly have a profound effect on the outcome of low back surgery. Patients with significant depression frequently express their depression as a complaint of low back pain. The reason for this is not clear, but certainly operating on these individuals will not alleviate their depression and will not stop their complaint of low back pain. The solution for these individuals lies in appreciating their problem, taking a careful history, and using antidepressant medication and psychotherapy rather than surgery. Within the same context compensation and litigation involvement appear to have such a profound effect on pain complaints and return to function after surgery that we no longer consider individuals with such a history appropriate subjects for surgery unless confronted with a cauda equina syndrome or progressive paralysis.

To summarize in terms of surgical success, patient selection remains the most critical factor, and the treating surgeon must have certain basic information if he or she is to adequately advise patients afflicted with lumbar disc disease. First, what is the natural history of the disease process? Second, does surgery alter the course of this disease? Both surgeon and patients must know not only the quality of the result that is to be expected after surgery but also how the surgical result compares to the relief of pain obtained simply by the passage of time. Third, what factors help to predict the patient who will benefit from surgery? Obviously, one may choose only those individuals who will experience excellent pain relief after surgery. However, it may be more important to predict those individuals who will not benefit from surgery. Too often the surgeon and patient are swept down the road toward surgical intervention simply because nonsurgical therapy has failed. Finally, the surgeon must appreciate which operation produces maximal benefit for the patient with a particular type of injury or disease.

As a result of advances in anesthesia, blood transfusion therapy, and diagnostic and intraoperative imaging techniques, surgical treatment—a standard discectomy—has become a reliable and safe procedure for the appropriately selected patient with a lumbar disc herniation. Most surgeons favor a laminotomy approach originally described by Semms[11] and Love[9] independently. This operation consists of removal of the ligamentum flavum together with the inferior margin of the proximal lamina on one side. Others favor a complete laminectomy. Herron and Pheasant,[5] in the January 1983 issue of *Spine,* reported on a series of patients treated with bilateral decompressive laminectomies and radical partial discectomies, partial facetectomies of the inferior and superior articular processes, and foraminotomies as indicated. They noted that the advantages of this procedure were the ability to recognize and deal surgically with all components of neural compression, the maintenance of segmental stability, and the prevention of neural compromise by further degenerative changes in the lumbar segment. They believed that this somewhat radical approach to a standard discectomy procedure is justified because it may be prophylactic, compensating for further anticipated changes. Each of these procedures may be viewed as a standard discectomy procedure.

The results of standard lumbar discectomies are good, but they could be better. Of those patients who are properly selected and properly treated, perineural fibrosis and scarring, as well as failure to evaluate for the presence of additional injury or disease such as lateral recess stenosis, remain a leading cause of surgical failures. It has been our experience with salvage surgery that neurolysis is a futile exercise. Those patients whom we have tried to salvage, and in whom perineural fibrosis was the primary concern, surgery was uniformly a failure. It is the prevention of this perineural and intraneural scarring that must be the key to success.

It has been shown in both clinical and laboratory studies that perineural scarring is related to three factors:
1. Mechanical trauma
2. Epidural hematoma
3. Contact between the dura and skeletal muscles

In questioning how often there are concerns other than disc herniation that may adversely affect the quality of the surgical result, Kirkaldy-Willis,[2] in analyzing 225 discectomy patients, found that 56% of the patients had concomitant lateral recess stenosis or lateral recess stenosis alone. Spengler[12] has reported that in his series of discectomy patients there is a 30% incidence of lateral recess stenosis, in addition to disc disease, requiring a limited medial foraminotomy at the time of surgery. An interinstitutional study of patients with a failed back surgery syndrome published by Burton[2] further dramatizes the issue. In over 800 failed back surgery patients seen over 1 year, the concomitant conditions of lateral recess or central stenosis accounted for 65% to 71% of failures, and postoperative arachnoiditis and epidural fibrosis were responsible for 12% to 24% of the failed cases.

Knowledge of these potential weaknesses of standard discectomy makes it possible for us to establish criteria for improving the procedure. Major criteria include (1) adquate removal of the offending disc material; (2) minimal retraction of the nerve root; (3) meticulous hemostasis; (4) evaluation for the presence of concomitant pathology; and (5) preservation of spinal stability.

The minor criteria that have been stressed by various authors incude (1) maintenance of epidural fat; (2) minimal muscle dissection; (3) decreased hospital stay; and (4) decreased postoperative pain.

MICROSURGERY TECHNIQUES

If means are available to meet these criteria, the operation is no longer a cookbook recipe, but a process that can evolve. The means for refining standard discectomy procedures may be present in microsurgical technique. Microsurgery requires proficiency in the use of a microscope, small incisions, meticulous hemostasis and precise removal of the diseased tissues. Several ingenious alternatives to standard discectomy have been reported in the past 5 years. These procedures can be grouped into one of two categories: (1) the percutaneous lateral discectomy technique as developed by Friedman[3] and Kambin[8]; and (2) the microsurgical discectomy techniques involving the use of the operating microscope, which have been performed with and without bone removal surrounding the interlaminar space.

PERCUTANEOUS DISCECTOMY TECHNIQUE

Friedman's technique involves positioning the patient in a lateral decubitus position on the operating table with the painful side down. Under fluroscopic guidance a skin incision is made just over the iliac crest, and a specifically designed speculum is inserted through the psoas muscle to the midpoint of the lateral part of the desired interspace. Using specially lengthened instruments, the annulus then is incised and the disc is removed piecemeal with pituitary rongeurs. At the time of his report, nine patients had undergone the procedure. Seven had clear radiculopathies with approciate radiographic findings, and they all had excellent relief of symptoms. Two patients had intractable low back pain, bilateral mechanical findings, and central disc herniations on radiographic examination. One experienced good relief, and one did not. Three of the patients had several days of paraspinal spasm after the procedure, and one complained of a lower extremity dysesthetic sensation that persisted for several weeks after the operation. It was Friedman's presumption that this resulted from damage to the lumbar sympathetic chain. The length of follow-up was 6 months.

Kambin reported on a similar technique for percutaneous discectomy with modified Craig needle biopsy instrumentation, followed by evacuation of the disc using simple aspiration and insertion of specially designed punch forceps. After 4 to 8 months of follow-up, all nine patients in his study were free of radicular symptoms. All patients were discharged within 2 to 3 days of the operation.

The authors reported that the potential advantages of these procedures were very similar to those of chemonucleolysis, that is, no lumbar incision, muscle stripping, or bone removal and the procedure frequently took less than 15 minutes. Minimal postoperative pain was encountered by the majority of patients in these studies, the overall hospital stay was shortened, and the epidural space was never violated. One potential disadvantage of the procedure in Friedman's study was that all patients underwent preoperative screening for the identification of aberrant and retroperitoneal structures that might lie in the projected surgical path. This involved performing a transaxial scan at the level of the upper iliac crest after giving the patient Gastrografin orally 4 hours before.

One patient was denied percutaneous discectomy because his abdominal CT scan revealed that his ascending colon was directly in the surgical path.

Although not encountered, the potential for injury to the abdominal vasculature and viscera, as well as the sympathetic, lymphatic chains, and lumbar plexus, is possible. Because of the height of iliac crest and the size of the instrumentation used, entry into the L5 interspace is impossible without drilling through the crest; therefore the procedure has not been performed for an L5-S1 herniation.

There are many potential complications associated with these procedures that prohibit their general use. It is possible, however, that as a longer follow-up and more experience is accrued by the individuals investigating these techniques, it may be possible to recommend percutaneous discectomy as an alternative to chemonucleolysis for the herniated disc that is not sequestered or extruded and if the patient's preoperative myelogram, CT scan, and x-ray films demonstrate no evidence of anomalous nerve roots, altered intraabdominal pathology, or anomalies of the osteoarticular structures.

MICROSURGICAL DISCECTOMIES

A microsurgical discectomy involves the use of the operating microscope during all or a portion of the procedure. A typical operating microscope for use in discectomy procedures should have the following features: (1) adjustable heads for both the surgeon and assistant; (2) 7.5 to 30 power zoom capability; (3) electronic foot control focusing; (4) a fiberoptic coaxial light source; (5) a foot pedal for X/Y access control; and (6) optional third head for camera and color video recording for documentation and teaching.

As previously mentioned, the technique is by no means standardized and the procedures can be divided into those in which a purely intralaminar approach is used and those in which a laminotomy is created, in addition to removal of the ligamentum flavum.

In 1978 Williams[13] was the first to advocate the microsurgical discectomy technique. He reported on 530 cases with a follow-up period ranging from 6 months to 18 months. His technique involved a purely interlaminar approach with no bone removed. After one procedure 91% of the patients were rated as achieving a satisfactory result. The 48 patients who were rated as unsatisfactory underwent repeat microsurgical discectomies. Of these patients 11 were ultimately listed as failures, for a total failure rate of 2.1%. Of the remaining 37 patients the diagnoses after the second procedure were listed as follows: recurrent herniations at the same level occurred in 8 patients; recurrent herniations at the same level but on the opposite side were found in 4 patients; and in 6 patients only adhesions were found. In 3 patients the surgery had been performed at the wrong level, and in the remaining 16 patients, the author described them as having peculiar nucleoid material protruding beneath the posterior longitudinal ligament; he gave the patients in this group a diagnosis that he termed the *undulating disc syndrome*.

Williams stated that the average stay for the patient undergoing a microsurgical discectomy procedure was 3.1 days compared to an average length of stay of 9.1 days for his laminectomy patients. The average surgical time was 37 minutes compared to 67 minutes for his routine discectomy patients.

Goald[4] in 1978 also reported on a 2-year follow-up study of 116 patients undergoing microsurgical discectomy using Williams's technique. It was noted that 10% of the patients had herniations at more than one level, 33% of the patients were compensation cases, and only 85% of the patients had positive neuroradiographic findings. He reported a surgical cure rate of 96% after one procedure. He again cited the advantages of reduced length of hospital stay and less surgical time as primary advantages. He reported on no complications, and at 1 year follow-up all of his noncompensation patients were working and 80% of the compensation patients were back at their original employment.

Hudgins[6] modified Williams's surgical technique by removing sufficient bone and ligamentum flavum laterally to be able to look down at the lateral edge of the nerve root. He reported on 200 cases with an average follow-up of 1 year. Of these patients, 10% had either a midline herniation or more than occasional bilateral leg pain and underwent bilateral procedures. Hudgins changed to a wider exposure because he believed that the interlaminar approach may lead to traction injuries to the nerve root and inadequate decompression. With adequate bone removal, concomitant evaluation for bony encroachment is facilitated. He classified 68% of the patients as achieving an excellent result, rated 20% as good, 8% fair, and 4% poor. In listing his complications, 3 patients developed an aseptic discitis that responded to conservative therapy and 11 patients developed recurrent herniation within 1 year's follow-up. He further stated that, while originally using Williams's technique, another reason he decided to change to the hemilaminotomy exposure was because many of his patients had more numbness after surgery than his previous standard discectomy patients.

Wilson and Harbaugh[14] compared 100 cases of microlumbar discectomy with sufficient bone removal to visualize the lateral border of the nerve root with 100 standard discectomy cases chosen retrospectively. Patient profiles and surgical results were similar; however, an excessive number of dural tears from the microdiscectomy procedure occurred early on, reflecting the definite learning curve involved in refining a new technique. In postoperative follow-up after 2 years the microsurgical technique was superior to the standard operation; their patients returned to work in less than half the time, and more patients required a second operation for recurrence with the standard discectomy. After microsurgical discectomy, recurrences and the failed disc syndrome were reduced to one half that occurring after the standard operation.

Let us examine how percutaneous lateral discectomy, microdiscectomy without bone removal as advocated by Williams and Goald, and microdiscectomy with bone removal as advocated by Wilson, Harbaugh, and Hudgins compare (see box).

Criteria for improving standard discectomy

Major
1. Adequate removal of disc material
2. Minimal retraction of nerve root
3. Meticulous hemostasis
4. Evaluate for concomitant pathology
5. Preservation of stability

Minor
1. Maintain epidural fat
2. Minimal muscle dissection
3. Decreased postoperative pain
4. Decreased hospital stay

The preservation of spinal stability is accomplished by all three techniques. In our experience significant portions of the facet joint can be excised at one level unilaterally without subsequent problems. When considering how each of the procedures affords minimal manipulation of neural tissue along with adequate exposure to the epidural space, we find that although percutaneous discectomy theoretically involves no direct contact with neural tissue the potential definitely exists for damaging neural tissue at any point from an intradural location all the way out to the lumbosacral plexus. As already mentioned, this is a relatively blind procedure and the hazards are significant. Williams's technique totally excludes any laminotomy.

As Hudgins and Wilson did, we strongly believe that after the ligamentum flavum has been opened sufficient bone removal from the inferior edge of the supradjacent lamina and the medial aspect of the facet joint should be performed to allow clear visualization of the lateral border of the nerve root. We believe the single most important measure of safety involved in this phase of the discectomy is clear identification of this lateral border of the root. The root may be stretched and tightly compressed over an extruded disc fragment, making this identification difficult. In addition, the root may be bound down by scar tissue provoked by a free fragment of disc tissue and the surrounding granulation tissue. If any doubt exists as to the true margin of the root, the dissection should be carried in a cranial and caudal direction to more normal anatomy. Once the nerve root is clearly identified, excision of the disc can be performed easily. To use the microscope for a restrictive exposure of the interlaminar space along with an excessively small incision is to be a slave to the instrument.

Absolute hemostasis and atraumatic technique are also of fundamental importance in the prevention of perineural fibrosis and scarring. With percutaneous discectomy the potential exists for damage to the great vessels. Williams stated in his article that blood loss with his technique is minimal and that if rupture of the epidural veins occurs bleeding will stop spontaneously when the herniation is decompressed.

We have been taught that preservation of the longitudinal intraspinal veins is a reasonable and achievable goal. Not only are the internal longitudinal veins preserved but also the small arteries and veins coursing along the nerve root itself, and a conscious effort is made not to strip the nerve root. To facilitate this, the use of magnification is a great adjunct in the performance of lumbar disc surgery. After using both the operating microscope and binocular loupes, we have found that binocular loupe magnification has proved most satisfactory. We recommend 2.5 or 3.5 magnification wide-angle lenses. The lenses can be adjusted by the manufacturer to a comfortable working distance for the surgeon. Coaxial illumination provided by a fiber-optic headlight is a must for adequate visualization during intraspinal surgery.

Overhead operating room lights simply do not illuminate the lateral recesses where the majority of disc injury or disease is found. Light weight headlamps such as this give excellent illumination.

Despite the gratifying results reported by the percutaneous discectomy advocates, the patient numbers were small and we would anticipate that in patients with large extrusions or sequestrated fragments failure would be inevitable. Williams believed that lumbar disc protrusion was not a disease of the whole disc but rather of the annulus alone. The fallacy of this deduction is evident when one compares his reoperation rate of 9.1% to the 5% rate in Hudgins's series and 4% in the series reported by Wilson. Lumbar disc protrusion is a disorder of the whole disc, and subtotal removal of the nucleus remains the better treatment. Once any free fragments are removed, we prefer to excise a large rectangular window of annulus centered beneath the nerve root. The purpose of the resection of this large window is to prevent late nerve root compression caused by collapse of the disc space and further buckling of the annulus. Through this large window in the annulus a radical disc excision can be performed with excision of the majority of the nuclear material. Large heavy-tipped pituitary rongeurs are used to prevent inadvertent instrument breakage. With good lighting and magnification, the anterior disc space can be visualized and excision of nucleus performed under direct vision. A surgeon should always be able to feel the instrument against bony end-plate if inadvertent puncture of the anterior annulus and injury to the great vessels are to be avoided.

Obviously, with percutaneous discectomy there is no opportunity to evaluate for concomitant injury or disease. It has been stated that the critical area of disc surgery lies in the epidural space. Magnification, whether it be by the operating microscope or loupes, should be used to facilitate the examination of this space and not to ignore it as Williams chose to do.

We believe that once excision of the nucleus has been completed attention should be turned to the course of the nerve root into the foramen, and a complete exploration of the foramina should be performed. This is done by palpation rather than direct visualization. A short and long Fraser elevator can be used. With this technique one should be able to recognize compression in the foramen caused by osteophytic overgrowth, pedicle migration, bulging of the annulus laterally, or lateral disc extrusion.

SUMMARY

We believe the factors that will determine the final outcome of microlumbar discectomy are the experience of the surgeon and assistant, knowledge of anatomy and pathomechanics, proper use of microinstrumentation, extensive laboratory practice, and most importantly proper patient selection. In terms of performance of the technique the prerequisites are adequate exposure, atraumatic dissection, and absolute hemostasis.

Finally we would like to point out that the poor results of lumbar disc surgery are not from incisional morbidity. To use the microscope simply for operating through a small incision and compromising neural tissue exposure is synonymous with being unable to distinguish the useful from the useless.

REFERENCES

1. Aitken, A.P., and Bradford, C.H.: End results of ruptured intervertebral discs in industry, Am. J. Surg. **73**:365, 1947.
2. Burton, C.V., et al.: Causes of failure of surgery on the lumbar spine, Clin. Orthop. **157**:191, 1981.
3. Friedman, W.A.: Percutaneous discectomy: an alternative to chemonucleolysis? Neurosurgery **13**:542, 1983.
4. Goald, H.J.: Microlumbar discectomy, Spine **3**:183, 1978.
5. Herron, L.D., and Pheasant, H.C.: Bilateral laminotomy and discectomy for segmental lumbar disc disease, Spine **8**:86, 1983.
6. Hudgins, W.R.: The role of microdiscectomy, Orthop. Clin. North Am. **14**:589, 1983.
7. Jockheim, K.A.: Lumbaler Bandscheibenvoefall, Berlin, 1961, Springer-Verlag.
8. Kambin, P., and Gellman, H.: Percutaneous lateral discectomy of the lumbar spine, Clin. Orthop. **174**:127, 1983.
9. Love, I.G.: Removal of protruded intervertebral disc with laminectomy, Mayo Clin. Proc. **14**:800, 1939.
10. Mixter, W.J., and Barr, J.S.: Rupture of intervertebral disc with involvement of spinal canal, N. Engl. J. Med. **211**:210, 1934.
11. Semmes, R.E.: Diagnosis of ruptured disc without contrast myelography and comment upon recent experience with modified hemilaminectomy for their removal, Yale J. Biol. Med. **11**:433, 1939.
12. Spengler, D.M.: Lumbar discectomy: results with limited disc excision and selective foraminotomy, Spine **7**:604, 1982.
13. Williams, R.W.: Microlumbar discectomy, Spine **3**:175, 1978.
14. Wilson, D.H., and Harbaugh, R: Lumbar discectomy: a comparative study of microsurgical and standard technique. In Hardy, R.W., editor: Seminars in neurosurgery: lumbar disc disease, New York, 1982, Raven Press.

CHAPTER 13

MICRODISCECTOMY

W. Bradford DeLong

Techniques of magnification and auxiliary fiberoptic lighting increase the ease and accuracy of surgical dissection and allow the surgeon to limit the amount of soft tissue trauma and bone removal.[11]

The terms *microdiscectomy*, *microsurgical discectomy*, and *microlumbar discectomy* have been popularized in the orthopedic and neurosurgical literature, as well as in the media, but there are two schools of thought regarding the meaning of these terms. Both schools agree that use of the operating microscope can limit the size of the incision and the amount of soft tissue dissection required to excise the herniated disc material.

There is disagreement concerning the amount of bone removal required and the degree to which degenerated disc material should be removed from the intervertebral space. One school believes that very little bone should be removed and that the disc space should not be curetted.[4,9] The other school is represented by Hudgins, who noted that patients in whom he used this technique had a higher incidence of postoperative numbness than those in whom he had used the standard partial hemilaminectomy technique.[5] He modified the more limited technique to include lateral bone removal and interspace curettage. He commented on a reoperation rate of 8% and 9% in two series that used the more limited bone excision and little interspace dissection,[4,9] and he compared these rates to a 5% reoperation rate in his own series (using the modified microsurgical procedure)[5] and to a 4% rate in the series of Wilson and Harbaugh, who removed degenerated disc material from the interspace, although they did not curette the interspace.[10] The success rates of the major microsurgical discectomy series reported range upward of 88%.[4-6,9,10]

I am aligned with Hudgins's thinking. I use the term *microsurgical discectomy* to mean the use of microsurgical techniques to create as small an incision as practical through which a "standard" discectomy is performed. Enough of the lamina is excised to gain access to the spinal canal overlying the disc space. Enough of the medial inferior and superior articular processes are excised to allow access to the disc lateral to the dural sheath of the involved nerve root. If the preoperative CT scan demonstrates the existence of lateral spinal stenosis, then further lateral resection is necessary. After the herniated portion of the disc is excised, degenerated disc material from the ipsilateral posterolateral quadrant of the disc is excised to minimize the chance of recurrent disc herniation.

PREOPERATIVE EVALUATION AND PREPARATION

Potential candidates for microsurgical discectomy will have sciatica. They may or may not have back pain as well. Very few, if any, individuals with back pain alone will experience a satisfactory result with a unilateral microsurgical discectomy.

Before our clinic considers an individual a surgical candidate, we try to relieve his or her symptoms with Robin McKenzie's protocol of therapeutic exercises.[7] This program demands active patient participation and develops an exercise regimen based on the behavior of the individual's symptoms in response to repetitive movements in a particular direction (flexion, extension, or side gliding). The individual is educated in body mechanics and postural awareness. Traction is used as necessary in the form of outpatient autotraction,[8] outpatient inversion gravity traction,[2] or inpatient gravity lumbar reduction.[3] Epidural injections, selective nerve root blocks, and nonsteroidal antiinflammatory agents are used as necessary to facilitate the therapeutic exercises and traction. In only a rare instance is narcotic medication prescribed, and then only for a very short time. Potential psychosocial problems are evaluated and a program of stress management utilized as indicated.

We rely on high-resolution CT scanning to define the injury or disease present. The CT scan should include sagittal and curved coronal reformatted images, in addition to the standard axial images. The axial images will depict the posterior disc margins, the lateral recesses, the configuration of the central canal, and the configuration of the zygapophyseal joints. The sagittal images present the nerve root foramina, the end-plate margins, and another dimension of the posterior disc margins. The curved coronal images are ideal for defining the exact position of migrated free disc fragments, and the surgeon who uses them regularly will soon find them to be an indispensable adjunct to planning the surgical approach.

Myelography is not required if the injury or disease demonstrated on a high-quality CT scan correlates with the clinical picture. If the CT scan demonstrates a unilateral herniated disc, the patient is a candidate for a microsurgical discectomy. If the CT scan demonstrates the presence of unilateral spinal stenosis, a disc fragment that has migrated away from the interspace, or an uncinate spur, a unilateral microsurgical approach can still be used, but the surgeon will have to deal with these conditions by extending the bone removal.

If the CT scan demonstrates central and/or contralateral spinal stenosis, central and/or contralateral disc herniation, spondylolisthesis and/or bilateral spondylolysis, or clinically significant multilevel disease, then a simple unilateral microsurgical discectomy will not suffice.

If a far lateral disc herniation is demonstrated on the CT scan, its removal is better accomplished by microsurgical techniques using a paramedian muscle-splitting approach or a more lateral muscle-elevating approach rather than the midline exposure described here.

It is unusual for an individual undergoing primary disc surgery to require a blood transfusion. However, most of our patients wish to reduce the chance they might receive a transfusion from an unknown donor to the lowest level. Therefore most of them provide two units of packed red cells for their surgery through autodonation or through the use of designated donors.

I routinely use prophylactic preoperative antibiotics and/or intraoperative antibiotics, usually one of the cephalosporin preparations.

OPERATIVE POSITIONING, INSTRUMENTATION, AND MEDICATIONS

The patient kneels on the Andrews frame, which provides optimal abdominal decompression (Fig. 13-1).

The Zeiss operating microscope is the standard of intraoperative magnification. For disc surgery, a 300, 350, or 400 mm objective can be used. The 300 mm lens attenuates the illumination less and provides a brighter field, but the 400 mm objective provides greater clearance for the manipulation of the instruments. I prefer the 300 mm lens, but some surgeons use the 350 mm option as a reasonable compromise. Either 12.5X or 16X high-eyepoint oculars can be used. An angled binocular should be used for lumbar spinal surgery. The binocular tube comes in focal lengths of 160 mm and 125 mm. The 160 mm option provides higher magnification, but it is longer and puts the surgeon farther from the surgical field. I prefer the shorter 125 mm binocular.

The OPMi I model, which I prefer, has manual magnification settings of 6X, 10X, and 16X. The actual magnification achieved is somewhat less than the settings indicate and depends on the selected combination of oculars (12.5X or 16X), objective (300 mm, 350 mm, or 400 mm), and binocular tube length (125 mm or 160 mm).[11] To achieve the full magnification indicated on the settings of the Zeiss OPMi I microscope, one would have to use 20X oculars, a 200 mm objective, and a 160 mm binocular tube length. The use of 16X oculars, a 300 mm objective, and a 160 mm binocular gives actual magnifications of one half the indicated settings—3X at a setting of 6X, 5X at a setting of 10X, and 8X at a setting of 16X.

I use the OPMi I model with 16X high-eyepoint oculars, an angled 125 mm binocular, and the 300 mm objective. This combination gives actual magnification of 2.5X at a setting of 6X, 4X at a setting of 10X, 6X at a setting of 16X, 10X at a setting of 25X, and 16X at a

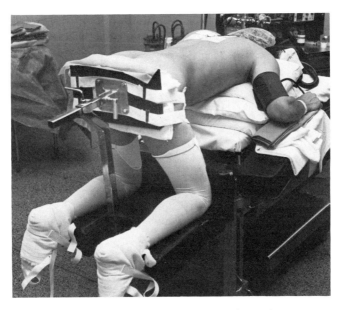

Fig. 13-1 Patient positioned on Andrews frame.

setting of 40X. At a setting of 16X (6X actual magnification), the field of vision is 33 mm wide.[11]

The OPMi II model has a power zoom magnification changer, which gives a range of actual magnification similar to the manual settings on the OPMi I.

The use of the Contraves electromagnetically controlled microscope stand makes the procedure much easier, but many community hospitals find the cost of this stand prohibitive.

The surgery will become unduly difficult if the microscope and the stand are not configured properly. If the Contraves stand is not available, a tall stationary stand should be used. The stand should be fitted with extra extension arms, and the microscope should be suspended from the extension arm by a fitting that allows the microscope to rotate in an oblique plane.

The operating microscope allows the use of a small incision, which limits soft tissue trauma and seems to decrease postoperative discomfort. Magnifying operating telescopes or loupes can be used, but the incision required is then somewhat larger, since these devices do not "compress" the interpupillary distance to the degree that the operating microscope does. Whichever method of intraoperative magnification is chosen, it is important to make the fascial incision off the midline to preserve the supraspinous and interspinous ligaments.[1]

The operating microscope has the additional advantage of allowing direct televised monitoring and/or videotaping of the procedure, although further miniaturization of television cameras will soon provide a monitoring device that can be attached to a surgeon's headband in combination with fiberoptic illumination.

Auxillary fiberoptic lighting increases the accuracy of surgical dissection. If the operating microscope is used, then internal fiberoptic lighting can provide brilliant coaxial illumination. If magnifying operating telescopes or loupes are used, then a fiberoptic headlight can be used to illuminate the surgical field in near-coaxial fashion. However, if loupes and a headlight are used instead of the operating microscope, the surgeon's comfort is decreased because of the weight of the devices and because of the head and neck position required to maintain focus and illumination.

It is important to use self-retaining retractors. To retract the paravertebral muscles, we use a narrow custom-made Taylor-type blade that attaches to the Scoville-Haverfield retractor. Countertraction is provided by a small double hook attached to the other side of the Scoville-Haverfield retractor. Alternatives are a regular Taylor retractor that has been cut to a narrow width (¾ inch) or the Williams microdiscectomy retractor. The nerve root is held medially by a Cloward self-retaining nerve root retractor, which is clamped to the Scoville-Haverfield retractor (Figs. 13-2 and 13-3).

Bipolar coagulation is essential to minimize the spread of the coagulating current to sensitive neural tissue. Standard discectomy instruments are used for the bone resection, nerve root mobilization, and disc excision.

Intraoperative Medications

Before making the incision, the skin is infiltrated with 0.25% Marcaine (bupivacaine hydrochloride) with 1/200,000 epinephrine.

The free fat graft is placed in 5 ml of Depo-Medrol (methylprednisolone acetate suspension, 40 mg/ml).

In the spinal canal, hemostasis is secured by the temporary application of Gelfoam (absorbable gelatin sponge, USP) soaked in thrombin, USP (1000 units/ml).

Before closure, 0.25% plain Marcaine without preservatives is instilled into the disc space and the exposed epidural space.

Microdiscectomy 127

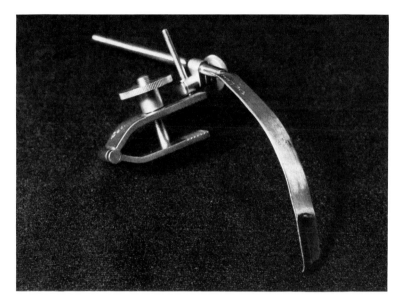

Fig. 13-2 Cloward self-retaining nerve root retractor.

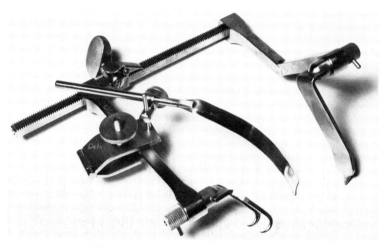

Fig. 13-3 Cloward nerve root retractor clamped to Haverfield-Scoville retractor. Double hook is placed in supraspinous ligament, and modified Taylor blade retracts paravertebral muscles.

INTRAOPERATIVE X-RAY FILMS

When utilizing a small incision for lumbosacral disc surgery, it is essential to use localizing x-ray films to confirm the level of the interspace being approached (Fig. 13-4). Attention to a few points will minimize the risk of being misled by the x-ray films.

The first localizing lateral x-ray film is taken before making the skin incision. It can be obtained either before or after the skin is prepared. The location of the involved interspace is estimated, and the skin over this point is prepared if full preparation has not yet been done. A 18- or 19-gauge spinal needle is used as a marker, with the stylet in place. A smaller needle may be difficult to visualize on the portable x-rays. The needle is inserted beside the spinous process at the involved level and advanced until it contacts the lamina.

The intervertebral space at L5-S1 lies directly anterior to the superior portion of the interlaminar space, but at L4-5 it lies anterior and superior to the inferior margin of the L4 lamina. At L3-4 the intervertebral space lies approximately anterior to the junction of lower and middle third of the lamina. It is well to keep these relationships in mind when placing the marking needle, since the surgical incision should be centered over the involved disc space rather than over the interlaminar space.

The marking needle is inserted perpendicular to the floor so that its relationship to the involved disc space can be easily determined on the portable x-ray film (Fig. 13-5). If the needle is angled superiorly or inferiorly, it is easy to become disoriented once the skin incision has been made.

If the needle is properly placed at the involved level, the site of the tip of the needle is marked by using a tuberculin syringe to inject 0.1 ml of indigo carmine through the needle. (Use indigo carmine, not methylene blue. Methylene blue is neurotoxic and has no place in the operating room when there is even the slightest chance it might be accidentally injected into the cerebrospinal fluid.)

The anatomic level of the involved disc space usually can be located by reference to surface anatomy. Preoperative x-ray films or CT scans will demonstrate the

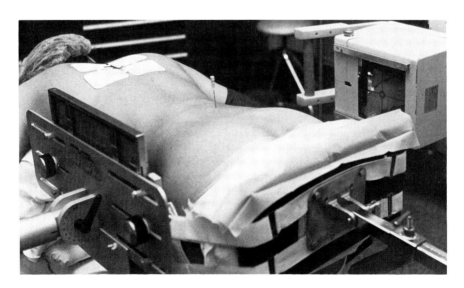

Fig. 13-4 Lateral localizing roentgenogram.

relationship of the intercrestal line to the involved disc space. The posterior iliac spine is at the level of the S2 spinous process. If the patient is obese or if a transitional vertebra is present, then a marking needle can be inserted at each of two levels and the proper one chosen for the indigo carmine injection.

After the lamina over the involved interspace has been marked with the indigo carmine, the needle is removed. Residual dye within the needle will leave a small blue dot at the site of the needle puncture to distinguish it from other skin markings.

If there is any doubt whatsoever about the level being approached after the self-retaining paravertebral muscle retractor has been placed, then a second localizing lateral x-ray film is taken. A clamp or other metallic marker is placed on the interlaminar soft tissue to confirm the correct level.

If the L5-S1 interspace cannot be defined on the films, the x-ray procedure must be repeated with better alignment and penetration.

If the patient has a transitional vertebra or if the intrasacral interspaces are well developed, it is easy to be misled by the localizing portable x-rays. In these cases the intraoperative x-rays must be closely correlated with the preoperative x-rays and CT scans.

OPERATIVE TECHNIQUE
Preparation

Under general anesthesia, the patient is positioned on the Andrews frame. The localizing x-ray film is taken. Preparation and draping are done. The site of the incision is marked with a sterile marking pen, 1 to 1½ inches long and centered over the involved intervertebral space. The surgeon stands at the side of the operating table opposite the involved nerve root to facilitate the lateral bone removal that is frequently necessary.

Exposure

Marcaine (0.25%) with epinephrine is injected before making the incision. Subcutaneous fat is removed to facilitate visualization into the depths of the operative field. It is placed in Depo-Medrol and used as a free fat graft in the epidural space at the conclusion of the operation.

The lumbodorsal fascia is incised 1 cm

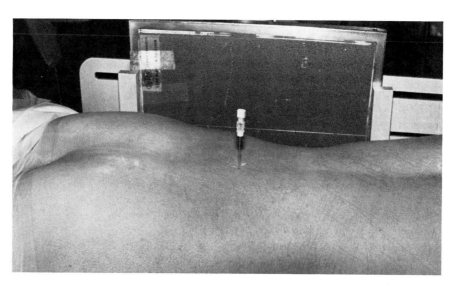

Fig. 13-5 To facilitate visualization on portable roentgenogram, an 18-gauge or 19-gauge spinal needle with stylet inserted is used as marking needle. It is inserted perpendicular to floor to facilitate anatomic orientation on roentgenogram.

lateral to the midline to preserve the supraspinous and interspinous ligaments.[1] The paravertebral muscles are mobilized subperiosteally and retracted laterally. Soft tissues are swept off the laminae, the ligamentum flavum, and the facet capsule. This portion of the dissection is done by the feel of the instruments. The interlaminar interval is carefully palpated; care is taken not to penetrate it accidentally. The tooth of the Taylor blade is engaged by the lateral edge of the pars interarticularis or by the lateral edge of the facet.

Bone Removal

The operating microscope is brought in. If a second localizing x-ray film is required, it is obtained at this time.

Remaining soft tissue is excised from the ligamentum flavum and from the facet capsule. The lateral aspect of the pars interarticularis is located. Enough of the pars is preserved to avoid sacrificing the inferior articularis process. The inferior rim of the lamina above is excised with an angled Kerrison rongeur or a straight chisel. The medial edge of the inferior articular process is removed with a straight chisel. The medial edge of the superior articular process is scored with a straight chisel to create a stress riser, and then removed with a 2 or 3 mm angled Kerrison rongeur.

The ligamentum flavum is picked up with vascular forceps and excised with a no. 15 blade or a no. 67 Beaver blade. The angled Kerrison rongeur is used to remove the superior rim of the lamina below and to resect remaining fragments of the ligamentum flavum.

If a free (sequestered) disc fragment has migrated away from the interspace, its location should be evident on the sagittal and coronal reformatted images of the preoperative CT scan. The bone resection may have to be extended superiorly or inferiorly to reach it.

Epidural fat is preserved, and the epidural veins are visualized and protected. They are not coagulated unnecessarily. Bleeding from them can usually be arrested by the temporary application of Gelfoam soaked in thrombin. If they must be coagulated, bipolar coagulation is used.

The dural sheath of the nerve root is visualized. The bone removal is extended laterally far enough to expose the posterior annulus well beyond the lateral margin of the dura.

If the preoperative CT scan or intraoperative exploration demonstrates the presence of a narrow neural foramen, the anterior aspect of the superior articular process of the vertebra below is removed with an angled Kerrison and/or curved Link rongeur. If an uncinate spur arising from the posterior aspect of the vertebral body is compromising the foramen, then it must be removed.

Exposed cancellous bone is coated with bone wax to discourage future spur formation and to decrease irritation of the adjacent nerve root.

Disc Excision

If all the bone removal can be accomplished before the herniated disc is excised, there is less likelihood of compressing the nerve root during medial mobilization. However, if a large disc herniation compromises the bone removal, it should be excised when encountered and the bone work finished later on.

If a sequestered disc fragment or a portion of an extruded disc is evident in the epidural space, it is removed before mobilization of the nerve root. The nerve root then is gently mobilized medially and held in place with the Cloward self-retaining nerve root retractor. If the herniated portion of the disc is contained by thinned out annulus and/or the posterior longitudinal ligament, these structures are perforated with a small dissector, such as a Penfield no. 4. A small stab incision (with a pointed no. 67 Beaver blade) may be required to facilitate entry into the annulus, but a large incision or wide resection of the posterior annulus is avoided. Often, herniated disc material will be extruded through the opening at that point and can be removed by grasping it with the disc rongeur. The opening then is gradually dilated until a disc rongeur can be inserted into the interspace itself.

Removal of degenerated material from within the disc space is generally confined to the ipsilateral posterior disc quadrant, although obvious loose and/or degenerated material is removed even if it lies in the anterior quadrant or across the midline. Cup curettes, ring curettes, Epstein curettes, and disc rongeurs are used, but no intentional attempt is made to remove the cartilaginous end-plates. Firm annular material is not removed unless it projects posteriorly into the spinal canal.

If the disc has herniated into the axilla of the involved nerve root, it may have to be initially approached medial to the nerve root. No attempt is made to retract the nerve laterally in these cases. Once the root has been decompressed by the removal of the herniated material, it can then be mobilized medially so the interspace itself can be approached lateral to the root.

After the degenerated disc material has been removed, the epidural space is very thoroughly searched for any additional disc material that may have migrated away from the interspace. Care is taken that additional disc material is not hidden between the posterior cortex of the vertebral body and the posterior longitudinal ligament superior or inferior to the interspace.

Closure

Before closure, 0.25% plain Marcaine without preservatives is instilled into the interspace and into the exposed epidural space. The free fat graft is gently laid over the exposed dura and nerve root. Marcaine (0.25%) is injected into the ipsilateral paravertebral muscles. There is no need to suture the muscles. The fascia, subcutaneous tissue, and skin are closed according to the surgeon's preference. I use interrupted synthetic absorbable sutures to close the fascia and subcutaneous tissue and stainless steel staples or sterile adhesive strips for the skin closure.

POSTOPERATIVE MANAGEMENT

Usually little or no narcotic medication is required. The individual begins ambulation the day of surgery or the next day. The day after surgery, gentle midrange therapeutic exercises are started in both flexion and extension. The individual leaves the hospital when he or she is ambulating comfortably and independently, usually on the third postoperative day.

The therapeutic exercise program is developed further after discharge. Walking and swimming are encouraged. The program of spinal education is continued. I encourage the individual to become involved in a formal conditioning program utilizing low-impact aerobic exercises and supervised weight training with a goal of making spinal exercise and general fitness lifelong habits.

SUMMARY

An individual is not considered a candidate for surgery until he or she has failed to improve with an aggressive program of nonsurgical therapy, including therapeutic exercises, gravity traction and/or autotraction, and epidural injection of steroids. Exceptions are individuals with progressive neurologic deficits or symptoms of cauda equina compromise.

The preoperative use of high-resolution spinal CT scanning with sagittal and curved coronal reformatted images will make myelography unnecessary in cases where the injury or disease clearly correlates with the clinical findings.

If the CT scan identifies the presence of

lateral spinal stenosis, the surgical plan is modified accordingly.

The use of the operating microscope keeps surgical trauma to a minimum and seems to increase postoperative comfort. The microscope must be properly configured or the surgery will become considerably more difficult than necessary.

Intraoperative localizing x-ray films are essential to identify positively the interspace being approached.

After the herniated portion of the disc has been excised, degenerated disc material is removed from the ipsilateral posterior quadrant of the interspace. The actual discectomy accomplished is similar to a "standard" discectomy performed without the microscope.

Postoperative management includes the use of therapeutic exercises, spinal education, and general conditioning with the use of low-impact aerobic exercise and supervised weight training.

REFERENCES

1. Balagura, S.: Lumbar discectomy through a small incision, Neurosurgery **11**:784, 1982.
2. Bastian, S., et al.: Clinical protocol for inversion gravity traction, Clin. Management **4**:18, 1984.
3. Burton, C.V.: The Sister Kenny Institute gravity lumbar reduction therapy program. In Finneson, B.E., editor: Low back pain, ed. 2, Philadelphia, 1980, J.B. Lippincott Co.
4. Goald, H.J.: Microlumbar discectomy: follow-up of 477 patients, J. Microsurg. **2**:95, 1980.
5. Hudgins, R.W.: The role of microdiscectomy, Orthop. Clin. North Am. **14**:589, 1983.
6. Maroon, J.C., and Abla, A.: Microdiscectomy versus chemonucleolysis, Neurosurgery **16**:644, 1985.
7. McKenzie, R.A.: The lumbar spine: mechanical diagnosis and therapy, Waikanae, New Zealand, 1981, Spinal Publications, Ltd.
8. Natchev, E.: A manual on auto-traction treatment for low back pain, Sweden, 1984, Tryckeribolaget i Sundsvall AB.
9. Williams, R.W.: Microlumbar discectomy: a conservative surgical approach to the virgin herniated lumbar disc, Spine **3**:175, 1978.
10. Wilson, D.H., and Harbaugh, R.: Microsurgical and standard removal of the protruded lumbar disc: a comparative study, Neurosurgery **8**:422, 1981.
11. Yasargil, M.G.: Microsurgery applied to neurosurgery, New York, 1969, Academic Press.

EDITORIAL COMMENTARY

Most of the authors of this text have found microdiscectomy of some value, but few found it of great value. Richard Rothman seldom uses microdiscectomy and has experienced no complications for the procedure. Some surgeons, such as Kirkaldy-Willis, state that they have never done the procedure although there may be a place for it. He also stated that "one cannot help suspecting that microdiscectomy is carried out too early and too frequently."

Hugo Keim has the classical impression, which I happen to share, that it is difficult to "fix a fine watch in an inkwell" or to "operate on a fine watch in a keyhole." He believes that good surgical exposure allows the surgeon to actually see the injury or disease. The slight increase in the length of the incision does not "significantly alter the healing time and ability of the patient to be up and about promptly."

Microdiscectomy to Vert Mooney "offers no specific advantage."

Leon Wiltse summarizes that "the headlight and magnification is at this time the most practical system for most surgeons. One can start with a small incision and enlarge to a classical laminectomy at any moment. I see no indication for slavishly adhering to the rule that no bone is removed and no incision of the ligamentum flavum or annulus fibrosis is done. The classical laminectomy is likely to remain the most widely used operation for decompression and discectomy." The disadvantages as listed by Leon Wiltse for microdiscectomy are that it is easy to "get lost and to miss a sequestrated fragment or even an extruded fragment. Damage to neural structures occurs more often in the hands of the less skilled surgeon because the approach is so small. Bony decompression is more difficult, and bony compression is a very common cause of pain. It is difficult to check the lateral canal through this small approach." Dr. Wiltse hastens to add that there is a big difference between microdiscectomy with and without the use of a microscope. The microscope allowing for extensive exposure and the ability to do some bony decompression.

It is our experience in the San Francisco Bay area and with the authors of this book that, in general, it is the neurosurgeons who have tended more toward microdiscectomy.

Since the major causes of excess failure in disc surgery are recurrent herniated disc and spinal stenosis, we tend to do a "little more" than a "little less." A larger exposure allows more disc to be removed, inspection for occult herniations, and decompression of potential areas of developmental spinal stenosis. The price of a longer scar, increased blood loss and slower recovery is minimal when compared to a failed spine surgery with months of extended disability, rehospitalization, and reoperation.

Only one of our authors has reported significant complications with this procedure.

Microdiscectomy among our authors was the least popular surgical procedure aside from posterior lumbar interbody fusion and chemonucleolysis.

Arthur H. White

CHAPTER

14

EXPOSURES FOR LUMBAR DECOMPRESSIONS AND FUSIONS

Charles D. Ray

SKIN MARKING AND SKIN INCISION

Marking the skin and underlying spinous process with an indelible dye is quite valuable to the surgeon. The deep injection into the inferior edge of the spinous process (or its adjacent interspinous ligament) at the level to be decompressed and the simultaneous injection of the overlying skin not only serves to better orient the skin incision and deep dissection but also may eliminate the mistake of operating at the wrong level or having to make an on-table localizing x-ray film during the surgical procedure. This is an intensely blue dye, isosulfan blue for lymphography (Lymphazurin 1%).* The injection of 0.7 ml into the deeper structures and 0.1 to 0.2 ml into the dermis should be performed within 4 to 8 hours before the start of surgery.

The radiologist (or whoever else might perform the injection) must be familiar with the anatomy of the patient's spine, that is, number of movable lumber segments, presence of congenital anomalies (especially partial lumbarizations-sacralizations), and whatever otherwise might be misunderstood between apparent radiologic anatomy and the location of the actual lesion(s). An order from the surgeon directing the radiologist as to level and location of the injection should be written on the patient's chart. For the marking, the patient is placed prone on the fluoroscopic table with the arms in a neutral position. Before removing the needle from its deep location, an x-ray film is made showing the location of the needle relative to the anatomy; this film must accompany the patient to the operating room. One should remember that the skin marking usually will be displaced caudad to the deep spinous process mark as the patient's thighs are flexed and remain in that position on the operating table. If a very broad or multilevel exposure is to be made, no marking usually is needed.

The size (length) of the skin incision is determined largely by the number of spinal segments to be operated on plus some

---

*Hirsch Industries, Inc., Richmond, Va.

additional length dictated by the depth to the target, flexibility of overlying tissues, difficulty of the procedure, and extent of lateral dissection expected. Cosmetic appearance of the final wound is heavily dependent upon the initial incision, method of retraction and technique of dealing with superficial bleeding. For a microdiscectomy, a short incision (about 2 to 3 cm) usually suffices, centered slightly cephalad to the dye marker.

For long incisions I find that one should "prick" the skin overlying the extreme dorsal spinous processes, that is, the upper and lower extent of the exposure, using the tip of the scalpel. A flat ruler or the edge of a long, straight osteotome is laid in correspondence with the two pricked marks; the no. 20 scalpel blade is plunged in and with a single, perpendicular cut, the marks are connected. Some prefer to preinject the dermis with a solution of 1% lidocaine with about 1:200,000 (or 1:400,000) epinephrine; this reduces skin margin bleeders. One may instead coagulate just below the epidermis with an electrosurgical knife (cautery tip), being careful not to burn the epidermis itself. The recent self-heated Shaw hemostatic (heated) scalpel is of value for bloodless opening of the skin, but I have not found it to be a distinct advantage for lumbar surgery.[6]

When one is planning a decompression with fusion and fat grafting, a single midline incision should be able to accommodate both the exposure and harvesting of the grafts; there is no need for a J or "hockey-stick" incision. By making the inferior end of the wound slightly longer (sometimes down to the S3 level), one can easily stretch the skin laterally with a Hibbs, Meyerding, or S-shaped Wiltse retractor or spiked Raylor retractor,* decapitate the posterior iliac spine (along a length of about 5 cm), then reach inside between the cortical tables and obtain a very substantial graft of pure cancellous bone. Cutting the cluneal nerves and detaching the gluteal muscles are avoided. The fat graft is obtained from the retrogluteal fat pad through the same incision. This combined technique is a distinct refinement over several earlier ones.

Just below the surface of the midline skin one can usually obtain an acceptable fat or fat-fascia (paratenon) graft of about 10 to 15 cc volume (adequate for a one level unilateral exposure). Incidentally, the globules of fat, no matter where they are harvested, should be left as intact as possible, since cutting across or rupturing them or letting them dry out usually will result in subsequent atrophy of the fat cells. (See Chapter 44.) In the virgin back a single piece of fat may be harvested by dissecting from beneath one or both sides of the skin margins at once, but such a graft should never be extensive for fear of creating a large void that subsequently will not close well. In the reoperated patient, there is no midline fat. Such cases usually have less bleeding in the wound margins. If any patient has recently taken moderate amounts of aspirin or any one of several nonsteroidal antiinflammatory drugs, the skin oozing may be difficult to stop at first; the application of stable retraction usually stops this, however. On reaching the dorsal fascia, one may gently sweep all the tissue away from the midline with a large blunt instrument (Cobb, Hoehn) so that the unique criss-crossing fibers of this posterior fascia may be seen. This represents the exact midline. Fascial perforating bleeders are coagulated.

I prefer to cut through the dorsal interspinous fascia and its underlying ligaments with an electrosurgical (ES) knife but not straight down along the center of the spines. Instead, closely spaced, parallel cuts are made leaving a narrow, central posterior band of interspinous ligament, the cuts being widened as one circles the

---

*CeDaR Surgical, Inc., Minnetouka, Minn.

lateral edges of the tips of the spinous processes. This remaining tough central strip permits a much tighter and more anatomic subsequent closure of the wound by reuniting the lateral fascia with this strip.

MUSCLE STRIPPING

A broad-bladed dissector (Cobb, Hoehn, or Cushing) is used to strip the muscle and fascia laterally away from the spinous processes and the laminas. In the far lateral region near the facet capsule the blade tip is pried posteriorly, hinged against the spinous process as one pushes ventrally with the handle. Tough fascial bands are cut with the ES knife. One side at a time is stripped away then packed with gauze, and then the second side is stripped. This "subperiosteal muscle stripping" technique often breaks the small arterial branches that pass dorsally through the pars interarticularis; they originate from the segmental arteries. They can be coagulated (the bipolar technique is preferred) or simply packed for a few minutes. The second side is also packed while the retractor is made ready.

Wound reopening and dissection in the previously operated cases is a different matter entirely. There is usually a dense layer of collagenous scar tissue that attaches to the spinous process, lamina, facet capsule and (if a fat graft is not present) posterior dural surface. However, if the patient has a viable, significant fat graft present, the dissection will proceed much easier and safer (avoiding dural tears). One should carefully study the CT scan to determine the level of the posterior dura relative to the posterior limit of the lamina and the facet joint. Each level to be reopened must be studied individually so that one is not suddenly surprised with "spring water and sphaghetti" emerging from the dissection. I have become greatly impressed with the speed and precision of scar tissue dissection and removal using a hot-wire cutter; this technique is discussed in detail in Chapter 21.

RETRACTION

Once the field has been opened and the invariate bleeders coagulated, especially those emerging from the spinous processes at the extremes of the wound length and the segmental branches, the retractor is placed. Selecting the retractor is a minor but important art; length and depth of the wound are the principal factors. Whether the dissection is unilateral or bilateral is important, as are relaxation of the muscles, time (length) of the procedure, and location (anatomic level) of the wound. Gentle bilateral exposure is obtained using a Scoville, Beckman, Tower, Gelpi, or cerebellar retractor, among others. Forceful, bilateral, far lateral retraction is best obtained, in my experience, with a large self-retaining MacElroy retractor. One should have on hand three sets of blades: long, medium, and short (although the latter is seldom used). The blade notch accommodates the iliac crest (more or less). Large, self-retaining retractors, or those exerting great force against the muscle, are likely to produce considerable postoperative muscle pain and possibly a compartmental syndrome in some cases. For unilateral exposures, Taylor retractors are popular but one must be careful with the placement of the tooth at the tip; further, it can be unstable and slip.[5]

Whether for a unilateral exposure or bilateral exposure at L5 to S1 and higher, I prefer to use a special retractor having two blunt teeth at the tip. I have developed a set of maleable retractors based on the same prying action as the Taylor; they are described in the following discussion.

FORCE-FULCRUM RETRACTORS

Only a few retractors use a prying method to achieve exposure. All retractors exert their force or power against the patient's muscle and skin; however, prying or force-fulcrum ones are unique in that the fulcrum is at the tip, deep within the wound, lodged against bone. One therefore does not "pull" on the instrument, in the sense of a free, hand-held retractor. The weight or counterforce is applied by attaching a gauze strip or band to the free end of the retractor; this gauze strip then is tied to a weight hanging off the edge of the operating table or may be tied elsewhere on the table itself. In this configuration the retractor acts as a second-class lever, that is, fulcrum at one end, weight at the opposite end, and power applied at the center. (A first-class lever is a center-fulcrum system, like a child's see-saw or laboratory balance; and a third-class, end-fulcrum system is like a claw nail-pulling hammer or the elbow-biceps-forearm system.) The most commonly used force-fulcrum or prying-type spinal retractor is the Taylor.[7] Another is the Bennett.

A variety of modifications have been made of the Taylor and other similar retractors and used over the years. The basic Taylor has a single, somewhat blunted tip or "tooth," which is held deeply in the wound by force with the fulcrum tip pressed against a prominence of bone. In spinal surgery this prominence is frequently the lateral margin of the facet joint or its junction with the pedicle. A two-toothed variation on the Bennett has been described.[2] Bell and Lavyne have published a similar modification of the tip of a standard Taylor retractor for use in spinal surgery.[1]

The Taylor is not malleable; nor are any of the other spinal surgery retractors. By accepted definition and present manufacturing specifications, force-fulcrum devices must be rigid, otherwise the prying action will be presumed lost. However, this is only relatively true. For example, one would not design or manufacture a malleable or flexible crowbar for prying purposes because the prying action apparently would be frustrated by inadvertent bending of the bar (shaft of the tool). Almost invariably, therefore, where malleability is an important characteristic for a retractor, it is reserved for those used for soft tissues, for example, the brain and the abdominal viscera.

Of course, malleability is a relative factor. It is a property of a material, usually a metal. As applied to surgical instruments, the term indicates that the device can be bent rather easily by hand, that is, special tools are not required. Therefore a truly malleable retractor is one that can be pre-bent to reach a particular depth, placed in the wound, removed, rebent and thus easily readjusted as the surgeon requires, without the need for any instruments other than gloved hands. Of course, the retractor should not be so soft that when weighted and pulled it might spontaneously bend and pull out of the wound. The principle value of malleability with these new retractors is to provide for variation in length and contour between the fulcrum (the tip caught deeply inside, against an edge of bone) and the power point (mass of muscle, edges of fascia, and skin). In contrast, the usual dual-bladed, self-retaining retractor systems provide for variable depths to the surgical target from the skin surface by using sets of removable blades having various lengths and widths.

The combination of malleability and force-fulcrum action, the principal elements of the present group of retractors reported here, has not formerly been made available in retractors.

STABILITY AT THE TIP

At the tip of the force-fulcrum retractor, where it is placed into the depths of the wound, some structural elements for stable anchoring must be provided; the shapes or characteristics of the tip must conform to—and provide stability by firm contact with—a bone structure (joint, shaft, process) or other convenient bony prominence. The single blunt tip of

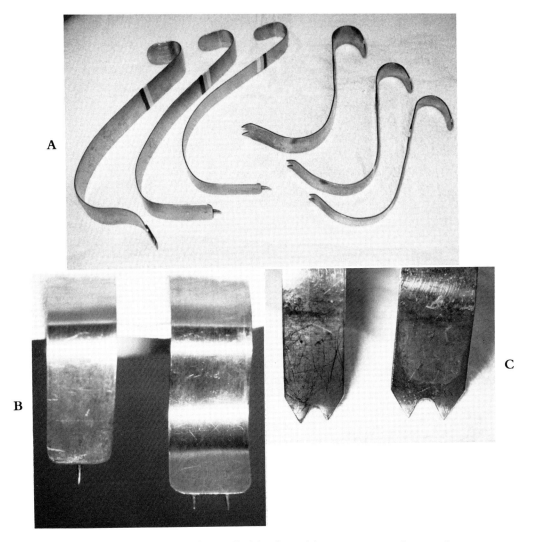

Fig. 14-1 A, Raylor (Taylor-like) malleable, force-fulcrum retractors for spinal surgery. Three on left have spikes (claws) on tips. Widest spiked Raylor (far left) has two spikes for use in larger exposures; this one also has an **S**-shaped reversal at spiked end for placement out along ilium while obtaining bone grafts. Three on right have two blunt teeth to place lateral to facet. Overall length of instruments when flattened out is about 30 cm. Bend in the handle (opposite end from the spike or teeth) permits tying a gauze strip; it is passed over side of operating table and weighted. **B,** Close-up of spiked (claw) type Raylors. Short but sharp spike is hooked into sacral bone, sacroiliac joint, or some bony prominence; gauze and weight are attached as above. Spike permits stable anchor for blade. This form is best used where no facet joint is available, for example, posterior to fusion mass or at L5 to S1 level and below. **C,** Two-toothed type, where the notch between teeth is hooked lateral to facet joint. This form of retractor is particularly useful at L4 to L5 level and above.

the standard Taylor is often quite unstable when placed lateral to a facet joint or a pedicle.[1] Therefore one of the versions of the present set of malleable retractors is provided with two tips (or teeth) that can be hooked laterally around the pedicle or other prominent structure (Figs. 14-1 and 14-2). I routinely use a narrow (2 cm wide) Raylor of this type during microsurgical discectomies performed with the patient under either general or local anesthesia; it has been used in many cases and has proved to be the easiest, most flexible and most quickly positioned retractor for this purpose.

As shown in Fig. 14-2, the notch between the two teeth of the tip of the retractor is placed just lateral to the facet joint; it provides a very stable but easily movable access to the surgical target. Where larger decompressions are to be performed, wider Raylor retractors (up to 6 cm) of the same type are employed. The counterweight used should not exceed 2 kg, regardless of the width of the retractor, otherwise the force against the facet joint might be sufficient to break the joint or pedicle, especially in patients with osteoporosis. (No such fracture has occurred to date in the use of these retractors by me or my associates.) If a wider exposure is required, more Raylors may be placed or a wide self-retaining unit may be needed.

Below the fifth lumbar level, further caudad along the sacrum, neither a one- nor a two-toothed retractor of the above type may be practical or stable, because

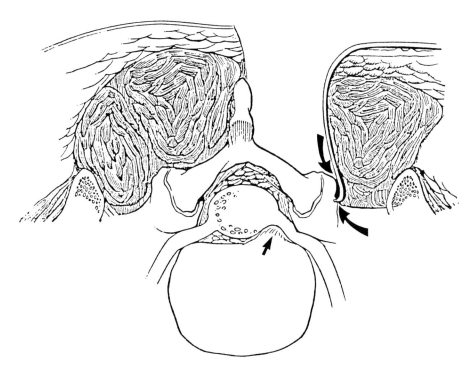

Fig. 14-2 Diagram of posterior aspect of lumbar spine with cross-section through L5-S1 disc space. Two-toothed Raylor retractor has been placed lateral to facet joint *(curved arrows)* and tied laterally to 1 or 2 kg weighted gauze band.[6] For simple discectomy, retractor is only 2 cm wide, therefore an incision of not much over 2.5 cm is required. One side alone may be opened, as shown here, or each side may be opened in turn. In case a higher level must be explored as well, short incision often can be "stretched" over nearly two segments (by moving the skin about and extending the fascial incision and subperiosteal stripping up or down as needed for deep exposure). Lateral herniated disc is shown on right, elevating and compressing the exiting L5 nerve *(small arrow)*.

an appropriate ridge or prominence of bone usually cannot be found against which to lodge the tips. For such applications, a spiked or claw-tipped Raylor is used. This type has one or more very sharp, slightly curved, hard stainless steel spikes or claws at the tip, the spikes are 9 mm long. One selects the retractor width and number of spikes largely depending on the requirements of the bony structures (greater or smaller distance between the posterior iliac spines), the depth of the surgical target, and the length of the incision. The spiked tip is gently pressed or driven by hand into bone, the sacrum or sacroiliac joint. The spikes then provide a remarkably stable fulcrum tip and make the far lateral retraction quite simple in most cases. The force needed to pull the muscles away from the center of the wound is quite low; 1 kg tied to the gauze strip usually suffices. Spiked retractors are also quite practical for exposure in a partial take-down of a fusion. For harvesting iliac bone for a fusion, a double-spiked retractor with a reverse S curve near the tip end can be placed far laterally, over the iliac crest; this instrument is shown on the far left in Fig. 14-1, *A*.

In typical bilateral procedures toothed or spiked retractors may be used for exposing one side at a time or both sides simultaneously. One must be careful that a spike is not placed so that it may slip into a sacral foramen or beneath a pars interarticularis. Having a set of the retractors in three widths, both double-toothed and single-spiked plus a very wide double spiked type (plus another wide, S-shaped unit), a total of eight, provides the spine surgeon with a family of instruments for most spinal applications. The major exceptions are those cases requiring far lateral procedures, that is, exposure to or beyond the margins of the facet joints.

In another application the paralateral approach (far-lateral access via the plane between the spinal erector group and the quadratus lumborum) successfully utilizes a two-toothed malleable retractor.[3,4] (See Chapter 18.) In this application the notched tip is placed dorsal then medial to the facet and the prying force is applied dorsally, the retractor being pulled by a weight from the opposite side of the operating table.

In my experience the force-fulcrum malleable retractors described here have proved to be quite useful in lumbar decompressions; in some cases more useful than any other retractors, including those developed for microdiscectomy.[8] They are very simple and easy to handle. With a small weight attached (usually 1 kg), adequate exposure is achieved via a much shorter wound than is customary with the usual self-retaining retractors. In addition, it is easy to loosen up on the weighted gauze band from time to time to allow momentary restoration of circulation to the retracted tissues or to move the retractor easily to another level, higher or lower.

REFERENCES

1. Bell, W.O., and Lavyne, M.H.: Retractor for lumbar microdiscectomy: technical note, Neurosurgery **14:**69, 1984.
2. Gross, H.P.: The bent Bennett (retractor), Clin. Orthop. **123:**105, 1977.
3. Ray, C.D.: The paralateral approach to lumbar decompressions, proceedings of the annual meeting of the American Association of Neurological Surgery, Washington, D.C., April 1983.
4. Ray, C.D.: Lateral spinal decompression using the paralateral approach. In Watkins, R.G., editor: Principles and techniques of spine surgery, Rockville, Md., 1987, Aspen Press.
5. Simpson, C.W.: (Comments) from: Bell, W.O., and Lavyne, M.H.: Retractor for lumbar microdiscectomy: technical note, Neurosurgery **14:**69, 1984.
6. Steichen, F.M., and Levenson, S.M.: The Shaw hemostatic scalpel: clinical use, advantages and limitations, Problems in Gen. Surg. **2:**11, 1985.
7. Taylor, G.M.: A simple retractor for spinal surgery, J. Bone Joint Surg. **28A:**183, 1946.
8. Williams, R.W.: Microlumbar discectomy: a conservative surgical approach to the virgin herniated lumbar disc, Spine **3:**175, 1978.

CHAPTER 15

PERCUTANEOUS NUCLECTOMY

James Morris Gary Onik

Recent reports of neurologic complications associated with chymopapain injections, as well as potentially serious allergic reactions, have caused considerable concern about its safety. As a result, there has been increased interest in percutaneous nuclectomy as an alternative.

This procedure involves mechanical removal of nuclear material and disc decompression rather than removal by enzymatic action. The method was first used by Dr. Hitjikata[2] of Japan in 1975. A clinical study was started at the University of California, San Francisco, in 1981. Kambin and Gellman[3] and Friedman[1] reported their experience in 1983.

As with laminectomy and chemonucleolysis, patient selection is extremely important. The criteria for using percutaneous nuclectomy should be very strict and must include two of the first four symptoms:
1. Sciatica—leg pain greater than back pain
2. Paresthesias in specific dermatomes
3. Straight leg raising 50% of normal or less
4. Wasting, weakness, sensory changes, or reflex alteration
5. CT scan or myelography that correlates with clinical findings
6. Must have failed to improve after 6 weeks of conservative therapy

Percutaneous nuclectomy is indicated when there is nuclear protrusion with some intact posterior annulus and not when there is extrusion or a free fragment. Presumably by removal of a portion of the nucleus, a void or partial vacuum is created, allowing the protruding nuclear material to recede into the central portion of the disc. This may then result in decreased bulging of the disc and reduced pressure or irritation of the adjacent nerve root (Fig. 15-1).

If there is an extruded or free fragment of disc material present, the procedure would be contraindicated. At times it may be very difficult or impossible to determine by CT or myelography if there is a free fragment. In such instances it has been found that CT after a discogram may aid in the diagnosis (Figs. 15-2 and 15-3). It is also likely that, with improvement of magnetic resonance imaging technology, more accurate differentiation of a herniation or free fragment and a contained disc can be made.

142 *Surgical Procedures*

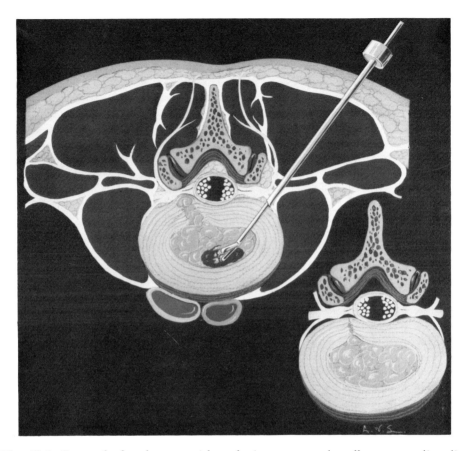

Fig. 15-1 Removal of nuclear material results in a vacuum that allows protruding disc material to recede into the central portion of the disc.

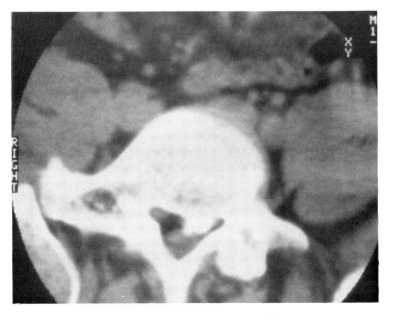

Fig. 15-2 Extruded fragment demonstrated by discogram–CT scan.

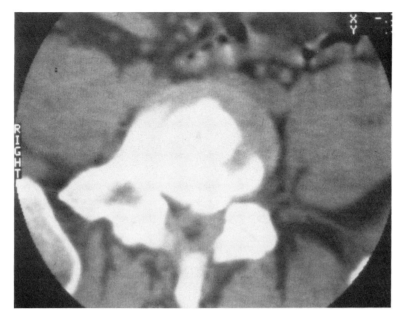

Fig. 15-3 Bulging or contained disc demonstrated by discogram–CT scan.

PROCEDURE

Percutaneous nuclectomy is performed with the patient under local anesthesia and in the lateral decubitus position. Biplane fluoroscopy is used to accurately monitor placement of the instruments. The approach is essentially the same as that used for placement of the needle for chemonucleolysis. The position of the involved disc, generally L4 to L5, is located by lateral fluoroscopy, and an entry point approximately 10 cm lateral to the midline (spinous process) is marked. The patient then is prepped and draped in the usual sterile manner. The skin and deeper tissues then are infiltrated with local anesthetic.

Originally, an 18-gauge trocar was inserted and directed anteriorly and medially to the posterolateral corner of the annulus. This position was confirmed by anteroposterior and lateral fluoroscopy. Progressively larger sleeves then were inserted over the first or guide sleeve until a 3 mm diameter cannula was situated against the annulus. An end-cutting saw then was used to cut a hole through the annulus. Small pituitary rongeurs then were used to remove pieces of nucleus pulposus tissue. This method was tedious and time consuming. For this and other reasons acceptance of the procedure has been slow. Large cannulas (up to 6 mm in diameter) have been used by Kambin[3] and Friedman.[1] Presumably, this involves some increased risk of nerve root damage.

Recently, a new automated nucleus aspiration probe has been used for percutaneous nuclectomy. The small size of the probe (2 mm in diameter) minimizes the risk of nerve root injury, and its automated action allows rapid removal of nuclear material. The technique for insertion of the aspiration probe (Nucleotome) is the same as outlined previously; however, the outer cannula is smaller—2.5 mm in diameter (Fig. 15-4).

The Nucleotome probe was developed by Onik and Surgical Dynamics, Inc., Oakland, California. It has an 8-inch, 2 mm diameter needle with a blunt-

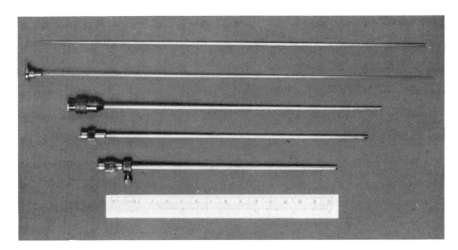

Fig. 15-4 Instruments used for insertion of the nucleotome.

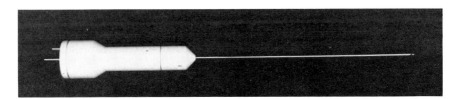

Fig. 15-5 Nucleotome.

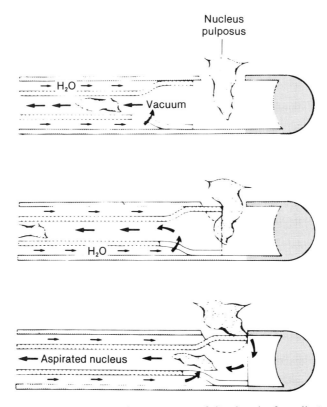

Fig. 15-6 Nucleotome aspiration probe. Diagram of distal end of needle in longitudinal section. Cutting sleeve within needle slices off any material sucked into port. Water for irrigation flows around cutting sleeve and is aspirated with disc material into center of hollow sleeve.[4]

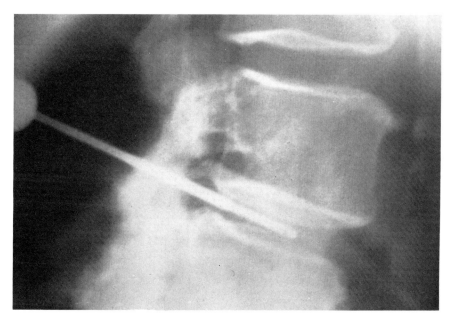

Fig. 15-7 Aspiration probe in place confirmed by fluoroscopy.

rounded closed end and a single-side port near its distal end (Fig. 15-5). The aspiration probe works as follows:

A cannula with its distal end sharpened to a surgical blade is fitted through the center of the outer needle. Suction is applied through the inner cannula, aspirating the nucleus pulposus into the port of the needle. The sharpened end of the inner cannula is then pneumatically driven across the port, thus cutting off the disk material. This material, suspended in saline that has reached the port by flowing distal between the inner cannula and the walls of the outer needle, is then aspirated through the inner cannula to a collection bottle. The cutting instrument operates at up to 180 cycles/min, enabling rapid aspiration of large amounts of material [Fig. 15-6].

When its position within the disk space has been confirmed, the probe is activated and gently moved back and forth within the disk space while suction is taking place [Fig. 15-7]. The aspiration line is monitored, and when no further material can be aspirated, the probe is rotated to change the orientation of its port before continuing. During the aspiration process, firm pressure is maintained on the cannula to ensure that it remains within disk space. When the flow of nuclear material decreases in the aspiration line, the probe is removed and a 50-ml syringe is connected to the cannula; suction is applied. The probe may then be placed into the disk space again and more material aspirated.[4]

DISCUSSION

Percutaneous nuclectomy appears to be a safe, well-tolerated alternative to laminectomy with discectomy or chemonucleolysis in carefully selected cases. The procedure is applicable to those patients having predominantly sciatica resulting from a bulging, contained disc and is not applicable to those cases where a free fragment is present.

The procedure is safer and has fewer potential postoperative complications than either laminectomy or chemonucleolysis. There is no epidural scarring, allergic reactions, or serious neurologic complications.

The potential problem of nerve root injury is minimized by use of local anesthesia, relatively small instrumentation, and careful monitoring with fluoroscopy. Anterior annular penetration is avoided by close monitoring and by the blunt rounded tip of the probe, which will not penetrate an intact annulus (cadaver studies).

At present the results of percutaneous nuclectomy in appropriate patients are

146 Surgical Procedures

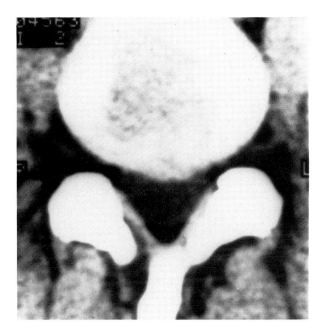

Fig. 15-8 CT of bulging disc preoperatively.

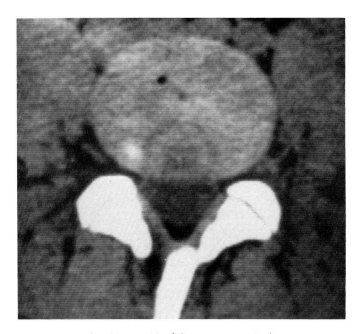

Fig. 15-9 CT of disc postoperatively.

comparable to those obtained with chemonucleolysis. There have been no prospective randomized double-blind studies. However, at this point, it does not seem reasonable to insert a cannula and do nothing.

The procedure is generally applicable for the L3-L4 and L4-L5 discs. With present instrumentation it is frequently difficult to adequately enter the L5-S1 disc, especially if it is deep set below the iliac crests. The aspiration probe, however, can be bent to a 90-degree angle while still operating effectively. Currently, curved cannulas have been developed that make the L5-S1 disc more accessible.

REFERENCES

1. Friedman, W.: Percutaneous discectomy: an alternative to chemonucleolysis, Neurosurgery **13**:542, 1983.
2. Hijikata, S.: Journal of Toden Hospital, **5**:5, December 1975.
3. Kambin, P., and Gellman, H.: Percutaneous lateral discectomy of the lumbar spine, Clin. Orthop. **174**:127, 1983.
4. Onik, G., et al.: Percutaneous lumbar diskectomy using a new aspiration probe, Am. J. Radiol. **144**:1137, June 1985.

EDITORIAL COMMENTARY

Although Robert E. Jacobson developed this method and has very likely performed hundreds of cases, he apparently has not yet published his observations and results. It appears that Hijikata was the first to publish a report on the method in 1975. A small number of other authors have described variations on this concept. At the L4-L5 space the procedure should prove reliable and relatively safe, but whenever the intercristal (between the iliac crests) line falls above the disc level to be operated on (it is usually one half to one full segment higher in males), the percutaneous route will be technically far more difficult. Therefore at L5-S1 the technique may prove to be impractical if not impossible to perform without high risk to intervening structures, for example, the L5 nerve and its confluence with the descending L4 nerve, various vessels, and even the bowel lying in the path to the disc. The reader should not overlook the potential use of chemonucleolysis as an alternative to this technique. Furthermore, for the far laterally herniated disc the surgeon may employ a paralateral approach. (See Chapter 18.)

As of February 1987 several authors in this book have had positive experience with this procedure. Leon Wiltse has had good success; he still uses chemonucleolysis, which he believes is more successful but should be used in smaller doses (0.5 to 1 ml).

Vert Mooney and his associates in Dallas and physicians at the St. Mary's Spine Center in San Francisco have replaced chemonucleolysis with percutaneous neclectomy. We find the procedure safe, easy, and certainly as successful as chemonucleolysis in well-selected cases.

Charles D. Ray
Arthur H. White

CHAPTER

16

LAMINECTOMY VS. LAMINOTOMY

Charles D. Ray

The lumbar laminotomy, which is often called a laminectomy, is the most commonly used surgical procedure for herniated disc disease. It is estimated that between 200,000 and 500,000 of these procedures are performed each year in the United States.[4,5] For relatively simple mechanical reasons the majority of the herniations occur at the L4-L5 level, and at the L5-S1 level slightly less frequently. Only about 2% of the herniations will be found at the L3-L4 or L2-L3 levels and then often because degenerative changes have already occurred with some degree of autostabilization in the space below them.

In about 95% of herniated nucleus pulposus (HNP) cases the rationale for surgery is based on moderate to severely incapacitating pain principally radiating into one leg, not infrequently producing severe back pain. With conservative treatment the acute condition may come and go, but in those patients who come to surgery the symptoms and signs persist. If the condition goes untreated, the pain will probably disappear but only after a long period of time, a condition termed *sciatic burnout*. Of course, such patients may be left with a noticeable or even marked weakness, muscular wasting, and lost or abnormal sensation. In most major nations, and to a growing extent in the rest of the world, it is believed that persistence of pain, disability, and ultimate loss of function is not acceptable; therefore the majority of patients who have such symptoms and who do not respond to conservative care are operated on.[5,8] Whether the patient might receive a protracted course of gravity traction, chymopapain or some other unusual procedure such as a percutaneous discectomy is not a matter of consideration here.[2,6] I am assuming that the patient is indeed going to have a surgical procedure, and I will therefore discuss the rationale for the method of exposure and dissection.

It is remarkable that many learned surgeons and non-surgeons, especially those experienced with patients who have HNPs, have rather clear-cut, rigidly formulated opinions about what is right or wrong in the treatment of such patients; they very often prove indifferent or even hostile toward suggestions or findings contrary to their own, closely held beliefs. For example, one such author stresses the value of wide exposure (with removal of very considerable bone) the routine use of, and even the necessity for, myelography and general anesthesia.[5] Similarly, there are rigid advocates of closed drainage, removal of ligamentum flavum or facet joints, interbody fusions, wide exposure of the nerve roots, and large fat grafts, among other favorite techniques.[2,4,8,9,16] In all probability these variations and concepts simply reassert that there are many roads that lead to Oz. It is difficult if not impossible to have controlled studies comparing the relative importance of these and other techniques, since the major variations occur as frequently among patients and their conditions as they do among the orientations and abilities of individual surgeons. There is a great deal of truth in the statement, "you do what is best in your own hands." Remarkably, most reasonable methods work well in someone's hands; I prefer to seek, use, and teach the techniques that work well in almost everyone's hands, however.

Fortunately, there are opportunities for considerable objectivity in lumbar discectomies with associated removal of bone and other structures. I had the personal good fortune to have learned neurosurgery at the hands of two great and practical masters, Raphael Eustace Semmes and Francis Murphey of Memphis. Their practice and teachings were the essence of parsimony and simplicity. As early as 1938 they decried the dependency on myelography for diagnosis, and they strongly advocated the values of disc surgery under local anesthesia,[2,16] which teaches the surgeon the gentle handling of tissues, usually permits patients to recover faster after surgery, and gives the surgeon the remarkable opportunity to investigate the particular pain-generating sources (sensitive tissues). For example, as the surgeon dissects along the ligaments, the posterior annulus, or the course of nerves, a part or all of the particular pain syndrome may be reproduced. On the other hand any of these structures may be essentially asymptomatic. Most of the sensitive tissues then may be blocked using precise local infiltration to further confirm the location of clinical pain. This information is invaluable for drawing meaningful correlations between diagnostic methods and clinical effects, in spite of a significant blood level of various medications used during the administration of local anesthetics.

In recent years, with the development of improved anesthetics and techniques, local anesthesia (even with adjunctive intravenous medication) fell by the wayside. However, there is now a reawakening of interest in local anesthesia for several important reasons. In my own practice I have rediscovered the virtues and values of this method, especially when combined with a light epidural anesthesia by indwelling microcatheter, for use in routine discectomies and a few of the more complex lumbar procedures. It is an easy technique to return to, if one has been trained in its use, but it can be most disturbing to everyone in the operating room if one is not comfortable with the procedural and humanistic details. Patients may squirm and occasionally cry out, but with the intravenous use of diazepam (5 to 15 mg) and fentanyl (5 to 10 ml) nearly all patients will do well and will have little recollection of the procedure (including the more difficult moments). The epidural anesthetic (10 to 20 ml of bupivacaine 0.5% without additive) adds an additional dimension of comfort to the patient.

I now refer to this technique as "deep paraspinal infiltration anesthesia" rather than "local anesthesia," since the latter has been interpreted as trivial or superficial by some patients, colleagues, and third-party carriers. Although this method is more difficult and slower to perform, it can be worth the trade-off because the patient can help to guide the surgeon to the symptomatic lesion. Procaine 1% without epinephrine is used because of its low toxicity, although some surgeons may prefer lidocaine ½% to 1%. Skin wheals are raised using bacteriostatic saline containing 0.9% benzyl alcohol, which is a weak anesthetic that produces no pain in injection; the procaine is injected with less pain through the wheals.

Nearly all of us enjoy the high state of development in radiologic, ultrasonic, or magnetic imaging, particularly the CT scanning method; therefore the dependency upon myelography is even less than it was in 1938. In fact, in spite of much debate, in adept hands there is seldom a need or reason to perform myelography on patients who have herniated discs. In a few cases it is important to inject a very small amount of contrast media into the lumbar thecal sac to perform a contrast-enhanced CT scan, especially in cases of previous lumbar surgery where there is a need to establish a differential diagnosis between a clump of extradural scar tissue or rehernation, or those rare cases where a conus lesion is suspected. Semmes and Murphey stressed that in the typical herniated disc, that is, where the symptoms of low back pain have been replaced by often severe leg pain with objective neurologic evidence of specific root involvement, there should be no justification for subjecting the patient to a myelogram. The reader should be reminded that iophendylate (Pantopaque) has always been a major cause of lumbosacral adhesive arachnoiditis; the decline in use of this agent has been important in reducing the incidence of this potentially dreadful complication.[2]

Semmes and Murphey stated that if the clinical history, signs, and changes in sensation and reflexes are congruent, "the odds are probably 100 to 1" that the presence or absence of the herniated disc, as well as its anatomic level, can be specifically judged sufficiently well to warrant surgery.[9,16] These comments were made long before CT scanning was available. However, it is most interesting to recall that Murphey pointed out the importance of exploring two disc spaces, to rule out the possibility of a missed or second lesion.[9] However, he did indicate that the chance of having a simultaneous herniation at two or more levels is very close to zero. In view of the diagnostic detail available with CT scanning, this need (to explore two levels) is clearly outmoded. The only remaining disc problems for which the CT scanner is presently deficient are those that are significant when the patient is in the erect posture (the "standup discs") or segmental instability (the "sore" disc). There are now some useful CT and MRI criteria for the latter but scarcely for the former (except in cases having a clinically significant subarticular stenosis acting as a "stand-up" entrapment).[14]

These two authors were (and many others still are) unable to deal with what may be called the "sore disc syndrome," since the cause was not clear. I expect that what they referred to is now known as a mechanical low back syndrome (MLBS) of either facet joint pain origin or discogenic pain resulting from segmental instability. The MLBS is often worsened by discectomy regardless of the surgical (or enzymatic) method used. In such cases, as one explores while performing a decompression with the patient under local anesthesia, the facet joint will be found to be abnormally tender to maneuvering, the annulus will be painful to palpation with a blunt hook, or both structures may be hypersensitive. Furthermore, curetting the disc space in the awake patient will reproduce the low back pain. These patients might ultimately receive facet nerve blocks or diagnostic discography and fusion to fully control the pain.

WHAT'S WRONG, AND HOW TO GET TO IT

In general, the important elements to consider in performing a decompression such as a discectomy are (1) removal of pressure from the neural element, (2) maintenance of stability of the spinal segment, (3) avoidance of injury, and (4) prevention of future problems. Other than ignoring the presence of lateral stenosis or the existence of segmental instability, fibrosis may remain a major cause of persistent postoperative problems. These elements will be discussed only briefly here; the reader is referred to Chapters 14 and 15 for more detail.

The real purpose of nearly all spinal surgery is to obtain relief from the compression or entrapment of neural tissue. As reported elsewhere, the most common cause for failed back surgery (in about 60% of the cases) is the presence of lateral stenosis that was unknown at the time of the original procedure.[1,2,4,10] It is therefore essential to have a CT scan that allows one to search not only for herniations but also for potential stenoses as well.

Since nearly all the structures of importance in these cases are posterior or posterolateral in location, there is rarely anything within the disc space itself that is of CT diagnostic importance. That is, making the CT scans directly through the disc space is not particularly helpful; the CT scan image of the relationship between the disc, the displaced nerve, and overlying bone is essentially the same whether or not the scanner gantry is tilted to parallel the plane of the disc space.[7] On the other hand, it is often very important to obtain parallel, contiguous, sequential scan cuts through all of the involved or suspicious segments.[3] No portion of the suspected lumbar spine should be overlooked. Furthermore, sequential scans allow parasagittal or other off-axis reconstructions to be made; these may be of particular importance in determining the presence of a significant lateral stenosis, confirmation of a free fragment, or the extent of the herniation.

To sacrifice this information to obtain "disc-oriented scans" indicates that the involved radiologist and surgeon are not fully aware of lateral stenosis. In the opinion of several, the persistence of disc-oriented scanning, leaving gaps in the anatomic data, remains a major myth among many who might otherwise deal more effectively with spinal diagnosis and treatment. In my practice, which specializes in lumbar spinal disorders, the majority of all CT scans sent to me with patient referrals must unfortunately be repeated primarily for this reason.

It is also very important for the surgeon to carefully study the CT scans and visualize the target lesion, as well as the intended path to reach it (Fig. 16-1). In a real sense, he or she must develop a mental three-dimensional image of the target, the involved nerve, the approach, and other nearby structures of importance (especially the pedicle and lamina). Three-dimensional reconstructions can now be provided by computer software working on composite images made from sequential scans. The reason for the three-dimensional imagery lies in the need for simplification of the complex relationships of the individual CT slices, and ultimately to make apparent an appropriate but narrow approach for dissection and removal of the lesion without excessive manipulation of the nerve or probable loss of stability in that lumbar segment.

152 Surgical Procedures

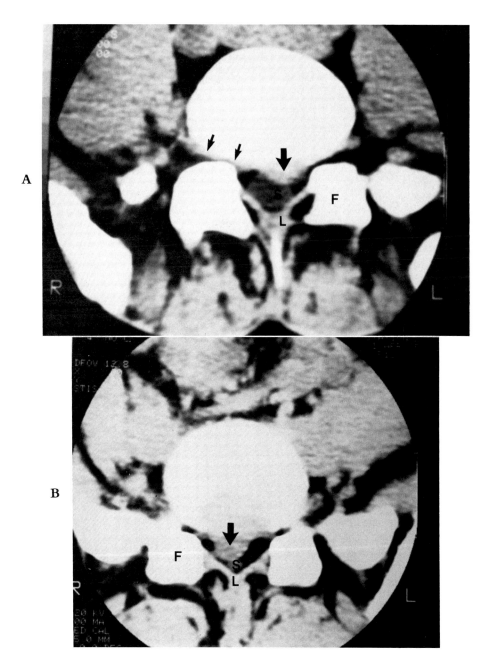

Fig. 16-1 **A,** CT scan at L5 to S1 level. In such a case, having no lesions at other levels or on opposite side, a one-sided microsurgical approach is used. Central and left-sided herniation *(large arrow)* displaces the S1 root and dural sac, *S,* towards the ligamentum flavum, *L.* Left facet, *F,* is normal, but right one is hypertrophic and compresses L5 ganglion against a disc bar or spur *(small arrows).* Bulge was presumably more prominent when patient bore weight, since leg symptoms were thus increased (this is the classical "stand-up" disc syndrome). **B,** Similar situation to **A,** but herniation is nearer midline; it was missed on previous CT scan by an apparently less experienced CT reader who interpreted the disc bulge as the dura itself. Remaining sac, *S,* is small and so dorsally positioned that disc does not appear to compress or displace it. However, patient had moderate bladder and bowel problems and pain in both legs on standing.

MECHANICAL INSTABILITY

There are many surgeons who feel that one can, with impunity, remove an entire facet joint during discectomy at a particular level. I do not agree with this. In keeping with the admonitions by Farfan and others, faced with an already potentially unstable disc segment (because of the HNP), removal of a facet joint at that level would be tantamount to cutting off two legs of a three-legged stool. This would potentially violate stability via the three-joint concept of Kirkaldy-Willis and others.[1,4] Furthermore, one should be certain in advance of the discectomy that there is no significant instability present, otherwise the patient might require both a decompression and fusion. Therefore, in the suspected case of MLBS with possible instability, one should clarify the differential diagnosis before discectomy, usually by a combination of injection procedures, namely, facet nerve injections at multiple levels possibly followed by MRI scanning and, in certain cases, by dynamic (saline acceptance) discography. If the facet injections largely abate the mechanically provokable pain, facet nerve blocks with a radio-frequency lesion generator are made, preferably before the discectomy (the patient will be better served than if the opposite sequence, that is, discectomy first, facet block second, is followed).[11,14]

When facet nerve injections and immediate interim mechanical (flexion-extension, rotation, side bending) testing of the patient show that the MLBS pain persists, saline acceptance injections into the suspected disc spaces are performed. This may be followed by contrast injections to view the internal disruption of the disc. The MRI scan will indicate which disc spaces are undergoing degeneration (dehydration) but not which ones are producing MLBS. The dynamic discogram remains the best method to determine specific reproduction of clinical pain at each segment. After the MRI has pointed out the degenerating segments, it is important to continue up the lumbar spine segments with the saline acceptance injections until one reaches an asymptomatic, normal segment. This will draw the upper limit of a possible stabilization procedure. One then must consider the potential both of discectomy at the herniated level with a clinically significant HNP, and of fusion to include the mechanically symptomatic, unstable segments.[14]

Usually the patients who are selected for this combination of procedures are those who have had an MLBS long preceding the onset of the herniation and in whom the low back–pain element continues unabated in spite of the onset of leg pain. Furthermore, these patients usually complain of back pain and leg pain that often act independently rather than in concert, as would a herniation alone. Let us now assume that instability is not an issue in the particular case and therefore proceed with a discectomy alone. The remaining considerations are those of the decompression and prevention of postoperative complications, for example, fibrosis.

Lumbar adhesive arachnoiditis (more commonly associated with the use of Pantopaque), probably occurs to a varying degree in many cases as a result of the surgical procedure itself. A more likely development from the surgery is epidural fibrosis and perhaps perineural fibrosis. At the present time, a free fat graft remains the best way to prevent potentially massive ingrowth of fibrosis pouring in from the overlying muscle that was injured by surgical dissection and retraction. (See Chapter 44.)

INCISION, DISSECTION, AND EXPOSURE

In nearly all cases of discectomy, especially if a microsurgical approach is used, the level of the incision should previously be marked on the skin and down into the spinous process at the involved level. This helps to prevent the need for a very large incision or an intraoperative lateral spinal x-ray film to search for the correct segment. Marking is done under fluoroscopic control a few hours before the decompression; 0.75 ml of Lymphazurin (1% isosulfan blue dye for lymphography)* is injected in the interspinous ligament immediately beneath the desired spinous process. As the needle is withdrawn, 0.1 ml of the dye is injected intradermally.

For a microdiscectomy, a short incision (about 2 to 3 cm) usually suffices, centered over the dye marker. Just below the surface of the skin one can usually obtain an acceptable fat or fat-fascia graft of about 10 cc. The globules of fat, no matter where the donor site, should be as intact as possible; cutting across them usually will result in atrophy later.

The incision into posterior fascia is made with an electric cautery knife (pencil), and the dissection is carried down to the level of the lamina (just on one side for a unilateral herniation) using a subperiosteal muscle-stripping technique. The muscle is swept away from the lamina laterally to the facet capsule with the use of a fairly broad elevator (a wide Cobb or Hoehn elevator) with caution not to plunge through the intralaminar space. Whether for a unilateral or bilateral exposure at L5-S1 and higher, I prefer to use a Raylor retractor† (see Chapter 14) having two blunt teeth at the tip.[12] The blade of this instrument is adjusted for the depth of the wound by bending it at an appropriate location along the blade. The two blunt teeth are placed just lateral to the mass of the facet joint (in patients under local anesthsia this will require an injection of additional anesthetic just lateral to the joint capsule). The Raylor then is attached to a dependent gauze strip to which, over the side of the wound, is attached a 1- to 2-kg hanging weight. This assembly will usually suffice for adequate exposure in all cases of lumbar discectomy. Should the exposure proceed further down to L5 to S1 or to the first sacral segment, a different form of Raylor retractor is employed. This latter unit has one or two very sharp spikes at the tip, curved inward to resist being dislodged during retraction. The spikes are gently pressed into the sacrum or sacroiliac joint lateral to the first sacral foramen and tied to a weighted gauze strip.

Excellent exposure can thus be obtained without the need for a long incision or very wide retraction as is usually required with the larger self-retaining retractors.[12,17] On reaching the lamina, one should carefully clean off the bone surface. As is shown in Fig. 16-2, with the use of a small curette (2 or 3 mm) one begins with the removal of the inferior attachment of the ligamentum flavum from the superior portion of the lamina below. The ligamentum then is detached from the more ventral surface of the lamina above. At this point small, far lateral superior and inferior laminotomies are performed using a small, sharp osteotome, a high-speed burr, and/or a Kerrison punch. The ligamentum then is detached from its more lateral shelf and retracted medially. With experience and caution the electric pencil can be used to clean connective tissue and much of the attachment of the ligamentum flavum from the dorsal surface of the lamina below. Furthermore, the lateral attachment of ligamentum to the medial facet capsule may be cut using the pencil. There may be some initial jumping of the leg, but this is probably never injurious to the anterior primary nerve. (In patients operated on under local anesthesia, for ex-

---

*Hirsch Industries, Inc., Richmond, Va.
†CeDaR Surgical Inc., Minnetonka, Minn.

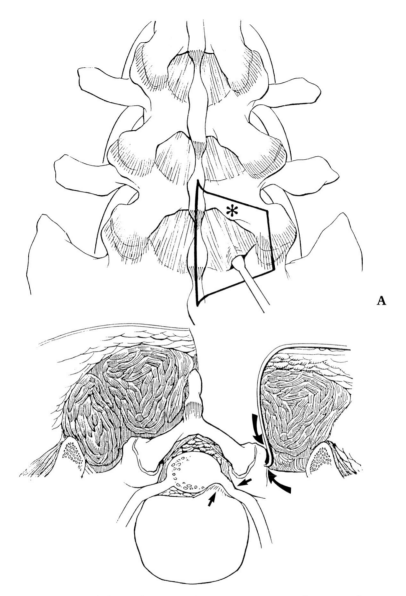

Fig. 16-2 A, Diagrams of a limited exposure laminotomy (essentially a microdiscectomy) at L5 to S1 space. A 2 cm wide Taylor-like retractor has been placed lateral to facet joint *(curved arrows).*[15] Lateral herniation and facet joint *(small arrows)* mutually compromise emerging ganglion. Small but adequate window of access *(asterisk)* is indicated by outlined area.

Continued.

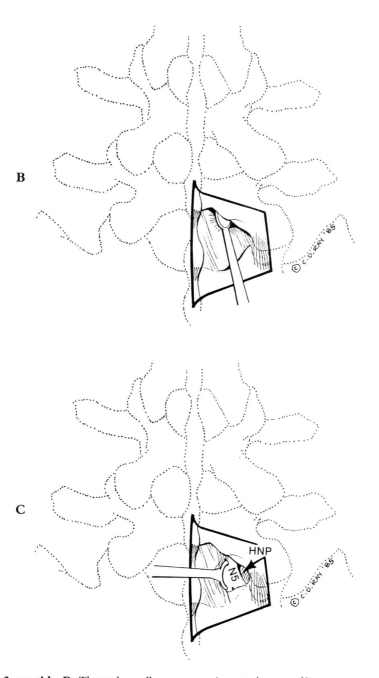

Fig. 16-2, cont'd B, Through small access superior attachment of ligamentum is dissected free from ventral surface of L5 lamina using curette, cutting edge facing dorsally. **C,** Laterally freed ligamentum is retracted medially revealing displaced, tightened L5 nerve root *(N5)*. Herniated disc *(HNP)* is now becoming visible. A small medial facetectomy is made to give exposure further lateral to root.

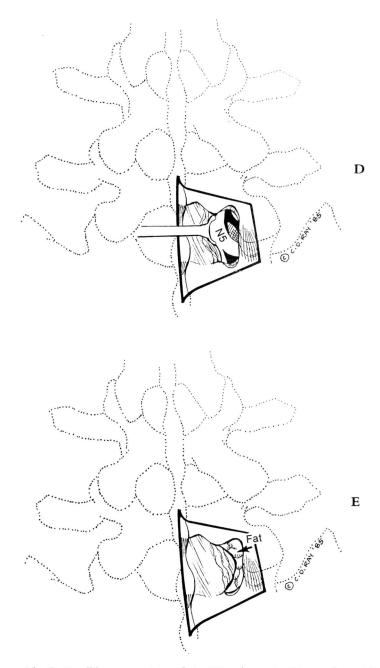

Fig. 16-2, cont'd D, Small laminotomies, inferior L5 and superior S1, together with medial facetectomy, usually provide excellent visualization and root mobility. Ligamentum remains largely attached. Herniation is now removed. **E,** Ligamentum is again laid over exposed dura; it has retracted since its elastic fibers (comprising about 80% of its bulk) shorten when detached from bone. A small fat or fat/fascia graft (about 5 ml) is placed near or around exposed nerve sleeve; a larger additional free graft (10 to 20 ml) will be placed over laminotomy site and wound closed.

ample, they will remark that the leg jump is not painful nor does it produce persistent effects, but is merely startling.) The margin of safety is large for electric cutting in the vicinity of an irritable or entrapped nerve in that it responds to the cutting current passed at some distance just as it responds to mechanical disturbance from a considerable distance. Furthermore, one sees muscular jumping almost exclusively when cautery-cutting around the facet capsule or synovium. This indicates hypersensitivity of the facet articular branch of the posterior primary nerve, producing paraspinous muscle contraction. (See Chapter 21.) The Kerrison rongeur or a small, sharp osteotome is used to take off elements of the lateral shelf of the ligamentum. This progresses until the medial aspect of the facet joint (especially the superior facet) itself is partially resected.

LAMINOTOMY VS. LAMINECTOMY

The decision as to whether there should be a large or small bony decompression, or one relatively more medial or lateral, should be based on preoperatively identified structures and lesions. A very good CT scan serves this function and helps guide the surgeon as well during the decompression itself.

To anticipate and routinely use a complete bilateral or a hemilaminectomy should be unthinkable. One should never follow a preset recipe for dealing with all lumbar decompressions. Most cases of herniated disc can be performed through a relatively limited laminotomy, although this becomes progressively more difficult as one goes more cephalad in the lumbar spaces; the size of the intralaminar space and laminar length are both markedly reduced in size above the L4-L5 level.

It seems to be a matter of discipline that many neurosurgeons will sacrifice large quantities of bone and even facet joints to obtain good neural decompression; however, many orthopedists prefer to maintain the bones and joints even though there may be left behind some moderate compromise of the nerve tissue. The only reasonable technique is an appropriate one, that is, appropriate to the patient's need, the anatomy, and the skill of the surgeon.[17]

DISCECTOMY

One should always have the CT scans available during surgery and should refer to them frequently. In this way small bony details will help to orient the surgeon to the exact location of the herniated disc and nerve, and to various clinically important elements of the patient's problems, for example, stenoses, spurs, disc bars, and facet chondromas.

Ordinarily, a small blunt hook or a Penfield no. 4 elevator may be slipped in between the lateral edge of the nerve and the medial edge of the partly resected facet joint; the nerve root is retracted medially (unless it is particularly tight and markedly displaced over the herniated disc) (Fig. 16-2, *C* and *D*). If the procedure is performed using local anesthetics, the patient will very likely complain about this maneuvering of the root and it may be necessary to inject about 0.25 to 0.50 ml of 0.25% bupivacaine (Marcaine) directly into the root for the patient to permit retraction of it. Nerve roots may be retracted with some vigor provided that one does not stretch them or the dura, the retraction must be gently applied, and it should be intermittent and never produce a visible, persistent indentation of the dura or nerve sleeve. The extent of benign tolerance to retraction has been shown many times through the performance of discectomy with the patient under local anesthesia. One should be cautious that the immediate preganglionic root is not retracted downward and medially simultaneously. The nerve is not particularly tender in many cases of central disc herniation or subarticular stenosis that lie caudal to the inferior laminotomy. Even with anesthetic injection into the nerve, if one is too vigorous with the manipulation, the patient will sometimes have sensory "breakthrough" and pain. If there is a major fragment or an extrusion easily approached, this should be removed first and an exploration begun in the nearby epidural space. This exploration is usually performed with a Murphey blunt nerve probe,* which is particularly helpful in searching for possible loose fragments, the presence of promontories not directly visible by the exposure, and for exploration of the medial aspect of the disc bar (or laterally, out along the neural foramen).

The laminotomy (or possible laminectomy) may be enlarged, but this should be done only as needed to gain adequate access to the disc material without undue traction on the nerve or dura. Should there be a more central, free fragment herniation, the material usually can be swept laterally with the Murphey hook and then pulled out. At times it is necessary to enter the annulus laterally to clean out the disc space material. Many surgeons make a fairly large window in the posterior annulus for this purpose. I believe it is quite unnecessary; a simple, linear up-down, axial, incision from one end-plate to the other suffices. One passes a curette inside the slit in the annulus, and with the use of various pituitary rongeurs the available degenerated nuclear material is removed. Clearly, it is not possible to remove the entire nucleus and even, for that matter, all of the highly degenerated material. There is always the risk that the nuclear remnants may degenerate and detach, creating a recurrent herniation. It appears that the incidence of reherniation is about the same for those cases in which a simple removal of all major fragments is performed and for those who have a vigorous clean-out of the disc cavity. I personally prefer a moderately good clean-out, if at all possible. Unfortunately, there is no way to determine whether a particular patient might experience a reherniation in the future. It may be useful to place a laminar spreader to further open the disc space to permit a more extensive curettage of the nucleus, particularly if the patient has been placed on a kneeling frame, which promotes lumbar extension (sway-back), to relax paraspinous muscles.

SUBARTICULAR STENOSIS AND THE "STAND-UP" DISC

If the superior tip of the lamina of the segment below moderately overhangs the disc space, this overhang should be removed by a small laminotomy to reduce the possibility of a subarticular entrapment. This stenosis occurs where the inferior margin of the disc, annulus, or bar posteriorly displaces and compresses the traversing nerve root (which may still be within the thecal sac) against the overhanging margin of the lamina (Fig. 16-3). This procedure can be particularly important in those discs that produce root compression signs when the patient stands and bears weight. The CT scan in such cases shows a rather narrow superior portion of the lateral recess and a rather cephalad riding rim of the lamina. If a hard posterior margin of the disc bar remains, it may be important to decompress this rim of bone spurs through the use of drift punches (impactors). I have developed impactors specifically for these and related spinal surgical applications.[12] (See Chapter 23.)

---

*Richards Manufacturing Co., Memphis, Tenn.

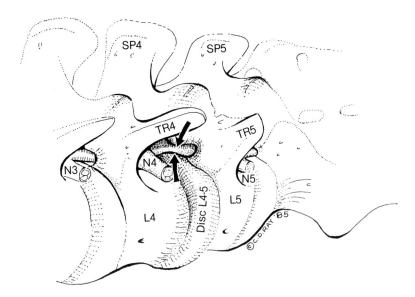

Fig. 16-3 Subarticular stenosis. Semitransverse view from high on left side. Indicated are L4 and L5 vertebral bodies, their respective dorsal spinous processes *(SP4, SP5)* and transverse processes *(TR4, TR5)*. Superior medial lamina of L5 overhangs HNP (at disc L4 to L5) catching traversing L5 nerve root in a squeeze *(arrows)*. In most cases definitive treatment is removal of laminar overhang, leaving disc annulus undisturbed and intact.

NERVE FREEDOM

At the conclusion of the discectomy the root should be freely movable (by at least a few millimeters). The root and ganglion are often enlarged and will continue to swell for a short period, immediately on decompression. The surface of the root sleeve may have congested veins, but one should resist the temptation to coagulate them, even if they bleed. Microfibrillar collagen material makes an excellent hemostatic agent for such bleeders, gelatin foam being outmoded. (See Chapter 44.) There are delicate fibrillar webs of connective tissue that are often found around the nerve sheath; they do not necessarily tether it during leg motion. If one performs a straight-leg extension while observing the root, it can be seen to move out the canal by a few millimeters but only when the leg raising approaches 90 degrees flexion. In general, it is best to obtain a sufficiently wide decompression of bone, away from the nerve tissue, such that a very small fat or fat/fascia graft might be placed between.

An additional means of estimating the degree of freedom from entrapment of the nerve in the lateral foramen is to pass a sterile, 2.5 mm (no. 8 French) disposable plastic feeding tube out the neural (more cephalad) portion of the foramen. Because of the remarkably open flexibility of the normal uncompromised perineural sheath, the feeding tube can often be threaded along it for a distance of many centimeters, perhaps as far as the sciatic notch. If the feeding tube hangs up in passage it may be due to a lateral compression, entrapment, or stenosis, or to some clinically insignificant far lateral–soft tissue band. One must therefore be careful not to overdiagnose a far lateral entrapment in the absence of supportive CT scan findings. Clear lateral passage for about 2 or 3 cm lateral to the foramen should suffice.

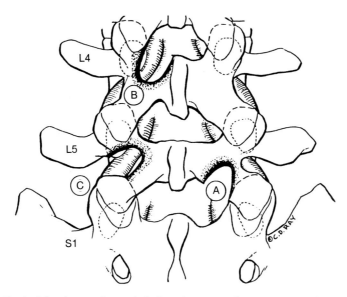

Fig. 16-4 Typical laminotomies and their primary applications. *A,* Inferior laminotomy (most common, for removal of HNP). *B,* Superior laminotomy (used in decompressions for subarticular stenosis but useful in certain cases of lateral stenosis to achieve good access to inferior medial aspect of pedicle). *C,* Lateral laminotomy (used for lateral stenoses and offending lateral osteophytes). I refer to this as a midline paramedial approach. After exposure is made to osteophyte, a bone impactor is usually used in decompression. See Chapters 21 and 23.

LAMINOTOMIES FOR LATERAL LESIONS

As indicated earlier, reaching and working effectively within the inaccessible zone ventral to the pars, with the maintenance or reestablishment of stability, can indeed be a technical challenge. If one attempts to do this via laminotomy alone, three approaches have been considered for such decompressions. As shown in Fig. 16-4, a laminotomy may be performed from below, *A,* which is the usual approach to a herniated disc; from above, *B,* the usual decompression for a subarticular stenosis; or from a lateral approach, *C,* for a lateral stenosis due to a spur, disc bar, or slippage. Although the first and second are by far the most common approaches used today, even for stenotic spurs, it is the third that may be the only appropriate one in most stenotic cases. This technique is somewhat more difficult, but must become a part of the spinal surgeon's repertoire. I have used this approach in a significant number of cases from a midline incision and refer to it as a midline paralateral laminotomy. It can be an excellent approach for the resection of the inferior aspect of the pedicle for stenosis. Of course, one must be careful to preserve enough of the pars to maintain mechanical stability. This is best determined from study of the anteroposterior spine films and scan films plus measurements of the lamina and pars during the operation.

EPIDURAL MORPHINE AND FAT GRAFTING

After the discectomy, epidural exploration, and foraminal probing have been completed, a morphine microcatheter is usually threaded up the epidural space (through a larger plastic feeding tube cut off at the tip); the external end of the microcatheter is brought out the flank through an 18-gauge needle.[15] If the procedure has been performed using epidural (or combined epidural/local) anesthesia, the microcatheter is already in place and will remain there for 3 days. A Milipore filter and an injection port are attached to the microcatheter. The patient is given 4 mg of morphine sulfate plus 10 ml of 0.5% bupivacaine (Marcaine) just at time of wound closure and then 2 to 4 mg of morphine alone via the filter and catheter every 8 to 24 hours afterward for the next 3 days. With this technique the patients ordinarily experience little or no postoperative pain and discomfort. They also rarely have the usual side effects (nausea, vomiting, orthostatic hypotension, ileus) that often occur with parenteral narcotics. In a number of cases epidural morphine may cause a generalized itching without rash and difficulty in voiding for a few hours after each dose. These side effects are related to the histamine-releasing effects of morphine and are sometimes controlled by a few doses of diphenhydramine 50 mg and cimetidine 300 mg given by injection or by mouth. If not controlled in this way, 0.1 to 0.3 mg naloxone by hypodermic will stop the side effects, although the analgesic effects will not be taken away.

The fat graft is placed around or beneath the portions of the ligamentum flavum that remain attached; the combination of low-reactive tissues together will remain as a posterior barrier to the ingrowth of fibroblasts from the under surface of the surgically injured muscle. The wound is closed in a standard multilayer technique using absorbable suture. A subcuticular stitch also of absorbable material (Vicryl or PDS) then is used to close the skin in a cosmetic fashion (this is the only part of the surgery that the patient and family can see, so good cosmesis is important).

SUMMARY

When the principles in this discussion are followed and the surgeon has had adequate experience to avoid excessive stretch or trauma to the root, patients will recover rather rapidly. Although most cases may have some immediate postoperative numbness and tingling rather globally in the leg (or both legs), these symptoms generally abate in a matter of a day or so. Early ambulation and the occasional use of oral or parenteral dexamethasone (in a rather large, decreasing dose over a period of 4 to 5 days, starting on the third or fourth postoperative day) may be helpful where there may be significant postoperative swelling of the nerve or ganglion.

The use of mild, adjunctive epidural anesthesia together with deep paraspinal infiltration using procaine 1% (local anesthetic) demands gentle handling and therefore provides an additional dimension of safety to the neural structures and valuable information for the surgeon. Its use should be considered for uncomplicated discectomies. In addition, ambulation shortly after the procedure, freedom from the usual postoperative pain (provided by the morphine catheter) and a small incision closed with a plastic surgical technique, contribute to a rapid, benign recovery and good physician-patient rapport.[15,16]

REFERENCES

1. Burton, C.V.: Diagnosis and treatment of lateral spinal stenosis: implications regarding the "failed back surgery syndrome." In Genant, H.K., et al., editors: Spine update 1984, San Francisco, 1983, Radiology Research & Education Foundation.
2. Burton, C.V.: How to avoid the "failed back surgery syndrome." In Cauthen, J.C., editor: Lumbar spine surgery, Baltimore, 1983, Williams & Wilkins.
3. Burton, C.V., et al.: Computed tomographic scanning and the lumbar spine. II. Clinical considerations, Spine **4**:356, 1979.
4. Cauthen, J.C.: Lumbar spine surgery, Baltimore, 1983, Williams & Wilkins.

5. Fager, C.A.: Lumbar disc disease—surgical treatment. In Hardy, R.W., editor: Lumbar disc disease, New York, 1982, Raven Press.
6. Friedman, W.A.: Percutaneous discectomy: an alternative to chemonucleolysis? Neurosurgery **13**:542, 1983.
7. Lifson, A., et al.: High-resolution computed tomographic scanning of the lumbosacral spine, Mod. Neurosurg. **1**:31, 1982.
8. Morris, J.M.: Surgical management of lumbar disc disease. In Genant, H.K., et al., editors: Spine Update 1984, San Francisco, 1983, Radiology Research & Education Foundation.
9. Murphey, F.: Experience with lumbar disc surgery, Clin. Neurosurg. **20**:1, 1973.
10. Pheasant, H.C., and Dyck, P.: Failed lumbar disc surgery: cause, assessment, treatment, Clin. Orthop. **164**:93, 1982.
11. Ray, C.D.: Percutaneous radio frequency facet nerve blocks: treatment of the mechanical low back syndrome (monograph), Burlington, Ma., 1982, Radionics Corporation. (Addendum published 1983.)
12. Ray, C.D.: New malleable force-fulcrum retractors for lumbar spinal surgery: technical note, Spine (in press).
13. Ray, C.D.: Bone impactors: new instruments for spinal decompression, technical note, Spine (in press).
14. Ray, C.D., et al.: Discogenic pain, segmental instability and the mechanical low back syndrome: diagnosis and treatment, Unpublished manuscript, 1987.
15. Ray, C.D., and Bagley, R.: Indwelling epidural morphine for control of post lumbar surgery pain, Neurosurgery **13**:388, 1983.
16. Semmes, R.E.: Ruptures of the lumbar intervertebral disc, Springfield, Ill., 1984, Charles C Thomas, Publisher.
17. Wilson, D.H., and Harbaugh, R.: Lumbar discectomy: a comparative study of microsurgical and standard technique. In Hardy, R., editor: Lumbar disc disease, New York, 1982, Raven Press.

EDITORIAL COMMENTARY

Our authors consider the classical laminectomy to be the procedure with the greatest value. It is performed the most often, and it is the most common procedure used by Richard Rothman. Most of us have experienced some form of significant complication with the procedure. As Vert Mooney points out "for the herniated or extruded disc this is the ideal approach, and as other statistics have demonstrated, resolves the problem in over 90% of the cases. This is the most successful surgical approach." Hugo Keim states that "I generally prefer the posterior approach for 95% of all spinal surgery." C.D. Ray finds "there are few indications for true laminectomies, laminotomies being almost exclusively preferred for simple laminotomies/laminectomies, single- or dual-sided. I much prefer microdissection."

Kirkaldy-Willis, Spangler and Burton, and others have found between 30% and 75% of their disc herniation patients had concomitant spinal stenosis. Analysis of our disc excision cases in 1977 disclosed that 75% of the cases had concomitant spinal stenosis. We therefore find that most of our herniated disc cases, if they require surgery, require a more extensive lumbar decompression. Simple herniated discs improve very well with conservative care and rarely need to have surgery.

Because of the high failure rate of discectomy secondary to recurrent herniated disc and lumbar spinal stenosis, we tend to do more extensive decompressions and fusions.

Arthur H. White

CHAPTER

17

EXTENSIVE LUMBAR DECOMPRESSION: PATIENT SELECTION AND RESULTS

Charles D. Ray

Among patient selection considerations for lumbar spine surgery, one must always remember that perhaps 95% of cases are operated on for subjective reasons, principally pain (claudication, dysesthesia, or pure discomfort).[4,8,14] The remaining small number of cases are chosen because of true (nonsubjective) weakness, autonomic effects (rarely), or other objective signs of functional loss. Therefore one must pay considerable attention to subjective complaints and their effects on the patient's life-style, for example, ability to work, effect on the family, economic elements, hidden strategies, legal implications, or secondary gain. No matter how carefully performed and exquisitely demarcated the diagnostic studies, in the final analysis it is pain that is the leading reason for surgery; one does not operate on x-rays but on people. We can only hope that the objective studies match the subjective complaints and thus clarify both diagnosis and treatment. If they are not congruent, the clinical plan is in trouble.

Criteria for the selection of individual cases for both categorically simple or extensive decompressions are relatively straightforward, although the subcategories of these criteria are complex and usually require considerable attention to detail, such as (1) significant knowledge about the patient, (2) excellent diagnostic studies that resolve the pathoanatomy in relationship with the clinical picture, (3) extensive clinical awareness and, (4) surgical experience of the surgeon and the team.[3]

PATIENT CRITERIA

When selecting patients largely based on information of subjective complaints, it is important that the structural changes, alterations of function, and patient complaints be congruent and logical. However, one must accept some variation in the recipe and not arbitrarily rule out the use of decompression simply because the symptoms do not quite match the surgeon's objectives and criteria. This is a plea for the surgeon to stretch his or her repertoire as new techniques and instruments emerge.

In general, a patient's age is not, of itself, a major factor. Far more important are the overall health, medical status, presence of possible intercurrent disorders, activity level, emotional and social factors and patient-perceived need. I have several times operated on patients in the eighth and ninth decades of life, provided they were in generally good health and relatively active, enthusiastic about the need for the decompression, and not inappropriately optimistic about potential outcome. A recent onset of inactivity caused by neurogenic claudication related to a lateral stenosis, for example, is not a limiting factor, as would be the case of a patient who has been markedly inactive and largely bedridden for some months or years. Of course, there is a trade-off between the severity of the problem and the general condition of the patient. That is, if the patient has a highly localized, rather easily decompressed surgical problem, although it may be advanced and the patient considerably disabled, the decompression might still be performed with the view that a return of function and comfort at an early date might well lead to a fairly rapid increase in activity level and rehabilitation.[1,4,5,8] Although a significant osteoporosis might be present, patients may still do quite well postoperatively, even including the performance of a limited fusion (although one would certainly exercise considerable caution in selecting patients with advanced osteoporosis and multilevel, clinically significant degenerative disease of the spine).

Marked obesity is usually a far greater contraindication to extensive spinal surgery than advanced age. When the patient is indeed very fat, it indicates either the possible presence of a metabolic disorder, a careless abandon about personal health care, or considerable restriction in activity. Encouraging the patient with a "carrot" of either losing weight or not being offered surgery may act as a test of commitment for postoperative cooperation in a program of recovery.[2] Furthermore, some evidence exists that preoperative reduction in fat intake over a matter of several weeks or a few months may well reduce the content of exogenous fat in the body. That is, when on a low-fat diet, the patient must synthesize fat from carbohydrates or protein. The recipient or host site for a fat graft during surgery may show less reaction to autogenous-grafted fat cells having a greater percentage of self-generated fat.

Patients should also be weaned from virtually all narcotics and all aspirin-containing medication for at least 2 weeks before the procedure. A similar interference in prostaglandin-related anticoagulation has similarly been reported with the use of other nonsteroidal antiinflammatory drugs.

Other important personal elements include the patient's emotional status, efforts toward secondary gain, amplification of symptoms, and a labyrnthine myriad of work-related and legal matters. Such elements may more than interfere with surgical outcome even in well-motivated cases.[8] However, one must not overlook those patients who might need to have, and would benefit from, extensive decompressions in spite of their personal disturbance; an old adage reminds us that "crazy people get sick, too." Part of the art of surgery clearly lies in patient selection and all the pertaining trade-offs.

Preoperative and postoperative preparation are quite important in order to maintain good spirits, a commitment to "get well," and a desire to participate in appropriate reactivation, although this may be painful at times. Patients who maintain a "here I am, you fix me" attitude will often not do well, regardless of age or infirmity.

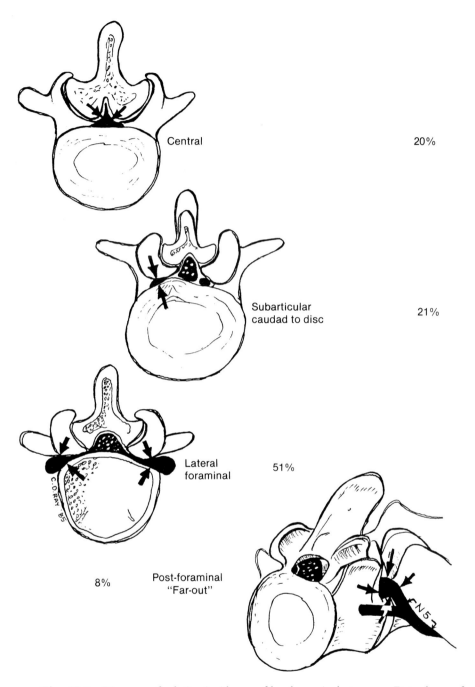

Fig. 17-1 Diagram of relative incidence of lumbar spinal stenoses. Data drawn from 100 consecutive cases in my practice devoted to lumbar spine surgery. Subarticular stenosis occurs at inferior margin of disc, where there is an overhang of lamina from below, affecting root passing over disc to emerge at next segment below. Lateral foraminal stenoses affect root emerging at that level. The "far-out" (alar-transverse process, L5 nerve impingement) stenosis is that described by Wiltse and associates.[15]

SITE SELECTION CRITERIA

Fig. 17-1 shows the location and relative incidence of the various forms of "spinal stenosis." The data for this figure were obtained from a consecutive series of 100 of my patients who required spinal surgery for stenosis. Central stenosis, as an isolated rather than merely primary diagnosis, is much less common than indicated here. It is usually seen in concert with other stenoses. Note that discectomy has not been included in this presentation.

TYPES OF LATERAL STENOSIS

It is a remarkably common misconception that the primary cause of lateral stenosis is the entrapment of a ganglion or nerve root between the cephalad tip of the superior facet and the inferior margin of the pedicle above.[14] This combination is rarely seen. One would expect that if this did occur patients would have recurrent root-compression signs (tingling, pain, or weakness in the appropriate dermatome) on hyperextension of the lumbar spine; they do not. Fig. 17-2 demonstrates this misconception. The most common cause of lateral stenosis is an "up-down" compression of the nerve or ganglion between the pedicle above and a disc bar or spur from below; patients often experience pain and weakness (real or sensory-inhibitory) after prolonged standing, weight bearing or walking.

The question has often arisen as to how a tight but adequate, immovable canal might suddenly become stenotic about the nerve that passes through. As an example, consider the case of a nerve passing in the tight gutter between a disc bar or uncinate process (on the posterolateral

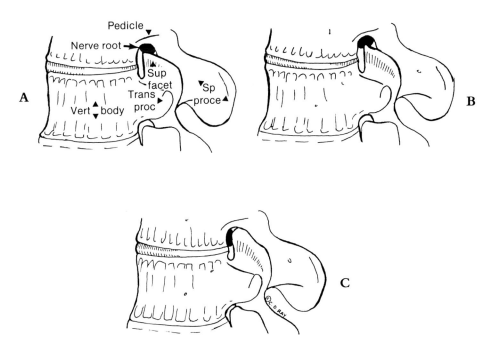

Fig. 17-2 Diagram showing current popular misconception regarding lateral stenosis. **A** and **B** show root being compressed by blunt or sharp tip of superior facet. This situation probably cannot occur except in rather rare case of synovial chondroma arising from facet capsule or traumatic subluxation. If this condition were to occur commonly, we should expect patients to complain of tingling, pain, or weakness on hyperextension, further pressing the nerve upward. Although **C** shows actual situation one encounters, it too is almost rare. See Fig. 17-3 for further discussion.

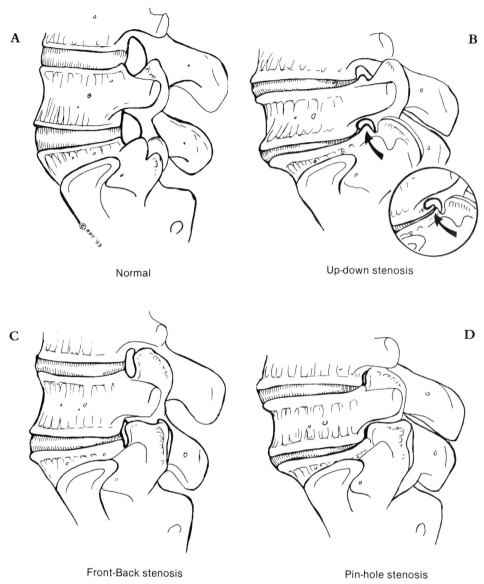

Fig. 17-3 The three types of lateral stenosis. **A,** Normal configuration, for comparison. **B,** Up-down stenosis caused by impingement of root or ganglion by osteophytic disc bar arising from S1 pressing nerve against pedicle of L5. In circled vignette impingement arises from uncinate spur of L5, S1, or both. This type and location (at L5-S1) represents about 90% of clinical cases of lateral stenosis. Disc space collapse with marginal osteophytosis or an uncinate spur, or collapse with degenerative spondylolisthesis, all commonly produce this type of stenosis. **C,** The front-back stenosis as presented in Fig. 17-2. Although it, too, more commonly occurs at L5-S1, it is sometimes seen with retrolisthesis, which can be found at higher lumbar levels. As indicated, this type is seen in only about 3% of stenoses, although it is incorrectly thought to be the most common type of lateral stenosis. **D,** A pin-hole or combined stenosis, representing an amalgam of **B** and **C**. This type also occurs most often at L5-S1, but about as infrequently as front-back type alone. In cases with severe disc space collapse at any lumbar level, this type can be found, however.

edge of the vertebral end-plate), pressing the nerve cephalad against the inferior aspect of the pedicle—both structures being elements of the *same* vertebral body. It is easy to appreciate a compression or stenosis created by opposing, restricting elements arising from adjacent, separate, movable vertebral bodies, but not between elements of the same one. Since the nerve moves in or out only a small amount even in extreme flexion of the leg, there can be only one primary explanation—edema. That is, the nerve must be tightly fitted between the opposing, immovable elements and then with a minor trauma, stretch injury, or a reversible pulsion effect from adjacent soft tissues (such as a disc or annulus), the nerve begins to swell; the canal size now becomes relatively inadequate, causing an avalanche of the stenosing effect. One could then expect vascular effects (hypoxia), and the late buildup of axonally transported substances leading to an hour-glass appearance of the compressed nerve. The nerve may not then escape these unrelenting pressures until the edema subsides, the nerve is decompressed, or the nerve and associated tissues in the canal begin to atrophy. In all probability, entrapment between moving elements probably causes pain without loss of function or electrophysiologic change; whereas when the stenosis is created between nonmoving elements, there should be loss of function and a change in electrophysiology of the nerve.

Perhaps surprisingly, the entrapment resulting from the nerve being pressed by a hypertrophic facet from behind forward against the dorsal surface of the vertebral body ("front-back" stenosis) is highly unusual, found more often at the L4-L5 level but occurring in less than 3% of all cases having lateral stenosis. I first suggested the terminology "up-down," "front-back," and "pin-hole" (or "combined") stenosis at the November 1983 meeting of the American Academy of Orthopaedic Surgeons in San Francisco, which served as the impetus for compiling this book. The anatomic relationships in these stenoses are shown in Fig. 17-3. In general, lateral stenosis occurs nine times out of ten at the L5-S1 level.[3,6,7,12]

THE INACCESSIBLE ZONE

Most nerve entrapment occurs in the vicinity of the pedicle. This has been referred to by Casey Lee as the "hidden zone." This area is relatively inaccessible as far as the preservation of anatomy during decompression is concerned (Fig. 17-4). The nerve root and ganglion are highly protected, since they are covered by bone, beginning with the medial aspect of the pedicle and then passing caudad to the pedicle (somewhat like a rope passing around a pulley). The four sides of the neural foramen consist of the superior pedicle, cephalad; the inferior pedicle of the vertebra below, caudad; the facet joint, dorsally; and the vertebral body, ventrally. The nerve occupies only the upper, ventral part of the foramen, however, in close proximity with the superior pedicle. After emergence from the foramen, the nerve may once again be vulnerable to compression or entrapment but at very few places.[6,7,15] Nearly all postforaminal stenosis occur at L5-S1; the most likely lying between the inferior (caudad) margin of the low-lying pedicle of L5 and the superior (cephalad) rim of the sacral ala. This is the "far out" compression as described by Wiltse.[15] Perhaps the last potential focus of compression of the fifth lumbar nerve, occurring even farther out than the "far out" entrapment given above, is found in a small triangular zone lateral to the disc margin at L5-S1; a disc bar or bulge at this point may press the nerve against the sacral ala, often as it joins the base of the pedicle of S1, as shown in Fig. 17-5.

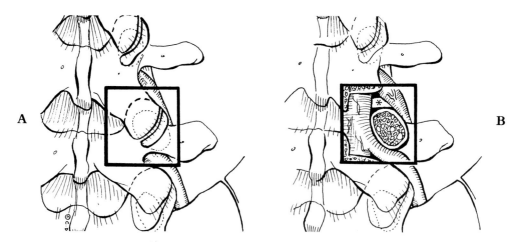

Fig. 17-4 The "inaccessible zone." **A,** Inside the boxed area, right lumbar 4 level, lies the zone, centered around pedicle. Most lesions of lumbar spine are found beneath (ventral to) laminas here. **B,** Facet joint and laminas have been removed in boxed area of **A.** Beneath are shown the L4 and L5 roots and the relationship of each to base of pedicle. Disc at L4-L5 is indicated at asterisk. Illustration is only for clarification of anatomy; a surgical decompression to this extent would likely produce some degree of instability, probably torsional.

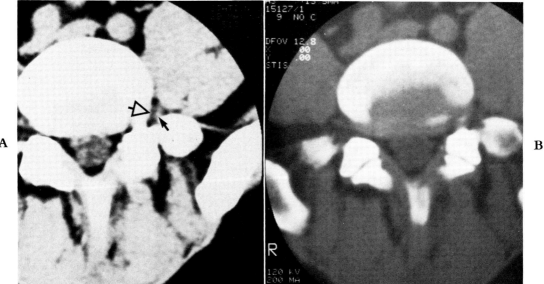

Fig. 17-5 Very far out (ventrolateral) stenosis with herniated disc impingement. This is a different lesion from that described by Wiltse and associates.[15] It occurs where L5 spinal nerve passes lateral to already osteophytic disc margin, just at "corner" by sacral ala. Presence of herniation, although slight, causes entrapment. This situation is not unlike a subarticular stenosis, where there is a considerable "massaging" effect caused by small herniation *(open arrow)* intermittently producing compression of nerve *(small black arrow)* in rigid confines of this narrow passage. **A,** Soft tissue and **B,** bone window CT images are shown. Case required direct nerve injection with anesthetic and contrast to identify lesion. Patient had been operated on elsewhere a few months earlier but was not helped (posterior midline disc exploration was negative, disc space was "cleaned out"). Direct decompression by paralateral approach led to remission of pain and disability.[10,11] Although uncommon, the potentiality of this lesion should be considered in cases of lateral stenosis at L5-S1.

With these considerations in mind, any decompression that is appropriate to the particular patient must address: (1) the location and extent of the lesion, (2) the overlying structures and approach to the lesion, (3) the presence or potential presence of segmental instability and, (4) the surgeon's experience with similar cases.

STABILITY OR INSTABILITY, THAT IS THE QUESTION

In many cases one is faced with the unfortunate combination of lateral stenosis, such as a spur in the foramen, and an open (not yet collapsed) disc space or a herniated disc at the same level. If in this situation the mechanical integrity of the facet is markedly disturbed or destroyed during the decompression or removal of the herniated disc, there is a very great chance that the patient will become clinically unstable with subsequent discogenic pain or recurrence of stenosis. In addition, in my opinion it is wrong to consider that one may remove either one of the facet joints in the presence of a fully open disc space, herniated or not. The complete destruction of even one facet may well produce torsional imbalance or instability, leading to a progressive degeneration of the disc annulus, nucleus, opposite facet, or all of these plus a regrowth of the stenosing uncinate spur or disc bar. One must therefore pick and choose among the various surgical approaches to satisfy the various conditions but make every attempt to maintain segmental stability. That is, one must always carefully consider the various surgical approaches that are best used in cases having a herniation, a stenosis, instability, or some combination of these.[4,5,9-11,15]

PUTTING IT ALL TOGETHER

Table 17-1 shows a matrix of combinations that, in my opinion, particularly suggest certain surgical procedures, and vice versa. One must remember the important factors in selecting a particular patient for a particular procedure, simple or complex: the patient's findings and status, the lesion, the anatomy, stability, the surgical approach, the surgeon's skill and familiarity, the operating team, the hospital setting and rehabilitation facility, follow-up plans, the patient's family, the patient's vocation, and other social, psychological, or legal factors.

An *unstable space* is defined as one in which the disc is still open, where there is a circumferential bulging of the annulus, some spurring (especially anterolaterally and uncinate), diastasis (wide opening) of the facet joints, slippage of the vertebra, a positive saline acceptance (and contrast) discogram, positive MRI dehydration of the disc, mechanical low back syndrome (probably responding well to bracing), and a positive flexion-extension study. A *moderately stable segment* has an open disc space, no displacement on flexion-extension, mild spurring, minimal MRI dehydration, and minimal low back pain. An alternative moderate stability has marked disc space narrowing and spur formation but some movement remains, for example, there may be gas in the disc space implying that it is dry but still moves (cavitates). A *very stable space* has largely collapsed, is fused, or calcified. Here, stability implies both present and future condition, that is, the space would not destabilize regardless of the removal of posterior spinal structures. Central and subarticular stenoses are not considered in Table 17-1; central stenoses are treated with midline laminectomies and removal of the spinous process, and subarticular stenoses usually require a superior laminotomy with undercutting of the adjacent superior facet and medial pedicle. (See Chapter 16.)

When these elements and circumstances are optimal, the overall results in a great variety of cases that require simple or extensive lumbar decompression or

Table 17-1 *Decompressions for spinal stenosis: indications and selection of approach*

Technique	Status of lumbar segment(s) having stenosis														
	Unstable (potential or actual)					Moderately stable					Very stable (autostabilized)				
	Lateral unilat.	Lat. bilat.	Cent. and HNP	Lat. and HNP	Lat. and new slip	Lateral unilat.	Lat. bilat.	Cent. and HNP	Lat. and HNP	Lat. and old slip	Lateral unilat.	Lat. bilat.	Cent. and HNP	Lat. and HNP	Lat. and old slip
Posterior "wedge"	N	N	N	N	N	±	±	N	N	N	Y	Y	N	±	Y
Paralateral unilat.*	Y	N	N	±	±	Y	N	N	Y	Y	Y	N	N	Y	Y
Bilat.*	N	Y	N	±	±	N	Y	N	±	Y	N	Y	N	Y	Y
Midline, plit fusion	±	Y	Y	Y	Y	N	Y	±	±	Y	N	N	±	Y	±
Neur arch autograft†	±	±	±	N	N	Y, UNI	Y	N	±	±	N	N	N	N	N
Pars autograft†	N	N	N	N	N	±, UNI	±	N	±, UNI	N	N	±	N	±, UNI	N

N, Not Applicable Y, Applicable. ±, Applicable in selected cases. Unilat., unilateral; bilat., bilateral; HNP, herniated disc together with the stenosis. New slip, Spondylolisthesis of recent (unstable) onset. Old slip, Spondylolisthesis of long duration (stable). Posterior "wedge," author's technique for removal of the neural arch en bloc. Midline plit fus, Midline approach for decompression and subsequent intertransverse process fusion. UNI, Unilateral applications (usual cases are bilateral).

*See Chapter 22.
†See Chapter 18.

discectomy will range between 80% and 90% good to excellent. No matter how hard one strives to improve on these numbers, as skill and experience increases one tends to take on more difficult cases; therefore the statistical outcome becomes a moving target, going ever upward. This does mean, however, that with time and experience, cases once thought to be prohibitively difficult, having a low yield of good results, will begin to enjoy better results. Therefore, if one's good results drift significantly above 90%, it usually indicates a significant limitation in one's practice or unwillingness to tackle new or more difficult problems. Clearly, there is an argument for each side of this coin, that is, to become more limited yet more skilled vs. broadening the scope to include progressively more difficult cases with their attendant risks. Unfortunately, it may take some years to know the real truth about surgical outcome, since many desirable or undesirable results may be slow to emerge.[8] In spine surgery it appears that the relative time constant for long-term follow-up should be at least 3 years and probably 5 years or more.

Regardless of the several, more personal factors just discussed, selected surgical procedures yield a better or worse outcome when used to address certain lesions. For some combination of lesions, particular techniques or approaches may involve a greater risk for potential nerve injury, a higher likelihood of progression or recurrence of the problem, and increased chances for postoperative segmental instability. Table 17-2 briefly reviews the procedures given in Table 17-1 and compares overall results. The reference to "transverse wedge" is my procedure for radical removal of the entire neural arch, en bloc, using sharp osteotome cuts across both pars and then decompression throughout the entire course of the neural foramen. The "neural arch graft," "lateral laminotomy" and "paralateral procedures are described in Chapters 16, 18, and 22. These tables show limited groups of a small but highly selected population of patients who have relatively advanced problems of the lumbar spine. Finally, although believed to be moderately representative, these data must be considered rather tentative, since some of the newer procedures have had limited use over the course of the last 5 years.

Table 17-2 *Procedures and results*

Procedure	% lumbar decompressions	% all surgicals	% good results*
Discectomy, midline	24	8	87
Paralateral decompression	26	8	67
Subarticular decompression	13	4	82
Transverse wedge	26	8	77
Lateral laminotomy	5	2	65†
Central laminectomy	5	2	80†
Neural arch graft	2	<1	67‡
All lumbar decompression	100	36	

Total surgical cases performed, 826. Implants and minor cases, 579. Total major cases (primarily lumbar decompressions, fusions), 247. All categories approximate only. All cases peformed by the author.
*Good/excellent results reported by patient and independent observers; some groups too small to be significant, however.
†Procedure modified during the course of this study period.
‡Note small number of cases. The mixture of cases changed considerably over the 3-year period of these observations.

After writing this chapter, I have developed and am collecting data on results of an entirely new approach to instability with stenosis;[13] that is, a method for drilling through the facet (11 mm diameter hole), decompressing the stenosing uncinate spur *through* the hole by impaction of the osteophyte, laying a small fat/fascia graft over the decompressed ganglion, and then driving a 12 mm diameter donor bone graft dowel into the hole. The facet is distracted first using a lamina spreader. The segment is decompressed and stabilized at the same time. A PLIT fusion may also be performed, if the spine has been highly unstable. This new procedure is showing excellent results.

REFERENCES

1. Bernick, S., and Caillet, R.: Vertebral endplate changes with aging of the human vertebrae, Spine **7**:97, 1982.
2. Burton, C.V.: How to avoid the "failed back surgery syndrome." In Cauthen, J.C., editor: Lumbar spine surgery, Baltimore, 1983, Williams & Wilkins.
3. Burton, C.V., et al.: Computed tomographic scanning and the lumbar spine. II. Clinical considerations, Spine **4**:356, 1979.
4. Cauthen, J.C.: Lumbar spine surgery, Baltimore, 1983, Williams & Wilkins.
5. Epstein, N.E., et al.: Degenerative spondylolisthesis with an intact neural arch: a review of 60 cases with an analysis of clinical findings and the development of surgical management, Neurosurgery **13**:555, 1983.
6. Heithoff, K.B., and Ray, C.D.: Principles of the computed tomographic assessment of lateral spinal stenosis. In Genant, H.K., et al., editors: Spine update 1984, San Francisco, 1983, Radiology Research & Education Foundation.
7. Kirkaldy-Willis W.H., et al.: Pathology and pathogenesis of lumbar spondylosis and stenosis, Spine **3**:319, 1978.
8. Pheasant, H.C., and Dyck, P.: Failed lumbar disc surgery: cause, assessment, treatment, Clin. Orthop. **164**:93, 1982.
9. Ray, C.D.: New techniques for decompression of lumbar spinal stenosis, Neurosurgery **10**:587, 1982.
10. Ray, C.D.: The paralateral approach to lumbar decompressions, (abstract 21-W), Proceedings of the annual meeting of the American Association of Neurological Surgery, Washington, D.C., April 1983.
11. Ray, C.D.: Lateral spinal decompression using the paralateral approach. In Watkins, R.G., editor: Principles and techniques of spine surgery, Rockville, Md., 1987, Aspen Press.
12. Ray, C.D., et al.: Lumbar lateral spinal stenosis: classification and etiology, Clin. Orthop. (In press) 1987.
13. Ray, C.D.: Transfacet decompression, facet dowel fixation, and PLIT fusion for lumbar lateral stenosis induced by instability, Clin. Orthop. (In press) 1987.
14. Semmes, R.E.: Ruptures of the lumbar intervertebral disc, Springfield, Ill., 1964, Charles C Thomas, Publisher.
15. Wiltse, L.L., et al.: Alar transverse process impingement of the L5 spinal nerve: the far-out syndrome, Spine **9**:31, 1984.

EDITORIAL COMMENTARY

Dr. Ray, in this chapter, makes a good case for doing lumbar fusions, even though this chapter is not about fusions. When a disc is removed, or a hypertrophic facet resected, what is going to keep future problems from developing? The collapse of the disc space, bulging of the annulus, and narrowing of the foramen are quite likely to create recurrent nerve root compression. Mechanical instability is also highly likely. If the pathology can be corrected and the segment held in a corrected position, future problems are much less likely to occur.

Dr. Ray states that his patients with isolated up-down stenosis do not have pain with hyperextension of the lumbar spine. We find that condition to be quite frequent, especially if the patient is held in an extended position for two or three minutes, as they develop increasing paraesthesia and leg pain.

Arthur H. White

CHAPTER

18

FAR LATERAL DECOMPRESSIONS FOR STENOSIS: THE PARALATERAL APPROACH TO THE LUMBAR SPINE

Charles D. Ray

Although most surgery of the lumbar spine utilizes a midline incision and approach, there are a number of important lesions best approached from a more lateral direction. The technique described here (referred to as a paralateral approach because it begins quite far from the midline, at an intermediate-lateral distance) has been successfully used in over 75 cases of far-lateral herniated intervertebral discs, lateral stenoses, or lateral osteophytes.[8,9] The indications for the approach procedure only include those cases having laterally placed lesions without significant additional lesions medial to the pedicle, as demonstrated on CT scans. Performing the procedure is relatively easy for most far lateral lesions above the fifth lumbar level, but it can be difficult, especially at first, at the L5-S1 level, particularly in cases that have high iliac crests (as is typical in most male patients).

Surgical approaches to lateral lesions have been used rather rarely in the past, that is, before the development of high-resolution CT scanning. The earlier radiologic techniques, plane, x-rays and myelography, are not useful for localizing most lateral lesions at or beyond the root sleeve or the ganglion.[1-6,14,15] CT scanning has also helped the surgeon to plan expeditious surgical approaches to these lateral lesions, for example, stenoses, herniated discs, disc bars, or spurs.[1-4,6,7,14] The Watkins paraspinal approach for posterolateral lumbar fusion was not intended to provide access to lateral lesions for decompressions.[16,17] Wiltse and others have modified the Watkins technique; Wiltse and coworkers[18] split the sacrospinalis muscle longitudinally to reach the lateral laminas, facets, and transverse processes.

The paralateral approach more completely preserves posterolateral structures, such as laminas, ligaments and facet joints, than does a midline approach to the same lesion. The newer approach requires small incisions, and the retractors are narrow (the force of retraction is also small). For these and other reasons, patients generally have much less postoperative complaint and leave the hospital sooner than they do after experiencing midline approaches to similar lesions. Bilateral paralateral approaches are clearly almost twice as difficult as unilateral approaches or as compared to exploring a second side through a midline incision. However, multilevel, single-side and bilateral paralateral approaches are reasonable procedures in selected cases. Since lateral stenoses are often bilateral, the choice between two paralateral or one midline approach depends on the clarity of the diagnosis, anticipated technical challenge, experience of the surgeon, and expected long-term stability of the decompressed segment. Such considerations are guided by the history, physical examination, and careful study of plane films, transaxial CT scans, and parasagittal reformatted images.* Parasagittal re-

*References 1, 2, 4, 6, 14, 15.

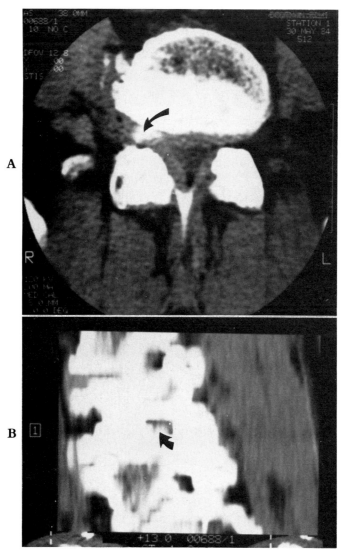

Fig. 18-1 **A,** Transaxial CT scan L4–L5 level; lateral stenosis from uncinate spur *(arrow).* **B,** Parasaggital reformatted image of **A,** showing up-down type lateral stenosis *(arrow)* caused by uncinate spur at L4–L5.

formatted images are almost essential to clarify the pathoanatomy. Sequential, parallel transaxial CT scans of 3 or 5 mm (or 5 mm slices with 2 or 3 mm overlap of the slices), are usually required. Reformatting then provides needed detail of the foraminae and exiting nerves (Fig. 18-1). Full-trunk (total body), cross-sectional scan images are also helpful for the study of muscle masses, fat deposits, fascial planes and ligaments, major vessels, and configuration of the iliac crests and sacroiliac structures (Fig. 18-2). Such slices are particularly valuable at the lum-

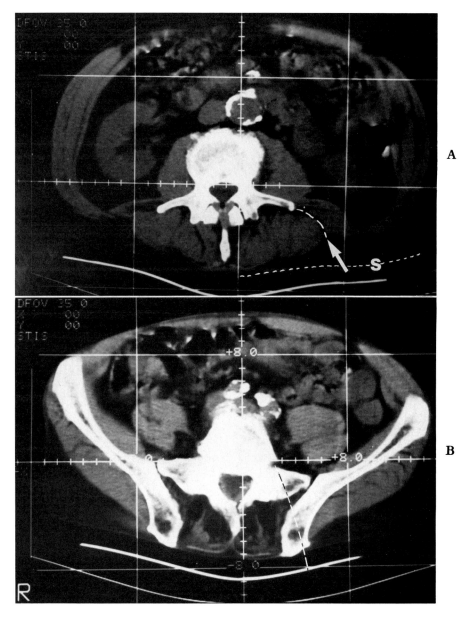

Fig. 18-2 **A,** Whole-body CT through L4 pedicles. Incision and path of dissection for paralateral approach are shown *(arrow and dashed line)* between quadratus lumborum and paraspinous muscles. Note that distance to lateral target from skin surface, *S,* is only slightly greater via paralateral approach than through midline. **B,** Whole-body CT at L5-S1 level. Portion of posterior iliac crest can be resected *(dashed line)* to gain improved access to paralateral target.

bosacral area, where access to the lesion and nerve may be hidden beneath the closely approximating transverse process of L5, the sacral ala, and the lateral facet and pedicle of S1. Portions of the iliac crest and the other structures mentioned immediately above might have to be resected along with overlying iliolumbar or iliotransverse ligaments to fully decompress a far laterally entrapped ganglion or lumbar spinal nerve. If the overall task is believed to be excessive, the surgeon may elect to approach the lesion by a posterior approach and prepare for a simultaneous fusion procedure.

PROCEDURAL CONSIDERATIONS

I believe that it is not only valuable but in many cases nearly essential to perform a paralateral approach while the patient is under local anesthesia with intravenous adjuncts (diazepam 5 to 15 mg and fentanyl 5 to 10 ml) or with a light epidural anesthesia using an indwelling microcatheter. In this way the patient can guide the surgeon (who is using a long 25-gauge exploring needle) to the nerve, often buried in a seeming mass of overlying muscle, ligament, bone, and scar tissue (in previously operated patients). Again, this is particularly true at the L5-S1 area. The patient is sufficiently awake so that he or she usually can clearly determine whether the nerve stimulated is the painful one, and yet there is little major discomfort (or memory of any). If the surgeon is unfamiliar with the use of "local and vocal" anesthesia or the patient is not suitable, then an insulated stimulating needle can be helpful to identify the nerve.* Of course, in the generally anesthetized patient stimulation only indicates the location of the motor portion of the nerve and does not demonstrate whether the particular nerve is the source of the clinical problem. This is especially true in cases of multilevel stenosis. In many cases it is wise to perform specific

---

*Neuro-Trace System for intraoperative nerve location, HDC Corporation, Mountain View, Calif.

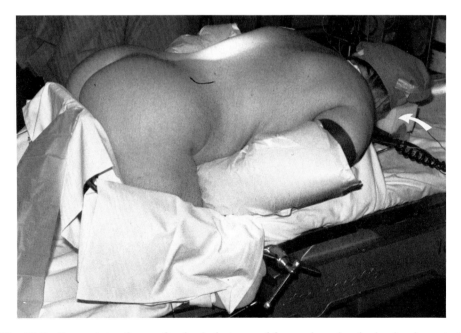

Fig. 18-3 Prone-sitting frame of author's design used for paralateral and other lumbar spinal surgical cases. Patient is face down on special forehead/chin rest *(white arrow)*, adjustable to permit normal lordosis of the neck. The paralateral incision is indicated.

root or ganglion injections under fluoroscopic control at some time before the surgery using 0.5 ml 0.25% bupivicaine to identify the exact symptomatic level.

Patients are usually operated on while they are in a prone-sitting position (Fig. 18-3). One should avoid extreme flexion of the thighs and spine, as with the tuck position, so that the paraspinous muscles are not drawn too tightly, otherwise retraction can be more difficult.[12] This is particularly notable with muscular males. I have developed a new prone-sitting frame for lumbar surgery particularly suitable for this and other types of decompression. The patient's lumbar spine is slightly hyperextended (abdomen hanging free), which greatly facilitates paraspinous muscular relaxation. If such a prone-sitting frame meeting these requirements is not available, the patient can be placed on a standard laminectomy frame.

Since exact location of the lesion level is absolutely essential, several methods for preoperative marking of the target have been tried but none is considered sufficiently reliable. An injection of 0.1 ml of isosulfan blue dye for lymphography (Lymphazurin 1%)* within 8 hours of the procedure into the skin overlying the x-ray image of the tip of the transverse process at the level to be explored may help placement of the incision but it is not reliable for target identification in the depths. Injection of a marker substance into a deep structure such as the transverse process itself has not proved useful. On plane lumbar films individual transverse processes usually show distinct characteristics (size, shape, spacing); with experience, the L5-S1 and L4-L5 levels can usually be easily identified by an exploring finger in the wound, searching for these characteristics.

Paralateral exposures require small incisions, usually 5 to 8 cm in length. The lateral placement is determined by measurement on the full body scan, extrapolating this to the patient's skin or by palpation for the junction of the spinal erectors with the quadratus lumborum. Once within the subcutaneous fat layer, a free fat graft of about 15 cc is taken; excess fat harvesting may result in a pocket that is difficult to close later. The fat graft is important to help prevent or reduce postoperative fibrosis around nerve and dura. One clears away the tissue overlying the deep fascia, at the valley between the muscle masses, and then cuts through this fascia with an electric hot-knife. If approaching the L5-S1 level, the fascia is detached from the iliac crest, saving enough of the muscular insertion to facilitate reattachment at the end of the procedure. If need be, portions of the iliac crest are cut off with a sharp, broad osteotome, and the bone is waxed. An exploring finger or thumb is slipped through the muscle layers to palpate and find the tip of the transverse processes. The exact anatomic level to be approached should now be clearly identified; if not, a cross-table lateral x-ray film at the operating table must be made using a metal marker inserted in the surgical wound.

At this point an operating microscope may be brought into use with a 250 or 300 mm working objective. Alternatively, surgical telescopes with a fiber-optic headlight may be employed; the procedure is usually faster with telescopes than with the microscope, since the set-up and maneuvering times are eliminated, but an assistant will not see the field very well. Usually a surgical assistant is not used, however.

Muscles are bluntly dissected off the transverse process (usually with some bleeding) and facet capsule using a large Cobb elevator. A modified two-toothed, malleable Taylor-like (Raylor)* retractor

---

*Hirsch Industries, Inc., Richmond, Va.

*CeDaR Surgical, Inc., Minnetonka, Minn.

is passed over the medial aspect of the facet and attached to a gauze strip passed off the opposite side of the operating table and lightly weighted (1 or 2 kg).[10] By and large, dissection to the target is simple digital separation of muscle fibers. A second Raylor, having a short, sharp, upwards curving spike at the tip, may be passed ventral to the transverse process and weighted externally. These two retractors usually provide adequate visual access to the deep target. In smaller patients a long double-bladed Scoville retractor may be placed in the wound and opened. In any case, the retraction is gentle.

One then begins the decompression by resecting along the inferior aspect of the superior pedicle or transverse process using an osteotome or a hot-knife (electrocautery pencil). In the depths of the small exposure dissection at the target level can be rather difficult but only for reasons of uncertainty as to the exact location of the nerve. This is the major advantage of local anesthesia, as mentioned above. Sometimes the most helpful structure that can be used to lead one to the ganglion is the neurovascular stalk, a medusa of small structures associated with the origin of the posterior primary division just at the distal portion of the ganglion. This medusa can bleed with conviction when cut and is usually the only such structure in the neighborhood to do so. One should also be on alert for branches of the segmental artery. Fig. 18-4 is a representation of the important anatomic elements as they lie within and lateral to a neural foramen. In the usual case all of these structures will be found and identified.

One must learn the appearance of iliolumbar ligaments and not be overly slowed by their dissection. The L5-S1 level procedures are particularly challenging because of the relative strangeness of the lateral anatomy, the limited exposure, and the deep dissection. One certainly does not have the impression of working in the "old, familiar" lumbar spine. The surgeon might well spend time in the anatomy laboratory before beginning to use this approach. The most challenging details occur while fully exposing and decompressing the course of the L5 nerve as it passes around the inferior aspect of its pedicle and descends into the pre-alar, medial pre-sacral, space. It is often best to burr away bone and ap-

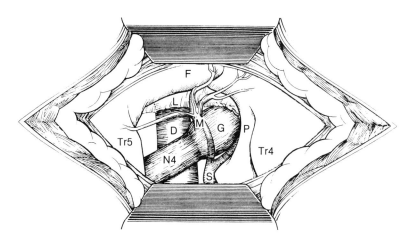

Fig. 18-4 Diagram of paralateral approach, right L4-L5 level. L4 to L5 disc margin, *D;* superior facet of L5, *F;* ganglion of L4, *G;* ligamentum flavum, *L;* neurovascular medusa of L4 posterior primary nerve branch, *M;* L4 nerve, *N4;* pedicle of L4, *P;* segmental artery, *S;* and the transverse processes of L4, *Tr4,* and L5, *Tr5.*

proach the nerve from its cephalad, caudad, or more medial aspect. The CT scan images should be at hand for continuous reference.

The usual bone-cutting instruments are employed, but they must be quite sharp, and somewhat longer and smaller than those ordinarily used with standard midline decompressions. Very little soft tissue or bone is removed, therefore one preserves the posterior supporting structures, mentioned earlier as a most important reason for this approach, especially where instability may likely become a problem if a more radical midline-posterior approach with extensive resection were to be used.

When the target level has been well identified and one has the appropriate surgical instruments, decompressions (especially those at or above the L4-L5 level) are usually rather straightforward and nearly bloodless.

ADDITIONAL CONSIDERATIONS

At L5-S1 and occasionally at L4-L5, a large, round iliolumbar ligament may be found overlying the nerve (Fig. 18-5). Such ligaments can participate in lateral entrapment of the ganglion or nerve. This may also happen at the L4 level or above with a particularly well-developed intertransverse process ligament.

Far lateral removal of disc fragments and a clean-out of the disc space may be slightly more difficult than the more familiar ones removed via a midline approach. On the other hand, free fragments have been found that virtually jumped out from between lateral muscle septae when approached and the muscles retracted. Since far-lateral herniations are nearly always missed except through the use of CT scanning, many of the herniations (usually at L3-L4) are of longer clinical duration with adhesions, and the nerve may well be swollen and tightly adherent over the disc space. Therefore it is not uncommon for postoperative symptoms to be somewhat slow to resolve. In the case of lateral osteophytes or uncinate spurs, most of them can be impacted (driven inward) through the use of special flat drift punches.[11] As discussed previously, the dissection often proceeds best by hollowing out cancellous portions of bone with an air turbine, cutting deep to a stenosing spur or other hypertrophic structure, and then collapsing the

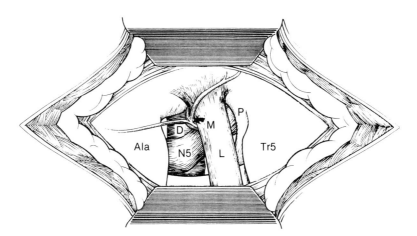

Fig. 18-5 Diagram of approach to the right L5-S1 space. L5 nerve, *N5*, and ganglion are trapped between lateral disc bar, *D*, or spur and an iliolumbar ligament, *L*. (See Fig. 18-7.) Posterior primary neurovascular bundle, or medusa, *M*, is displaced caudad around ligament. Also indicated are pedicle, *P*, and transverse process of L5, *Tr5*, and sacral ala.

remaining shell of the offending spur or cortical bone—using small curettes or the impactors—away from the nerve or ganglion.

Closed drainage is generally used for 24 hours to remove any delayed oozing of blood that may occur from the fat donor area, cut-muscle bundles or bone surfaces. Tamponade of bleeding is less easily achieved in the soft, lateral tissue spaces than between the tough ligamentous and muscular layers as found at the lumbar midline. The extradural instillation of morphine via an indwelling microcatheter is almost routinely used for postoperative pain control.[13] Morphine (4 mg) without preservative plus 5 ml of 0.5% bupivacaine (Marcaine) is instilled at the time of closing the wound. Very often patients require little or no additional narcotic except for a few oral doses. There is remarkably little postoperative pain in the typical case, and much less nursing care is required. In addition, the hospital stay is 1 to 3 days shorter, especially where local anesthesia has been employed, than with the usual midline case. Patients have generally returned to regular activities earlier than have comparable patients operated on by an appropriately more destructive midline approach.

In Figs. 18-6, 18-7, and 18-8 a few typical preoperative and postoperative scans are shown that demonstrate paralateral decompressions with rather minimal removal of segments of bone, ligaments, and other structures. The placement of fat grafts is also shown.

In general, this technique has served its intended purpose of providing a direct approach to the lesion with sparing of posterior stabilizing lumbar structures. Clearly, the paralateral approach is anatomically more appropriate to the lesion size and location than is the usual midline approach to an equivalent lesion. In the first 50 cases that I operated on using this approach, 35 (68%) had good to excellent results, 10 (20%) had minimal improvement, and 6 (12%) had no improvement. Most of the latter cases had nerve degeneration and fibrosis. No cases were rated as worse by the individual examiners (or the patients themselves) during follow-up visits. Postoperative follow-up time varied from 0 to 32 months (mean, 5.8 months). Five cases (10%) required additional surgery in some way related to the original problem; in most of these the decompression had been less than optimal (see box). The majority of the 50 cases (except those with herniated discs) had rather difficult and long-standing stenotic problems; this contributed to a somewhat lower percentage of good-to-excellent results than might have been anticipated if the cases had decompressions with fusions via midline approaches. It is expected that these numbers will improve with the evolution of new instruments and greater experience. It is fair to conclude that, in most of the cases selected for the paralateral approach, decompression without destabilization can be achieved. This might not have been so if the same lesion were approached using a standard midline technique with a more extensive removal of posterior supporting structures. The approach can be clinically and professionally rewarding, although it often presents a significant technical challenge to the surgeon.

ACKNOWLEDGMENTS

I have developed a prone-sitting surgical frame, special retractors, dissectors, small osteotomes, and cortical bone impactors now used with this and other procedures for decompressive surgery of lateral spinal stenosis,[10-12] available from CeDaR Surgical, Inc., Minnetonka, Minn. I wish to express my appreciation for the CT scanning assistance shown by Drs. Kenneth Heithoff and James Moyle; also for technical work on the images performed by Ms. Barbara Hess RT(R), Department of CT Imaging, Abbott-Northwestern Hospital, Minneapolis, Minn. Photographs were made by David Pickop and Kevin Gracie; graphic assistance provided by Bob Doig and Christie Marlene Ray.

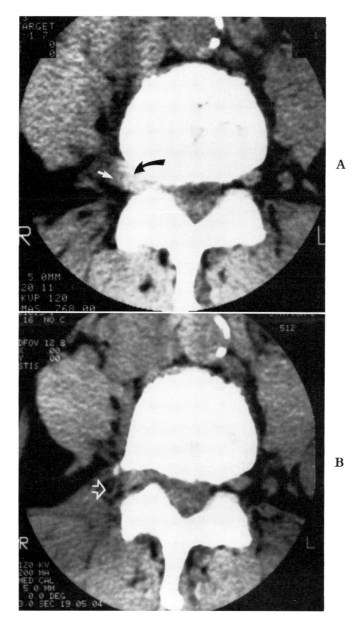

Fig. 18-6 **A,** Preoperative CT scans, and **B,** postoperative CT scans of far lateral extruded disc *(long arrow)* at right L4–L5 space elevating and compressing nerve *(short arrow).* Small fat graft is indicated *(open arrow).*

184 Surgical Procedures

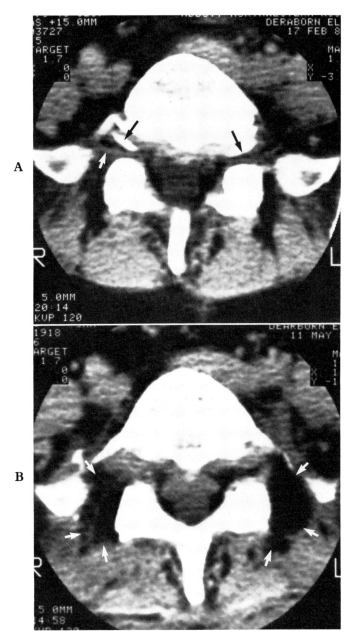

Fig. 18-7 CT scans of bilateral disc spurs with lateral stenosis and an entrapment of the L5 roots beneath tight iliolumbar ligaments. **A,** Preoperative scan at L5 showing bilateral stenosis and spurs *(black arrows)*. Portion of constricting iliolumbar ligament is best seen on right *(white arrow)*. (See also Fig. 18-5.) **B,** Postoperative scan showing wide bilateral paralateral decompression of spurs, resection of medial portions of sacral alae and fat grafts *(white arrows)* dorsal to the decompressed L5 nerves.

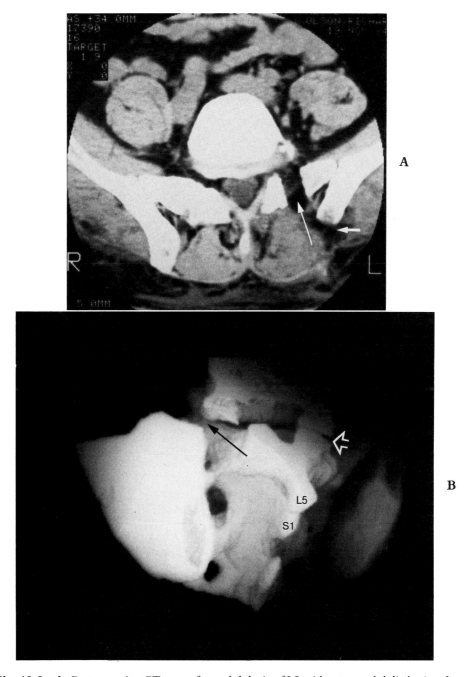

Fig. 18-8 A, Postoperative CT scan of spondylolysis of L5 without spondylolisthesis, after paralateral decompression. Portion of left iliac crest *(short arrow)* has been resected to permit improved approach *(long arrow)* to stenosis. **B,** Postoperative "three-dimensional" reconstruction of **A.** L5 and S1 spinous processes are marked; view is slightly from left, and direction of paralateral approach is indicated *(long black arrow)*. Pars defect is clearly indicated *(open arrow)*. (Courtesy Drs. Kenneth Heithoff and James Moyle; technical work on the images by Ms. Barbara Hess RT(R), Dept. of CT Imaging, Abbott-Northwestern Hospital, Minneapolis, Minn.)

> **Paralateral approach to lumbar decompressions***
>
> Summary: 50 cases; 23 females, 27 males; age range, 29 to 75 years; average age 51.3 years.
>
> Levels: L3-L4, 13 cases (10 discs, 5 stenoses)
> L4-L5, 24 cases (12 discs, 13 stenoses; 5 also spondylolistheses)
> L5-S1, 26 cases (2 disc, 24 stenoses; 8 also spondylolistheses)
> (11 cases had a second level decompression; 10 cases, bilateral)
>
> Results: 34 (68%) cases had good to excellent results.
> 10 (20%) cases had minimal improvement.
> 6 (12%) cases had no improvement (fibrotic nerves).
> No cases were worsened.
>
> Follow-up: range, 0 to 31 months; average, 14 months (April 1985).
>
> *All cases diagnosed by clinical picture and CT spine scanning; 12 cases also had direct injection of the involved nerve (or ganglion) using 0.2 to 1 ml 0.25% Marcaine as a screening technique.

REFERENCES

1. Burton, C.V., et al.: Computed tomographic scanning and the lumbar spine. II. Clinical considerations, Spine **4:**356, 1979.
2. Glenn, W.V., et al.: Multiplanar display computerized body tomography applications in the lumbar spine, Spine **4:**282, 1979.
3. Godersky, J.C., et al.: Extreme lateral disc herniation: diagnosis by computed tomographic scanning, Neurosurgery **14:**549, 1984.
4. Heithoff, K.B., and Ray, C.D.: Principles of the computed tomographic assessment of lateral spinal stenosis. In Genant, H.K., et al., editors: Spine update 1984. San Francisco 1983, Radiology Research Education Foundation.
5. Kirkaldy-Willis, W.H., et al.: Pathology and pathogenesis of lumbar spondylosis and stenosis, Spine **3:**319, 1978.
6. Lifson, A., et al.: High-resolution computed tomography scan of lumbosacral spine. In Contrast media in computed tomography, Amsterdam, 1981, Exerpta Medica.
7. Ray, C.D.: New techniques for decompression of lumbar spinal stenosis, Neurosurgery **10:**587, 1982.
8. Ray, C.D.: The paralateral approach to lumbar decompressions, (abstract 21-W), Proceedings of the annual meeting of the American Association of Neurological Surgery, Washington, D.C., April 1983.
9. Ray, C.D.: Lateral spinal decompression using the paralateral approach. In Watkins, R.G., editor: Principles and techniques of spine surgery, Rockville, Md., 1987, Aspen Press.
10. Ray, C.D.: New malleable, force-fulcrum retractors for lumbar spinal surgery: technical note, Spine (In Press), 1987.
11. Ray, C.D.: Bone impactors: new instruments for spinal decompression: technical note, Spine (In Press), 1987.
12. Ray, C.D.: A new kneeling attachment frame system for spinal surgery, Neurosurg. (In press), 1987.
13. Ray, C.D., and Bagley, R.: Indwelling epidural morphine for control of post lumbar surgery pain, Neurosurgery **13:**388, 1983.
14. Ray, C.D., and Heithoff, K.B.: Techniques for decompression of lumbar spinal stenosis "guided" by high-resolution CT scans, Mod. Neurosurg. **1:**31, 1982.
15. Ray, C.D., et al.: Lumbar lateral spinal stenosis: classification and etiology, Clin. Orthop. (In press), 1987.
16. Watkins, M.B.: Posterolateral fusion of the lumbar and lumbosacral spine, J. Bone Joint Surg. **35A:**1014, 1953.
17. Watkins, M.B.: Posterolateral fusion in pseudarthrosis and posterior element defects of the lumbosacral spine, Clin. Orthp. **35:**80, 1964.
18. Wiltse, L.L., et al.: The paraspinal sacrospinalis-splitting approach to the lumbar spine, J. Bone Joint Surg. **50A:**919, 1968.

CHAPTER 19

FAILED POSTERIOR SPINE SURGERY

Arthur H. White   Ken Hsu

The perfectly selected spine surgery patient who receives the absolutely appropriate surgery, which is perfectly performed in a total-care setting, has an excellent (95%) probability of returning to "normal."

Unfortunately, such perfection is seldom present. For every patient that we have of a classic nature there are myriads of patients with low back pain without classic symptoms. We do not all have ideal diagnostic and rehabilitation capabilities. Our surgeries are frequently done by one surgeon without an entire multidisciplinary team.

What are we to do with all of the patients that we are not absolutely certain we can help with surgery? Are they simply relegated to decreased activity and a changing of their jobs? At what point can we give a patient hope of continuing his or her current occupation through surgery? How important is it in our society to allow individuals to continue an active athletic existence?

DISCUSSION

Spine surgery frequently fails because we have failed to appreciate some aspect of the case. Before the advent of CT scans we failed to recognize lateral herniated discs and lateral spinal stenosis. When we don't do discograms we fail to recognize internal disc disruption and degeneration at the levels adjacent to our fusions. We do not have a good method of determining which laminectomy patients are going to suffer postoperative instability of a symptomatic nature. We fail to recognize which patients have low pain tolerance and high psychologic involvement. We fail in our successes because of our lack of rehabilitation.

There are some failures that seem unavoidable. Arachnoiditis and epidural fibrosis are examples. Internal fixation occasionally fails. Normal discs at adjacent levels to fusions can also fail. Patients who seem to be psychologically stable and strong can convert to drug addicts and chronic pain patients after surgery. Most of these failures, however, can be avoided by thorough preoperative multidisciplinary evaluation; by doing the surgery as one step in the rehabilitation process; and by using all of the diagnostic tools available to us to make an accurate diagnosis and arrive at the surgical procedure that has the highest possibility of success.

In diagnosing low back pain once a spinal surgery has failed to give success, the "water becomes muddy." It is harder to rehabilitate patients in the face of pain. It is harder to sort out the psychologic subjective symptoms from the organic physical symptoms. The surgery is more difficult to perform and more fraught with complications such as dural tears, instability, and arachnoiditis.

The process of evaluation for the failed surgical patient should be a multidisciplinary one. There is no one professional who has all of the skills of psychology, surgery, rehabilitation, pain control, and diagnostic testing.

The worst person to make the decision on reoperating in a failed surgery case is probably the surgeon who did the first surgery. He or she has "blinders on," wants to correct the failure, and has an ego that is too involved to make a totally objective, clear decision. He or she may be part of the team who makes the decision but should rarely make the decision alone.

The more diagnostic tests that point to a single accurate diagnosis, the more likely we are going to have a success with a specific surgery. If the patient's history and physical examination are consistent with a herniated disc, the EMG is positive, and the myelogram or CT scan are positive, we are probably on the right track. If the patient responds appropriately to the diagnostic blocks and is psychologically stable in psychologic testing, we have an even greater likelihood of success. If we add to all the preceding a good conservative-care program to which the patient responds appropriately but does not become cured, we have done just about all that we can do to verify the diagnosis. We have exhausted anything aside from surgery that might make the patient better. If these precepts hold for a primary surgery, they become doubly important in failed spinal surgery patients.

Diagnostic tests become more difficult to interpret when the patient has had previous surgery. It is hard to differentiate on myelogram new disc disease from scar tissue. It is similarly difficult with CT scans, but with the use of myelographic contrast material or intravenous contrast material, scar tissue can be better differentiated. The advent of the MRI may give us even better tools for differentiation of scar tissue from disc and neural tissue. The EMG is able in many instances to differentiate new from old neurologic involvement. The diagnostic blocks are hard to interpret because of uneven flow of injected material and difficulty of placing needles around fusions and areas of scar tissue. However, with persistence and multidisciplinary evaluation in an inpatient setting a probable diagnosis and decision for or against surgery can be made with accuracy.

The rehabilitative efforts in the failed back surgery patient takes much more time and effort. It has to be accepted by those paying the bills that time and money spent on physical and psychologic rehabilitation before reoperating on a failed surgery patient is well spent. Without such rehabilitation efforts the second, third, and fourth surgery would usually fail.

As with all spine surgery there is no one technical procedure that will work on the failed spine case. There are some general guidelines, however. Broader decompressions will usually be performed because of the frequency of postoperative spinal stenosis. Fusions will frequently be added because of the possibility of pain being caused by the instability from many or wide decompressive laminectomies. Internal fixation will frequently be used because of the need for additional stabilization in the face of deconditioning, obesity, weakness, and osteoporosis.

If one can be absolutely certain of the source of the pain from failed spinal surgery, a smaller surgery with a more direct approach can be used. As stated previously, however, it is hard to determine with absolute certainty that the patient's pain is coming from a certain area of spinal stenosis or recurrent herniated disc. We cannot be certain that there is not instability pain, facet joint pain from the same level, or degenerative disc pain from the level above a recurrent herniated disc. Therefore we are more prone on "redo operations" to do more rather than less, to be more stable than less stable, and to deal with all sources of pain rather than take the risk that there will be anything left undone to explain pain that continues after this "last surgery."

As many as 30% of laminectomy surgeries fail because of spinal stenosis or recurrent herniated disc. In our spine center nearly every failed spine surgery patient that we see has some degree of significant spinal stenosis or recurrent herniated disc material adjacent to copious amounts of scar tissue. In patients whose first surgical laminectomy was accompanied by a fusion, only 8% of the patients develop postoperative stenosis or recurrent herniated disc. Therefore it may be reasonable, at least from a statistical standpoint, to do a fusion at the time of the first surgery. It is even more reasonable to do a fusion at the time of a second surgery. The second surgery requires more bony decompression and therefore a higher risk of instability. In planning for failed spine surgery patients, we therefore almost always plan to do some form of fusion. We first give our attention to the areas of spinal stenosis that usually require a complete facetectomy on at least one side. To visualize and remove a recurrent herniated disc it is necessary to remove bone lateral to the previous decompression to get into a normal tissue plane and then retract the nerve root and scar tissue to visualize the disc.

Thus the technique to be described next is one for decompressive laminectomy, foramenotomy, and recurrent herniated disc removal. We routinely do a fusion after this procedure. The type of fusion again depends on many factors. If there is gross instability or great concern about stability, we will use pedicle screws and Steffee plates. If there is minimal concern for stability and we are only working with one level, a simple intertransverse fusion may be adequate. Between these two extremes of fusion stabilizing procedures lie the Knodt rods and Harrington rods with variable amounts of intersegmental wiring. Anterior interbody fusions are done if there is no significant pathologic finding in the vertebral canal.

TECHNIQUE

A midline incision is made through or excising the old scar. This is carried down to a safe (5 mm) distance from the dura as gauged by the exposure of the adjacent lamina. Soft tissue dissection is then carried laterally at this safe level, leaving several millimeters of scar tissue or fat overlying the dura (Fig. 19-1). This soft tissue is removed from the facet joints and then the same plane is carried to the transverse processes of the levels to be fused (Fig. 19-2). This gives a wide exposure of the full width of the dura, facet joints, and transverse processes. The bone remaining on the lamina and facet joints is totally cleared of all soft tissue, and the plane of attachment of the epidural scar to the facet joint or lamina is clearly defined. It is rarely easy to dissect the plane between the dura and posterior elements. This is usually scarred severely (Figs. 19-3, 19-4, and 19-5), and blunt or sharp dissection in this area results in dural tears or nerve root injury. Therefore we use a chisel to remove laterally approximately 1 cm of what is left of the lamina, facet joint, or pars interarticularis that can then be retracted medially (Figs.

190 *Surgical Procedures*

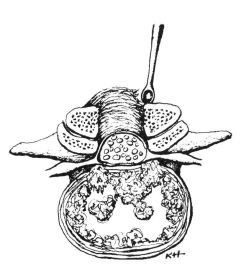

Fig. 19-1 Scar tissue overlying dura at previous laminectomy site.

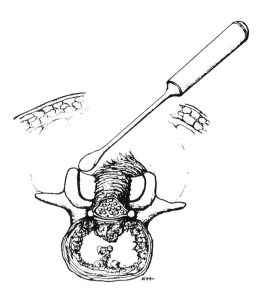

Fig. 19-2 Scar tissue removed from facet joints and transverse processes with periosteal elevator.

Fig. 19-3 Epidural scar encroaching laminectomy site and intervertebral foramen.

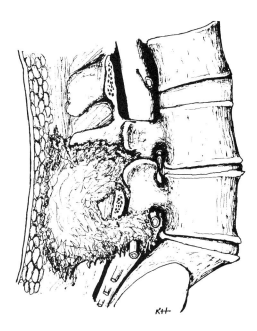

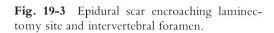

Fig. 19-4 Developing plane between scar tissue and facet with sharp curette.

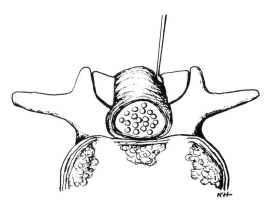

Fig. 19-5 Blunt dissection of plane between dura and facet.

19-6 and 19-7). Once this bone has been separated from the remainder of the posterior elements, it can usually be dissected free without damaging the dura (Figs. 19-8, and 19-9). Under this removed bone we find a nerve root with normal tissue planes (Fig. 19-10). We can then complete our foramenotomy adjacent to this route throughout its course. If the next level is to be explored, we then follow the dura around the pedicle to the next spinal nerve and similarly perform a foramenotomy there. This same technique is done bilaterally.

At this point the spinal nerve is frequently found to be adhered rather densely to the underlying recurrent herniated disc. It is again very hard to retract the nerve from this dense scar tissue, but an attempt is made to do so. If this is resulting in too much trauma to the root, no further attempt is made to create a plane. The disc is then entered lateral to the nerve, and disc material is removed from under the root from within the disc (Fig. 19-11). Down-cutting curettes are helpful in this situation (Fig. 19-12). The same procedure is done from the opposite side, which has frequently not had previous surgery and therefore is much easier. On both sides the disc is followed laterally and removed at its most lateral extent in

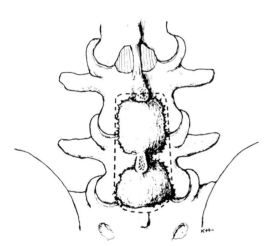

Fig. 19-6 Area of bone to be removed around previous laminectomy sites.

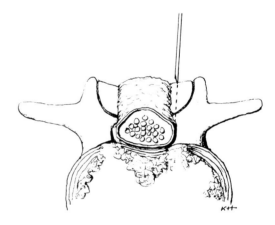

Fig. 19-7 Chisel being used to create new plane lateral to scar tissue.

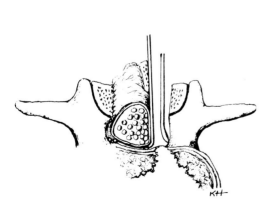

Fig. 19-8 New plane of dissection bluntly developed as dura is retracted.

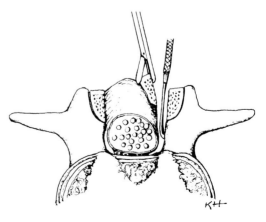

Fig. 19-9 Adherent bone fragment used for traction as new plane is bluntly developed.

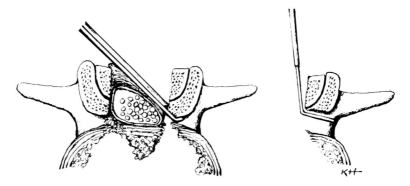

Fig. 19-10 Lateral recess and intervertebral foramen enlarged and probed.

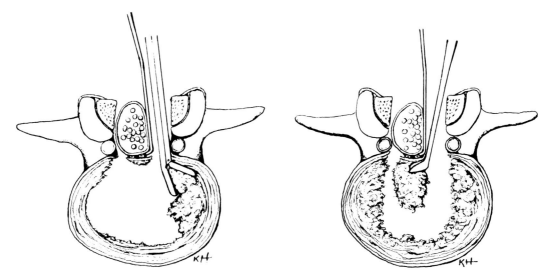

Fig. 19-11 Disc material removed with pituitary ronguer.

Fig. 19-12 Down-facing curette used to free disc fragments for removal.

the intervertebral foramen, visualizing and assuring that the next most proximal nerve adjacent to the disc is not in any way entrapped or in danger of being entrapped with further collapse of the disc space.

All possibly involved spinal nerves now lie free of any external compression from disc, scar tissue, or bony impingement. If there is any question about the integrity of an adjacent disc level, it too is exposed and evaluated by direct observation and palpation with a blunt dissector. Any abnormality found is corrected, and then a decision is made as to whether that level needs to be fused. All available preoperative information is used in making this decision, including the CT scan, discogram, and flexion-extension views, as well as the surgical findings.

By this time at least one inferior facet and one half of a superior facet has been removed to allow adequate visualization of the nerve root as it passes through the intervertebral foramen. Frequently, multiple levels at both sides have been similarly decompressed. The likelihood of future instability, future collapse of disc spaces, fractures of the remaining facets and pars interarticularis, and recurrent herniated discs are so probable that fusion must now be considered. The type of fusion will depend on (1) the needs for further distraction by the use of Knodt rods or Harrington rods, (2) the presence of lamina to which could be attached interlaminar wires, (3) the need for immediate and rigid fixation with pedicle screws and plates or (4) the adequate exposure to do an interody fusion. In cases where no immediate instability is suspected, but when there is some concern that progressive instability or stenosis will redevelop over a long period of time, a simple intertransverse fusion may be entertained. The techniques for these various fusions have been described extensively in other chapters in this book.

There are many variations on the technique for surgery on the failed surgery patient, and there are innumerable complications to this type of surgery. These surgeries take much longer than routine first operations. Infection rates are higher, and the risk increases with the use of internal fixation. Tears in the dura occur at least one time in ten of these "redo operations" and in some series as often as every other case. With the dural tears come the complications of postoperative pseudomeningiocole, cerebral spinal fluid fistulas, and potential meningitis. Each form of internal fixation carries with it its own complications. Sacral Harrington and Knodt hooks can irritate the S1 or S2 nerve roots and can even break through the S1 lamina in osteoporotic patients. Alar hooks can irritate the L5 spinal nerve, which passes in close proximity. Proximal hooks can produce spinal stenosis and symptoms at the upper end of the fusion. Pedicle screws can break the pedicle on insertion, can work free, can cause late fractures of the pedicle, or cause fracture of the screw with loosening of the plate.

The extensive dissection and exposure of the dura leads to copious amounts of postoperative epidural fibrosis. The trauma of multiple myelograms and surgery can also lead to arachnoiditis. With the removal of major portions of the posterior elements, bone graft placed over the transverse process can migrate or "grow" into the vertebral canal or over decompressed nerve roots. Most of these complications can be avoided by anticipating their advent. Having a well-coordinated surgical team that has done this type of surgery many times before, together with all of the equipment available to change procedures at any time during the surgery, can keep complications to a minimum.

The results of redo surgery on failed spine surgery ranges from 50% to 80%, depending on the nature of the underlying disease. It is well known that the success with surgery drops rapidly with each additional surgical attempt. The ultimate aim in many of these complex cases is not to return a patient to normal, but simply to get them out of bed. These complex patients usually have combinations of diseases—including osteoporosis, obesity, and spinal stenosis—and have had several operations. They have become so deconditioned that they are virtually house- or bed-bound. Expecting these patients to return to normal activity is feasible. With a multidisciplinary approach and surgery as described with multilevel decompression and internal fixation, we are able to return 80% of them to ambulatory status.

Some spine surgeons are finding it necessary to do both anterior and posterior surgery on these complicated reoperation patients. An anterior interbody fusion may be enough in some cases to stabilize a spine that does not have too severe a stenosis or herniated disc problem in the vertebral canal. If the anterior stabilization is not adequate, then a posterior decompression and further fusion may be necessary. Some surgeons do both the anterior and posterior procedure at the same sitting or within a week of each other. At our spine center we are finding that a single surgery is adequate posteriorly with the newer forms of internal fixation of pedicle screws and plates. If fusion is not accomplished or a screw breaks and pseudarthrosis develops, a further posterior surgery can be performed or an anterior procedure could then be done at the one level that seems to be symptomatic. It is not unusual in these complex cases with multiple etiologies to have to do additional procedures if the internal fixation becomes loose or the disease becomes symptomatic at the next most-proximal segment.

If the next level above a fusion becomes painful, it is one of our most frustrating and perplexing problems. Despite the use of discograms preoperatively and extensive use of back school, the segment adjacent to a multilevel fusion all too frequently becomes painful. This pain seems to emanate from degenerative segment disease caused by the rigid immediate fusion with internal fixation that creates a large stressful lever arm.

When the level next most-proximal to a fusion begins the degenerative process, various symptoms can arise. Pain is frequently referred from these areas to the sacroiliac region. Frequently, however, pain is also referred anteriorly into the lower abdomen, groin, or upper thigh. Tenderness, hypersensitivity, or referred pain can be elicited by palpation or heavy percussion over the involved area. Relief of signs and symptoms can be created by a high lumbar epidural block or selective nerve root block in the area of involvement. Sometimes facet blocks will give relief of pain. A discogram at this newly involved level usually will be positive. A CT scan demonstrates the hypertrophic facet changes, bulging or herniated discs, and spinal stenosis. An EMG may become abnormal.

When the clinical picture is unquestionable, the appropriate tests are positive, and the patient has not responded to conservative care, surgery may be necessary. In such a case the biomechanic factors are more complicated than when there has been no previous fusion. With this situation the increased lever arm of forces makes fusion of that level more difficult to produce. Internal stabilization is helpful. The fixation can be as simple as using a Knodt rod between the L3 lamina and the upper end of the fusion mass. A hook site can be created in the previous bone fusion mass without difficulty. This is not as stable as placing a hook beneath the lamina of S1. Further stability can be obtained by using a wire passed through the fusion mass and around the lower hook.

Decompression of the next level in question usually requires considerable resection of the facet joints and their hypertrophic synovium and capsule. The ligamentum flavum often is hypertrophied or buckled. The disc is usually protruding. The nerve roots are traced out into the intervertebral foramen and under the previous fusion. Stabilization is accomplished with whatever internal fixation is necessary. There is, of course, still the great problem of loss of lumbar lordosis. If previous lordosis had been lost at lower levels and now may be lost at a new level, it would be wise to maintain the lordosis with some other form of fixation. Steffee plates are an ideal method of maintaining lordosis. Screws are placed through the fusion mass at the level of the pedicle and then at the next level to be fused. The plates are fashioned to maintain the lordosis. Special screws are necessary to angle into the pedicle in such a way as to not violate the next level above the one to be fused. The Wiltse pedicle screw fixation device, the Edwards modular system, and Frymoyer's Vermont internal fixator may also be equally usable in this situation.

CHAPTER

20

DISC HERNIATIONS LATERAL TO THE INTERVERTEBRAL FORAMEN

Michael R. Zindrick   Leon L. Wiltse   Wolfgang Rauschning

Since the classic description of Mixter and Barr,[21] intervertebral disc herniaton posteriorly into the central vertebral canal and subsequent neural compression has been a well recognized cause of low back pain and sciatica. However, decades of failed back surgery and persistent pain testify to the myriad of other causes of similar symptoms that can exist in the face of a normal myelogram.[18,19,22,26] Dandy[5] recognized almost 50 years ago that symptomatic disc herniations could be "concealed" from conventional myelography. MacNab[18] described the "hidden zone" lateral to the dural sac extending under the facet joints and into the foramen as being a potential location of unseen pathologic conditions. With further refinement of our diagnostic radiographic skills and better understanding of pathologic conditions of the low back, many other causes of neural compression have subsequently been identified.*

Although it was not well recognized before the routine use of the CT scanner, disc herniations lateral to the intervertebral foramen can compress the nerve root ganglion and the spinal nerve, causing symptoms and findings similar to classic central vertebral canal pathology.[1,25] Multiple terms have been used to describe this entity: the lateral disc, the far lateral disc, the posterior lateral disc, the extreme lateral disc, and the extraforaminal disc.† Often these terms are used interchangeably to describe disc herniations that occur laterally within the cen-

---

Supported by research grant no. 517-84, Long Beach Memorial Hospital Medical Center, Long Beach, Calif.

*References 9, 11-14, 16, 17, 19, 20, 26.
†References 1, 2, 6, 9, 11, 14, 16, 17, 19, 20, 22, 24, 26.

tral vertebral canal, within the foramen, and laterally beyond the lateral border of the intervertebral neural foramen.

This chapter discusses disc herniation existing lateral to the intervertebral foramen with or without medial extension into the foramen. The anatomy, pathology, classification, and clinical and radiographic findings of disc herniations lateral to the intervertebral foramen are discussed and treatment options are described.

ANATOMY

The intervertebal foramen, or nerve root canal, is a true three-dimensional cylindric structure with an entrance and exit. The width of the canal is determined by the pedicles that form the cephalad and caudal borders. The medial entrance to the nerve root canal has previously been termed the *entrance zone,* or subarticular zone, while the lateral portal has been called the *exit zone.* The area within the intervertebral canal is termed the *pedicle zone* (Fig. 20-1).

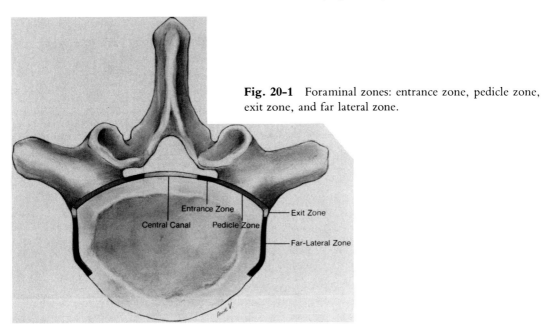

Fig. 20-1 Foraminal zones: entrance zone, pedicle zone, exit zone, and far lateral zone.

Fig. 20-2 A, Axial section through L4-L5 intervertebral disc with marked internal disruption and cleft tracking from center of disc to posterolateral aspect, where it tracks underneath outermost (intact) layers of annulus fibrosus. L4 spinal nerve is firmly stretched over the posterolateral disc bulge *(1).* L3 nerve lies more anteriorly but still in close contact with lateral disc margin *(2).* Overlying psoas major muscle, including some tendinous (aponeurotic) strands, occupies angle between disc, transverse process, and quadratus lumborum muscle (unyielding?) *(3).* Note also marked degenerative changes in facet joints with tropism. **B,** Close-up coronal section through pedicles at L3-L4 level. The thecal sac with two nerve roots of the cauda equina snugly follow medial aspect of pedicle *(1).* The dorsal root ganglion *(2)* lies immediately under the pedicle of L3 *(3).* Level of intervertebral disc is marked with dotted line. Laterally, in foramen muscle strands attach to pedicle *(arrow).* Segmental arteries and veins lie in vicinity of this muscle. Postganglionic L3 nerve tracks caudally to lateral aspect of pedicle below *(4).*

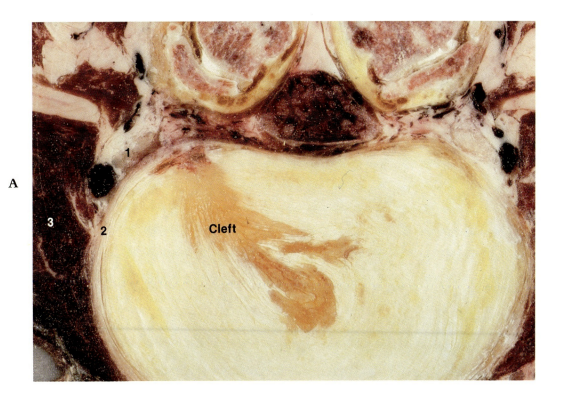

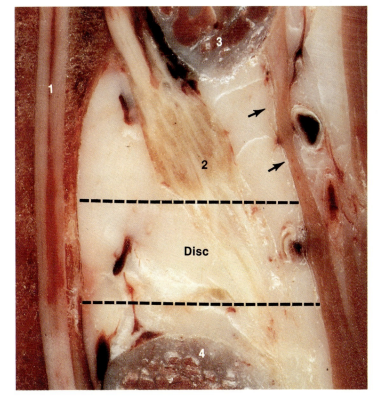

C

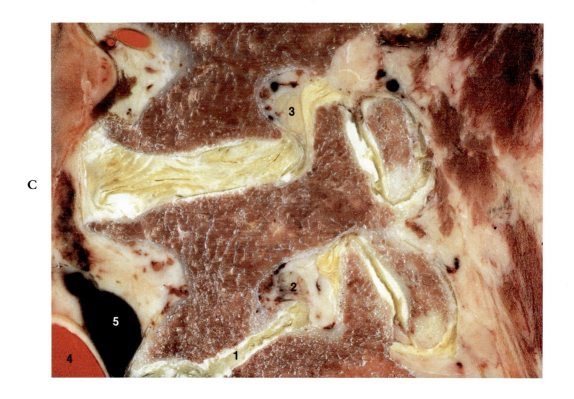

D

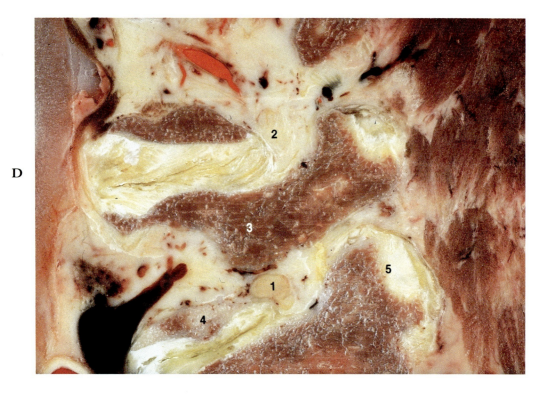

The dural sac extends laterally to the level of the spinal nerve ganglion. The ganglion begins to form within the nerve root canal and often extends laterally to a point beyond the exit zone of the nerve root canal. Beyond the ganglion the spinal nerve begins. The segmental neurovascular structures traverse the foramen in close proximity to the cephalad pedicle. At the level of and beyond the exit zone the nerve root ganglion and then the spinal nerve pass over the posterolateral margin of the intervertebral disc as these segmental structures pass ventrocaudal (Fig. 20-2).

Herniations within the central canal often compress the nerve root from the level below the interspace of herniation (Fig. 20-3, A). As herniations extend laterally, the chances of compressing the nerve root exiting at the level of herniation increase. In herniations far lateral in the lateral extraforaminal zone the exiting nerve root is often the only structure compressed. In this situation the neural compression occurs either within the foramen or beyond it laterally once the spinal nerve has exited (Fig. 20-3, B). The extradural nerve is bound by ligamentous attachments within and beyond the foramen that tether it to the inferior pedicle and annulus, making the nerve susceptible to compression from lateral herniated disc material in this lateral zone.[9,30,33]

CLASSIFICATION

Disc herniations can be divided into those occurring within the central canal, those occurring within the intervertebral foramen, and those occurring laterally beyond the intervertebral foramen (Fig. 20-4). Herniations that occur within the central canal either can be in the midline (central disc herniations) or can occur laterally within the canal off to one side. Herniations can extend from the central canal laterally into the entrance zone of the foramen, exist completely within the foramen, or extend laterally from within the foramen. Lateral extraforaminal herniations can occur just outside the foramen and further anterolaterally to 90 degrees (Fig. 20-5). Anterior herniations can occur, but they play no role in production of radicular leg symptoms.[4]

INCIDENCE

Although the exact incidence is not known, in reported series of disc herniations, lateral extraforaminal herniations occurred in 1% to 11.7% of cases.[1,17,22,24] The true incidence is most likely on the lower end of this range, because many

---

Fig. 20-2, cont'd **C,** Sagittal anatomic section through lower lumbar spine at level of lateral portion of L4 and L5 root canals. Dorsal root ganglion of L4 and postganglionic fifth spinal nerve lie at upper posterior aspect of discs and on top of a spondylotic circumferential bony ridge. Note subluxation of facet joints caused by loss of disc height, especially at lumbosacral level. Ligamentum flavum (facet joint capsule) buckles into root canal but does not compress nerve. *1,* L5 to S1 disc; *2,* L5 (postganglionic) spinal nerve; *3,* L4 ganglion; *4,* common iliac artery; *5,* common iliac vein. **D,** Sagittal anatomic section immediately lateral to lumbosacral root canal. Fifth spinal nerve is located in narrow bony niche delimited superiorly by base of transverse process and inferiorly by bony spondylophytic ridge. At this location disc herniation, especially free fragment dislodged superiorly, may compress nerve against inferior aspect of transverse process. A large disc fragment must migrate superiorly because the upper surface of the ala of the sacrum and the anterior aspect of the upper articular process of the sacrum would force disc material to migrate superiorly. *1,* Fifth lumbar nerve; *2,* fourth lumbar nerve; *3,* transverse process of L5; *4,* spondylophytic ridge lateral at lower end-plate of L5; *5,* superior articular process of S1.

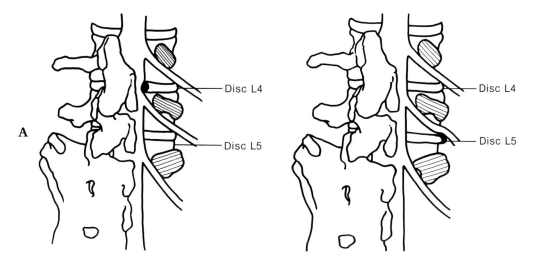

Fig. 20-3 **A,** Central canal herniations typically compress nerve from level below and spare nerve exiting at level of herniation. **B,** Lateral extraforaminal herniations compress nerve exiting at same level and typically go undetected by myelography.

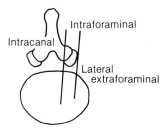

Fig. 20-4 Disc herniation can occur within central neural canal, within foramen, or laterally beyond foramen.

authors have combined all forms of laterally located disc herniations with those extending lateral to the exit zone of the foramen.[17]

LOCATION

The most commonly reported level of lateral extraforaminal herniations is the L4-L5 disc space[1,17,22,28] (Table 20-1). Herniations above the L4-L5 level occur more frequently than at the lumbosacral level. Abdullah suggested that because of the high incidence of lateral herniations above the L4-L5 disc space compared to the relatively rare occurrence of intracanal herniations at these more proximal levels, it was four times more likely that a herniation proximal to the L4-L5 disc space would be of the lateral variety.[1]

CLINICAL APPEARANCE AND PHYSICAL FINDINGS

With a few exceptions the clinical appearance of a patient with a lateral extraforaminal disc herniation is typically like that seen in classic, more medially located herniation within the central canal.

Although any adult age-group can be affected, most authors who report average age have described a slightly older population than typically seen with central canal herniations, with the reported average age ranging from 44 to 57 years.[1,22,33]

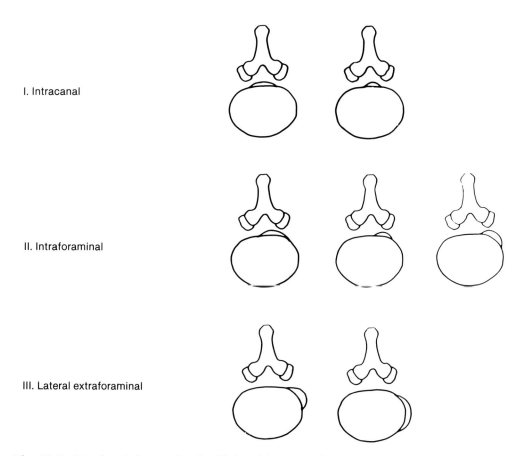

Fig. 20-5 Disc herniation can be classified as (1) intracanal: *a*, central disc or *b*, lateral to midline within central canal; (2) intraforaminal: *a*, extending into foramen from central canal, *b*, totally within foramen, or *c*, extending from within foramen lateral extraforaminally; (3) totally lateral to exit zone of foramen. Purpose of this classification system is to determine from preoperative CT scans where surgical decompression should be best directed, either to within the canal using classic laminectomy approach or extraforaminally.

Table 20-1 *Level of lateral extraforaminal herniations*

Author	No. of patients	L5-S1	L4-L5	L3-L4	L2-L3
Abdullah, et al.	24	0	18	1	5
Epstein, et al.	12	3	5	4	0
Godersky, et al.	12	5	5	2	0
Jackson and Glah	16	4	8	4	0
Nelson and Gold	10	8	2	0	0
Zindrick, et al.	39	7	25	7	0
TOTAL	113	27	63	18	5

Although in some cases rotational motion appears to be the mechanics of injury, commonly no clear-cut incident can be implicated as the causative factor.[1,22] After the initial period when both leg pain and back pain exist, the back pain component may subside, leaving buttock and leg pain to predominate.[1,9,22,25,33]

Most frequently, symptoms are monoradicular unless the medial extent of the herniation compresses the root from the level below the herniation. If biradicular findings cannot be explained in this manner, multiple-level pathologic conditions must be ruled out. Severe radicular symptoms that are more intense than those typically seen with central canal disc herniations may occur; these symptoms have been attributed to direct compression of the posterior spinal root ganglion.[1] The most common findings are quadricep weakness, decreased patellar reflex, and decreased sensation in the L4 dermatome. Herniations that occur at more proximal levels will appear similarly with a more proximal dermatome sensory deficit. Herniations that occur at the L5-S1 level appear with typical L5 root compression findings.

Straight leg raising is often found to be negative, as would be expected in upper lumbar level herniations. Femoral stretch examination may be negative. If previous disc surgery has been unsuccessful, the disc often was described as normal at the time of surgery and/or the next superior level was explored[1,17,25,33] (Fig. 20-6).

RADIOGRAPHIC FINDINGS

Normal myelographic examination in the face of radicular symptoms and clinical findings is the hallmark of disc herniation lateral to the intervertebral canal. The myelographic dye cannot extend laterally beyond the level of the spinal root ganglion because the dural sac ends at this point. The nerve root can only be visualized laterally to the level of the entrance zone of the intervertebral foramen.

Before the advent and refinement of the CT scanner, discography was the only method to visualize herniations that were out this far laterally.[1,22,25] The dye injected into the intervertebral disc can be seen to extravasate beyond the pedicles in the anteroposterior projection and may be seen to concentrate at the posterior margin of the disc in the lateral projection

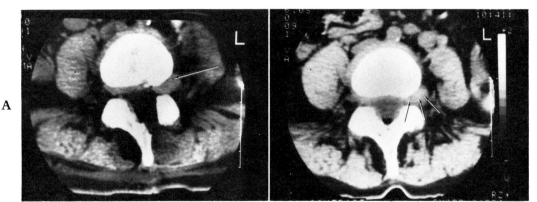

Fig. 20-6 A, This 58-year-old white woman with radicular leg pain and quadriceps weakness underwent standard laminectomy and discectomy. Disc appeared normal at time of surgery; after surgery there was no change in patient's symptoms. **B,** Reevaluation of preoperative CT scan shows lateral disc herniations to be unchanged by routine laminectomy approach. At reexploration carried out lateral to foramen, an extruded disc fragment was removed. After the second surgery the patient's leg pain was relieved.

(Fig. 20-7). Reproduction of radicular pain may occur, although not consistently.[1,22,25]

The CT scanner displays the anatomy of the extraforaminal area well.* The typical finding is of a focal bulge of material of disc density, laterally into and beyond the foramen. Loss or displacement of the epidural fat is seen in the foramen and lateral to it. Asymmetry exists between the nerve root and epidural fat of the contralateral side. Often the fragment is seen to be extruded and can be seen extending above and below the disc space on adjacent tomographic images.* Multiplanar reconstructions are especially good at delineating the extent of the lateral herniation away from the disc space in the cephalad, caudal, and anteroposterior directions[28] (Fig. 20-8). The disc material and the extent of the herniation can be further delineated if discography is used in combination with CT scanning of the involved level[2] (Fig. 20-9).

To aid further in diagnosis, the spinal nerve at the level in question can be blocked extraforaminally under fluoroscopic control with a local anesthetic agent. The level of the compressed nerve is confirmed if during the period of sensory and motor block the patient's pain is relieved.

The differential diagnosis of material that is seen extending laterally beyond the foramen includes conjoined nerve roots, enlarged ganglion, neurofibroma, primary schwanoma, and metastatic neoplasm. The patient's history, the results of examinations (such as plane x-rays and myelography), the existence of vertebral body or pedicle bony destruction or erosion, and soft tissue masses extending into the paraspinal muscles can help to differentiate these entities from lateral extraforaminal disc herniations.[9,10,19,26]

---

*References 2, 9, 11-14, 16, 17, 19, 20.

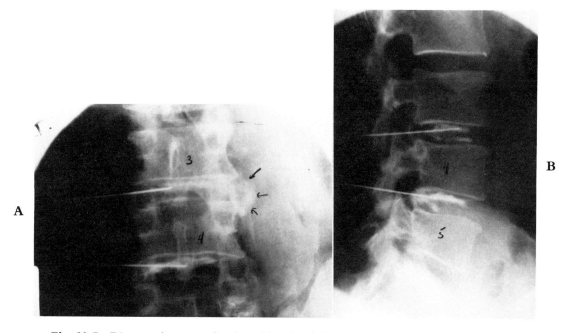

Fig. 20-7 Discography can outline lateral herniated disc material. **A,** Anteroposterior view. Note lateral extent of contrast material beyond pedicle. **B,** Lateral view. Contrast material concentrated just below level of posterior longitudinal ligament.

202 *Surgical Procedures*

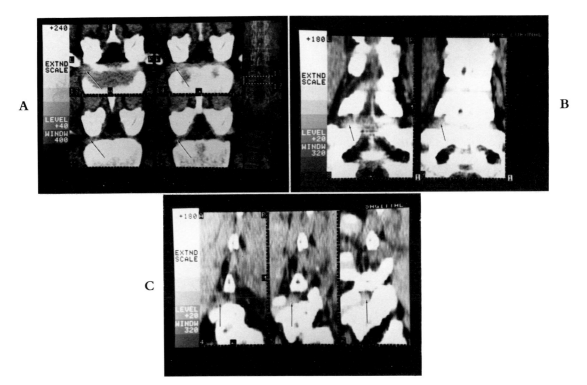

Fig. 20-8 CT scans with three-dimensonal reconstruction. **A,** Axial plane; note left-side disc herniation filling lateral extent of foramen and extending beyond the exit zone foraminally. **B,** Curve coronal reconstructions beginning posteriorly. Left-sided L5 herniation is seen laterally even at sequential CT images at level of vertebral body. **C,** Saggital plane reconstructions progressing from left to right. Note prominent disc material lateral to forming foramen.

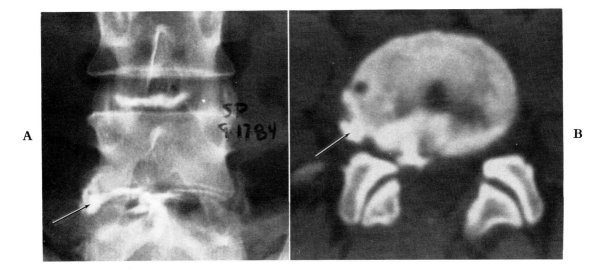

Fig. 20-9 CT scan can be combined with discography to facilitate delineation of lateral disc herniation. **A,** Discogram demonstrating lateral contrast material. **B,** Follow-up CT scan cut through level showing lateral extent of contrast.

TREATMENT OPTIONS

As with all forms of sciatica, the first approach is conservative. These modalities include, for example, bed rest, antiinflammatory medication, and pelvic traction. Although little clinical data is available, in my experience these herniations can improve clinically with conservative measures. If symptoms persist despite an adequate trial of conservative methods, treatment options that remain include chemonucleolysis or surgical resection of the disc material that is causing the neural compression.

Chemonucleolysis can be expected to be effective only if the enzyme can get to the herniated nucleus material. Chemonucleolysis is contraindicated if there are obvious extruded or sequestered fragments as seen on CT scan. If the protrusion is still felt to be in continuity with the disc space, discography, performed as a separate procedure, can help determine if the enzyme can reach the lateral extent of the herniation. If contrast material cannot outline the lateral extent of the disc herniation, then the enzyme cannot be expected to reach the pathologic condition and will be of no benefit.[28]

The standard laminectomy approach within the central canal may not uncover the lateral disc herniation.[1] In fact, often when the disc is viewed from this approach it may appear normal.[1,22,28,33] To address the lateral neural compression, dissection must be carried out laterally, into and beyond the foramen. The previously presented classification of disc herniation can assist in determining preoperatively which surgical approach is needed to adequately decompress compromised neural tissue. If the herniation exists within the canal, a standard laminectomy approach can be used. If the pathologic condition exists laterally within the foramen and beyond, the surgical dissection must be carried out laterally to expose this area.

There are three surgical approaches: (1) the nerve root can be followed out laterally by unroofing the neural foramen,* (2) the dissection can be done laterally along the facet using a midline incision,[1,6,24,28,29] and (3) a lateral paraspinal approach can be used to gain exposure to the exit zone and the most lateral extent of the foramen and spinal nerve and ganglion.[32,33]

The first surgical approach is least desirable; resection of the facet joint can in some cases result in segmental instability and progressive back pain. If this approach is used, a fusion of the involved level should be considered at the same time.

The second surgical approach, first described for exposing the spinal ganglion during ganglionectomy, involves obtaining adequate lateral retraction to pass anteriorly over the facet joint.[24,29] Often a small amount of bone resection of the lateral aspect of the facet is required to facilitate exposure (Fig. 20-10).

The third surgical procedure differs from the second in that the dissection is directed laterally by splitting the plane between the multifidus and the longissimus muscles (Fig. 20-11). The need for often difficult lateral retraction, as in the second procedure, is not a problem. Once the level of the facet joint is reached, the dissection should remain close to bone (Fig. 20-12). The spinal nerve and spinal ganglion are directly beneath the intertransverse ligament, and great care is needed to prevent damage to these structures during exposure. Cauterization should be done cautiously and with only a bipolar type of cautery. To prevent any risk of thermal injury to neural structures, oxidized refrigerated cellulose (Surgicel†) can be packed into the area of bleeding and removed at the

---

*References 1, 2, 6, 15, 20, 22, 24, 28.
†Johnson & Johnson, New Brunswick, N.J.

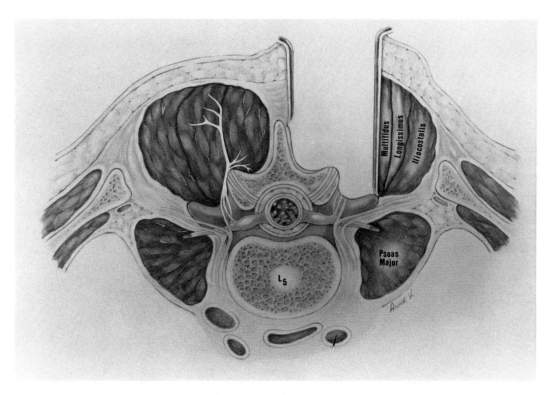

Fig. 20-10 Far lateral dissection and exposure using midline incision.

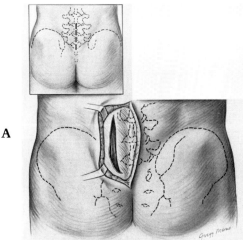

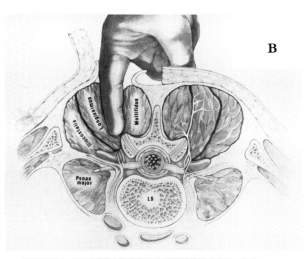

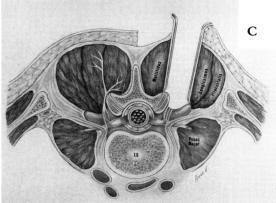

Fig. 20-11 Paraspinal approach. Using a midline skin incision a fascial incision is made 1 to 1.5 cm lateral to midline. **A,** A plane is identified between longissimus and multifidus muscles. **B,** Muscle splitting is carried out to level of facet between these two muscles. Plane can be identified by inserting a finger between muscle bellies. **C,** With retractors in place, both the central canal and lateral to the foramen can be approached.

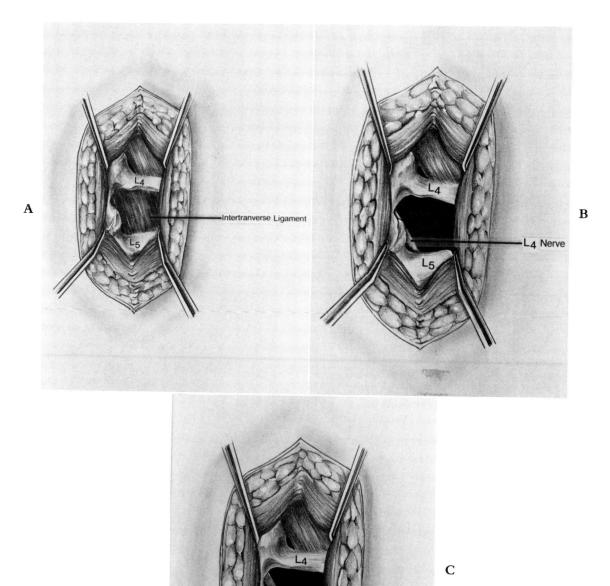

Fig. 20-12 Surgeons view of L4-L5 level lateral extraforaminal area through paraspinal approach. **A,** Intertransverse ligament between L4 transverse process and L5 transverse process. **B,** With intertransverse ligament removed, L4 nerve is seen. **C,** L4 disc and nerve are better visualized with resection of lateral edge of L5 superior articular facet. Hemilaminotomy of L4 and resection of ligamentum flavum can be performed also to expose the dural sac and L4 to L5 nerve roots within central canal.

completion of the decompression. Once the nerve or ganglion is exposed, it can be gently retracted either cephalad or caudad as needed to expose the disc material underneath it. Often the disc material is found to be extruded, and fragments can be first removed before entering the disc space. The neural structures are more easily retracted once extruded material is removed. The annulus then can be incised to allow further decompression of the disc space. If the lateral herniation exists at the L5-S1 level, the proximal aspect of the sacral ala is often resected to facilitate exposure.[33]

For all surgical procedures postoperative care is similar to that of classical laminectomy and discectomy, or fusion if performed.

SUMMARY

Disc herniations that cause neural compression can exist laterally into the foramen and beyond. The symptom complex is similar to classical central canal herniation with the exception of more persistent monoradicular symptoms of greater severity than back pain and involvement of more proximal spinal levels. Discography and CT scanning are the best methods of delineating the lesion, whereas myelography is often negative. If conservative treatment is unsuccessful in relieving symptoms, chemonucleolysis or surgical decompression can be used. Discography outlining the lateral extent of the herniation may be used to predict if the enzyme can reach the lateral extent of the herniated disc material. Surgical procedures should be aimed at directly addressing the location of the injury or disease. Dissection should be done that spares resection of the facet joint and pars interarticularis while preserving stability of the involved segment.

REFERENCES

1. Abdullah, A.F., et al.: Extreme lateral lumbar disc herniations: clinical syndrome and special problems of diagnosis, J. Neurosurg. **41**:229, 1974.
2. Angtuaio, E.J., et al.: Computed tomographic discography in the evaluation of extreme lateral disc herniation, Neurosurgery **14**(3):350, 1984.
3. Aronson, H., and Dunsmore, R.H.: Herniated upper lumbar discs, J. Bone Joint Surg. **45**:311, 1963.
4. Cloward, R.B.: Anterior herniation of a ruptured lumbar intervertebral disc: comment on the diagnostic value of the discogram, Arch. Surg. **64**:547, 1952.
5. Dandy, W.E.: Concealed ruptured intervertebral disks: plea for elimination of contrast medium in diagnosis, JAMA **117**:821, 1941.
6. Ebeling, U., et al.: Zur Diagnostik und Therapie Lateraler Bandscheibenvorfalle, II, Einteilung, Pathomechaniismus der Entstehung, Radiologischer Nachweis und Chirurgische Zugangswege Neurochirurgia **26**:80, 1983.
7. Eckardt, J.J., et al.: Extraforaminal disc herniation simulating a retroperitoneal neoplasm, J. Bone Joint Surg. **67A**:1275, 1985.
8. Edgar, M.A., and Park, W.M.: Induced pain patterns on passive straight leg raising in lower lumbar disc protrusion, J. Bone Joint Surg. **56B**:658, 1974.
9. Epstein, N.E., et al.: Far lateral lumbar disc herniation: diagnosis and surgical management, Neurol. Orthop. **1**:37, 1986.
10. Falconer, M.A., et al.: Observations on the cause and mechanism of symptoms production in sciatica and low back pain, J. Neurol. Neurosurg. Psychiatry **11**:13, 1948.
11. Fries, J.W., et al.: Lateral L3-4 herniated nucleus pulposus: clinical and imaging considerations, Comput. Radiol. **8**(6):341, 1984.
12. Gado, M., et al.: Lateral disk herniation in the intervertebral foramen: differential diagnosis, Am. J. Neuroradiol. **4**:598 1983.
13. Godersky, J.C., et al.: Extreme lateral disc herniation: diagnosis by computed tomographic scanning, Neurosurgery **14**(5):549, 1984.
14. Haughton, V.M., et al.: A prospective comparison of computed tomography and myelography in the diagnosis of herniated lumbar disks, Radiology **142**:103, 1982.
15. Jackson, R.D., and Glah, J.J.: Extreme lateral and foraminal disc herniations, diagnosis and treatment, Paper presented to the International Society for the Study of the Lumbar Spine proceedings, Dallas, May 1986.

16. Kornberg, M., et al.: Computed tomography in the diagnosis of a herniated disk at the L5-S1 level, Spine **9**(4):433, 1984.
17. Leonardi, M., et al.: CT evaluation of the lumbosacral spine, Am. J. Neuroradiol. **4**: 846, 1983.
18. MacNab, I.: Negative disc exploration, J. Bone Joint Surg. **53A**(5):891, 1971.
19. Matozzi, F., et al.: Correlate anatomic and CT study of the lumbar lateral recesse. Am. J. Neuroradiol. **4**:650, 1985.
20. Mikhael, N.A.: High resolution computed tomography in the diagnosis of laterally herniated lumbar discs, Comput. Radiol. **7**(3):161, 1983.
21. Mixter, W.J., and Barr, J.S.: Rupture of the intervertebral disc with involvement of the spinal canal, N. Engl. J. Med. **211**:210, 1934.
22. Nelson, M.D., and Bold, L.H.A.: CT evaluation of intervertebral foramina lesions with normal or non-diagnostic myelograms, report of ten cases, Comput. Radiol. **7**:(3):155, 1983.
23. Novetsky, G.H., et al.: The extraforaminal herniated disk: detection by computed tomography, Am. J. Neuroradiol. **3**:653, 1982.
24. Osgood, C.P., et al.: Microsurgical ganglionectomy for chronic pain syndromes, J. Neurosurg. **45**:113, 1975.
25. Patrick, B.G.: Extreme lateral ruptures of lumbar intervertebral discs, Surg. Neurol. **3**: 301, 1975.
26. Pheasant, H.C.: Sources of failure in laminectomies, Orthop. Clin. North Am. **6**(1):319, 1975.
27. Postacchini, F., and Montanaro, A.: Extreme lateral herniation of lumbar disks, Clin. Orthop. **138**:222, 1979.
28. Schmidt, V.R.C., and Poll, W.: Lumbale Bandscheibenvorfalle IM Diskogramm, Fortschr, Rontgen Str. **130**:85, 1979.
29. Scoville, W.B.: Extracranial spinal sensory rhizotomy, J. Neurosurg. **2**:94, 1966.
30. Spencer, D.L., et al.: Anatomy and significance of fixation of a lumbosacral nerve root and sciatica, Spine **8**:672, 1983.
31. Williams, A.L., et al.: CT recognition of lateral lumbar disk herniation, A.J.R. **139**:345, 1982.
32. Wiltse, L.L., et al.: The paraspinal sacrospinalis-splitting approach to the lumbar spine, J. Bone Joint Surg. **50A**:919, 1960.
33. Zindrick, M.R., et al.: Symptomatic disc herniation lateral to the intervertebral foramen, Paper presented to the proceedings of the International Society for the Study of the Lumbar Spine, Dallas, May 1986.

EDITORIAL COMMENTARY

Over 90% of the possible lumbar far lateral entrapments occur at the L5-S1 level. Perhaps a more common cause may not be due to the compression of the nerve between the inferior portion of the transverse process of L5 and the ala of S1, as described by Wiltse. Instead, it may occur where the nerve crosses the annulus laterally, where there may be an associated disc bar arising from the superior lateral lip of S1. This rigid ridge (especially when there is an overlying, movable annular bulge) may press the nerve against the ventral surface of the medial ala. I refer to this as a ventrolateral stenosis; there is a true canal involved that has bony margins (with the lateral limit made of the triangular, inferior extension of the intertransversus ligament as it passes along the presacral lateral gutter toward the sacral notch) through which the nerve descends. This entrapment can be shown by the CT scan; it can be functionally studied further with the use of local anesthetic injected into the involved spinal nerve or structurally studied by injection of radiopaque contrast material into the sciatic sheath as it emerges through the foramen. The latter technique is particularly clarified through the use of a digital subtraction, fluoroscopic image–amplifier system.

Charles D. Ray

CHAPTER

21

METHODS OF TISSUE DISSECTION AND RESECTION IN LUMBAR SURGERY

Charles D. Ray

Tissue dissection is quite different in patients who have not had previous lumbar surgery compared to those patients who are reoperated on. In patients who have not had previous surgery, fascial planes are cut, and muscle is bluntly parted or stripped, although when necessary muscle must be cut away from bone. However, in patients with residual scar tissue from previous surgery almost all dissection is sharp, except for stripping the scar tissue away from bone, when dissection is preferably blunt.

Generally, in patients who have not had previous lumbar surgery the dissection should remain in fascial planes, intramuscular planes, or at the midline. Whenever possible, coagulate a bleeding vessel first, then cut it (otherwise the cut stump of the vessel will retract, burying itself in surrounding tissues, thus producing a much larger crater of charred coagulum to control). Finally, use the bipolar coagulator forceps often, but keep it flooded with irrigating saline while coagulating. Remember too that none of the bipolar coagulators is absolutely balanced, that is, one tip coagulates more effectively than the other (due to an electrical current leakage from one blade). Therefore, when coagulating very tightly or near a nerve or the dura, determine in advance which blade may be the hottest and place it on the side of the vessel away from the nerve or dura. Furthermore most vessels passing through fascial planes are part of a neurovascular bundle (nerve, artery, and vein) so that as one cuts or coagulates any one of these, all three are coagulated. It is particularly important to avoid burning primarily sensory nerve branches where a painful neuroma could result; therefore do not coagulate a bundle (such as a cluneal nerve) unnecessarily. On the other hand, blunt dissection tears vessels and small nerves, sometimes breaking them at a distance from the dissection itself. Thus the best combination is sharp dissection along separable planes, coagulating and cutting as one goes.

ELECTROSURGICAL CUTTING AND DISSECTION

Electrosurgery dates back to the last century. It became widely accepted through the development of a practical surgical unit (a virtual Marconi-like transmitter unit with internal spark gaps and a transformer unit not unlike that in a neon sign system) by W.T. Bovie in 1928 and publications by Harvey Cushing in 1931.[12] There had been few serious studies of the effects of electrosurgical cutting and dissection, especially as it compared with the use of scalpel blades and scissors. However, since the development of practical surgical lasers, there is now considerably more published material on electrosurgical methods and devices.* Electrosurgical radiofrequency (RF) current is applied via tips attached to insulated handles; the RF energy is concentrated into a small area of a volume conductor (body fluids and tissues). The frequency is so high that little stimulation of muscle or nerve occurs even at high RF voltages (20 to 40 volts). As the current flows across tissue fluid, there is rapid boiling, dessication, and then charring as the temperature soars. Clotting rapidly forms, and shrinkage of dessicated cells produces a mechanical closure of small vessels (up to about 3 mm in diameter). Since thermally injured tissue heals largely by removal of the carbonized tissues, this process is slower than after simple surgical resection with steel instruments.[1,2,8,12,20]

Although several authors have reported an initial delay in wound healing from electrosurgical (ES) cutting compared to scalpel cuts, this difference is found primarily in the early stages of healing; the difference no longer is apparent after 1 month. Regardless of cause, however, initial delay may promote increased wound contracture.[19] A comparative study of these modes of cutting in the gastrointestinal tract of rats showed no difference in strength of anastomoses and no histologic lag in healing between them.[2,20] Helpap and associates found prolonged tissue healing associated with the use of an ES knife compared to the use of a surgical scalpel in the cutting of abdominal organs or the incision of tissues.[10] However, the difference appears to be closely related to the resorption of carbonized tissue components. In addition, it was believed that both electrosurgical or thermosurgical tissue damage may lead to a granulomatous tissue reaction. They proposed that this may be related to denaturaton of protein with autologous antibody formation, the magnitude of the subsequent reaction depending largely on the volume of tissue thermally denatured.

In clinical applications, after initial skin opening with a standard scalpel, I prefer to incise the posterior fascia and deeper tissues with an ES knife (that is, electrocautery knife, diathermy knife, electric pencil) and then to dissect down to the level of the lamina (if a unilateral herniation, just on one side) using a subperiosteal, muscle-stripping technique. The muscle is swept away from the lamina laterally to the facet capsule with the use of a fairly broad-bladed instrument, for example, wide Cobb or Hoehn elevator, with caution not to plunge through the intralaminar space, especially possible at L5-S1. (See Chapter 14.)

With experience and caution, the ES knife can be used to clean connective tissue and much of the attachment of the ligamentum flavum from the dorsal surface of the lamina below. Furthermore, the lateral attachment of ligamentum to the medial facet capsule may be cut using

---

*References 1, 2, 4, 8, 12, 19, 20.

the ES knife (or a small osteotome). There may be some initial jumping of the patient's back muscles while dissecting with the hot knife laterally, but this response usually arises from the posterior primary division branches innervating the facet capsule and multifidus muscles; it is never injurious to the anterior primary nerve. (Patients who have had a local anesthesic, for example, will remark that, while the surgeon is cutting or coagulating with the electrosurgical unit, the paraspinous muscle jump is not painful and has no persistent effects; it is merely startling.)

The margin of safety is generally quite large for electric cutting in the vicinity of an irritable or entrapped anterior primary nerve; it responds to cutting current passed at some distance just as it responds to mechanical disturbance from a considerable distance (as with fist percussion of the low back). Nevertheless, caution should be exercised to prevent damage. The most useful ES cutting tip (both for incising and for excising) in spinal surgery is the hot wire loop, discussed in detail later.

LASER CUTTING OF SOFT TISSUES

The laser (acronym for light amplification by stimulated emission of radiation) is a coherent (parallel waves, single wavelength), highly intense electromagnetic beam in or near the visible light spectrum. The beam is generated by exposing a large number of electrons to a very high level of energy in a gaseous, liquid, or solid medium.[17] Since the emission is coherent, it behaves somewhat differently from mixed or "white" light sources. The lasers most often used in surgery are carbon dioxide gas (middle infrared, invisible beam), neodymium-YAG (ytrium, aluminum, garnet) (invisible, near infrared), and the ruby-argon (visible) laser. To provide visibility to the invisible beams, a helium-neon (He-Ne), pilot-light beam is usually added. The important parameters of the beams are power output, beam density (focused or nonfocused) and length of exposure time. The particular wavelength also affects the mode of action on the particular tissue. Since infrared energy is absorbed by water, the intracellular water traps the beam and the entire cell is vaporized by the high temperature that results. The amount or content of the resultant temperature is known as heat, that is, energy mass or power delivered.[16]

Lasers as now used for the dissection (cutting), resection (removal), vaporization, and welding together of tissues comprise a recent art of considerable importance in several surgical disciplines. Unlike electrosurgery, where the electromagnetic energy (radiofrequency, diathermy, or microwave) is conducted through a medium (tissues, fluids, blood) via the line of least resistance in any and all directions at once (volume conduction), the laser can be precisely directed and controlled (even computer controlled) regarding all of the parameters plus three-dimensional deflection of the beam. The major advantages of laser surgery over conventional scalpel-and-scissors techniques are (1) most tissues (except bone, with its low water content) cut well; (2) there is much less bleeding of tissues and little focal edema; (3) small vessels (even up to 6 mm in diameter, if the vessel is clamped and cut at the clamped margin) are both cut and sealed at once; and (4) peripheral nerves cut by laser do not develop neuromas.[2,22,23] However, despite the remarkable potential that laser surgery has for certain applications, its use in spinal surgery is rather limited, except perhaps for the resection of certain tumors, cutting tracts of the cord, coagulation of vascular structures—including malformations—and possibly the dessication of connective tissue or the disc nucleus and annulus. Laser cutting of the bony structures of the spine (discussed later in this chapter) has as yet shown no virtues (except for narrowness of the cut) that are more important than mechanical hand cutting or the use of powered rotary tools.

COMPARISON OF ELECTROSURGICAL AND LASER RESECTION OF TISSUES

If the tissues are thick and slow to cut by laser or by ES knives, thermal damage is more likely to occur, which will impair healing. Thermal charring or carbonizing of tissue appears to be the major undesirable side effect of both ES knife and laser beam dissection. However, Fry and associates have shown that both laser and ES dissection and excision cause comparable thermal damage, when carbonization of tissue is held at a minimum.[8] Tissue injury typically extends away from the cut to about 0.5 to 1 mm. They found that initial wound healing delay was, in general, greatest following laser excision, slightly less with ES cutting, and shortest after scalpel excision.

Bellina and coworkers found that CO_2 laser cutting produces less tissue injury to the peritoneal mesothelium than ES cutting.[2] Laser cuts showed an absence of adhesions. They also noted that tissue damage and healing in either mode of cutting was most closely related to the degree of tissue carbonization. Histologically, wound healing was similar in both neodymium-YAG laser and standard ES cautery, although the latter was more destructive of regular collagen.[2] At 60 days after incision there was less collagen content of the pigskin wound margins from laser cuts than those of normal skin, suggesting that the laser may also be useful in scar and keloid removal. After 60 days the collagen content was normal in cautery-cut specimens. Although the basic effects of the laser beam on tissues are similar to those of electrocautery, the damage to wound edges can be negligible with the laser and therefore much less than that of gross electrocauterization.

Skin cut with a laser showed a greater tensile strength in the early healing period than skin cut with a surgical steel scalpel, perhaps because of the marked hyperemia, active cellular proliferation, and absence of hematoma in the incision line made with the laser.

Among others, Moreno and associates found a delay in the onset of epidermal migration of reparative cells rather than a decreased rate of epidermal migration as the primary contributor to the slower epitheliazation of CO_2 laser–induced skin wounds.[7,15] Other factors in promoting better skin healing after laser cuts relate to keeping tissues cool and devoid of atmospheric oxygen (which contributes to the charring) by surrounding them with inert gas and mechanically removing carbonized tissue before wound closure. The argon laser produced less subsequent necrosis, infection, and inflammation than did conventional electrocautery on coagulated lesions of the oral mucosa, as reported by Sanders and coworkers.[20] They also noted a minimal osseous reaction during coagulations of tissue overlying bone (also discussed later).

REOPENING AND RESECTING WITH "THE POOR MAN'S LASER"

As discussed previously, the extreme temperature of the laser, which literally evaporates the tissue, is an attractive concept. As a substitute for the expensive and potentially dangerous laser device during lumbar spinal surgery, I have experimented with a "revival" of the technique of cutting tissue with an ES hot wire loop. For many years hot-cutting loops have been used for the resection of bloody tumors (meningiomas, prostatic tissue, hepatomas, hemangiomas), cutting (conization) of the cervix, and removal of selected skin lesions.

The process of tissue resection and healing after ES cutting is rather like that of the CO_2 laser.* To this end, the wire must be of small diameter (about 0.25 mm); the RF energy is therefore highly concentrated so that the surface temperature of the wire, as it cuts through the tissue, is also quite high, but the heat mass effect is low. Thus tissue is at once both effectively vaporized and partly coagulated, but the temperature rise of adjacent tissue is kept to a minimum. Therefore this process does indeed resemble laser cutting. The hot wire–loop cuts were made at an RF intensity of 400 to 500 watts per cm^2; the resulting high temperature of the wire, with low heat imparted to the tissue, minimizes carbonizing of the tissues. This level of energy requires setting the cutting current close to maximum, with a moderate blend of coagulating current as well. Fortunately, in the animal studies cited previously there appears to be a minimal osseous reaction to applied energy—laser or electrocautery—in coagulations of tissue overlying bone.[5]

I have conducted a histologic comparison of cold (scissors, scalpel) and hot (ES wire loop) cutting of typical tissues (muscle, connective tissue, and fibrotic epidural scar tissue) encountered during laminectomies and reopenings for secondary decompression. Tissues from four patients were sampled after hot-loop cutting without nitrogen gas overflow, and tissues from two were sampled after loop cutting with an overflowing envelope of pure nitrogen gas. The gas was delivered through a Millipore filter, filling the deep wound and directed at the cutting loop. Histologic sections (10% formalin fixed, hematoxylin and eosin stained) in the nonnitrogen bathed cases showed a zone of minimal small-vessel occlusion and tissue denaturation extending to a depth of about 1 mm in muscle and connective tissue and 0.5 mm in collagenous scar tissue. Some carbonizing was seen along the cut margins (probably related to a slowing or stopping of the hot wire as it cut through the tissues). Wherever this occurred, the histologic changes extended to about 2 mm and 1 mm depth, respectively, for the different tissues beneath this char. In the nitrogen bathed cases the char formation was reduced or eliminated but only along the margins of the resected tissues, whereas the buried or deep tissue changes (not exposed to atmospheric oxygen) penetrated to the same depth, with or without nitrogen overflow.

The standard neurosurgical suction tip brings in a cooling flush of air around the loop cutter, but it also delivers atmospheric oxygen. A flush of saline, as is needed during bipolar coagulation, cannot be used because it would dissipate the cutting energy from the tissue and cause boiling of the saline solution. An inert gas bath over the hot wire loop cutter yielded no distinct improvement in the technique.

Microphotographs of the cut surfaces, especially of scar tissue, made during the cutting process (with or without nitrogen overflow) show minimal apparent change in the tissue surface; the cut margins were clean and dry (nonbleeding). Only scattered char was seen. On the other hand, if one uses a standard, wide-bladed ES knife, the carbonization build-up and sticking of the tissue to the knife is marked. Similarly, localized unipolar coagulation produces deep (several millimeters) charring and tissue damage. Remarkably, the high temperature in a confined volume of tissue renders the thin wire loop virtually self-cleaning, rather like a high temperature, self-cleaning

---

*References 1, 2, 4, 8, 19, 20.

electric oven. This can be further demonstrated by allowing a char to build up on the loop (using it for coagulation alone), then cutting through intact tissue; the char on the surface will be cleaned away from the loop and loosely left behind on the cut tissue margin.

The cutting loop is attached into a standard coagulation unit handle (Fig. 21-1). In my experience this technique of cutting is the most helpful method for reopening scar tissue in patients who have had previous lumbar surgery. It is also unsurpassed for cleaning the lamina, transverse process, or lateral surface of the facet capsule in preparation for a fusion, regardless of whether the patient has had back surgery before. Bony surfaces can be cleaned of all tissue, leaving behind a virtually academic and photogenic dissection. The loop cuts fat poorly. Certainly, it does not cut bone at all. Unfortunately, it cuts vessels and nerves all too easily, although the loop is quite useful for coagulating the resultant bleeding vessels. Larger vessels should be coagulated distal to an applied hemostat.

When cutting scar tissue with a hot wire, one should study the CT scan carefully to determine the location of and depth to nerves and dura, relative to easily identified bony prominences, for example, the laminas, facets, and osteophytes. These structures serve as limit guides to prevent sudden, unfortunate surprises, namely, cutting through the dura or a significant nerve. Loops about 1.2 cm (½ inch) in diameter appear to be best suited for cutting applications. Most spine surgeons will be pleased at the way in which tissue (especially collagenous scar tissue) can be removed with this technique. Of course, a void is created by the removal of scar tissue mass, but the healing and filling of this void appear to be little different from those seen after the use of other techniques, for example, cutting with a rongeur, especially when a fat graft has been placed, as shown on CT scan follow-up studies on a few representative cases.[18]

Although several manufacturers produce loops for their own electrodissection electrocautery–RF generator systems, I am investigating loops of various sizes, shapes, angles, and metal alloys for specific applications in spinal surgery.[18]

CUTTING BONE

The present major methods for cutting bone are (1) rongeurs, punches, and shears; (2) sharp osteotomes, chisels, and curettes; (3) rotary, high-speed burrs or drills; (4) reciprocating saws; and (5)

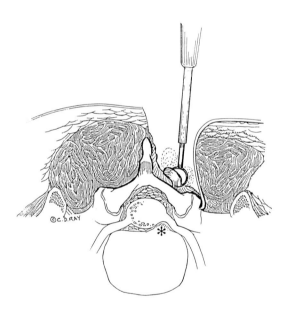

Fig. 21-1 Diagram of cross-section at L5-S1 level during process of reoperation, long after wound healing and scar formation. The hot wire RF cutting loop (attached to standard ES coagulation-cutting knife handle) is shown dissecting flap or slab of scar tissue away from dorsal surface of lamina and facet capsule. Smoke that evolves is suctioned away. Bleeding vessels can also be coagulated with the same loop. An ES knife handle with built-in, finger-operated switches is preferred. Loop is attached to long extension. Herniated disc is shown at asterisk; it displaces and entraps emerging root. Unilateral exposure is held open using two-toothed Raylor (malleable, Taylor-like) retractor passed lateral to facet joint and pedicle. (See Chapter 14.)

rasps and files. In general, if a prominent process or a relatively flat bone is to be cut, an opposing jaw cutter, for example, a rongeur, can be placed on both surfaces of the bone and the cutting, rather like a pinching or shearing process, removes the bone. Less accessible, more complex surfaces, or surfaces where one cannot place opposing cutter blades on opposite sides of the bone, are best cut with osteotomes, chisels, high-speed burrs, or a combination of these. Reciprocating saws are best used in deep, narrow slitting or slotting applications. Rasps are seldom used in spinal surgery, since rather little shaping of surfaces or edges of bone is required. In general, one must learn the particular virtues of each method of cutting so that it can be employed as needed. The surgeon should particularly learn how to cut bone "with" and "across" the "grain" of bone much as is done by a skilled carpenter or cabinet maker when cutting wood. Indeed, the lumbar surgeon would be well advised to take a short course in, or take up the hobby of, wood carving or cabinet making. In general, I believe that osteotomes and chisels of various widths, angles, and curves are the most useful instruments of all for cutting bone, provided one is exquisitely familiar with their uses and limitations and the instruments are sharp. Dull cutting instruments are a potentially great hazard in surgery.

Growth, ossification, or stress lines determine the "grain" of the bone (and wood as well), and one must be very familiar with this and the particular instruments that work best for each cutting need. For example, the grain of laminas parallels their relatively flat surfaces in the anteroposterior plane and parallels their superior and inferior edges in the cephalocaudal plane. Cuts made along the caudal to cephalic direction will cut across the grain and will more likely create fracturing perpendicular to the direction of the cut; when using an osteotome or chisel this may wedge the instrument within the cut. It is better to cut parallel with the grain, but this may splinter the bone if the ends of the cut have not been notched or slotted in advance. Cutting in the anteroposterior direction into a superior facet or pedicle (with the grain) will easily snap the bone apart, whereas cutting across the pedicle (whose grain resembles an upright dowel of wood) will more likely cause it to be crushed or broken off at its junction with the vertebral body.

When high-speed burrs or drills are used the grain plane is not as important (except at bone edges where the burr should be positioned to cut against or into the remaining bone and not to cut so that it will "kick up" an edge, cutting away from edge of the bone mass). Again, the surgeon's time would be well spent in practicing on dowels and flat surfaces of hardwood. (An especially good wooden cutting model is the junction of a branch with the trunk of a small tree.)

NEWER METHODS FOR BONE CUTTING: SONIC CURETTE, LASER, WATER JET

The sonic curette is a somewhat larger-appearing curette system that has removable shanks with various cutting tips.* The sonic unit is powered by a pair of piezoelectric crystals mounted inside the handle of the curette; these crystals deliver (at about 10 watts of energy) fine, axial vibrations (0.001 to 0.002 mm movements) of the shank at a frequency of about 25 kHz. Various shanks screw into the sterilizable hand-held generator unit. Several sizes and configurations of cutting tips are available. Effectively, the pulses of fine movement decrease the mechanical resistance of the curette cutting edges at contact with the margins or

---

*Quintron Corporation, Galena, Ohio.

surfaces of bone. Particularly useful is the right-angle curette tip for the undercutting of the superior facet in a laterally stenotic foramen, the straight tip for undercutting the lamina in cases of central stenosis,[3] or deep against vertebral end-plates in preparation for posterior interbody fusions.[13] Perhaps of more importance in the application of this instrument is the sharpness of the cutting edges; a dull sonic curette cuts bone no better than an ordinary dull bone curette. This not-inexpensive instrument is not widely used among spine surgeons.

The use of a high-powered laser for cutting bone is as yet in developmental stages. Clayman and associates, in a study of rabbit bone healing after osteotomy by rapid superpulsed (SP) and continuous-wave (CW) CO_2 (infrared) lasers, showed that the former of these two modes required less energy (power) for bone cutting.[5] In addition, when the narrow zone of tissue necrosis that inevitably occurs adjacent to the laser cuts was debrided, healing was similar for both laser modes (SP and CW) and showed a normal, orderly progression. The SP mode was operated at 4,000 watts but with pulse widths of only 50 to 200 msec and repetition rates of 83 to 225 per second. The CW laser was used at 10 to 20 watts with a one second "on" time. Although the wattages are vastly different between the two, the ultrashort SP pulses deliver less actual energy (in joules, 5 vs. 20) than the CW laser. It was important to bathe the tissue with a continuous stream of nitrogen gas at the cutting site; this inert gas "envelope," as discussed earlier, serves both to cool the tissue and to reduce oxidation (char formation).

Through tissue responses of rabbit tibia to osteotomies performed by SP laser, CW laser, and high-speed burr, Small and coworkers found that, although bone healing occurred in all three modalities, there was a delay in healing after either mode of laser osteotomy.[21] At the present time the role of the laser in bone cutting is unclear, but a few points emerge: laser cuts are much narrower than those of a mechanical saw or burr and there is much less bleeding from the bone margins. The laser may therefore be particularly useful in applications where strict hemostasis is required.

A more recent yet potentially useful development in cutting techniques employs a very fine stream of water under extremely high pressure; typically 55,000 pounds per square inch (about 3700 atmospheres).[11] The superpressure water jet has been used commercially to make very fine, nondistorting cuts through soft and hard composites, plastic foam, firm rubber, hard stone, or even hard steel. The application of this method for cutting bone is now being investigated.[11] Of course, any cutting force must have a counter force to balance it; if the water jet is not dissipated as it passes to the opposite side of the cut bone, there will surely result major soft tissue destruction. In all fairness, however, this comment also applies to the potential use of the high-powered laser for cutting bone. Clearly, the technical details still must be worked out for both of these potentially useful methods for resecting bone and soft tissues associated with the spine.

ACKNOWLEDGMENT

I wish to thank Dr. William Foley, pathologist, Department of Clinical Pathology, Abbott-Northwestern Hospital, Minneapolis, Minn., for his assistance in preparing and interpreting the tissue samples used in the investigative portion of this chapter. Appreciation is also extended to my associate, Dr. Alexander Lifson, who remarked, during a discussion about my experiments in electrosurgical cutting of tissue, that I should try the "old fashioned" loop cutter as was used in the removal of meningiomas of the brain; clearly, this suggestion was the key to reevaluating the use of this mode of cutting, discussed in detail in this chapter.

REFERENCES

1. Arnaud, J.P., and Adloff, M.: Electrosurgery and wound healing: an experimental study in rats, Eur. Surg. Res. **12:**439, 1980.
2. Bellina, J.H., et al.: Carbon dioxide laser and electrosurgical wound study with an animal model: a comparison of tissue damage and healing patterns in peritoneal tissue, Am. J. Obstet. Gynecol. **148:**327, 1984.
3. Burton, C.V.: How to avoid the "failed back surgery syndrome." In Cauthen, J.C., editor: Lumbar spine surgery, Baltimore, 1983, Williams & Wilkins.
4. Castro, D.J., et al.: Wound healing: biological effects of Nd:YAG laser on collagen metabolism in pig skin in comparison to thermal burn, Ann. Plast. Surg. **11:**131, 1983.
5. Clayman, L., et al.: Healing of continuous-wave and rapid superpulsed carbon dioxide laser-induced bone defects, J. Oral. Surg. **36:**932, 1978.
6. Cochrane, J.P., et al.: Wound healing after laser surgery: an experimental study, Br. J. Surg. **67:**740, 1980.
7. Finsterbush, A., et al.: Healing and tensile strength of CO_2 laser incisions and scalpel wounds in rabbits, Plast. Reconstr. Surg. **70:**360, 1982.
8. Fry, T.L., et al.: Effects of laser, scalpel and electrosurgical excision on wound contracture and graft "take," Plast. Reconstr. Surg. **65:**729, 1980.
9. Hall, R.R.: The healing of tissues incised by a carbon-dioxide laser, Br. J. Surg. **58:**222, 1971.
10. Helpap, B., et al.: Reaction of bone marrow after cryo- and thermolesions on internal organs, Cryobiology **22:**168, 1985.
11. Helwig, D.: 55,000-psi water jet cuts better than steel, Popular Science **227:**76, 1985.
12. Lawrenson, K., and Stephens, F.O.: The use of electrocutting and electrocoagulation in surgery, Aust. N.Z. J. Surg. **39:**417, 1970.
13. Lin, P.M.: Posterior lumbar interbody fusion technique: complications and pitfalls, Clin. Orthop. **193:**90, 1985.
14. Mester, E., et al.: Effect of laser rays on wound healing, Am. J. Surg. **122:**532, 1971.
15. Moreno, E., et al.: Epidermal cell outgrowth from CO_2 laser- and scalpel-cut explants: implications for wound healing, J. Dermatol. Surg. Oncol. **10:**863, 1984.
16. Ray, C.D., editor: Medical engineering, Chicago, 1974, Year Book Medical Publishers, Inc.
17. Ray, C.D.: Principles of electricity and electronics. In Ray, C.D., editor: Medical engineering, Chicago, 1974, Year Book Medical Publishers, Inc.
18. Ray, C.D.: Improved R-F hot-wire loops for dissecting and resecting tissues, especially deep, collagenous scar, Unpublished data, 1987.
19. Rosin, R.D., and Exarchakos, E.H.: An experimental study of gastric healing following scalpel and diathermy incisions, Surgery **79:**555, 1976.
20. Sanders, B., et al.: Comparison between laser photocoagulation and electrocautery on surgically-induced wounds of the oral mucosa, J. Oral Med. **34:**65, 1979.
21. Small, I.A., et al.: Observations of carbon dioxide laser and bone bur in the osteotomy of the rabbit tibia, J. Oral Surg. **37:**159, 1979.
22. Tauber, C., et al.: Fracture healing in rabbits after osteotomy using the CO^2 laser, Acta Orthop. Scand. **50:**385, 1979.
23. Walter, G.F., et al.: The effects of carbon dioxide- and neodymium YAG-lasers on the central and peripheral nervous system and cerebral vessels, J. Neurol. Neurosurg. Psychiatry **47:**745, 1984.

CHAPTER

22

EXTENSIVE LUMBAR DECOMPRESSION: AUTOSTABILIZATION AND OTHER VARIATIONS

Charles D. Ray

THE PROBLEM

Lumbar decompressions, especially in cases having lateral stenosis, might well result in destabilization of the segment resulting from removal of bone, joints, or ligaments.[1,4,5] This may occur in the process of exposure or in the performance of the decompression itself.[12] Extensive decompressions performed from a posterior midline approach in the lumbar spine, in order to reach an entrapped nerve, are sometimes deceptively easy to perform. However, in a significant number of these cases instability has resulted. Although such a loss of stability is unusual in most spinal surgery, when it occurs it can be most significant and debilitating. Postoperative instability is highly unlikely in cases having advanced autostabilization from collapsed, degenerated disc spaces. Nonetheless, there are many patients with lateral stenosis where the disc space is not yet collapsed; a freshly herniated disc that must be removed may even be present.

I shall define instability as a painful, disabling, motion-related disorder of one or more vertebral segments related to some loss of mechanical integrity of the structural components in that segment. Usually, there is a combined loss of several components producing the instability. They include the disc annulus, the facet joints, the pedicle, the lamina (especially the pars interarticularis), the ligaments, and the dorsal spinous processes. Loss of mechanical integrity that is painless, nondisabling, or otherwise asymptomatic is excluded by this definition.

When correcting instability, the usual fusion methods produce loss of mobility in that segment, therefore restabilization leads to the potential for a new set of problems. To avoid iatrogenic instability one may choose (1) decompression designed to avoid the likelihood of destabilization, (2) decompression and waiting to see if instability occurs later, or (3) decompression and intersegmental fusion during the same procedure. The present approaches addresses the potential problem by the first choice, namely, methods to avoid instability in certain cases where the usual midline approach would likely dictate simultaneous decompression with intersegmental fusion.

Selby[14] has pointed out that all surgical techniques should have the following mechanical characteristics.

1. Good anatomic dissection, good hemostasis, adequate exposure
2. Gentle handling of the tissue
3. Good instrumentation to shorten the procedure and achieve good results
4. Versatility in surgical approaches as needed by the pathologic condition, including the consideration for resultant instability
5. Meticulous postoperative care with early, well-planned rehabilitation

THE INACCESSIBLE ZONE

The majority of nerve entrapments occur in the vicinity of the pedicle. This has been referred to by Casey Lee as the "hidden zone" (Fig. 22-1). Because of this inaccessibility, the nerve root and ganglion are well protected or covered by bone, beginning with the medial aspect of the pedicle, passing inferior to the pedicle (somewhat like a rope passing around a pulley). The four sides of the upper part or true neural foramen consist of the segmental pedicle, cephalad; the next inferior pedicle of the vertebra below, caudad; the facet joint, dorsal; and the vertebral body, ventral.[2] After emergence from the foramen, the nerve once again may be vulnerable to compression or entrapment, but at very few places.[12,15]

Clearly, one well-established means for dealing with this surgically is to perform the decompression and wait to see if instability occurs or, alternatively, to perform the decompression and a fusion during the same surgical procedure. At the L5-S1 level, where most stenoses are found, there is often a preexisting relative stability of the vertebral segment. This occurs in the presence of large transverse processes projecting in close proximity to the sacral alae or sacroiliac junctions. In such cases one will ordinarily

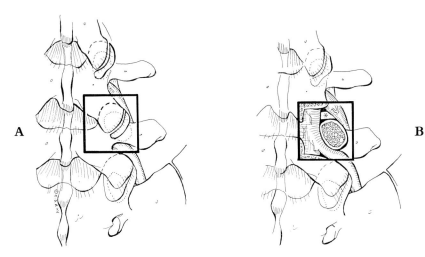

Fig. 22-1 The "inaccessible zone." **A,** Zone lies inside boxed area, right lumbar 4 level, centered around pedicle. Most lesions of lumbar spine are found beneath (ventral to) laminas here. **B,** Facet joint and laminas have been removed in boxed area of **A.** Beneath are L4 and L5 roots and the relationship of each to the base of the pedicle. Disc at L4-L5 is indicated at asterisk. A surgical decompression of this extent would likely produce some degree of instability, probably torsional (where the body of L4 might rotate away or to the left, hinged about remaining left facet joint).

find short, tough, and well-developed iliovertebral or iliotransverse ligaments.

The degree of stabilization offered by these ligaments is, of course, uncertain, although it is likely to be much more than one would find at higher levels. Therefore "taking a chance" of subsequent destabilization by extensive posterior decompression has some logic, albeit quite limited, but only at the L5-S1 segment and only when the self-stabilizing details just discussed plus considerable narrowing of the disc space may be found. In all probability, however, such cases would continue to develop a significant and clinically symptomatic spondylolisthesis.[1,4,5] On the other hand, if one is anticipating the performance of a fusion at the end of the decompression, one should have already performed magnetic resonance imaging and possible intradiscal saline acceptance and contrast discography to ascertain that there is no instability at the level above and below that to be fused. This sequence of considerations, rather like falling dominoes, is cumbersome and raises questions about what amounts to prophylactic surgery. There can be considerable argument on all sides regarding these details.

BACKGROUND OF THE CONCEPT

The idea of single- or multiple-level laminectomies with preservation and restoration of the removed segments has been described by a number of authors. Perhaps the most extensive work has been performed in the cervical spine. Japanese authors Tanaka and associates,[16] Tsuji,[17] and others have described careful, rather elaborate techniques for cutting the lateral neural arches, removing them together with their attached ligamenta flava and then, subsequent to the decompression procedure beneath the en-bloc multiple laminectomies, returning and restoring the arches as autographs. Raimondi[6] also touched on this concept and further mentioned the potentiality of such a restoration for the lumbar area.

Another technique, reported by Kaiwa and coworkers,[3] uses screws placed through the lamina and transected pars into the pedicle. Although good ultimate fusion and stabilization have been reported, this would appear to be a technically difficult task. Considering that the cross-sectional diameter of the pars is relatively small, one would expect that virtually all of the cancellous portion would be occupied by the screw, probably interfering with some ultimate stability of the fusion. Furthermore, one would expect that the development of callus ventral to the pars might produce or regenerate a significant stenosis.

NEURAL ARCH AUTOGRAFT

In a previous report I described a new technique that involved taking a completely free graft of a split neural arch with subsequent restoration.[7] An improved method now has been developed and is described here. In the search for nondestabilizing techniques that allow surgical resection of lateral stenosing lesions (bone spur or disc bar), with or without simultaneous removal of a herniated disc in the presence of a disc space of essentially normal height, the neural arch autograph technique was developed. The technique has three principle stages: preparation and splitting of the neural arch in a transverse fashion with preservation of facet stability, resection of the stenotic lesion (and removal of the disc or whatever else might be additionally required), and replacement of the split portion of the resected arch as a reattached bone graft for restabilization.

Before deciding on the arch autograft procedure, one should examine the size and slope (vertical angle) of the lamina at the involved level. That is, if the lamina is narrow (cephalocaudad) and has a considerably oblique tilt relative to the long axis of the spine, it might be feasible to perform an ordinary laminotomy and then cut beneath the lamina with a sharp, curved (Cloward) osteotome to perform the decompression without need for an autograft. A Cloward spinous process spreader may be helpful in making the approach to the entrapment more ample. However, if the lamina is both wide (cephalocaudad) and relatively flat (paralleling the vertical axis of the spine), the arch autograft as presented here or a lateral approach may be needed to reach the entrapped nerve.

SURGICAL PROCEDURE

The surgeon should carefully examine the CT scans to determine the plane of the facets; that is, if the joints are relatively sagittal in orientation, as is generally seen above the L4 level, this method requiring bisection of the facet would probably be

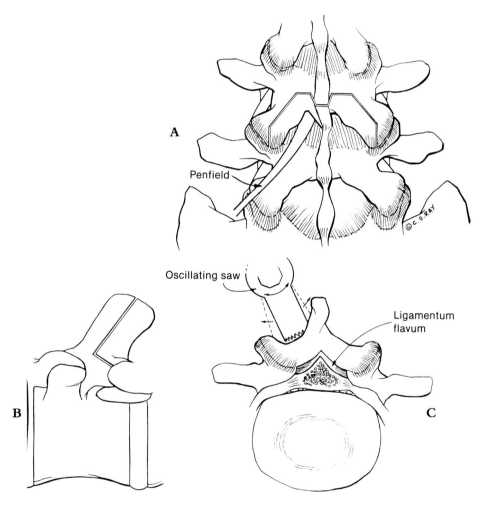

Fig. 22-2 Neural arch autograft technique. **A,** Area to be cut has been marked *(double line)* on facets, laminas, and dorsal spinous process. A Penfield elevator no. 2 is being passed beneath the lamina, dissecting away ligamentum flavum very close to base of spinous process. The elevator will remain in place to protect dura during cutting of arch, first on one side, then the other. **B,** Parallel lines showing lateral aspect of the cut through the spinous process and lamina. **C,** Transection of neural arch using powered oscillating saw. Spinous process is cut on a slope through its long axis. Dura and roots are protected medially, and cephalad shelf of superior facet protects them laterally. Cuts through facet joints are carefully selected to prevent weakening of lateral lamina and pars.

undesirable. There would be little or no anteroposterior bearing surface remaining, in which case slippage would be likely. There should be a generous exposure utilizing wide retraction and a clean posterior dissection of ligamentous structures made before cutting the bone. I have developed special force-fulcrum retractors* for performing this and other lumbar procedures.[11] Dura and nerve must be visualized, protected, and checked frequently.

The technique is diagramed in Figs. 22-2 through 22-4. The ligamentum flavum is dissected free from beneath the arch in one small area bilaterally, and the dura is displaced ventrally and protected near the midline with a Penfield no. 2 elevator. Since the dorsal surface of the superior facet is the ventral limit of the lateral cut, no dural protection is needed there. With the tissues cleaned off of the lamina and dorsal spinous process, a sterile gentian violet skin marker is used to mark the bone for the exact location of all cuts. An oscillating saw* with a thin, 1 cm wide blade is used to carefully cut through the marked lines, cutting across the lamina and spinous process, as shown in the diagram, then downward to bisect the facets. The cut that transects the spinous process is angled to follow its center line. One should measure before cutting—and measure and listen to the saw while cutting—so that the superior facet is injured as little as possible by the facet cut. In addition, one should avoid saw chatter or wandering; the blade will need careful orientation during the cutting process. Finally, one must be careful not to cut free any piece of the facet or pars, because this may destroy the intent of the procedure and leave behind a bone fragment that might not reunite. As illustrated, as much of the attached ligament as possible is left intact. This cutting process requires about 5 minutes to complete, so careful planning and execution of the saw slots is essential. The lateral corners of the slots may require slight additional cutting

---

*CeDaR Surgical, Inc., Minnetonka, Minn.

*3M Co., St. Paul, Minn.

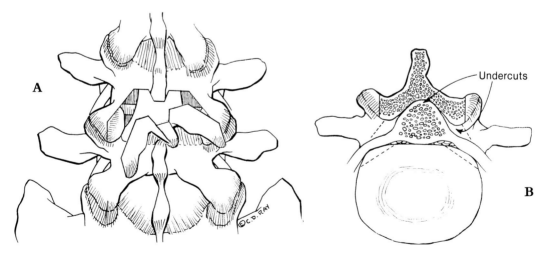

Fig. 22-3 A, Inferior piece of transected arch, shaped like a segment of a hexagon, still attached to its ligamentum flavum. Interspinous ligament is swung aside for exposure of the tip of superior facet, inferior aspect of pedicle, and lateral disc space. Exposure is the same as an extensive laminotomy. **B,** Undercutting of facets and lateral vertebral body is now performed as needed. In cases also having central stenosis the superior, attached arch segment may now be trimmed and enlarged ventrally.

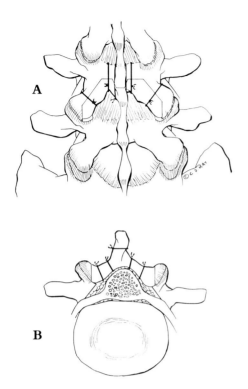

Fig. 22-4 A, Cut piece of arch is returned to position and secured with wire (see text). **B,** Segments of fat graft were placed over exposed dura and roots before restoring the arch. After fusion and regrowth of autograft, strength of arch is restored.

with a thin, small osteotome (such as the 5 mm curved Cloward osteotome) to effect complete separation of the segment. This cut arch segment piece resembles a portion of a hexagon.

Once the segment is freed, it is mobilized laterally as shown. The facet capsule will be stretched or even separated, but good displacement is easily achieved. The interspinous ligaments are remarkably flexible, especially with the patient positioned in slight extension on the table. (I have developed a special kneeling or prone-sitting frame for this and other spinal procedures.)[10] A Cloward spinous process spreader* may be used to obtain even greater visibility beneath the laminas, but one must be careful not to fracture the base of the already thin spines.

---

*Codman, Inc., Boston, Mass.

One can now trim, cut, impact, or otherwise approach the spur or disc bar as needed; good access is now available to medial portions of superior facets, inferior pedicles, posterior disc spurs, or even to central stenoses. The disc may also be resected. (The long-term results of such a combined procedure together with disc removal are not yet known). A small fat graft is placed dorsal to the dura and exposed nerve sleeves, with caution that no fat or other tissue separates the neural arch segment as it is reattached.

The neural arch piece is now very firmly anchored back into its original anatomic position with double strands of 24-gauge (0.4 mm) stainless steel wire. The wires are passed around the spinous process and on both laminas. Passing wires around the lamina and pars laterally has been abandoned, because two cases have had slippage of the wire into the facet space with resultant irritation of that joint and in two other cases the tightening of the wires has fractured the pars. In five earlier cases strands of no. 2 (0.4 mm) heavy monofilament nylon were used with success. Clearly, the pars is more fragile than it was originally, therefore the patients wear a brace for 4 months to prevent hyperextension. Fig. 22-5 shows preoperative and postoperative CT scan images of a typical case.

MAINTAINING GRAFT VIABILITY

It is worth repeating a few comments to emphasize the importance of careful planning for this procedure. When one transects the neural arch, one effectively cuts off most of the vascular supply to the removed bone. The principle arterial supply to the neural arch arises from a branch of the segmental artery, which penetrates into the pedicle and then traverses the pars interarticularis to enter various structures that are attached to or part of the neural arch, including the dorsal spinous process, the laminae, and the

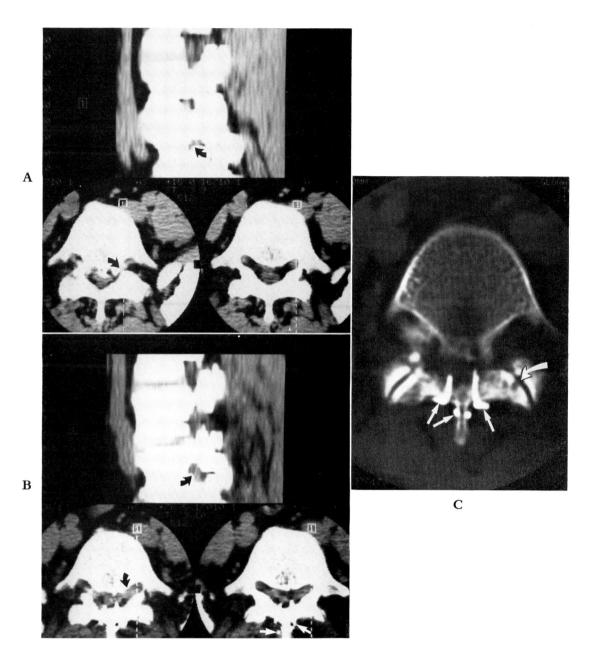

Fig. 22-5 Preoperative and postoperative CT scans of neural arch autograft procedure. **A,** Up-down lateral stenosis (present bilaterally) shown at arrows. Upper image is a parasaggital reconstruction showing clarity in displaying lateral stenosis. **B,** Postoperative scan of same area showing decompression *(black arrows)*. Laminar and spinous process wires are indicated *(white arrows)*. **C,** Postoperative transaxial CT scan showing wires placed around laminas and spinous process *(short arrows)*. Small portion of one saw slot is also seen *(long arrow)*.

inferior facet joints. There are other significant perforating arterioles entering the arch via the spinous process and laminae. Venous drainage is equally multiple but principally through the dorsal spinous process. Some circulation reaches the arch via the attached ligaments; therefore these are carefully preserved. In none of the 12 cases performed to date has bony atrophy of the arch occurred. The neural arch autograft is an interesting and satisfying procedure where one can remove bone, shape the structures, and then replace the piece without the need for a bony allograft or intersegmental fusion. However, cases must be selected carefully.

UNILATERAL ARCH AUTOGRAFTING

In six cases a sawed notch has been taken out of a hemilamina and subsequently replaced, as outlined previously, to reach and decompress a unilateral spur. This procedure was performed in patients who had an open disc space or herniation; the variation has also proved to be satisfactory in maintaining pars strength. In one such case there was a subsequent fracture of the remaining pars, but with wearing of the back brace the fracture subsequently reunited and the mechanical symptoms stopped. One other case required subsequent decompression and intertransverse process fusion for stabilization. Careful consideration of the anatomy is important in selecting these cases. This unilateral variation is worth trying in certain cases to obviate intersegmental fusion.

TRANSECTION OF THE PARS WITH AUTOGRAFT FUSION

An additional technique has been developed and tried in three cases: a frank transection of the pars bilaterally has been performed, the intact neural arch mobilized, the stenotic lesion resected, and the pars restored. This technique is illustrated in Figs. 22-6 through 22-9. Varia-

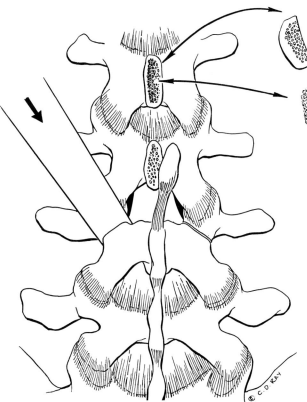

Fig. 22-6 Pars autograft technique. Spinous process of L2 has been cut off and split *(upper arrow to side)*; some cancellous bone has been scooped out of remaining stump *(lower arrow to side)*. Spinous process of L3 is cut off closer to its dorsal tip and interspinous ligament has been left attached. Pars of L4 is carefully cut with a sharp osteotome angled toward inferior cortical margin of pedicle. Depth of cut to root is carefully monitored with small, blunt probe in medial aspect of foramen. Cut is angled as much as possible. (This procedure has been used in only a small number of cases; its utility is not yet clear.)

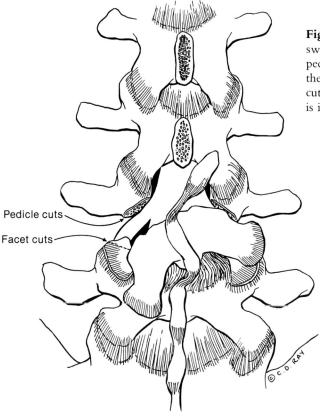

Fig. 22-7 Intact neural arch has now been swung aside to expose inferior margin of pedicle and superior tip of superior facet; these structures may now be trimmed or cut. Note that ligamentum flavum of L4-L5 is intact.

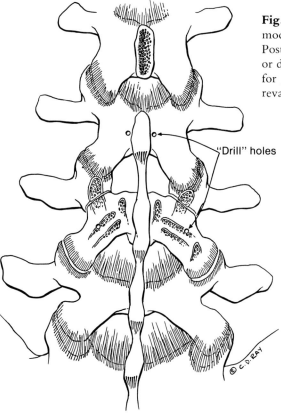

Fig. 22-8 Drill holes are made to accommodate wiring of arch back into place. Posterior surfaces of laminas are scarified or decorticated in selected areas, not only for placement of bone chips but also for revascularization of neural arch.

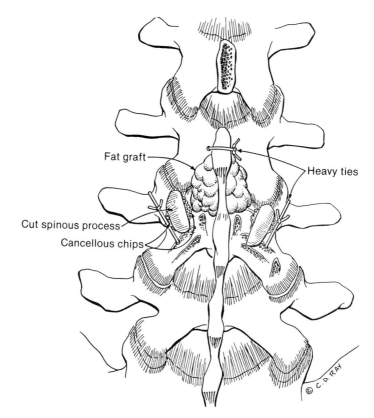

Fig. 22-9 Arch is restored. Heavy ties of 22-gauge stainless steel wires hold bony segments in place. The cut spinous process is laid, cancellous portions together, against scarified pars. Available bone chips are placed. Wiring is placed for maximal stability and will require some maneuvering on ventral surface of lamina to prevent root compression. A fat graft is placed only over exposed dura at L3-L4, leaving posterior surface of L4 so it will interface with muscle. Patients will wear a brace for 4 months to prevent lumbar hyperextension.

tions of this technique, perhaps with the cutting of the pars closer to the inferior margin of the attachment to the pedicle, might improve on the process of fusion and again reduce the likelihood of a callus arising ventrally on the pars causing a late foraminal stenosis. One case required additional lateral decompression due to this latter complication. Two of the three cases appear to have reunited; it is too early to judge the other. Fig. 22-10 shows the postoperative CT scans of such a pars autograft fusion case. Insufficient cases and time are available to evaluate the effectiveness of this technique. The effect of facet capsular tearing, required for mobilization of the arch, is also unknown.

OTHER APPROACHES AND ANOTHER LOOK AT LAMINOTOMY

As indicated earlier, reaching and working effectively within the inaccessible zone ventral to the pars, with the maintenance or reestablishment of stability, is indeed a technical challenge. If one attempts to do this via laminotomy alone, three types may be considered for such decompressions. As shown in Fig. 22-11, the laminotomy approach may be from below, *A*, which is the usual approach to a herniated disc; from above, *B*, the usual decompression for a subarticular stenosis; or from a lateral approach, *C*. Although the first and second are by far the most common approaches,

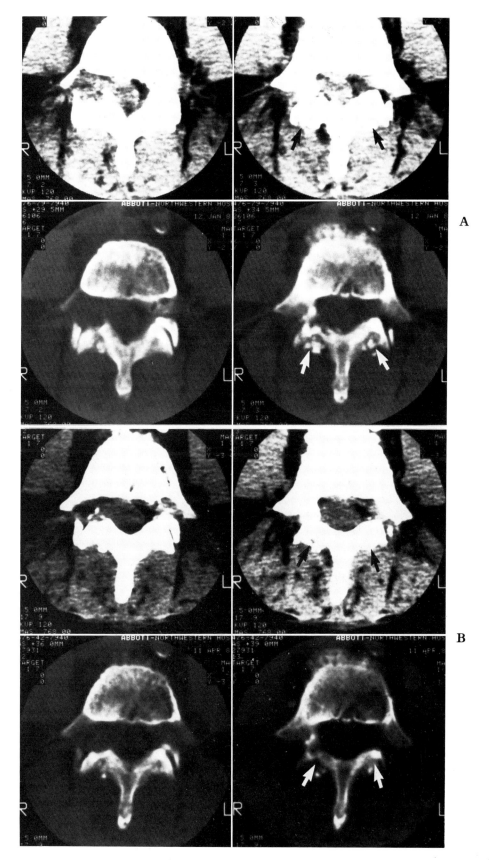

Fig. 22-10 Postoperative CT scans on a patient having had a pars autograft. **A,** 2 months postoperative films showing cut spinous process and other chips lying against laminar surface *(small arrows)*. Bone and soft tissue window (contrast) scans shown. **B,** 14 months postoperative CT scan of same area. Further redevelopment of an intact pars is shown (somewhat better seen on the left).

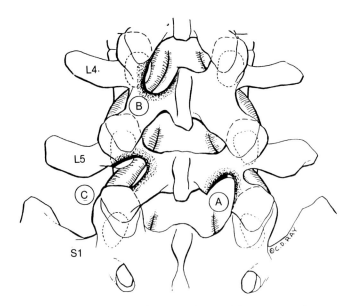

Fig. 22-11 Three laminotomy approaches. *A,* The usual laminotomy for removal of herniated disc. Access to root and ganglion of L5 are not good; pars has been made quite thin. *B,* Laminotomy from superior aspect of L4. This is the usual approach for a subarticular decompression, in this case, of L4 root passing over the L3-L4 disc bulge. Access to pedicle or to lateral spurs is also poor. *C,* Lateral laminotomy showing excellent access to inferior aspect of pedicle, lateral disc margin (with potential spurs or bars). Pedicle is again thin, however, although there is good attachment across neural arch to the other hemilamina. This paramedian approach is preferred for certain lateral stenotic problems (see text).

even to stenotic spurs, it is the third that may be the only appropriate one in most cases. This technique is technically more challenging, but it must become a part of the spinal surgeon's repertoire. I have used this approach in a significant number of cases from a midline incision and therefore refer to it as a paramedial decompression.

In the performance of this laminotomy the electric knife (cautery pencil) is used rather freely, although there may be some occasional stimulation of the motor portions of the spinal nerve. Several patients have had surgery under local anesthesia and have remarked that the jumping of a leg while the surgeon is cutting near the nerve is neither accompanied with nor followed by pain; therefore there is little likelihood of nerve damage, even when the hot knife is but a few millimeters away from the ganglion. Again, experience is required to make this approach work.

The retraction that I use is provided by the new malleable variations of Taylor retractors developed for this and other spinal procedures.[11]* It is important to clean the connective tissue and muscular attachment away from the lateral lamina to fully appreciate the lateral aspect of the pars and associated anatomy.[14] One carefully identifies the dorsal rim of the foramen (ventral dimension of the pars) with the use of a small blunt hook passed lateral to the pars and into the foramen. There is a significant neurovascular bundle or "medusa" that arises from or just distal to the ganglion. A small artery making up part of this medusa will bleed with conviction; it is the only structure to do so in this area. Bipolar coagulation

---

*CeDaR Surgical, Inc., Minnetonka, Minn.

should be used, but not too close to the ganglion, otherwise one runs the risk of possible postoperative dyesthesia. A small sharp osteotome or high-speed burr is used to remove the lateral portions of the lamina. Since the foramen is usually quite tight, it is important not to use a large Kerrison rongeur for this far-lateral laminotomy. Instead, small, curved or straight curettes may be used to break the remnant bone, thinned out by burr or osteotome cutting, away from the underlying nerve. Once the foraminotomy is made, the spur or other source of stenosis is addressed. An excellent method for reduction of these small structural lesions is via impaction, discussed in detail in Chapter 23. For an additional far-lateral approach to similar but more extensive lesions, see Chapter 18.[8,9]

Since writing this chapter, I have developed and applied clinically an entirely new approach to decompressions for stenoses arising from instability-induced uncinate spur formation.[13] The method involves spreading the facet joint (by laminar distraction), boring an 11 mm hole through the facet, emerging exactly dorsal to the spur. After impacting the spur (see Chapter 23) and decompressing the ganglion and nerve *through* the transfacet hole, a small fat/fascia graft is placed dorsal to the ganglion and then 12 mm homologous bone graft dowels are driven into the holes, immediately stabilizing the segment in distraction. A PLIT fusion is also usually placed.

REFERENCES

1. Epstein, N.E., et al.: Degenerative spondylolisthesis with an intact neural arch: a review of 60 cases with an analysis of clinical findings and the development of surgical management, Neurosurgery **13**:555, 1983.
2. Heithoff, K.B., and Ray, C.D.: Principles of the computed tomographic assessment of lateral spinal stenosis. In Genant, H.K., et al., editors: Spine update 1984, San Francisco, 1983, Radiology Research & Education Foundation.
3. Kaiwa, S., et al.: Enlargement of the lumbar vertebral canal in lumbar canal stenosis, Spine **6**:381, 1981.
4. Kirkaldy-Willis, W.H., and Farfan, H.F.: Instability of the lumbar spine, Clin. Orthop. **165**:110, 1982.
5. Kirkaldy-Willis, W.H., et al.: Pathology and pathogenesis of lumbar spondylosis and stenosis, Spine **3**:319, 1978.
6. Raimondi, A.J. and Gutierrez, F.A.: Reconstruction of the posterior vertebral arch and laminotomy for intraspinal surgery. In Ransohoff, J., editor: Modern technics in surgery—neurosurgery, Mt. Kisko, New York, 1979, Futura Publishing Co.
7. Ray, C.D.: New techniques for decompression of lumbar spinal stenosis, Neurosurgery **10**:587, 1982.
8. Ray, C.D.: The paralateral approach to lumbar decompressions, (abstract 21-W), Proceedings of the annual meeting of the American Association of Neurological Surgery, Washington, D.C., April 1983.
9. Ray, C.D.: Lateral spinal decompression using the paralateral approach. In Watkins, R.G., editor: Principles and techniques of spine surgery, Rockville, Md., 1987, Aspen Press.
10. Ray, C.D.: A new, improved kneeling attachment for spinal surgery, Neurosurgery. (In press), 1987.
11. Ray, C.D.: New malleable force-fulcrum retractors for lumbar spinal surgery: technical note, Spine (In press), 1987.
12. Ray, C.D., et al.: Lateral lumbar spinal stenosis, classification and etiology, Clin. Orthop. (In press), 1987.
13. Ray, C.D.: Transfacet decompression, facet dowel fixation and PLIT fusion for lumbar lateral stenosis induced by instability: a new technique, Clin. Orthop. (In press), 1987.
14. Selby, D.K.: When to operate and what to operate upon, Orthop. Clin. North Am. **14**:577, 1983.
15. Semmes, R.E.: Ruptures of the lumbar intervertebral disc, Springfield, Ill., 1964, Charles C Thomas, Publisher.
16. Tanaka, H., et al.: Surgical treatment for the ossification of the ligamentum flavum: wide en-bloc laminectomy, Jpn. J. Orthop. Trauma Surg. (Seikei Saigai Geka) **23**:779, 1980.
17. Tsuji, H.: En-bloc laminectomy, Jpn. J. Orthop. Surg. (Seikei Geka) **29**:1755, 1978.

CHAPTER

23

LUMBAR DECOMPRESSION OF OSTEOPHYTES, SPURS, AND BONY ENCROACHMENT

Charles D. Ray

BONY ENTRAPMENT

Among the major causes of spinal stenosis or entrapment of neural tissues are hyperostoses, bone spurs, disc bars, and other bony and calcified ligamentous excrescences.[1,2,3] When the bone spur is a mixture of calcified and soft tissues along the lateral margins of a disc bar, for example, the removal of this source of stenosis, entrapment, or root irritation may be a technical challenge.

By and large the surgeon must be guided primarily by what the patient says, what the examination shows, and what the diagnostic tests (especially the CT scan) reveal. When the surgeon reaches the lesion and surveys the status of the involved tissues (for example, the nerve, dura, ligament, joints, bone) additional judgments must often be made. By definition, the lesions creating the stenoses lie tightly pressed against the nerve root or ganglion. That is, from the spinal surgeon's point of view the most important bony lesions lie beneath the lamina or facet where the root and ganglion pass, on the opposite side of the nerve structure from one's posterior approach. The skills of the spinal surgeon are probably tested more by the lesions that lie within this inaccessible zone than in any other way. The process of removing an offending bony lesion without damaging the nerve or creating a new (or potential) problem (instability, scarring, loss of function, chronic pain) is difficult enough in itself; but when the lesion lies in an inaccessible area the matter is made even the more complex.[1]

SURGICAL METHODOLOGY

There exists a virtual mosaic of surgical tools that perform remarkable tasks in the cutting of hard and soft tissue. The number, kind, complexity, and cost of these instruments increase at regular intervals. This review discusses a few representative, relatively simple instruments used for the removal of bony excrescences,

---

Impactors and related instruments described in this chapter are manufactured by CeDaR Surgical, Inc., Minnetonka, Minn.

simple lesions that may nonetheless have severe effects. There are relatively few methods of cutting bone, although there are many various versions of the instruments that are used for this purpose.

The cutting, fracturing, chipping, shaving, or removal of bone prominences by the use of sharp-bladed, striking instruments (osteotomes, chisels, or gouges) may be particularly valuable when removing parts or surfaces that cannot be cut with opposing-blade cutters (shears, rongeurs, punches). (See Chapter 21.) This situation is particularly true for cutting (or starting a cut edge) on laminas, pedicles, facets, or vertebral bodies, that is, on relatively massive spinal structures. Bony margins may be struck-cut or split in immediate proximity with nerve or dura and yet not injure them. However, other instruments are needed to clean away this cut or splintered debris. A curette, sometimes difficult to use because the mechanical fulcrum point needed to get the appropriate cutting leverage is not available, may be well suited to scoop out this debris. In additioin, curettes often seem (or actually are) too dull for significant cutting—especially where one is confronted with relatively flat surfaces. However, they are particularly useful for detaching softer tissue from hard tissue. Thus scraping a ligament or small osteophyte from a flat bony margin is often best performed with a curette. Opposing-blade cutters, for example, rongeurs, scissors, shears, or punches, are particularly suitable to thin bone when the plane is perpendicular to the direction of instrument jaw closure. This would seem to limit these tools, but when used in combination with other cutters (osteotomes, turbines), these biting, shearing instruments are among the most useful. A remaining class of cutting tools, the hand-operated, reciprocating files and rasps or the hand-rotated reamers, have had little application to spinal surgery, much less to the removal of osteophytic processes.

High-speed turbines are clearly important tools for cutting into flat or massive surfaces, although they are at the same time especially (potentially) hazardous where nerve tissue is close at hand. The cutting range (limits of free motion) of the burr should be braced or otherwise controlled at all times to prevent chatter, runaway cutting, or plunging of the burr. Although it is a relatively recent instrument, high-speed cutting of hard tissues with a burr has become a basic skill required of spinal surgeons. The cutting burr places little pressure against the bone that is being cut, the burr does not cut soft tissues well, it tends to "wrap up" filamentous or stringy tissue, its energy is imparted against the bone as heat production, and it requires a flood of fluid to keep its cutting edge cool; however, it is fast and clean. There are many bony entrapments that cannot be approached by the turbine, since it puts the nerve or dura too much at mechanical risk. Sometimes the burr is used to undermine an entrapment, and curettes or punches are used to break away the remaining shell of the entrapment.

IMPACTION

Impaction has been used very little for the relief of bony excrescences. Impactors (rather like modified drift punches) allow one a direct attack on a bone spur or prominence so that it may be simply "driven away" from the nerve. The concept of decompression by the use of impaction (or compression) of a bony excrescence is certainly not new. The practical application of this technique is, in keeping with the design of other types of surgical instruments, highly dependent on the mechanical and structural characteristics of the tools. That is, the impactors must be shaped and sized such that reaching the lesion and impacting it, strik-

232 *Surgical Procedures*

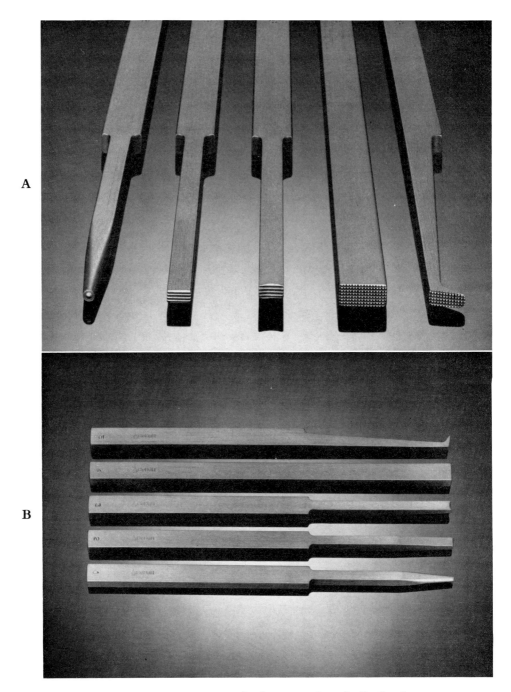

Fig. 23-1 Bone impactor instruments for decompression of offending bony excrescences, disc bars, or osteophytes. **A,** Full-length view of impactors; overall length is 25 cm. **B,** Close-up view of tips of impactors showing small rounded, small rectangular, and curved tip (to fit the contour of the pedicle), large rectangular, and footed types. Note that all have nonslip knurling on the bone-striking surfaces to prevent slippage when impacting bone. Large rectangular impactor is also used to drive bone fusion dowels and bone chip tamper for fusions. The toe of the footed impactor is passed beneath (ventral to) the dura or an entrapped ganglion to decompress by impaction of an osteophyte. (See also Fig. 23-3, **B.**)

ing the free-end instrument with a mallet, must be safe, practical, and stable. The tip that is applied to the bone spur should not slip off during impaction, otherwise it could traumatize the neural tissue. In addition, if the impactor is too large for the task, it may produce a significant, albeit momentary, compression of the nerve. This would be particularly true if the impactor were to become wedged between the bone and a nerve during the impaction. If the impacting instrument is too small, the result consists of multiple small fractures along the surface that may remain adjacent to the neural tissue. In general, the impaction technique has been best performed when the remaining bone surface is relatively smooth, preferably cortical (rather than cancellous), and relatively free of ragged connective tissue or ligament.

The instruments used for this technique (Fig. 23-1) are specifically designed for use in surgical decompressions of the spine.* The first, is a round tip instrument (2.5 mm diameter) for driving or fracturing smaller segments of a spur, which may then be impacted with a larger instrument or removed as small fragments, as with a curette; the next has a small, squared-off tip for straight-line impaction of disc bars or spurs. The third impactor is specifically designed with a curved, sloping, angled end surface that fits quite well against the usual contour of the inferior aspect of a lumbar pedicle. Since a great number of stenoses involve the inferior and medial aspect of the pedicle, especially that at L5, this impactor is often used. The fourth impactor of the set is a much larger instrument for compressing still greater surfaces or driving bone plugs during a fusion procedure. Perhaps the most important impactor of the group is the fifth one shown, the footed impactor. The toe of this device is passed beneath (ventral to) the dura or root to remove osteophytes. All of these instruments have machined, nonslip tips to reduce the likelihood of slippage from the surface that is driven or impacted. Fig. 23-1, A shows the impactors in full view; they are 25 cm in length and are made of an anodized hard aluminum alloy. Other shapes of impactors are under development.[4]

SURGICAL APPLICATIONS FOR IMPACTION

The spinal surgical procedures for which these impactors are most commonly used involve lateral stenosis. As discussed previously, portions of the superior, lateral, or inferior lamina must be removed to reach and decompress the offending osteophyte and free up a compromised nerve or ganglion. Approaches from a far lateral direction (see Chapter 18) may spare most of the posterior and lateral structures in order to reach the root, ganglion, spinal nerve, or the stenosing bone spur or disc bar.[2,3]

A rather common form of stenosis occurs where the pedicle forces the root or ganglion downward against a disc bar or spur. At times it is preferred to remove the bar or spur, but there are a number of indications for the impaction of the inferior portion of the pedicle itself. For this application there is a specific impactor designed for the inferior pedicle (see Fig. 23-1). From a midline approach, it is brought against the inferior edge of the pedicle from an acute angle; the tip is sloped to optimize the approach to, and impaction of, the pedicle. In Fig. 23-2 a midline approach to a lateral stenosis involving the pedicle (cephalad to the nerve), the facet (dorsal to the nerve root), the vertebral body and spur (ventral to the nerve structure) is shown. In this situation, after completion of a dorsal decompression, the inferiomedial cortex of the pedicle is "moved away" from

---

*CeDaR Surgical, Inc., Minnetonka, Minn.

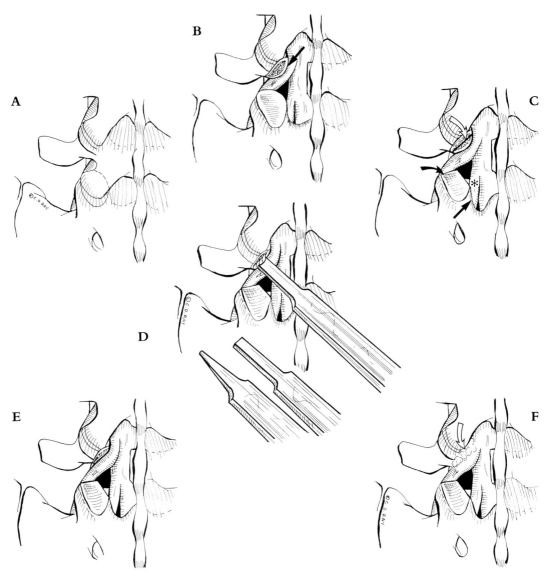

Fig. 23-2 Impaction for decompression of inferior pedicle. **A,** Exposure of left sided L4-L5 and L5-S1 is diagramed. **B,** Full left hemilaminectomy has been performed, showing tight situation of L5 nerve as it passes around its pedicle *(arrow)*, somewhat as a rope would pass around a pulley. Exposures are ordinarily not this extensive. Disc space should have been found to be quite stable so that total facetectomy will not destabilize the segment. **C,** Tip of the superior facet *(curved black arrow)* at S1 has been cut. Inferior pedicle *(open white arrow)* has been cut across (slotted) with an osteotome. S1 root passing over L5-S1 disc margin is indicated by asterisk. (If subarticular stenosis of L5-S1 were present, the location of an appropriate decompression is indicated by the straight black arrow.) **D,** Impactor, shaped to fit inferior curve of pedicle, is tapped with nylon mallet, aiming upward and laterally, driving cortical portion of pedicle away from root, allowing it to relax. Root is carefully protected from possible pinching by impactor as it is struck. Two other types of impactors (see Fig. 23-1) are also shown. (Also see Chapter 16.) **E,** Root is now relaxed as it passes around impacted pedicle. If need be, more of pedicle can be resected and impacted. Exposure is often sufficient to permit exploration and impaction of possible disc spur or bar at L5-S1 level. **F,** Small fat graft has been placed between impacted pedicle and L5 root/ganglion.

the nerve root and ganglion by first cutting through the cancellous portion with an osteotome and then impacting the hard cortical portion into the partially resected cancellous portion, loosening the nerve. Thus the nerve has been relieved from its being drawn tightly around the inferior pedicle rather like a rope passing around a pulley, and it now presents a more-or-less smooth cortical bony surface against which the root will lie.[1]

A more extensive application for the technique arises where one must cut off the posterior portion of a pedicle (cut like a stump); the cut, bleeding stump of bone is waxed, and the cortical margins are impacted or "folded inward," leaving a relatively smooth cortical margin. No other noncutting surgical instrument is presently available to accomplish this task. A further refinement of this decompression technique is to provide sufficient space between the neural tissue and the impacted bony surface so that one may place in between them a thin layer of free-fat globules or a small wrap of fatty paratenon (either of them acting as an insulating or isolating free-fat graft).

An excellent application for impaction is along the posterior ridge of a disc bar. After removal of a bulging herniated disc (especially one that is partly calcified) the surgeon may find that a rigid ridge remains quite prominently beneath the traversing nerve root or dural sac. In most such cases impaction is a reliable means for displacing the offending osteophyte or disc bar away from the nerve, usually leaving behind a relatively smooth surface (Fig. 23-3).

In many patients with lumbar lateral stenosis one must perform a posterior unroofing of the nerve structure. Such a procedure often is accompanied by a further need for decompression of the dorsal disc margins because of an associated osteophyte or bar. Impaction has proved to be a superior method for this, especially by using a footed impactor, passed ventral to the dura or nerve to drive away the osteophytes.[5] Since the disc bar is a mixture of crumbly bone and ligamentous tissue (for example, the annulus), the turbine burr cannot well address the problem. Sometimes the spur can be wedge-cut with an osteotome and removed by scraping with a curette, but ragged tissue still remains. If the nerve is far enough away, a small cautery tip (or the bipolar tip) may be used to dessicate the remaining frayed tissue. Impaction can be a preferred means to address this

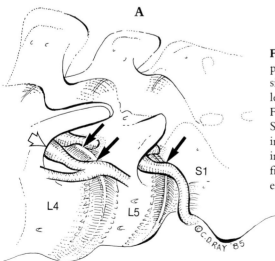

Fig. 23-3 Lateral approach to impaction of pedicles and disc bars or spurs. Shown are left side of vertebral bodies at the L4, L5, and S1 levels. **A,** Tight pedicle situation, as shown in Fig. 23-2, is indicated by open arrow at L4. Similar compression is located at L5 but not indicated with an arrow. Disc bars and spurs are indicated by solid arrows, covered with annular fibers so that they appear as smooth mounds elevating spinal nerves, L4 and L5.

Continued.

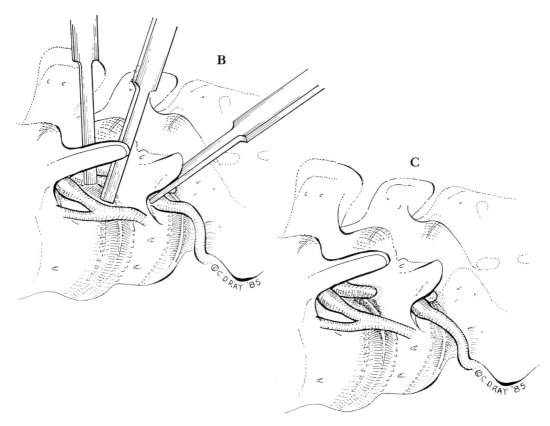

Fig. 23-3, cont'd B, Impactors being used to decompress nerves by driving spur or bar into the vertebral body. Impaction of inferior aspect of pedicle of L5 is shown; this has already been done at L4 in this diagram. A footed impactor (Fig. 23-1) is particularly useful for impacting spurs beneath the dura, ventral to a ganglion or a spur inside a foramen. **C,** Postimpaction situation showing relaxed position of L4 and L5 nerves as they now pass over impacted bony ridges, caudad to impacted pedicles.

friable mass with a relatively clean result. In a rather similar application the disc bar and step-off of a spondylolisthesis may be impacted so that the nerve roots passing over the step will be relaxed. Such a maneuver can be added to a fusion to reduce the acutely localized displacement that presses against the ventral surface of the dural sac. Sometimes one may find that localized decompression is easier to perform where the cortical surface is first fractured by one of the impactor instruments and the remaining bone fragments lifted or curetted out. Other shapes of impactors may be developed to address other elements of complex decompressions.

REFERENCES

1. Ray, C.D.: New techniques for decompression of lumbar spinal stenosis, Neurosurgery **10:** 587, 1982.
2. Ray, C.D.: The paralateral approach to lumbar decompressions. (Poster session, abstract 21-W) Am. Assn. Neurol. Surg., Proc. ann. meet, p. 191, April, 1983.
3. Ray, C.D.: Lateral spinal decompression using the paralateral approach. In Watkins, R.G., editor: Principles and techniques of spine surgery, Rockvill, Md., 1987, Aspen Press.
4. Ray, C.D.: Bone impactors: new instruments for spinal decompression: technical note, Spine (In press), 1987.
5. Ray, C.D.: Transfacet decompression, facet dowel fixation and PLIT fusion for lumbar lateral stenosis induced by instability: a new technique, Clin. Orthop. (In press), 1987.

SECTION THREE

FUSION

CHAPTER 24

HISTORY OF SPINAL FUSION

Hugo A. Keim

Fred Houdlette Albee was born in Alna, Maine on Friday, April 13, 1876. He was the son of a farmer and the eldest of seven children. The family was quite poor, and it was difficult for the Albees to raise their children in the rugged countryside of Maine, especially during long and difficult winters. At an early age Albee was intrigued by the art of "tree grafting," which he learned from his grandfather, Charles G. Houdlette, who was the local fruit-tree grafter in his community.[3] The precision and attention to detail that was necessary to perform successful tree grafting was of great interest to young Albee, and he delighted in seeing successful transplants of apple shoots to cherry trees and pear shoots to apple trees.

Albee went to Lincoln Academy at Newcastle, Maine, which was 6 miles from Alna, and attended Bowdoin College where he graduated with a Bachelor of Arts degree in 1899. During his senior year he became the right tackle of the "All Maine" college football team, an honor that he cherished. His physical stamina, which he perfected during years as an athlete, was of great benefit to him during his later years as a hard-working surgeon.

Albee continued his studies at Harvard University, where he received a scholarship in anatomy. After Havard he went to the Massachusetts General Hospital, where he interned. Through a series of fortunate coincidences, he met a physician who had a practice in Waterbury, Connecticut, where through the kindness of Dr. Charles Ogilby he became an assistant at the orthopedic clinic at the New York Postgraduate Hospital. There, he became close friends with Henry Ling Taylor, who helped him secure an appointment at the Hospital for Ruptured and Crippled on East 42nd Street as a radiologist. He was most interested in the future of radiology and quickly saw its ramifications and importance in the field that was ultimately to become orthopedic surgery.[8]

In February 1907 he married Louella

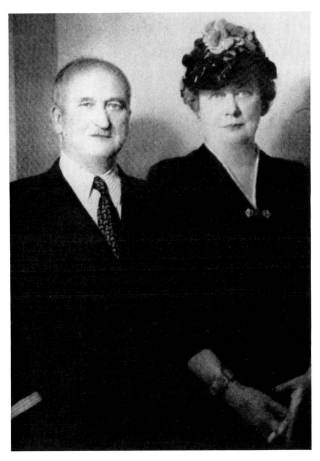

Fig. 24-1 Dr. and Mrs. Fred Albee. They had a long and happy marriage during which she gave him great emotional support, which helped him in his studies and research.

Berry, and in 1908 he was elected to the chair of orthopedic surgery at Cornell Medical College in New York City (Fig. 24-1). He was then 32 years old. While at Cornell, Dr. Albee met Professor S.P. Beebe, who was in charge of the animal hospital there. He also met Dr. James Ewing, who was doing considerable work on the blood of sheep. Both of these men helped Albee get involved in bone-graft transplantation from different species of animals, and he soon learned that trying to transplant bones from a sheep to a dog or vice versa was not desirable. The autogenous graft (an original Albee idea) proved to be the most dependable of his early experiments. As a result of these experiments Albee soon decided to try transplantation of graft material from an extremity of an animal to the spinal vertebra, this procedure laid the foundation for what is now known as the "Albee bone graft" method of spinal fusion.

The experimental work that Albee did in animals in 1910 and 1911 was to fuse the spine. The satisfactory and revealing results of these experiments was reported at a meeting of the American Orthopaedic Association held in Cincinnati, Ohio, on May 15, 1911. Unfortunately, Dr. Albee did not publish this report in a medical journal. If it had been published, it would have prevented the controversy over whether it was Russell Hibbs or Fred Albee who performed the first spinal fusion.

Hibbs *published* his work on fusion of the spine on May 28, 1911, 13 days after Dr. Albee *verbally reported* his spinal fusion technique at the orthopedic meeting in Ohio. The two operations, however, were at different locations in the spine. This sparked the controversy concerning who was the actual originator of the spinal fusion technique.[11]

There is no doubt, however, that the basic methods of "bone grafting" were solely the product of Albee's experiments and research. His further experimental work on dogs, sheep, and rabbits soon convinced him that local fusion of the spine was not the best method; therefore he created his first bone graft. This work was published on September 9, 1911.[2]

Hibbs, who became a surgeon at the New York Orthopaedic Dispensary and Hospital in 1898 at age 23, was born in Birdsville, Kentucky in 1869. After graduation from Vanderbilt University in 1888 he entered the University of Louisville Medical School, where he received his degree in 1890. At that time the course in medical school consisted of two 6-month series of lectures. After this meager preparation, Hibbs began medical practice. He soon moved to Texas, where he did general medical practice, visiting his patients on horseback. He quickly became convinced that he needed more training, and in 1893 he went to New York in search of a hospital internship. There, he secured an appointment at the Polyclinic Hospital; his duties included the attendance of obstetric cases in patient's homes, and it is doubtful that he obtained any worthwhile experience in the operating room. The following year, in 1894, he became a house surgeon at the New York Orthopaedic Dispensary. Although he had no particular interest in orthopedics at this time, it seemed to be the best available opportunity. That he became a skillful surgeon and introduced many surgical procedures that were to transform the nature of orthopedics and place it on a real surgical basis is extraordinary.

The appointment of Hibbs to be the chief of the hospital at this time was providential (Fig. 24-2). Before this time, there was little encouragement for applying surgical procedures to the correction of deformities and stabilization of joints. The results of infection were so severe that the treatment of these conditions was limited largely to the use of braces and gymnastics. At this time, however, surgical techniques were being improved and the occasion had arrived for applying them to orthopedics.

Dr. Charles F. Taylor, who started the New York Orthopaedic Hospital and Dispensary, along with Theodore Roosevelt (the father of President Theodore Roosevelt) and the Board of Trustees, saw the need for a dispensary to aid the many crippled people inhabiting New York at that time. Tuberculosis was rampant because of poor sanitary habits at numerous dairies in the city and the total lack of hygienic supervision and medical care of indigent people.

After Dr. Taylor, Dr. Newton M. Shaffer became the chief of the New York Orthopaedic Dispensary in 1874. Both he and Taylor were ultraconservative and had no training in surgery. In 1891 Shaffer said that the only surgery performed at the institution was on patients who also needed special mechanical treatment before and after surgery.

All other patients who did not need special orthopedic care were sent to general hospitals. Taylor and Shaffer were basically "leather and buckle" physicians, who believed that the correction of orthopedic deformities could be performed satisfactorily with the use of external supports such as braces. Shaffer believed strongly that joints and limbs could be straightened and saved by properly applied mechanical treatment. If this

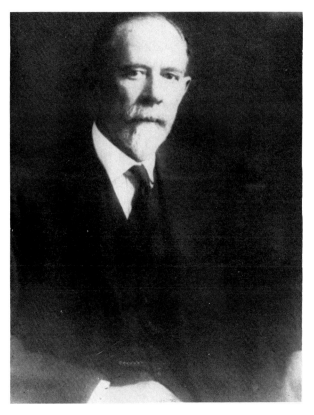

Fig. 24-2 Russell A. Hibbs at the height of his career. He performed the first spinal fusion on a human being in January 1911.

could not be done, the patient should be transferred to a general surgeon. He stated that the surgeon who amputated the leg or reduced the fracture, repaired a dislocation, and applied a hip splint on the same day was not likely to advance orthopedic science. Thus the function of an orthopedic surgeon should be to fill a space not occupied by a general surgeon. Surgical treatment should be secondary to mechanical treatment; conservative treatment was important overall.

Because of an unfortunate occurrence in December of 1900 Dr. Shaffer tendered his resignation to the Board of Trustees of the New York Orthopaedic Dispensary and Hospital. The board appointed Hibbs acting chief, but at age 29 Hibbs stated that he needed the full confidence of the medical staff and that he would take the position only as full director and chairman. Thus he was subsequently appointed to that position. The Trustees gave further evidence of their confidence in Hibbs in January 1902 by increasing his salary to $2000 per year.

Hibbs observed that in the relatively few instances in which Pott's disease or tuberculosis of the spine actually was cured a fusion of the vertebra took place spontaneously.[10] He reasoned that if a fusion could be induced early in the disease the cure could be accomplished much sooner, and severe kyphotic deformities could be prevented. He devised a procedure that could accomplish this by experimenting on dogs; it consisted of breaking down the spinous processes and facet joints so that they came in contact with each other and grew together in a bony bridge to join the vertebra. Hibbs performed the first spinal fusion on a human being on January 9, 1911.[1] After Albee described his procedure for implanting a bone graft, Hibbs and Albee developed a rivalry concerning who first conceived of the principles underlying the operation, because both procedures were described in the same month.

From the beginning, Hibbs foresaw that his operation might be useful in the treatment not only of Pott's disease but in other deformities of the spine as well, and he entitled his first paper on the subject "An Operation for Progressive Spinal Deformities: A Preliminary Report of Three Cases from the Service of the Orthopaedic Hospital."[5] He was proved correct by the application of spine fusion to a number of other conditions, including scoliosis, spinal fractures, and painful conditions in the lumbar spine.[6,7]

The success of the procedure in the treatment of tuberculosis of the spine soon became evident, and at the Orthopaedic Hospital it became the routine treatment. Other papers followed as more and more cases accumulated. One paper, "The Treatment of Vertebral Tuberculosis by the Fusion Operation: A Report of 210 Cases," appeared in the *Journal of the American Medical Association* in June 1918. Another paper, by Hibbs and Joseph Risser, on the result of 286 cases appeared in the *Journal of Bone and Joint Surgery* in October 1928. In addition to his excellent work on the spine, in 1909 Hibbs described the technique for fusing the knee that utilized the patella as a graft between the tibia and the femur and included removal of the cartilage only from the joint surface, thus sparing the epiphyseal centers. This procedure was also used successfully in cases of tuberculosis of the knee. His report, "Tuberculosis of the Knee Joint in the Adult in which Operations Were Done, Eliminating Motion by Producing Fusion of the Femur and Tibia" was published in the *New York Medical Journal* on May 19, 1917.

The marked success of these operations by both Hibbs and Albee were apparent to all in the New York area. The dispensaries were no longer filled with patients making repeated visits for the adjustments of braces and dressing of tuberculosis abscesses. In a great majority of cases the patients were cured of the disease, enabling them to resume normal and active lives. However, the idea of operating on tuberculous joints met with almost universal opposition by other orthopedic surgeons. Many of them were from the conservative school and foresaw all kinds of harmful results from such surgery. They argued that (1) it was unnecessary, and (2) it was dangerous, because it would result in spread of the disease. Although these statements were fallacious, it was many years before the increasing number of good results and the willingness of younger surgeons to try new methods finally led to general acceptance of this treatment.

The controversy over the treatment of tuberculosis of the spine prompted the American Orthopaedic Association in 1921 to appoint a commission, consisting of Doctors E.G. Brackett, W.S. Baer, and J.T. Rugh, to investigate the subject. They asked various surgeons to give them reports on the results and personally visited a number of clinics. Their report, published in the *Journal of Orthopaedic Surgery* in October 1921, stated that there was only one clinic (the New York Orthopaedic Hospital) where accurate records were kept and a follow-up system was maintained. They gave qualified approval of the operation and stated that there was no foundation for many of the fears that had caused opposition to it. Before this time Hibbs had been denied membership in the American Orthopaedic Association. He was prevented from joining that prestigous society until

1921, when a committee of the American Orthopaedic Association established a commission to investigate his results with spinal fusion. At that time they strongly recommended that he be elected to membership, which was done unanimously. Ultimately, the New York Orthopaedic Dispensary and Hospital merged with what is now called the Columbia-Presbyterian Medical Center.

In her book Marie Benyon-Ray states:[4]

Albee isn't all there is to Orthopaedic surgery, any more than Freud is all there is to Psychiatry. But there has been no greater single contribution than his. He discovered bone grafting and applied it to many different types of deformity; he invented many of the techniques and tools for bone grafting and worked out many of its laws, such as the law that only human bones, preferably from the patient himself, could be used to repair the human skeleton.

And at last the medical profession was willing to admit that here was a new science, but not that Albee was its prophet. Many Orthopaedists chose another man to be their hero, Dr. Russell Hibbs, a horseback doctor from Tennessee, who rose to be Surgeon-in-Chief of the New York Orthopaedic Hospital. He was a modest man; and Albee was never noted for his sweet humility.

They don't deny Albee the bone-graft, but they claim for Hibbs the first spine fusion and the immobilizing of a joint to give a useful member with infantile paralysis. If the medical profession disputes, who are we to step in and settle the bout? Albee or Hibbs, the victory is still ours.

Of historical interest is the fact that Albee's Institution, The Hospital for Ruptured and Crippled, affiliated with Cornell University, eventually became the Hospital for Special Surgery, and the principles that Albee espoused are still in constant use on a daily basis.

Russell Hibbs continued his dynamic leadership as a teacher and surgeon at the New York Orthopaedic Hospital until his death at age 63 on September 16, 1932.

The following is a case history of the fourth person in the world to have a spinal fusion performed by Russell Hibbs and who was examined in the Orthopaedic Hospital and Dispensary with a 71-year follow-up.

E.M. was first brought to the New York Orthopaedic Dispensary when it was located on 59th Street in New York City in July 1911. At that time, he was thirteen years and ten months of age and had a proven tuberculous abscess of the lumbar spine. The abscess had drained spontaneously in the inguinal region on the right on two occasions and the boy was emaciated and quite ill. He was seen by Dr. Hibbs who suggested a posterior spine fusion.

The boy's mother and father argued with each other about the merits and risks of the proposed surgery, but on August 1, 1911, the mother carried the boy into the hospital and agreed to surgery. The patient was placed on a ward immediately next to patient E.Q., who had been the first patient in the world to have a spinal fusion. His surgery had taken place on January 9, 1911, On August 4, 1911, E.M. had his surgery performed. The fusion consisted of stripping the paraspinal muscles from the posterior elements of L5-S1. The spinous processes were divided and intertwined with each other. No bone graft was used. No blood was transfused and the patient made an uneventful recovery after several months of bedrest. He was followed in the New York Orthopaedic Clinic yearly and was recently admitted at the age of eighty-one with a benign tumor of the left sixth rib. During the past years, he had developed diabetes mellitus and had a large ventral hernia following an appendectomy in 1964. He claimed to have almost no back pain and had never had any difficulties since his surgery [Figs. 24-3 and 24-4]. His life was spent doing many types of work and he had married and successfully raised several children.

Because of the work by Hibbs and Albee there was a new dimension to the surgical treatment of tuberculosis of the spine. Drainage of tuberculous lesions had been advocated from the time of Hippocrates, who observed beneficial effects obtained by surgical decompression of tuberculous abscesses. In 1770 Percival Pott advocated this procedure as his "method of cure" and the disease now bears his name. More than a century later the French surgeon Menard again renewed the idea of drainage of these abscesses because he found that in so doing, remission from paraplegia might ensue.[9]

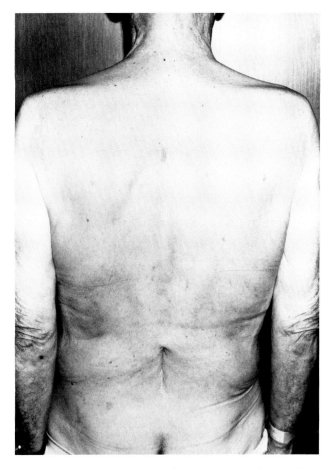

Fig. 24-3 Patient E.M. at age 81. He was the fourth person in the world to undergo a spinal fusion, which was performed on August 4, 1911.

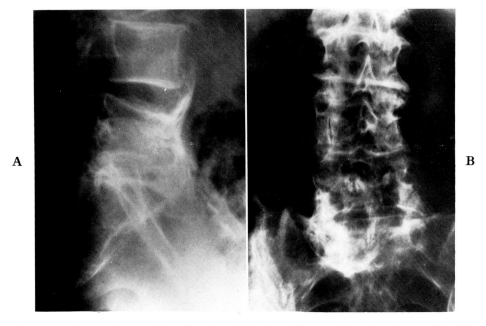

Fig. 24-4 **A,** Lateral x-ray film of patient E.M. taken 68 years after spine fusion of the fifth lumbar vertebra to the sacrum. Notice the anterior bridging of bone at L4 and L5. **B,** anteroposterior view showing fusion of L5 to S1.

However, such drainage procedures were hazardous until effective antibiotic therapy was available. Bacterial superinfection of drainage sites was all too common.

Before the work of Hibbs and Albee no previous successful surgical attack had been made on the deformity of Pott's disease. The principles laid down by Hibbs remain valid, despite the controversy that has arisen since introduction of effective antituberculous drug therapy. Today with the advent of drugs, as well as surgery, the treatment of tuberculosis in most modern countries has resulted in an effective and certain cure for the disease. Over 70 years after E.M.'s operation by Dr. Russell Hibbs, the insight that both Hibbs and Albee had in the conceptualization of spine fusion is still apparent.

After the original concept of lumbar spine surgery by both Hibbs and Albee the technique was improved upon by Joseph Risser, who succeeded Hibbs as the chief of the spinal service at the New York Orthopaedic Hospital. Risser used several modifications, especially the resection and impaction of bone grafts into the facet joints at all levels to give better fusion to those areas. In 1953 Dr. Melvin B. Watkins, on the same staff, conceived of using the bilateral-lateral approach to the lumbar transverse processes. He devised his own surgical exposure and used the iliac crest from each side as bone graft material, which he secured to the transverse process with a short screw in most instances (Fig. 24-5). Dr. Watkins published his paper on two occasions.[13,14]

After 1956 Dr. Keith McElroy at the New York Orthopaedic Hospital improved on the bilateral-lateral technique by devising many new instruments to

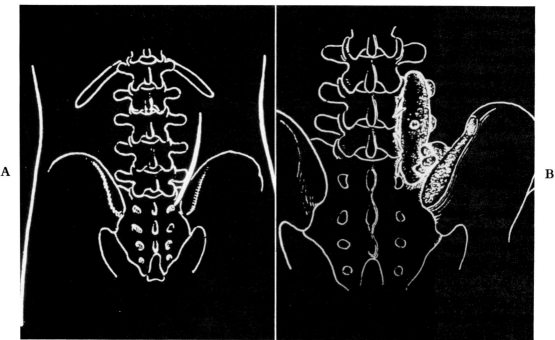

Fig. 24-5 A, Paraspinal surgical approach advocated by Dr. Melvin B. Watkins in 1953. Dr. Watkins would use two such incisions, one on each side of the spine, for bilateral-lateral fusion. **B,** Illustration of use of the iliac crest and screwing it to one of the transverse processes after proper decortication and preparation for fusion.

make the surgery easier and obtain more uniform results from fusion. McElroy's instruments and his insistence on good surgical preparation before the fusion have led to an extremely high fusion rate. Since that time everyone trained at the New York Orthopaedic Hospital of the Columbia-Presbyterian Medical Center has learned to use these techniques. Many thousands of patients have had the bilateral-lateral fusion (Chapter 26). The effectiveness and stability of this widely used and biomechanically sound fusion technique have been clearly demonstrated. A success rate of 90% can be safely anticipated by surgeons who are properly schooled and experienced in the sound application of these principles.[12]

REFERENCES

1. Adams, F.: The genuine works of Hippocrates, New York, 1929, Wm. Wood Co.
2. Albee, F.H.: Transplantation of portion of tibia into spine for Pott's disease: a preliminary report, JAMA September 9, 1911.
3. Albee, L.B.: Doctor and I, Detroit, Michigan, 1951, S.J. Block Company.
4. Benyon-Ray, M.: How to conquer your handicaps, Indianapolis, 1948, The Bobbs-Merrill Co., Inc.
5. Hibbs, R.A.: An operation for progressive spinal deformities: a preliminary report of three cases from the service of the orthopaedic hospital, New York Med. J. **93:**1013, 1911.
6. Hibbs, R.A.: A report of fifty-nine cases of scoliosis treated by the fusion operation, J. Bone Joint Surg. **6:**3, 1924.
7. Hibbs, R.A., et al.: Scoliosis treated by the fusion operation: an end-result study of three hundred and sixty cases, J. Bone Joint Surg. **13:**91, 1931.
8. Howorth, M.B.: Evolution of spinal fusion, Ann. Surg. **117:**278, 1943.
9. Menard, V.: Causes de la paraplegie dans le mal de Pott. Son traitement chirugical por l'ouverture directe du foyer tuberculeux des vertebres, Rev. d'orthop. **5:**47, 1894.
10. Pott, P.: Remarks on that kind of palsy of the lower limbs which is frequently found to accompany a curvature of the spine and is supposed to be caused by it. Together with its method of cure, vol. 1, In Medical classics, Baltimore, 1936, Williams & Wilkins.
11. Smith, A., DeF.: The New York Orthopaedic Hospital, New York, 1966, J.B. Watkins Co.
12. Truchly, G., and Thompson, W.A.L.: Posterolateral fusion of the lumbosacral spine, J. Bone Joint Surg. **44A:**505, 1962.
13. Watkins, M.B.: Posterolateral fusion of the lumbar and lumbosacral spine, J. Bone Joint Surg. **35A:**1014, 1953.
14. Watkins, M.B.: Posterolateral bone-grafting for fusion of the lumbar and lumbosacral spine, J. Bone Joint Surg. **41A:**388, 1959.

CHAPTER 25

THE EFFECT OF METABOLIC BONE DISEASE ON SPINAL FUSION

†Frank L. Raney, Jr.   Felix O. Kolb

As orthopedists it is important that we understand—particularly when dealing with the back—when bone is normal and when it is abnormal. The patient who does not form bone in a normal manner will not heal a fracture and will not heal a fusion. It is imperative that we learn how to determine in advance whether patients are able to form bone in a normal manner so that they can heal a fusion. It is important that each of us has the ability to do a satisfactory screening procedure to determine whether we need a metabolic bone expert to help us.

Dr. Raney now has every patient on whom he is going to do a fusion seen by a metabolic bone specialist to do a preoperative metabolic bone workup and give appropriate metabolic treatment if it is indicated. The patient's metabolic bone state is always normalized, or at least stabilized, before a fusion is done. Dr. Felix Kolb, an endocrinologist and metabolic bone expert, has developed a metabolic bone workup that is outlined in detail in this chapter. Initially, a set of screening tests is done. If they show an abnormality, then the metabolic bone expert is called in to study and treat the patient further. The first tests ordered are a complete blood count (CBC) with differential, a sedimentation rate, a blood chemical panel (usually a JMAC-23) a parathyroid hormone assay, a vitamin D assay, and, if there is any need, a protein electrophoretic pattern. A 24-hour urine test is ordered for calcium, phosphorus, creatinine, and, if gout is suspected, uric acid. The creatinine is measured to be certain that an equivalent specimen is obtained each time. An AP x-ray film of the hands and a lateral film of the skull are ordered. A technetium bone scan is usually ordered, and spinal bone densitometry is measured either by the dual photon or CT scan method; the bone mineral content at the radius is measured by the single photon method. Once this set of screening tests is completed, it can be decided whether a more complete workup is needed. If these tests are all within normal limits, one can feel fairly

†Deceased.

certain that the metabolic bone state is not out of order. However, if Dr. Raney plans to do a fusion himself, he requests a metabolic bone expert to review the findings to determine whether further testing needs to be done.

Metabolic abnormalities related to the spine are graphically illustrated by a series of patients with pseudoarthrosis. Dr. Raney reviewed the spine fusions he did over a period of 10 years and found that 66 of these had a pseudoarthrosis. Of these, 41 had been referred for repair of already established pseudoarthroses performed elsewhere, whereas 25 of these were pseudoarthroses after fusions Dr. Raney had done. Of these 66 patients, 35 were found to have metabolic abnormalities. Not all of the 66 patients were given a bone metabolic workup, because Dr. Raney was not aware initially that metabolic abnormalities were of such great importance. As the importance was appreciated, more and more of the patients were metabolically evaluated.

Of the 66 pseudoarthroses treated, 47 completely healed, and at the time of the analysis four more were under treatment for their metabolic bone defect before contemplated surgery. Four had been seen for evaluation only and were not treated. Four had been lost to follow-up, one had died, one had decided against surgery, and five were not healed but were still under treatment.

The categories of bone abnormalities most often recognized are (1) untreated menopause with osteoporosis, (2) malabsorption syndrome from either a bowel defect or after gastric or bowel surgery with osteomalacia, (3) phosphate depletion from excessive use of antacids not containing calcium or phosphorus with resultant osteopenia, (4) vitamin D abnormality in either absorption, liver conversion, or kidney conversion with resultant failure to grow and mineralize bone, and (5) excessive use of tobacco and alcohol.

Metabolic bone treatment is geared to the patient's needs. If patients are deficient in hormones, they are given hormone replacement. An optimal calcium and phosphorus intake is usually given. Vitamin D_3 (calciferol) is also given, and if it is found that hydroxylation of the Vitamin D is not occurring in the liver, patients are placed on Calderol, which is the 25-hydroxylated form of Vitamin D. Some patients are given fluoride. In patients who are taking antacids in great amounts that do not contain calcium or phosphorus, antacids that do contain calcium and phosphorus are substituted (for example, calcium carbonate and phosphalgel). Patients with more complicated reasons for their metabolic disturbances are studied in detail by our metabolic bone specialist, usually Dr. Kolb, with evaluation of thyroid function, parathyroid function, adrenal function, pituitary function, liver function, kidney function, and estrogen and testosterone levels. Appropriate treatment for any abnormalities found is then carried out. Bone biopsy after tetracycline labeling has been used in a good many instances to further assess the bone dynamics.

It is our finding that measures to correct the metabolic abnormalities almost always speed up the healing of previously failed fusion, and have increased the success rate of either future revisions or new fusions. We have become convinced that patients who are going to have a fusion procedure should have a metabolic bone workup. The outline of the metabolic bone workup is as follows. (See Chapter 38.)

METABOLIC BONE WORKUP
I. Blood tests
  A. CBC and sedimentation rate
  B. SMAC-23, for overall view of metabolic state
  C. Parathyroid screen
  D. 25-Hydroxy vitamin D screen

E. Protein electrophoretic pattern if indicated
II. 24-hour urine tests
   A. Calcium
   B. Phosphorus
   C. Creatinine
   D. Total hydroxyproline
   E. Uric acid
III. X-rays
   A. AP of hands for bone resorption
   B. Lateral skull for hyperparathyroidism
   C. X-ray films of involved area
IV. Bone scan—technetium (^{99m}TC methylene diphosphate)
V. Bone densitometry
   A. Dual photon or CT scan of the spine
   B. Single photon for radius
VI. Calcium loading
   A. Oral calcium 1500 mg per day for 3 days. At end of second day, repeat 24-hour urine test for calcium, phosphorus and creatinine
VII. Bone biopsy in some cases, usually after tetracycline label

Additional Details Concerning Reasons for and Interpretation of Metabolic Bone Tests

I. Blood
   A. CBC and sedimentation rate to determine if inflammatory or neoplastic process is present
   B. SMAC-23 to give overall view of metabolic state
      1. Tests for calcium, phosphorus, alkaline phosphatase, total protein, albumin, globulin, albumin/globulin ratio, 25-hydroxy vitamin D, and parathormone level to assess metabolic bone state
      2. Blood urea nitrogen (BUN), creatinine, BUN/creatinine ratio, and electrolyte panel (sodium, potassium, chloride, and HCO_3) to assess kidney function
      3. Serum glutamic-oxaloacetic transaminase, serum glutamic-pyruvic transaminase, alkaline phosphatase, and total bilirubin to assess liver function
      4. Cholesterol and triglycerides to assess fat metabolism
      5. Glucose to assess glucose metabolism for diabetes
      6. Uric acid to assess for gout
      7. T4 and T3 by radioimmunoassay, free thyroxine index and thyroid stimulating hormone to evaluate thyroid function
      8. Luteinizing hormone, follicle stimulating hormone and prolactin to evaluate pituitary and gonadal function
      9. Cortisol to evaluate adrenal function
      10. Estrogen or testosterone levels to evaluate gonadal function
II. 24-hour urine tests
   A. Calcium
      1. Low
         a. Osteomalacia from malabsorption of calcium or lack of vitamin D
         b. Low bone turnover state
      2. High
         a. Hypercalciuria
         b. High turnover state
         c. Hyperparathyroidism
   B. Phosphorus
      1. Low
         a. Poor absorption
         b. Inadequate Vitamin D intake
         c. Phosphate depletion

from excessive antacid use or poor kidney function
  C. Creatinine, indicates appropriate specimen has been obtained and that renal function is adequate; if creatinine level remains the same from one test to the next, it indicates like specimens are being compared
  D. Hydroxyproline, indicates high or low turnover state because hydroxyproline is breakdown product of bone matrix
III. X-ray films
  A. X-ray films of involved area
  B. AP hands—preferably on industrial film
    1. Resorption of bone from radial side, especially of middle phalanges, indicative of hyperparathyroidism
    2. Assesses cortical thickness of metacarpal (cortical bone loss)
  C. Lateral x-ray film of the skull
    1. Determines if lamina dura present
    2. Assesses size of sella turcica (posterior clinoids gone with severe demineralization).
    3. Evaluates mineralization of skull; ("salt and pepper" skull in hyperparathyroidism, or in severe osteoporosis or myeloma)
IV. Bone scan (technetium)
  A. Persistent hot spot in fusion over 1 year old indicative of delayed fusion or pseudoarthrosis
  B. Bright scan of skeleton with pale kidneys indicative of osteomalacia
  C. Symmetric lesions indicative of pseudofractures as seen in osteomalacia
  D. Bright bone and kidneys—high turnover state
  E. Pale scan—low turnover state
  F. Scattered or asymmetric lesions—cancer or Paget's disease
V. Bone densitometry
  A. Evaluation of amount of mineral in spine
    1. Dual photon method very accurate and reproducible
    2. CT scan method measures primarily trabecular bone
  B. Evaluation of amount of mineral in radius
    1. Single photon method, evaluates primarily cortical bone
VI. Calcium loading
  A. Oral calcium 1500 mg per day for 3 days; at end of second day repeat 24-hour urine test for calcium, phosphorus, and creatinine
    1. Low urinary calcium indicative of malabsorption
    2. Usually no malabsorption problem if low urinary calcium normalizes
    3. If urinary calcium becomes excessively high, patient is an overabsorber and overexcreter (hypercalciuric); occurs in about 10% of patients
VII. Bone biopsy
  A. Usually, iliac crest undecalcified biopsy preceded by a single or double tetracycline label; most commonly done when osteomalacia is suspected, but also helps to differentiate low turnover from high bone turnover states

CHAPTER

26

THE TECHNIQUE OF THE BILATERAL-LATERAL LUMBAR SPINE FUSION

Hugo A. Keim

In the hands of accomplished surgeons very difficult surgical techniques look extremely simple. During my early training I would marvel at the speed and ease with which some of my teachers, who were gifted surgeons, would perform an arduous procedure. The procedure was deceptively simple to the novice, but the complexities of performing a similar surgical procedure by myself soon became evident. It is obvious that attention to detail and frequent repetition of these details make a surgical procedure appear surprisingly simple and easy. Over the past 25 years I have been trying to determine exactly what it is about lumbar spine fusions that can lead to overall success rates as low as 40% to 50% in some reported series and as high as 95% in other series, although they are reported by men of equal ethical repute. What then is the difference between the techniques employed by these different groups of surgeons? It is exactly the fine attention to detail that enhances the success rate and contributes to reproducibility of results in case after case, *if* the principles are strictly observed.

During my resident years at Northwestern University in Chicago I was fortunate to have Dr. Robert T. McElvenny as one of my mentors; Dr. McElvenny had been trained by Russell A. Hibbs. After some years on the staff of the New York Orthopaedic Hospital McElvenny joined the staff of Northwestern University, where he performed incredibly accomplished spine surgery for the remainder of his career. He was considered by many to have been the "Picasso of the spine," and it was fortunate for me as a resident to have been associated with him and to have observed the many techniques that he had learned from the master, Russell A. Hibbs.

Subsequently, I joined the staff of the New York Orthopaedic Hospital and was fortunate enough to spend time with Drs. Frank E. Stinchfield, Theodore R. Waugh, Melvin Brent Watkins, and Keith B. McElroy. These men had also learned through the lineage of Hibbs how

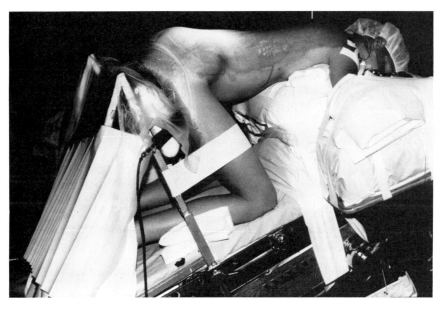

Fig. 26-1 Patient in kneeling position before surgery on Hastings laminectomy frame. The main advantage of this frame is to keep abdomen free during surgical procedure, thus decreasing intraabdominal pressure and controlling venous bleeding.

to do the posterior lumbar spine fusion, and through the work of Watkins, who perfected the bilateral-lateral spine fusion, I was able to distill in my own mind the minute details that make the bilateral-lateral spine fusion successful if certain principles are observed.

Aside from the usual workup and preparation, all patients are placed in the operating room in the kneeling position on a Hastings laminectomy frame. These frames are now standard in most operating rooms and permit the abdomen of the patient to be free throughout the entire procedure, thus decreasing the amount of venous pressure on Batson's plexis surrounding the vertebral bodies (Fig. 26-1). Bleeding is therefore restricted, and with the use of hypotensive anesthesia the field remains relatively dry in most cases, although the lumbar spine is a highly vascular area.

I generally use the midline incision; however, in cases of previous infection I will use the lateral incision, which can be used bilaterally according to Watkins. This bilateral-lateral incision to the transverse processes has been advocated by Dr. Leon Wiltse, who has used it very successfully for the treatment of spondylolisthesis in a large number of cases.

In the routine midline incision a very superficial skin incision is first made, and the area is injected with approximately 1500 ml of 1:500,000 epinephrine solution to try to avoid bleeding of the small vessels immediately under the dermis. Next the incision is deepened to the fascia; immediately, self-retaining retractors are inserted to stretch out the skin and stretch the multiple small bleeding vessels that are usually encountered.

The incision is carried directly over the tips of the spinous processes from the lower limit of the spinous process of L3 (for a two-level joint fusion) to the midsacral area by electrocautery. The electrocautery is used in the "cutting" mode throughout the procedure. Even bleeding vessels are cauterized with the cutting mode only and not the "coagulation" mode. This seems to cause less tissue reaction and is much quicker than the coagulation mode. With the cautery, the incision is carried down to the lamina in between each of the spinous processes so that the intraspinous ligament is divided at the same time that the approach is made directly through and along the entire crest of each spinous process. Using Cobb elevators, the paraspinal muscles are then stripped off of each side of the spine while those muscles are then retracted with two long, thin Hibbs retractors in the hands of a strong assistant. Each side is worked on alternately; a sponge is packed directly in one side while the other side is being developed. This role is reversed frequently so that bleeding is generally controlled by the tamponade effect of the sponges. Very little cauterization is required throughout these stages with effective use of the sponges.

As the facet joints are exposed the Cobb elevator sweeps the paraspinal muscles directly away from their adherence to the capsular structures. The tip of the Cobb elevator then seeks out the transverse process of L4 and L5. At this point great care must be taken not to break off this process or in any way damage the intertransverse membrane, which traverses from one transverse process to another. The importance of this membrane cannot be too strongly emphasized, since it is really one of the main keys to successful spinal fusion. The membrane is actually quite thick and supports the bone graft on top of each of the transverse processes after they have been decorticated (Fig. 26-2). Penetration of this intertransverse membrane causes absorption of the graft by body fluids anterior to the transverse processes, and I believe it is a main cause for graft resorption and failure of the fusion, leading to nonunion.

With assistance of good retraction, working first on one side and then on the other, the transverse processes can be gradually brought into adequate view. At this point a deep retractor is extremely helpful, since it is very strong and the blades at the top of the retractor are much narrower than those on the business end, which helps to hold the paraspinal muscles away from the transverse processes (Fig. 26-3). Sometimes there is some difficulty in inserting the retractor if the paraspinal muscles have not been adequately separated from the transverse processes; occasionally, the blades have to be applied inside the incision first and then brought up to the arms of the retractor and secured in place before complete retraction can occur.

Once the transverse processes of L4 and L5 have been adequately identified and the retractor is in place, attention is focused to getting maximal exposure of each of the transverse processes on both sides while carefully maintaining the integrity of the intertransverse membrane. At this point it is helpful to resect the facet joints of L4 and L5 bilaterally. It gives much better visualization of the transverse processes and eases decortication of those processes. The facet joints are usually resected using a power osteotome.* With the use of this impact osteotome the facet joints are resected in a matter of minutes (Fig. 26-4). A radical resection is done at this time, since there is no reason to save any articular cartilage of these facet joints.

After resection, all bone and capsular tissue are removed using a double-action rongeur and attention is focused on decorticating the transverse processes. This can be done best by the use of an extremely sharp curette. All sharp surgical instruments are honed before each and every surgical case. It is imperative that the curettes, as well as all osteotomes, be sharpened before every case, since even

---

*Stryker Corp., Kalamazoo, Mich.

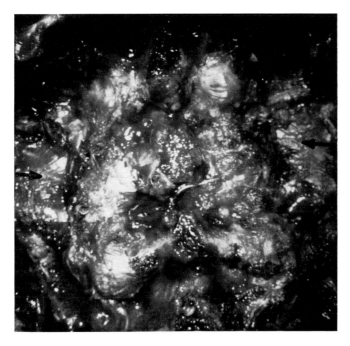

Fig. 26-2 Intertransverse membrane is illustrated between the transverse processes of L4-L5. Dark arrows point directly to thin membrane, very distinct anatomic entity between transverse processes of each lumbar vertebrae. It is most important not to perforate this membrane during the transverse process exposure. Bilateral-lateral bone graft is placed directly on decorticated transverse processes and is held in place anteriorly by this membrane.

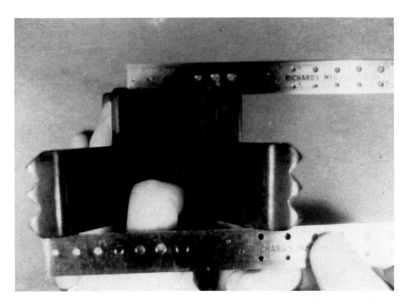

Fig. 26-3 Spinal retractor used in lumbar spine surgery was originally designed by Dr. Keith McElroy. Note that end deepest in wound is much wider than opening as it enters wound posteriorly. In this illustration, retractor is facing the reader. (Richards Manufacturing Co., Memphis, Tenn.)

254 *Surgical Procedures*

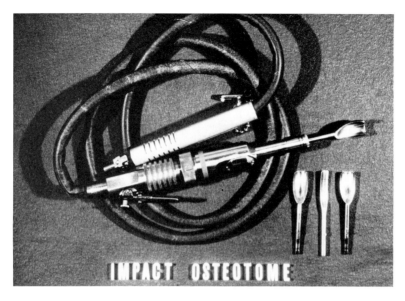

Fig. 26-4 Nitrogen-powered impact osteotome for use in decorticating spine and obtaining iliac bone graft. This tool makes the entire decortication and harvesting procedure much simpler. Blades are interchangeable and are sharpened before each operative case. (Stryker Corp., Kalamazoo, Mich.)

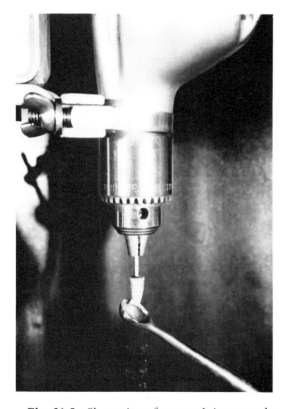

Fig. 26-5 Sharpening of curette. It is extremely important to sharpen curette cup on inside, as well as outside. Great care must be taken not to shave off the entire edge. Curettes must be sharpened before each surgical case, since autoclaving will dull edges.

autoclaving dulls the edge of these instruments (Fig. 26-5). A sharp instrument is much safer than a dull one; this is especially true of curettes. It is because of dull curettes that most transverse processes are broken. Too much downward pressure is applied on the transverse process in an attempt to decorticate it, and this of course is one of the main causes of nonunions. Do not use a periosteal elevator, since downward pressure can easily fracture the process (Fig. 26-6).

With the use of the sharp curette, the approach to decortication is made at the *lateral* portion of the transverse process itself (Fig. 26-7, *A*). The curette starts laterally at the bulbous tip of the transverse process and moves in toward the midline at the base of the L4 transverse process. One must be very careful, when pulling the curette medially and sweeping it upward, not to damage the capsule and articular area of the L3-L4 joint. However, there is a large surface of cortical and cancellous bone that can be exposed immediately superior to the base of the transverse process along the edge of the superior facet joint of L4, which in-

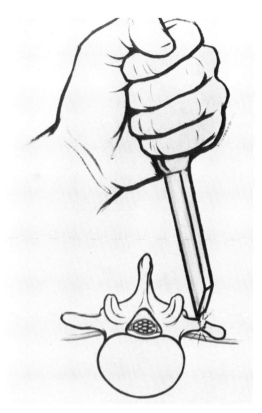

Fig. 26-6 Illustration of need to prevent breakage of transverse processes. These structures are extremely important in supporting the bone graft. Transverse process of L4 is usually smallest of five lumbar vertebrae, and great care must be taken to preserve it by avoiding downward pressure. This is especially important during subperiosteal elevation, as well as decortication.

creases the fusion surface by approximately 30% to 40% on each transverse process (Fig. 26-7, *B* and *C*). This is an extremely important detail for preparation for the fusion, since this extra exposed articular surface on both sides of the superior face of L4 gives 30% to 40% additional area to which the bone graft can adhere during the healing process. Naturally, if the fusion is to extend up to L3, the L3-L4 facet joint will be excised; the same concept applies to the transverse process of L3 with preservations of the L2-L3 facet joint and capsule.

These techniques can be safely used with fusions all the way up to T12 without undue difficulty. In my hands many four- and five-level fusions have been performed with successful union rates. However, long fusions using the bilateral-lateral technique generally need immobilization in a lumbar orthosis that includes one leg to above the knee. Attention then is focused to the transverse process of L5, which is easy to decorticate because the facet joint at that level has already been resected.

With the use of any extremely large curette, approximately the size of a nickel (Fig. 26-8), the lateral gutter of the sacrum and iliac wing is then very aggressively decorticated and freed of all soft tissue and cortical bone. This should be done in a very gradually inclined plane so that no "step defect" occurs that can later lead to greater stress and nonunion. If a very gradually inclined plane is decorticated in this level, it allows for better biomechanical stresses to be applied to the fusion area. These lateral gutters on both sides can be further augmented with the nitrogen-powered impact osteotome, and the areas can be deepened to furnish good acceptance to the bilateral-lateral bone graft that will soon be applied. Many times these areas bleed rather generously; therefore attention should be focused on stopping individual bleeders—especially small arteries and clusters of veins. These are often found in the sacral foramina and should be cauterized promptly and effectively to prevent prolonged bleeding. After preparation of the bilateral-lateral gutters, the wound is then very tightly packed with sponges and attention is focused on obtaining the autogenous iliac bone graft.

Generally, I take the right-sided crest, since I am right handed and stand on the patient's left side during surgery. For many years, Dr. Frank E. Stinchfield has believed that if a patient has right leg sciatica, one should take the opposite iliac crest for a bone graft because then the patient can differentiate between the

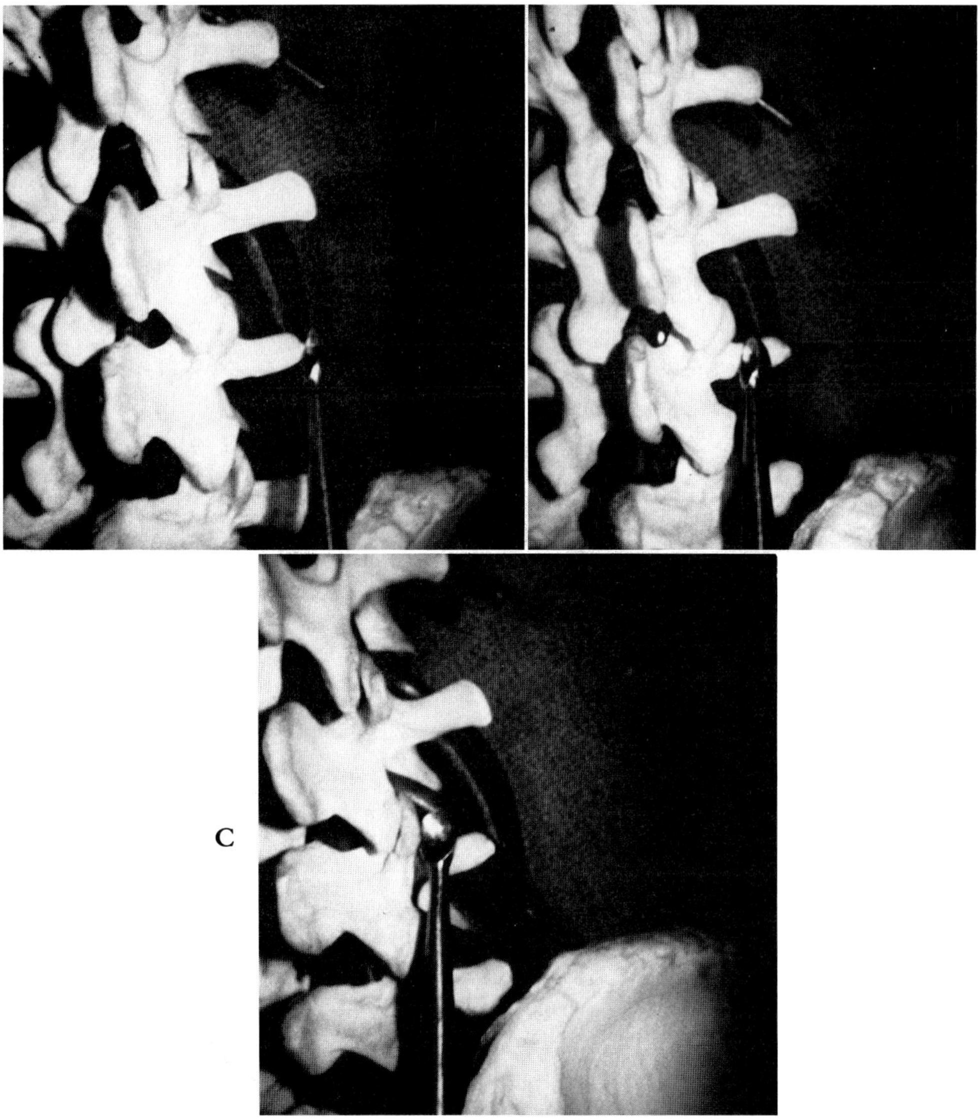

Fig. 26-7 **A,** Illustration indicates in sequence how transverse processes should be decorticated from lateral border moving toward medial area. **B,** Process has been swept near midline. **C,** Curette is used to roll up the side of superior articular facet of that particular vertebra. This increases fusion area of transverse process and vertebra by approximately 30%, and is the most important step in securing a solid spinal fusion.

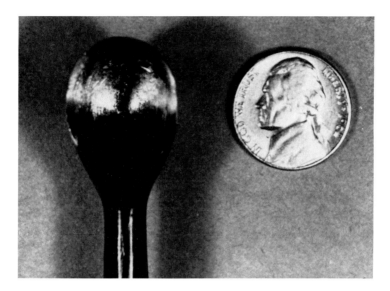

Fig. 26-8 The size of large curette used to make iliac gutters bilaterally. It has an extremely large cup and is sharpened before every surgical case.

donor-site pain from the preoperative sciatic pain. This is quite a good idea, and many surgeons trained by Dr. Stinchfield have continued this practice.

The iliac graft is approached through exactly the same midline incision. There is no need to make a separate incision to the iliac donor area. The second incision results in an ugly scar, which is wide, unsightly, and usually divides the clunial nerves leading to troublesome numbness over the buttocks. The first incision down the midline is absolutely straight; it is not curved to either side because it is not necessary to obtain the iliac crest bone graft if the proper retractors are used.

As soon as the cutting electrocautery is used to start the dissection toward the right iliac crest, two towel clips are placed in the skin to elevate this layer and make retraction easier. Once the large flap is elevated, the two long, thin Hibbs retractors then are inserted in place of the towel clips and the skin is retracted so that the iliac crest becomes completely visible. Upon palpation of the iliac crest with the left index finger, the electrocautery wand in the cutting mode then is brought directly down the midline of the iliac crest for most of its excursion. This dissection is facilitated with the use of the Cobb periosteal elevator. It is most important to be cautious in elevating the gluteal muscles from the iliac crest by strict adherence to the contours of the crest, so that one does not push forward directly in the gluteal muscles and cause increased bleeding. If a very careful subperiosteal dissection of the iliac crest is made followed by packing with a large sponge, very little bleeding is encountered. Naturally, care must be taken not to bring the Cobb elevator in direct contact with the sciatic notch, where the superior gluteal artery and its plexis of veins reside.

After elevation of the gluteal muscles from the iliac crest a large retractor, designed by Theodore R. Waugh,* is inserted and pressure placed in a downward and outward direction to completely expose most of the posterior iliac wing (Fig. 26-9). Large amounts of cortical and cancellous bone can be harvested from the

---

*Zimmer USA, Inc., Warsaw, Ind.

258 *Surgical Procedures*

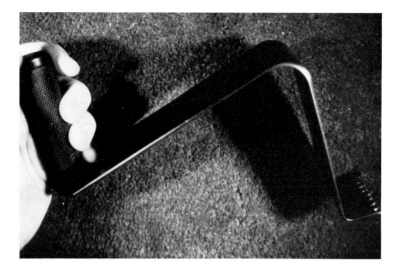

Fig. 26-9 Iliac crest retractor originally designed by Theodore R. Waugh, which holds iliac muscles completely away from crest and allows large amounts of cortical and cancellous bone to be harvested by the impact osteotome.

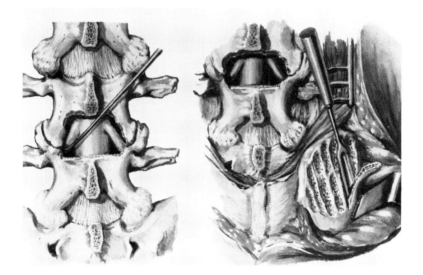

Fig. 26-10 Decompression done by midline approach. Nerve roots are completely freed of all bony, cartilaginous, and soft tissue pressure in entire neural canal and followed through their exit in intervertebral foramen. Iliac crest then is removed completely down to the inner table, making numerous small matchstick-size grafts of cortical and cancellous bone available.

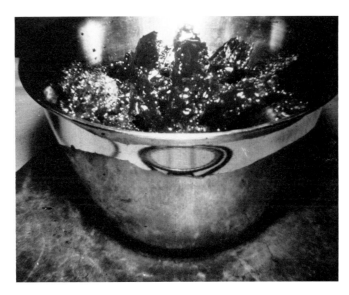

Fig. 26-11 The amount of cortical and cancellous bone that can be obtained from iliac crest of average patient. It can easily fill a bone cup and provides adequate graft material for a very massive bilateral-lateral spine fusion.

iliac crest (Fig. 26-10) with the impact osteotome. As much bone as possible is removed directly down to the inner table, practically penetrating the sacroiliac joint, so that large volumes of both cortical and cancellous strips are taken (Fig. 26-11). These strips then are cut further into even smaller matchstick-size strips by an assistant so that they can be later interwoven to obtain a very uniform and thick autogenous bone graft. Once the graft has been completely obtained, a plug of bone wax is uniformly spread throughout the areas of cortical and cancellous decortication to cut down on bleeding along the donor site. (Be certain to obtain a history of bee allergies on all patients before using bone wax, since it can be extremely allergenic in patients who are allergic to bee stings.)

After the application of the bone wax a large piece of doubled-up Gelfoam is spread over the entire iliac crest and rubbed into the interstices of the bone to further aid in coagulation of all bleeding points. At this moment there should be almost no bleeding from the iliac donor site; the area should remain quite dry unless veins have been injured, in which case sometimes they may need to be individually cauterized. A sponge is left in place in this area for later removal and closure over hemovac drains. Attention then is focused to the main midline dissection.

By this time, when the McElroy retractor is again inserted into the midline, the wound should be relatively dry because the tamponading of the sponges has taken effect. If the patient is to have a spinal decompression for spinal stenosis at this point, I then use the impact osteotome to thin down the lamina, which will need to be removed by rongeurs, so that they are as thin as possible and can be removed piecemeal with ease. This is one little step that makes the laminectomy much easier and less traumatic both for the patient and for the surgeon. By thinning the lamina with the impact osteotome, much additional good bone can also be obtained for the subsequent fusion procedure.

If the patient has a herniated disc that is

to be treated by disc excision and fusion, the disc approach can be made at this point and the disc can be excised. If the patient has spondylolisthesis, the arch of the affected vertebra can be completely excised and the nerve roots freed of all encroachment by the cartilagenous debris around the pseudarthrosis of the spondylolysis or spondylolisthesis. If the patient is to have a bilateral-lateral decompression for central and lateral recess stenosis, this procedure can be facilitated by an approach at the sacrum using a broad-based transverse osteotome, driving it directly downward so that a flap of the superior edge of S1 can be elevated along with the ligamentum flavum of L5 to S1. The dura and its epidural fat is promptly exposed, and a Hurd retractor is inserted by an assistant to protect the dura from injury (Fig. 26-12). This technique is actually quite safe if the osteotome is very wide and driven downward with care.

With the Hurd retractor in place and with proper guidance by a trained assistant, the principal surgeon uses a large double-action rongeur and removes the arches of L5, L4 and any other level as required. The decompression can be done rather widely and directly out to the remainder of the facet joints from inside the neural canal. Because the lamina have been thinned previously by the use of the osteotome, there is very little effort required to effect this total laminectomy and decompression. After this step, a 45-degree angle Kerrison can be used in all peripheral areas of the site for decompression and to trace the nerve roots bilaterally out of their intervertebral foramina; thus the decompression can be made safely and completely.

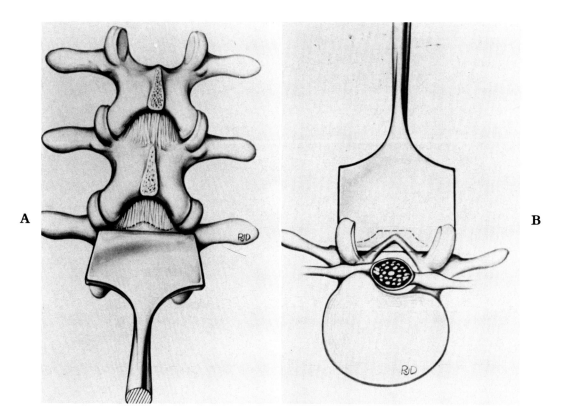

Fig. 26-12 **A** and **B,** Technique used to expose thecal sac by cutting superior border of either sacrum or L5 to gain exposure to dura. A very broad osteotome must be used, and care must be taken to drive it gingerly down to the dura only.

It is extremely important to be aware that sometimes large discs are in a most lateral position (described by Wiltse as the "far out syndrome"), and the nerve root must be very carefully observed so that it is adequately decompressed throughout the length of its entrapment. The most common mistake in this type of spinal decompression is to decompress only centrally and not to proceed far enough laterally through the intervertebral foramen with adequate freeing up of each nerve root. It is not adequate merely to pass a probe or rubber drain through the intervertebral foramen, because CT scan studies by experts such as Kenneth Heithoff from Minneapolis have shown that the nerve root lives in the superior-medial aspect of each intervertebral foramen. Thus merely passing a probe or catheter through the foramen does not at all ensure that the nerve root is adequately decompressed, falsely misleading the surgeon into thinking that the job is done, when in reality was stopped far too short of adequate nerve-root decompression. Once this procedure has been performed, attention then is focused on placing several layers of very thick Gelfoam directly over the midline decompressive site. Sometimes it is advantageous to use a fat graft, although this is an area of great controversy. Some surgeons believe that fat grafting may cause complications, whereas others believe that it prevents the ingrowth of scar tissue. I generally will use a fat graft on people who are having their second, third, or fourth operative procedure but on a "virginal" spinal approach, I usually use two or three layers of thick Gelfoam stacked on each other, completely covering the laminectomy defect so that no piece of bone graft can wander into the neural area during closure of the wound (Fig. 26-13).

With the Gelfoam safely in place the bone graft then is added in large quantities as superiorly and bilaterally as possible with very direct compaction and pressure by the surgeon's fingers to lace and intertwine the juxtaposed pieces of bone, providing a uniform mesh of graft material on both sides (Fig. 26-14).

The bone that is impacted should resemble a suitcase handle on each side of the spine when completed. At this point the retractor can be safely released and very slowly removed. It is a good practice for the surgeon to keep his or her fingertips in the wound, holding the graft firmly lateral to keep it from spreading to the midline as the retractor is gently withdrawn. Once the retractor has been removed from the wound, the surgeon's fingers can again push small fragments of bone outward and away from the midline so that closure of the paraspinal muscles does not cause fragments

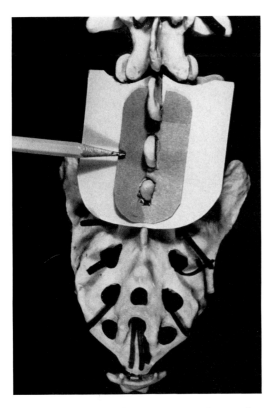

Fig. 26-13 Dark area, the amount of bone that can be decompressed for a very major spinal decompression for central and lateral recess spinal stenosis. Lighter shaded drawing, area to be fused by bilateral-lateral spine fusion using autogenous iliac bone graft.

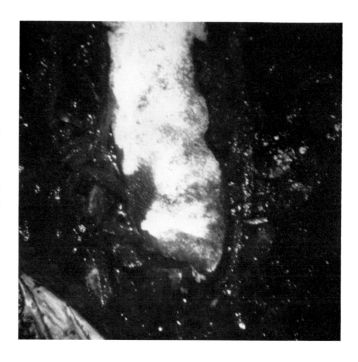

Fig. 26-14 Insertion of several layers of very thick Gelfoam in central decompressed area after total laminectomy and bilateral foraminotomies at multiple levels. Bone graft then is impacted around both sides of the transverse processes to effect bilateral-lateral lumbar spine fusion.

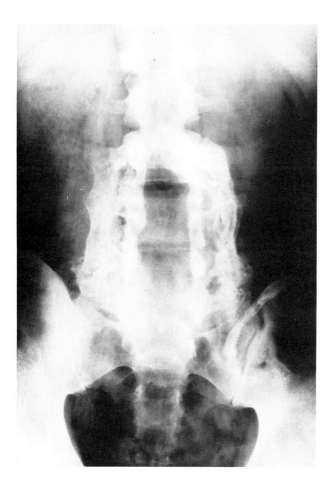

Fig. 26-15 X-ray film of three-level lumbar spine fusion using bilateral-lateral technique. Note central area of massive decompression for both central and lateral recess spinal stenosis.

to shift into the midline area. Two medium-sized hemovac drains then are inserted at this point and brought out to bellows suction. A heavy compression dressing is applied and is generally changed on the third postoperative day along with removal of the hemovac drains, which have an additional drain in the donor site brought to a separate bellows.

Postoperative ambulation should begin as early as the patient will allow. There is really no advantage in starting ambulation within the first or second day because it is very stressful, especially on older patients. It is better to allow patients to stablize for 2 or 3 days and then start them sitting at the edge of the bed and eventually have them up with a walker. Most patients leave the hospital 5 or 6 days after a simple posterior fusion or 8 or 9 days after a wide spinal decompression and bilateral-lateral fusion combination (Fig. 26-15).

After surgery, patients are given a soft lumbosacral corset with metal stays. It has been well established that spinal bracing does not prevent pseudarthrosis; a rigid spinal brace can actually predispose to nonunions because it increases the lever arm at the lumbosacral junction. Therefore rigid spinal braces such as the chair-back are to be avoided. The patients are, however, given a lumbosacral corset with metal stays for a period of 6 months. This corset is used mainly to remind the patient that he or she has had surgery, because at three and four months after surgery many persons tend to be far too aggressive and sometimes injure their backs injudiciously. The lumbosacral corset does not need to be worn in the house, around-the-clock use is discouraged. I tell patients to use it for a 6-month period whenever they leave the house.

Patients are seen 6 weeks after surgery, at which time they are instructed to start physical therapy with abdominal and lumbar muscle strengthening exercises and to attend a postoperative back school, which teaches them proper body mechanics and appropriate lifting techniques. The patients are taught to squat and never to bend forward or stay stooped for long periods. Most patients resume work 2 to 3 weeks after surgery. They can resume sexual activity shortly after their hospital discharge. Patients can drive a car 4 to 6 weeks after arriving home, although I advise them that if they have a flat tire they should leave the changing of the tire to someone else. Patients are seen again 6 months after surgery, at which time x-ray films, which usually show an immature fusion mass on both sides, are taken. The patients are informed at this time that the fusion consists of soft woven bone, and although it seems solid, it will be a further 2 years before hard cortical bone will take its place. Therefore the patient must protect and *gradually* stress the fusion over that period of time. The patient is given an increased list of activities and encouraged to be more active with sports such as tennis and swimming. Very aggressive sports such as downhill skiing are discouraged. Patients are further seen at 1½- and 3-year intervals after surgery, at which time further x-ray films are taken (Fig. 26-16).

My experience with over 1800 lumbar spine fusions, as well as the experience of my predecessors and teachers at the New York Orthopaedic Hospital, attests to the efficacy of the bilateral-lateral lumbar spine fusion. Many surgeons trained by Drs. Watkins, McElroy, Stinchfield, and Waugh can also attest to the principles that are discussed in this chapter.

The work of Albee and Hibbs, which started before 1911, has certainly withstood the test of time. Thousands of spinal fusions that originated from their experience have been performed with great

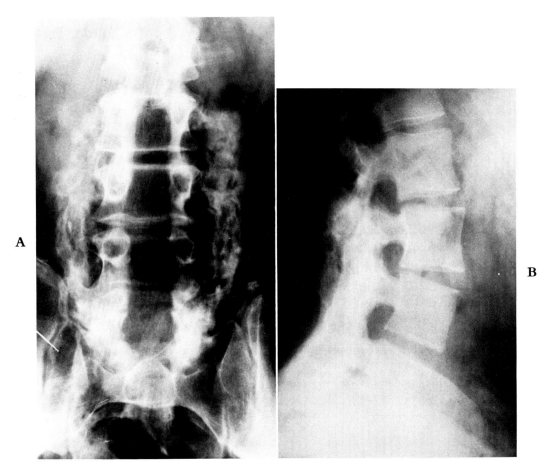

Fig. 26-16 Illustration of AP and lateral four-level vertebral spine fusion. **A,** Fusion extends adequately from tips of transverse processes directly down to sacrum bilaterally. Midline is left completely open and has been filled in with several layers of Gelfoam. **B,** Very solid spine fusion can be seen posteriorly using massive amounts of cortical and cancellous autogenous iliac crest bone.

success. It is unfortunate that surgeons who have not obtained adequate training and who have not paid attention to the specific details that will lead to these successes have made reports of large series of nonunions. This is not the failure of the surgical procedure; it is really the failure of the technician involved. The surgeons who have learned these techniques properly can certify that in a two-level spine fusion the fusion rate is usually between 90% to 95%. In cases where the fusion needs to be extended to three or four levels the success rate drops to approximately 80%. This is still extremely high, especially if on higher level fusions the patient has immobilization to include one leg to the knee in a removable orthoplast brace with adequate lordosis built into it. With the advent of metal fixation and the concomitant surgical complications, we must not forget the wisdom of proper surgical techniques to effect a lumbar spine fusion. It is this return to principles and adherence to detail that can teach new surgeons that a well performed bilateral-lateral lumbar fusion can be a highly successful surgical procedure.

CHAPTER

27

POSTERIOR INTERTRANSVERSE FUSION: INDICATIONS, PATHOMECHANICS, AND RESULTS

Ronald J. Wisneski   Richard H. Rothman

Of all the imprudences dared by man in his brazen reach for ascendancy, the most arrogant was the decision to stand up, to eschew his all-fours, and, piling his vertebrae one atop the other, to thrust himself erect. . . . Better to have maintained our low profile, content to nose among the droppings of mastodons—for it is swollen, bunched, succulent, honed down, gibbous, hummocky, knobbed, sagging, adroop, warped, tipped, and tilted that we are made to wage life, slouching toward our infernal copulations and our eternal reward. Such is the revenge of bone.[26]

Richard Selzer

In his essay on bone Dr. Selzer[26] poetically describes the age-related and pathologic postures that the vertebral column of *Homo sapiens* sometimes assumes as a reward for being the only erect bipedal mammal with a lordotic lumbar curvature. This curvature clearly allows gravity to exert significant shearing stresses, particularly on the last two lumbar intervertebral discs.

In the orthopedic surgeon's quest to straighten the crooked and mechanically unsound vertebral column—and thereby alleviate pain and incapacitating deformity—we can trace the history of spinal fusion procedures back to New York City in 1911 when Hibbs and Albee[2,14] introduced their posterior spinal arthrodesis techniques. With only minor modifications the Hibbs fusion operation remained the standard technique for over a half a century. Originally, the Hibbs fusion was indicated for the treament of certain cases of scoliosis and Pott's disease. During the past 65 years, however, the indications and technique for spinal arthrodesis have broadened considerably. At present there is no question in spinal surgery that is so charged with emotion, or frequently so devoid of reason, as the selection of the proper patient for spinal fusion. An abundance of articles describing the use of spinal arthrodesis as a primary, secondary, or adjunctive surgical treatment has appeared within the last 2 decades. In the lumbosacral spine the key concept surrounding all of the indications for surgical arthrodesis is the demonstration of symptomatic instability.

THE PATHOMECHANICS OF SPINAL INSTABILITY

White and others[36] have defined clinical instability as "the loss of the ability of the spine under physiologic loads to maintain relationships between vertebrae in such a way that there is neither damage nor subsequent irritation to the spinal cord or nerve roots and, in addition, there is no development of incapacitating deformity or pain from structural changes." In physics an unstable structure is one that is not in an optimal state of equilibrium. In the spine the structures involved in static and dynamic equilibrium are the muscles, the ligaments, the intervertebral disc complex, the congruous articular surfaces of the facet joints, and the osseous components.

It is a useful concept to consider these components within the construct of the functional spinal unit or motion segment,[35] which is defined as the smallest segment of the spine that exhibits biomechanical characteristics similar to those of the entire spine. The motion segment consists of two adjacent vertebrae and their connecting soft tissue structures. Each functional spinal unit is capable of rotational angulation and translatory motion in three planes. Rotation is possible in the coronal, sagittal, and transverse planes. Translation can occur vertically or horizontally in either a front to back or side to side motion.

Each of the regions of the vertebral column has an upper limit for each of these motions that may be considered normal. Viewed as a whole, however, the clinical range of motion of the entire spine is a composite of the individual motion-segment units, which in turn are governed by the specific geometry of the osseous components and the restrictive forces of the soft tissues. In biomechanical terms this interconnection of multiple motion segments is termed the *coupling behavior* of the spine.

White and others[36] have given us a list of guidelines in evaluating angulatory and translatory movements in the spine. In a normal state a modest amount of angulation occurs, but very little translatory movement exists. The spinal motion segment–unit, as shown by Gertzbein and Tile,[10] does not move about a single fixed center of rotation but rather a centrode, that is, a locus of instantaneous centers of rotation. In a physiologic state the centrode for any given motion segment falls within the posterior one half of the disc. With degenerative disc disease the centrode changes in flexion and extension are considerable and create marked shearng forces parallel to the plane of the disc, as well as abnormal tensile stresses at the points of ligamentous attachment. MacNab[19] coined the term *segmental instability* to describe this process. He hypothesized that abnormal tension on the anterior fibers of the annulus that attached to the paradiscal margins of the vertebral body just distal to either side of the interspace leads to the radiographic appearance of traction spurs. We are well aware that, as with other degenerative changes noted on routine lumbosacral spine films, the appearance of a traction spur does not imply the concomitant presence of symptomatology. Because of the human body's viscoelastic and remodeling properties, equilibrium can be maintained by compensating for the wear and tear phenomena that are concomitant with aging.

There is little information concerning why certain patients develop back pain and others do not. The evidence is much clearer when one considers spinal stenosis or radiculopathy from a disc herniation in terms of the compromised space in the spinal and nerve-root canals, which produces restricted motion of the neural elements and direct compression effects. In contrast to the precision with which we are usually able to define nerve-root compression, it is most difficult to define the anatomic origin of lumbago with any degree of precision. The pain from segmental instability may be related to the soft tissue structures exceeding their viscoelastic limits, thereby stimulating pain-sensitive mesenchymal structures. The acute attack of lumbago may correspond to actual tears of the soft tissue structures, facet arthritis, or herniation of the disc through the outermost fibers of the annulus. Many of these structures receive their afferent nerve supply via the sinuvertebral nerve. Pedersen[123] has shown that the individual sinuvertebral nerves are actually connected by an ascending or descending series of connected fibers. Therefore, since there is an overlap in the levels of the sinuvertebral nerve ramifications, it is possible that lumbago from instability occurring at a single motion segment may involve more than one recurrent branch of the sinuvertebral nerve. This anatomic factor may explain the poor results of fusion procedures performed for lumbago in the past.

The Biomechanics of Fusion

Because our knowledge of the pathomechanics of the unstable spinal motion segment has expanded, we are able to pursue a more scientfic approach to the analysis of which factors contribute to an increased incidence of solid fusions. We should point out again that the vertebral column is not a totally inert structure but can remodel and adjust its patterns of motion in accordance with the viscoelastic properties of living tissue.

As yet, no completely reliable method of spinal fusion has been developed. Each of the procedures will to a certain degree alter the coupling behavior of the vertebral column and be associated with its own unique incidence of complications and pseudarthroses. These factors, of course, must be weighed against the potential for the fusion technique to alleviate the impairment that has occurred in a symptomatically unstable spine. Table 27-1 illustrates the advantages and disadvantages from a technical standpoint of the three most common fusion techniques used in the lumbar spine. The concept of rigidity relates to the stiffness produced in the motion segment by the fusion mass. In general, the closer the fusion is to the centrode of the motion segment, the greater the stiffness achieved. Theoretically, the interbody fusion technique should have the greatest rigidity and the posterior fusion the least.

Table 27-1 *Technical comparison of lumbosacral fusion techniques*

	Interbody fusion	Posterior fusion	Posterior intertransverse process fusion
Rigidity	Highest	Lowest	Intermediate
Area of recipient site (contiguous surface for grafting)	Low	High (but not contiguous because of the interlaminar spaces)	High
Low vascularity	Variable	Low	High
Rotatory and translatory stability	Low	Low	High
Surgical complication rate	High	Low	Low

In practice, however, the interbody fusions have not held up as expected, possibly as a result of the tendency for graft collapse, as well as the impaired vascularity of the vertebral end-plates. If the posterior fusion mass is extended to include the laminas and facet joints, as well as the spinous processes, the rigidity is proportionally increased. However, this has in some cases led to the complicating factor of iatrogenic spinal stenosis from bone overgrowth, producing spinal canal and foraminal encroachment. The intertransverse process fusion is superior to the posterior fusion technique in that it considerably increases the area moment of inertia, so that greater stability is obtained in axial rotation and lateral bending.

RESULTS OF POSTERIOR INTERTRANSVERSE PROCESS FUSION

Unfortunately, there are few reports of comparative analyses of the various fusion procedures. One such study that stands out, however, was performed by MacNab and Dall.[20] They reported on the results obtained by three techniques of spinal fusion: anterior interbody fusion, posterior fusion, and intertransverse process fusion. The only result assessed was the achievement of a solid fusion. The analysis of results obtained (Table 27-2) showed that the incidence of pseudarthrosis after intertransverse fusions was significantly lower than in the other two methods employed. The authors suggested that the low incidence of pseudarthrosis could be explained by the large contiguous bone surface available for grafting, spanning the transverse processes, lateral surfaces of the articular processes, and intervening isthmic regions. In addition, the local vascularity in the region of the transverse process is abundant and therefore may hypothetically enhance the rate of neovascularization of the donor graft material.

Many authors have described techniques of posterolateral fusion that vary as to surgical exposure and the type and placement of bone grafts (Table 27-3). Originally, the technique was advocated as a secondary procedure in patients with pseudarthrosis or posterior element defects. As experience accumulated, however, it becomes apparent that the technique was valuable as a primary procedure in many disorders of the lumbosacral spine, particularly spondylolisthesis.

In 1939 Campbell[7] described his method of exposure, which utilized the posterolateral region of the lumbosacral spine in conjunction with fusion of the sacroiliac joint. Watkins[34] described a technique in 1953 that employed an incision lateral to the erector spinae and sacrospinalis musculature, followed by retraction of the muscle mass toward the midline until the transverse processes of L4 and L5 were palpable. After decortication of the exposed transverse processes and sacral alae, a full thickness graft from the iliac wing was obtained, split in two, and then impacted into firm contact with the exposed bony surfaces. Follow-up results of 52 patients treated by this method, 40 of which had undergone at least one previous surgical procedure, demonstrated a success rate of 82%. Adkins[1] used a midline approach with subperiosteal elevation of the muscles out to the level of the tips of the transverse processes and placed autogenous tibial grafts as blocks between the transverse processes. In 29 cases he achieved a solid fusion in 83%. Truchly and Thompson[31] modified Watkins's technique by using slivers of bone graft rather than large blocks, two separate posterolateral incisions, and no attempt at facet articulation disruption. Solid fusion was obtained in 92% of two-level fusions and 100% of lumbosacral fusions in 43 patients so treated. Kelly[17] also modified Watkins's approach by placing precisely fitted blocks of fibular bone as struts between

Table 27-2 *Incidence of pseudarthrosis**

Type of operation	Number of cases	Pseudarthrosis	%
Anterior interbody fusion	54	16	30
Posterior fusion	174	30	17
Intertransverse fusion	138	10	7

From MacNab, I., and Dall, D.: J. Bone Joint Surg. **53B**:628, 1971.
*Two segment fusions (fourth lumbar to first sacral) for degenerative disc disease.

Table 27-3 *Posterolateral fusion results*

Author	Year	No. of cases	% solid fusion L4 to S1	L5-S1	Floating*
Adkins	1955	29	83		
Watkins	1959	52	82		
Truchly and Thompson	1962	43	92	100	
Kelly	1963	32	44	100	
Wiltse	1968	49	79	97	
Dawson, Lotysch, and Urist	1981	58	91	100	55
Urist and Dawson (allogeneic bone)	1981	40	86	75	

*One segment fusion above L5-S1.

the transverse processes and the spinous processes of his 32 patients. In 14 patients who had single-level fusions, solid arthrodesis occurred in all. In the 18 patients with two-level fusions, 44% were solid at all levels.

In 1972 Stauffer and Coventry[29] reported on the Mayo Clinic experience with posterolateral lumbar spine fusion. Their technique used the midline approach to the spinal column and a subperiosteal exposure of the lamina, the joints between the articular processes, transverse processes, and alae of the sacrum. Partial thickness cortical and cancellous bone grafts were removed from one posterior iliac crest and placed in the lateral gutters, on the transverse processes and sacral alae, and across the laminas posteriorly. The overall clinical success in their series of 177 patients was 81%, and the overall fusion rate was 80%. Furthermore, they compared the posterolateral fusion results with a retrospective group of patients treated with anterior interbody bone grafting and found that 72% of those with a solid posterolateral fusion had good clinical results, whereas only 55% of those with a solid anterior interbody fusion had good clinical results.

In 1968 Wiltse[37,38] described a new approach to the transverse processes. In contrast to Watkins's approach, which passed lateral to the sacrospinalis, Wiltse used a trans-sacrospinalis approach, believing that the transverse processes and lateral masses are reached more directly and that blood loss is minimized. In his series of 35 patients (33 with spondylolisthesis), solid fusion was achieved in 97% of cases. In 14 patients undergoing two-level fusions through this approach, failure of fusion occurred between L4 and L5 in two and in both levels in one. This gave an overall failure of 21%. Using the midline approach, which was otherwise similar to Wiltse's, Dawson[18] reported on his experience with 58 patients. The overall clinical success rate was 92%. Solid fusion occurred in 100% of patients undergoing lumbosacral fusions and in 91% of patients undergoing two-level fusions. Fusions that did not include the sacrum (floating fusions) had a significantly lower rate of success in achieving a solid arthrodesis (55%). In a companion article, Urist and Dawson[33] reported on the results of 40 intertransverse process spinal fusions performed across two or three vertebrae in four cases of fracture/dislocations in the dorsal lumbar region and 36 cases of degenerative joint and disc disease, including spinal stenosis and spondylolisthesis of the lumbosacral segments. Arthrodesis was performed with a composite of autolyzed antigen-extracted allogeneic bone and local autologous spongiosa bone. Overall, there were over 80% excellent and good results; the pseudarthrosis rate was 12%. Urist and Dawson[8] concluded that, although autologous bone is the ideal bone for graft, allogeneic bone may serve as a useful substitute, particularly when one desires to avoid the complications of excision of massive amounts of bone graft from the iliac crest.

Thomas and coworkers[30] compared the effect of intertransverse process fusion with anterior and posterior spinal fusion in experimental laminectomy operations on guinea pigs and dogs. Their conclusions again favored the intertransverse process fusion technique, since it avoids the iatrogenic complications of spinal stenosis and facetal arthritis. An excellent rate of solid arthrodesis with the intertransverse process fusion far above that of the anterior and posterior techniques was again documented.

These biomechanical considerations, in addition to the abundant supporting clinical evidence, have caused us to use the posterior intertransverse process fusion as our procedure of choice in primary fusion procedures in the lumbosacral spine, as well as in occasional cases of salvage spine surgery.

INDICATIONS FOR POSTERIOR INTERTRANSVERSE PROCESS FUSION
Degenerative Disc Disease

It has become evident to students of the lumbar spine that the primary goal of low back surgery is the relief of mechanical nerve-root compression and sciatica. For the most part patients find their low back pain annoying but tolerable. When a patient has back pain that is so severe that it results in disability, the surgeon must carefully consider whether it is the back pain per se or the patient's psychosocial complexion that is the cause.

Again, it is most difficult to define the anatomic origin of lumbago with any degree of precision. As clinical research on spinal surgery expands, our experience has shown that only rarely is spinal fusion indicated and necessary for degenerative disc disease.

Segmental Instability

The presence of segmental instability at a disc space is manifested radiographically by traction spurs, facet and vertebral body subluxation, and disc space narrowing. The patient who has these symptoms with incapacitating low back pain, who has failed an adequate course of conservative treatment, and who has no emotional, compensation, or litigation issues clouding the clinical picture, may be a candidate for primary arthrodesis. However, these patients should be thoroughly evaluated before surgery to exclude the occult neoplasm, metabolic disorder, or rheumatoid/rheumatoid-variant arthropathy. In addition, Boumphrey[5] suggests routine discography to demonstrate that normal discs are present above and below the proposed fusion site. In my practice it is rare to find such a patient; therefore my predominant mode of therapy is based on conservative measures.

Isthmic Spondylolisthesis

Children with asymptomatic spondyolysis or grade I spondylolisthesis should in general be managed conservatively, although risk factors for progressive slippage may warrant early aggressive intervention. Young children with spondylolisthesis are at greater risk for progression, and females are at greater risk than males. Other risk factors include the existence of spina bifida occulta, a trapezoidal lumbar vertebra (high lumbar index), a dome-shaped sacral end-plate, and a high slip angle (see box).

If conservative management fails, a child who has a grade II or less spondylolisthesis is managed surgically with an in situ bilateral-lateral fusion from L5 to the sacrum. Wiltse[16] believes that there is rarely, if ever, any indication for posterior decompression in children, since he has observed resolution of neurologic symptoms—including footdrop—following successful arthrodesis. A laminectomy alone (Gill procedure) is absolutely contraindicated in children, because progressive slip will occur without concurrent fusion.[18,22]

Fusion usually is indicated in children with greater than grade II slip, regardless of symptoms, because of the risk of progression. It should be noted that progression of slips can be observed even after a successful fusion (Table 27-4).

Treatment of adults differs little from that of children, except that the older adult is more likely to have concomitant effects of degenerative disc disease and hypertrophy of the fibrocartilaginous defect in the pars, producing true radicular symptoms. Myelography is routinely performed before surgical intervention in the adult. Surgical fusion of spondylolysis in the adult must be tempered by the realization that chronic low back pain

Risk factors for progression of spondylolisthesis

Age (skeletal immaturity)
Sex (female risk greater than that of male)
Spina bifida occulta or posterior element dysplasia
Low lumbar index (trapezoidal vertebral body)
Dome-shaped sacral contour
High slip angle

Table 27-4 *Incidence of progression after successful fusion*

	Ratio	%
Newman[21]	9/24	38
Bosworth[4]	14/73	19
Laurent and Osterman[18]	10/91	11
Boxall and others[6]	9/34	26
AVERAGE		19

may be the result of degenerative lumbar disc disease, which is not responsive to lumbosacral fusion. In older patients (more than 30 years of age) who have low back and radicular symptoms with normal myelograms, bilateral-lateral fusions to the sacrum are sufficient combined with simple postoperative immobilization in the form of a lumbosacral corset or molded polypropylene thoracolumbosacral orthosis. In the presence of both radicular signs and symptoms decompression of the L5 root alone may be considered, although results are improved with concomitant bilateral-lateral fusion (Table 27-5). If foraminotomy is performed unilaterally in young adults, immobilization in a single leg, pantaloon spica cast is used after surgery for at least 3 months to minimize further slip in the postoperative period. If bilateral foraminotomies are necessary, postoperative management should include immobilization in a two-leg pantaloon spica with bed rest for 3 months, because the risk of

Table 27-5 *Clinical success of surgical treatment of spondylolisthesis*

Procedure	Overall success (%)
Gill procedure only[11,22]	75
Posterior fusion[4,12,18,32]	80
Bilateral-lateral fusion[3,4,13,27]	85
Gill plus bilateral-lateral fusion[4,8,25,27,33]	85
Anterior fusion[4,9,15,28]	75

progressive slip in the early postoperative period is high. In our experience, however, it is unusual for bilateral foraminotomies to be required in adult isthmic spondylolisthesis.

Degenerative Spondylolisthesis

In the adult with degenerative spondylolisthesis and symptoms of spinal stenosis, the issue is less clear regarding the need for a fusion procedure in addition to decompression of the compressed elements of the cauda equina. Rosenberg[24] studied the epidemiology of degenerative spondylolisthesis in 20 skeletons in 200 patients and confirmed its common occurrence between L4 and L5. He believed that with an unduly stable lumbosacral joint more stress is placed on articulations between the fourth and fifth vertebrae. Decompensation of that disc and its ligaments adds to instability, hypermobility, and degenerative disease of the articular processes. The degenerative changes cause wear and tear, deformation of the articular processes, and ultimately allow for its slipping until the isthmus of the slipped vertebra abuts on the upper margin of the superior articular process of the vertebra below.

In our practice, unless there is significant radiculopathy, these patients are treated conservatively. If radiculopathy is present and documented myelographically, then we recommend decompressive laminectomies and selective medial facetectomies to unroof the nerve-root canal at the levels involved. We reserve performing a concomitant floating intertransverse process fusion for the younger patient (less than 60 years old), the patient over 60 who is physiologically quite active, or the patient who at the time of decompression requires bilateral foraminotomies at the same level.

Indications for Posterior Intertransverse Fusion in Secondary Operations

The establishment of an accurate diagnosis in patients with failed spinal surgery is a difficult task that calls for great judgment on the part of the physician. In addition to the many painstaking steps that are necessary before deciding to embark on salvage back surgery, the surgeon can delineate certain clear indications for spinal fusion at the time of reoperation.

The first of these is the presence of a neural arch defect that was not stabilized at the primary operation. A second indication for spinal fusion is the presence of significant back pain after disc excision. Assuming no other pathologic process is producing the back pain, and one is able to define a localized degenerated segment, one might hope for success in patients who have localized disc degeneration. This is among the more tenuous indications for repeat spinal surgery and spinal fusion. The difficulty in defining the origin of low back pain is, of course, the factor that precludes confidence in operating on these patients.

Iatrogenic instability produced through the intervention of the surgeon at the time of the primary procedure is the third indication for spine fusion. With a more complete knowledge of the condition of the spine and a more radical exploration of the nerve roots, the spinal surgeon will often find it necessary to resect facet joints, complete laminas, and occasionally pedicles. Although resection of these elements is often necessary to achieve nerve-root decompression, the resultant spine may be quite unstable. These situations demand fusion.

After a simple disc excision certain patients will also develop instability. Statistical analysis of this problem would indicate that extensive motion after discectomy will tend toward persistent pain, whereas restriction of interspace motion will tend toward a more satisfactory result. We define anatomic instability to be when a bilateral foraminotomy is performed at a disc space or in the presence of demonstrable radiographic instability as described earlier.

A fourth and also controversial indication for spinal fusion is the presence of a recurrent protrusion at a previously operated disc space. When we are called on to reexplore a nerve root and disc space that have had previous surgery, it is not uncommon to find a mixed type of disease or injury. Usually, fibrosis is present about the dura and nerve root, extending well into the foramen. The protrusions at the disc space itself may consist of both a bulging annulus and nuclear material. Varying amounts of bone will have been resected at the time of primary or secondary laminectomy. We believe it is necessary to perform a radical exploration of the nerve root, which often entails an extensive laminectomy and radical foraminotomy. At this juncture the amount of instability created is difficult to evaluate. In an attempt to render a definitive operation, we will usually perform a posterior intertransverse fusion at the completion of the decompressive portion of the operation.

SUMMARY

As yet, no completely reliable method of lumbar fusion has been found. Therefore each surgeon should be equipped with the knowledge and techniques to choose and perform any of the standard fusion procedures that may be indicated for the management of acute and chronic disabling conditions of the lumbosacral spine. The posterior intertransverse process fusion may be considered a multipurpose, reliable procedure indicated for a wide range of spinal disorders and has been shown to have a rational biomechanical basis and a low pseudarthrosis rate. The prerequisites for a surgeon performing this procedure include a sound body of knowledge relating to the pathophysiology and natural history of spinal disorders and adequate training to acquire the technical skills and judgment required for excellence in the actual performance.

REFERENCES

1. Adkins, E.W.D.: Lumbosacral arthrodesis after laminectomy, J. Bone Joint Surg. **37B:** 208, 1955.
2. Albee, F.H.: Transplantation of portions of the tibia into the spine for Pott's disease, JAMA **57:**885, 1911.
3. Blackburn, H.S., and Belikos, E.P.: Spondylolysthesis in children and adolescents, J. Bone Joint Surg. **59B:**490, 1977.
4. Bosworth, D.M., et al.: Spondylolisthesis: a critical review of a consecutive series of cases treated by arthrodesis, J. Bone Joint Surg. **37A:**767, 1955.
5. Boumphrey, F.R.S.: Fusion in the lumbar spine. In Seminars in neurologic surgery—lumbar disc disease, New York, 1982, Raven Press.
6. Boxall, D., et al.: Management of severe spondylolisthesis in children and adolescents, J. Bone Joint Surg. **61A:**479, 1979.
7. Campbell, W.C.: Operative orthopaedics, St. Louis, 1939, The C.V. Mosby Co.
8. Dawson, E.G., et al.: Intertransverse process lumbar arthrodesis with autogenous bone graft, Clin. Orthop. **154:**90, 1981.
9. Freebody, D., et al.: Anterior transperitoneal lumbar fusion, J. Bone Joint Surg. **53B:**617, 1971.
10. Gertzbein, S.D., et al.: Centrode patterns and segmental instability in degenerative disc disease, Spine **10**(3):257, 1985.
11. Gill, G.G., et al.: Surgical treatment of spondylolisthesis without spinal fusion, J. Bone Joint Surg. **33A:**493, 1955.
12. Henderson, E.D.: Results of the original treatment of spondylolisthesis, J. Bone Joint Surg. **48A:**619, 1966.

13. Hensinger, R.N., et al.: Surgical management of spondylolisthesis in children and adolescents, Spine **1**:207, 1976.
14. Hibbs, R.A.: An operation for progressive spinal deformities, N. Y. Med. J. **93**:1013, 1911.
15. Hodgseon, A.R., and Wong, S.K.: A description of a technique and evaluaton of results of anterior spinal fusion for deranged intervertebral disc and spondylolisthesis, Clin. Orthop. **56**:133, 1968.
16. Jackson, D.W., et al.: Spondylolysis in the female gymnast, Clin. Orthop. **117**:68, 1976.
17. Kelly, R.P.: Intertransverse fusion of the low back, Trans. South. Surg. Assoc. **74**:193, 1963.
18. Laurent, L.E., and Osterman, K.: Operative treatment of spondylolisthesis in young patients, Clin. Orthop. **117**:85, 1976.
19. MacNab, I.: The traction spur: an indicator of segmental instability, J. Bone Joint Surg. **57A**:663, 1971.
20. MacNab, I., and Dall, D.: The blood supply of the lumbar spine and its application to the technique of intertransverse lumbar fusion, J. Bone Joint Surg. **54**:1195, 1972.
21. Newman, P.H.: Surgical treatment for derangement of the lumbar spine, J. Bone Joint Surg. **55B**:7, 1973.
22. Osterman, K., et al.: Late results of removal of the loose posterior element (Gill's operation) in the treatment of lytic lumbar spondylolisthesis, Clin. Orthop. **117**:121, 1976.
23. Pedersen, H.E., et al.: The anatomy of lumbosacral posterior rami and meningeal branches of spinal nerves (sinu-vertebral nerves), J. Bone Joint Surg. **38A**:377, 1956.
24. Rosenberg, M.I.: Degenerative spondylolisthesis, J. Bone Joint Surg. **51A**:467, 1975.
25. Rosenberg, N.J., et al.: The incidence of spondylolysis and spondylolisthesis in nonambulatory patients, Spine **6**:35, 1981.
26. Selzer, R.: Mortal lessons: notes on the art of surgery, New York, 1976, Simon & Schuster, Inc.
27. Sherman, F.C., et al.: Spine fusion for spondylolysis and spondylolisthesis in children, Spine **4**:59, 1979.
28. Sorensen, K.H.: Anterior interbody lumbar spine fusion for incapacitating disc degeneration and spondylolisthesis, Acta Orthop. Scand. **49**:269, 1978.
29. Stauffer, R.N., and Coventry, M.B.: Posterolateral lumbar fusion, J. Bone Joint Surg. **54**:1195, 1972.
30. Thomas, I., et al.: Experimental spinal fusion in guinea pigs and dogs, Clin. Orthop. **112**:363, 1975.
31. Truchly, G., and Thompson, W.A.L.: Posterolateral fusion of the lumbosacral spine, J. Bone Joint Surg. **44A**:505, 1962.
32. Turner, R.H., and Bianco, A.J.: Spondylolysis and spondylolisthesis in children and teenagers, J. Bone Joint Surg. **53A**:1293, 1971.
33. Urist, M.R., and Dawson, E.: Intertransverse process fusion with the aid of chemosterilized autolyzed antigen-extracted allogeneic (AAA) bone, Clin. Orthop. **154**:97, 1981.
34. Wadkins, M.B.: Posterolateral fusion of the lumbar and lumbosacral spine, J. Bone Joint Surg. **35A**:1014, 1953.
35. White, A.A., and Punjabi, M.M.: Clinical biomechanics of the spine, Philadelphia, 1978, J.B. Lippincott Co.
36. White, A.A., et al.: Spinal stability: evaluation and treatment, Instructional Course Lectures, The American Academy of Orthopaedic Surgeons, vol. 30, St. Louis, 1981, The C.V. Mosby Co.
37. Wiltse, L.L., and Jackson, D.W.: Treatment of spondylolisthesis and spondylolysis in children, Clin. Orthop. **117**:92, 1976.
38. Wiltse, L.L., et al.: The paraspinal sacrospinalis-splitting approach to the lumbar spine, J. Bone Joint Surg. **50A**:919, 1968.

EDITORIAL COMMENTARY

Posterior lumbar intertransverse process fusions are the most common fusions used by the authors of this text and the second most common procedure used overall. All of the authors found this procedure to be of great value, including Richard Rothman who, although he rarely does a fusion, does find this type of fusion to be the most clinically successful and biomechanically appealing. A few have experienced significant complications with the procedure.

Posterior intertransverse fusion is the most common fusion that I do, and I use this procedure in at least 50% of the lumbar surgeries that I perform. After extensive decompression, there is frequently gross instability and certainly potential long-range instability and recurrent stenosis. Our controlled series of fusions vs. nonfusions after decompressions in San Francisco has not proved that fusions are more successful in the short term.

Kirkaldy-Willis does not take fusions lightly. When he does a fusion he usually uses the intertransverse fusion. He finds this fusion "gives the best results for (1) instability proven by dynamic lateral radiographs, (2) degenerative spondylolisthesis, and (3) isthmus spondylolisthesis. Before considering this operation, I want to exhaust all possible conservative measures of treatment and be reasonably certain that the psychologic state of the patient is satisfactory."

John Frymoyer made the following editorial comment about fusions. "The water is even more muddied when one faces the issue of spinal fusion, the techniques of which comprise approximately one half of this book. Despite the strongly held beliefs the authors of chapters may have for a specific fusion technique or the use of fixation devices, the critical question is whom should we fuse in the first place. The basic principle that leads to the consideration of fusion rests in the concept of spinal instability, that is, the patient's spine is presently unstable, the patient's spine has a high risk of becoming unstable, or the operation being performed has produced either instability or a high risk of it in the future. We talk glibly about segmental instability, and a few of us have tried to classify it into specific types and perhaps even into specific syndromes. In reality, we have no truly satisfactory definitions—a point emphasized by the inability of an international symposium to reach consensus on what constitutes segmental instability."

Vert Mooney makes some cogent comments about fusions. "There are two levels of analysis of fusion procedures. The first is the conceptual rationale, and the second is the technical difficulty to achieve a fusion at this biomechanically and anatomically complex site. Conceptually there are three reasons for fusion. The first is the demonstration of true painful mechanical instability such as related to spondylolysis or single-level severe degenerative/posttraumatic instability. The second reason is surgically created instability created by the extent of surgery appropriate to achieve total relief of neural impingement and pressure. Surgery for degenerative spondylolisthesis is a good example. The third reason for fusion is the most controversial—the painfully incompetent disc, perhaps even on a chemical basis, as suggested by Harry Crock. The syndrome of disc disruption is the classification of some of these cases. Whereas the first two categories have good justification by experience and in the literature, the third—the painfully incompetent disc—remains to be further clarified by better study and more precise follow up experience."

For the first two categories my own preference is the reliable transverse process fusion. The expectation of a successful fusion is over 80% in the previously unoperated or unfused patient. It is ideally suited for categories one and two. The third category requires disc replacement by bone graft. This, although anatomically appropriate, is technically difficult. In the lumbar spine, with the wide gap between vascularized bone (the vertebral bodies), the time necessary for vascularization of the disc replacement is usually many months. Thus the morbidity of the procedure in terms of delay of normal function may last as long as 6 months. Even the surgical systems that offer excellent mechanical stability at the time of disc replacement still cannot achieve the solidity necessary to have speedy vascularization. The spine surgeon's inability to achieve immobilization of the lower two lumbar motion segments by orthotic devices is an aspect of this problem. Apparently in Japan it is expected that a spica cast would be used—our patients would have difficulty accepting the severity of this postoperative course.

Another aspect of the fusion problem is donor bone. The larger the amount of bone necessary to achieve fusion, the greater the morbidity and persistent pain of the patient. Thus the temptation to use bank bone or other alternative is very significant. My experience with bank bone has been varied. Sometimes the bone supplied is excellent, strong cancellous bone with associated cortical margins. On other occasions the bone is quite porotic with thin cortices and thin trabeculae. At this time we have no studies comparing the rate of incorporation and rate of fusion of bank bone vs. autogenous donor bone. I prefer to compromise and use some of each.

I have no doubt that the future improvement in expectations and effective care in the lumbar spine will be by the use of internal fixation. Pedicle screws certainly offer this opportunity. We are so early in the learning curve of this approach to stabilization that failures can be expected as we learn various "dos and don'ts." On the other hand, just as fracture care throughout the rest of the skeleton improved once we had appropriate internal fixation equipment, our rates of fusion and our postsurgery morbidity will be favorably changed with better internal fixation systems. I am very enthusiastic about this innovation.

I believe that the posterior interbody fusion has offered the least appealing approach. Whereas the anterior approach—accomplished with the assistance of a qualified general/vascular surgeon—is easy, rapid, and reliable, the posterior approach is technically demanding, potentially hazardous, and requires extensive surgical time. It also bears the significant additional potential of adding morbidity to the surgical procedure due to prolonged retraction of the intolerant neural tissues. Therefore I do not believe that this is a favorable procedure.

I still use fat grafts in most of my patients, although I really have no clear-cut impression that they offer a better postoperative and long-term course than the use of Gelfoam. I have experienced one severe complication from a fat graft of a cauda aquina lesion; thus care to avoid "stuffing" the graft must be taken.

It must be recognized that the use of fusions still remains controversial for degenerative disease. Our inability to measure the degree of pain and the degree of dysfunction before surgery and the changes after surgery are the source of the confusion. There is sufficient evidence to identify the natural history of degenerative spinal disease so that efficacy of fusion treatment can be demonstrated, as long as we have a population to which similar criteria of pain and disability measurement have been applied. This is the goal for research in the future.

Leon Wiltse says of posterior lumbar intertransverse fusions: "It is my opinion that the posterior lumbar intertransverse process fusion is the gold standard of lumbar spinal fusion operations. The fusion rate is high and the complication rate extremely low when the spinal canal is not violated. Several levels can be done with little added danger. Decompression can be added as necessary. The original Hibbs fusion was strictly a posterior fusion. The facets were partially excised and strips of bone turned over onto themselves, so that a fusion took place across the area between the laminae. This can still be done in addition to the intertransverse process fusion. The facets can be partially excised if the surgeon prefers. The outer faces of the superior articular processes and other parts of the lateral mass should be very carefully denuded of soft tissue and decorticated. The transverse process must be carefully decorticated, thus using every square millimeter of available bony surface.

I do not believe the anterior surfaces of the transverse processes should be denuded of soft tissue. There is danger to the nerves and circulation to the transverse process is compromised. The upper aspect of the sacral ala should be decorticated, and I like to turn a flap of bone in a cephalad direction from the superior surface of the ala. This flap is based anteriorly.

Some surgeons believe that fusing the laminae may cause spinal stenosis. I do not subscribe to this. However, if a large laminectomy has been done with bone laid over the laminectomy defect, bone may grow anteriorly and impinge the spinal canal. Likewise, if pseudarthrosis results, the constant motion can cause bony growth anteriorly. Also, bone may grow anteriorly at the top of the fusion. I base my conclusion that bone does not grow anteriorly if the ligamentum flavum is intact on the observation that bone never grows anteriorly into the sacral canal after posterior fusion that has involved decorticating 2 or 3 cm of the upper sacrum.

Concerning excision of the facet cartilage, if there has been no midline decompression and the laminae are virtually intact, I take a needle-nosed rongeur and excise the posterior one third of the facet and pack pure cancellous bone into this area. If there has been a midline decompression, one does not want to take away even this amount of bone since the patient needs that stability. Many surgeons object to excising the facet cartilage at all because they believe it destabilizes the spine. This is certainly a valid point.

One can use either a midline approach to do the posterior lumbar intertransverse process fusion or the paraspinal approach. A midline approach is better if one is to do a bilateral decompression, excising the spinous process and both laminae. Many surgeons prefer the midline approach because they are more comfortable with the anatomy of the approach.

I prefer the paraspinal approach, especially if I have to decompress far laterally.

I find no difficulty doing a simple discectomy, if I wish, through this paraspinal approach. And of course if one wishes to remove a far lateral disc, out beyond the pedicles, the paraspinal approach is probably necessary."

Augustus White and Kirkaldy-Willis do not favor internal fixation for standard lumbar disc and stenosis surgery. Hugo Keim finds his posterior intertransverse process fusion very successful without the use of internal fixation.

Most of our authors, however, find internal fixation of some or great value, although half of them have experienced significant complications. Among the authors of this book internal fixation is used more frequently than anterior or posterior interbody fusions.

Leon Wiltse summarizes my thoughts on internal fixation quite well:

"As the population gets older, more need exists for massive decompression in the treatment of spinal stenosis. There can be central canal stenosis, but more often there is also a component of lateral canal stenosis. There can even be far lateral stenosis where the nerve is caught between the transverse process and the ala of the sacrum. Many of these patients with severe spinal stenosis have associated progressive lumbar degenerative scoliosis. If the necessary extensive decompression is done, they collapse further. The need for internal fixation is great, and it is not limited to the lower two or three segments. Often the need for internal fixation extends clear up to the thoracolumbar area or higher. Along with degenerative scoliosis and spinal stenosis, especially in older women, there is usually osteoporosis. This makes internal fixation more difficult because the bone is so soft that the device does not hold well. However, the need for stability in these cases is even greater.

Harrington rods have not done well in the lumbar spine. They tend to eliminate the lordosis. One, of course, can bend the rods and wire them to the laminae if there are any laminae left. It is also possible to wire them around the pedicles. This is somewhat hazardous and requires considerable skill. In the osteoporotic spine the wires are likely to cut out.

Luque rods do better but are difficult to attach to the sacrum. If there also has been a midline decompression, there is difficulty looping the wires around the pedicles. Likewise, the wires tend to cut through the soft bone in osteoporotic spines.

Efforts are being made to use large pedicle screws with fairly deep threads to get a better hold on the soft bone. If these screws can be just a little smaller than the actual diameter of the pedicles, they hold quite well, even in the osteoporotic spine. One does have to be careful not to get the screws so big that they cut out of the pedicles. Unfortunately, the cauda-cephalad diameter of the pedicles is considerably greater than the transverse diameter, so the screw tends to toggle. In these osteoporotic spines, if the screw can be brought down through the pedicle and partially through the anterior cortex of the body, they hold much better. However, there is more danger to the vascular structures when one brings the screw to the anterior cortex of the vertebral body.

In putting in rods or plates there is some likelihood of damage to the facet at the point where the fusion area joins the unfused area. This facet should be kept intact and undamaged, since we are depending on this juncture to remain strong and painless. If the screw can be brought in from the lateral side of the superior articular process of the last vertebra to be fused and angulated medially, damage to the facet can be avoided fairly well.

If one gets good internal fixation, the patient can be up immediately with relatively little need for external support.

A disadvantage of this system is that there is a fair amount of danger to vascular and neurologic structures in inserting these large screws. A high degree of skill and training is required. Great care must be taken that the screw is placed properly the first time. If it has to be replaced, especially in osteoporotic bone, it will usually have lost its holding power. Injecting methylmethacrylate may restore the strength of fixation.

Putting in screws and plates or rods takes an extra 1 ½ to 2 hours. If this time is added to 1 or 2 hours used in making this approach and decompressing the spine, and another 45 minutes fusing the spine, these operations can stretch to 5 hours. If homologous bone could be used to good advantage in the spine, the operating time would be shortened. Our experience has not been good with homologous bone in the spine of the elderly person. Homologous bone mixed with autologous bone seems to work well for children, but children's spines usually fuse anyway so we don't really know what part the homologous graft played. We can, however, look forward with optimism to the availability of acceptable allograft in the next decade.

Another disadvantage of present internal fixation devices is that they use a lot of the graft area that could be used for bone graft. After a decompression there is not a great deal of graftable area left, and if this area is further encroached upon by rods or plates the fusion may fail. This is a fairly serious problem. We try to overcome it by tamping cancellous bone everywhere possible, especially under the internal fixation device.

There is great need for methods that enable us to decompress the stenotic spine adequately and still maintain stability. I believe this is possible if we can develop a posterior internal fixation device that is safe and acceptably easy to put in. The need is immense."

Arthur H. White

CHAPTER 28

SPONDYLOLISTHESIS

James Reynolds

The treatment of spondylolisthesis by in situ fusion requires an understanding of the types of spondylolisthesis. Wiltse, Newman, and MacNab[5] classified spondylolisthesis into five types: dysplastic, isthmic, degenerative, traumatic, and pathologic. I will describe the type and method of in situ fusion of each of the first three.

DISPLASTIC SPONDYLOLISTHESIS

Dysplastic spondylolisthesis is the only true congenital spondylolisthesis. The articular process of S1 is hypoplastic and permits the forward subluxation of the inferior articular process of L5. The lamina of L5 may be intact or may be hypoplastic. With the lamina intact, the neural elements are more susceptible to injury. The lamina, moving forward because of partial dislocation, will compress the cauda equina. The inferior articular process of L5 will compress the S1 root. Patients present the typical picture of hamstring tightness and pelvic waddle, and peculiar to this group is walking on their toes on one side or the other with an inability to place the foot flat. These patients are younger than most of my patients, with symptoms relative to the leg and gait abnormalities.

One patient of mine had a paraspinal fusion and was kept in bed 2 months. A solid fusion was obtained and long term follow-up is perfectly normal. A second patient, who was 6 years old at the onset of symptoms, fused at 11 months after surgery. However, it took 26 months for the hamstring tightness to resolve. The patient was normal in all other ways and eventually became an all-star pitcher in Little League.

A third patient was a grade III. She had obtained a solid fusion through a paraspinal approach done at another hospital. Despite this, she could never stand with both feet completely flat. A midline decompression and a release of the filum terminale completely relieved her symptoms in a few weeks.

The fourth patient had a grade III spondylolisthesis with severe S1 deficit. Through the paraspinal approach one side was decompressed by removal of the inferior articular process of L5, and a paraspinal fusion was performed. This seems to be the best procedure for congenital spondylolisthesis with symptoms of hamstring tightness gait abnormality.

ISTHMIC SPONDYLOLISTHESIS

Isthmic spondylolisthesis is type II. The symptoms related to this type of spondylolisthesis usually are found in the early adolescent and the middle age of life. I have studied a group of 24 high-grade (grade III and IV) spondylolisthesis patients treated by in situ fusion through a paraspinal approach. Much controversey has occurred with regards to the method of measurement, recently described by Wiltse and Winters.[4]

The two significant measurements of these patients were anterior displacement and saggital rotation. Anterior displacement is described as a percentage of the displacement of L5 on S1. The saggital rotation is the rotation of L5 over the anterior portion of S1. The average anterior displacement before surgery was 73%. The range was 50% to 100%. After surgery, the progression was 0.55%. The average saggital rotation was 26% with a progression of 1% after surgery.

The indications for surgery were (1) 96% had severe pain, (2) 8% showed progression of their slip as well as having pain, and 54% had neurologic findings that included motor, sensory, and/or reflex changes. One third of these patients had back pain only, one third had their pain evenly distributed between back and leg, and one third had only leg pain. Neurologic involvement was found in 13 patients. After surgery the average time for pain reduction was 4½ months. Total resolution of neurologic findings occurred in 8 patients, and 5 patients had mild residuals of their preoperative neurologic findings. Of these patients 3 had a mild decrease in the ankle jerk persist and 2 patients had a single grade loss of EHL strength. All patients were not aware of any weakness. Immediately after surgery 4 patients had a very mild transient increase of neurologic symptoms. All resolved rapidly to preoperative status.

Hamstring tightness was present in 21 patients. In 19 patients this resolved in an average of 7½ months. Two patients required a longer period of time for their hamstring tightness to resolve. One was the 6½-year-old boy (previously mentioned) with congenital spondylolisthesis, whose fusion was solid at 11 months and with hamstring tightness resolved at 26 months. The second was a 13-year-old boy whose pain resolved at 6 months. His fusion became solid at 41 months and his hamstring tightness resolved at 44 months.

The various factors—age, sex, amount of anterior displacement, amount of saggital rotation, or the length of symptoms—were not predictive of the end result. The patients who had only leg pain or neurologic deficits were less likely to obtain an excellent result. Of five patients with persistent neurologic symptoms, three were rated good.

The levels of fusion made no difference. There were 14 one-level fusions, 9 two-level fusions, and 1 three-level fusion. The multilevel fusions were done if the angle of L4 to L5 to the horizontal was greater than 50 degrees or the transverse process of L5 was small.

The technical aspects of the procedure have been previously described,[3] but several points are worth reiterating. The ala is the "lighthouse" to this approach. The skin is incised from L3 to S2 in the midline. The subcutaneous tissue is reflected off the lumbodorsal fascia with a Key elevator. Two fingers from the midline the fascia is incised at the level of the spinous process of L4, extending it distally to the sacrum and curving the distal portion of the incision medially. The plane between the paraspinal muscle is split bluntly, and the ala is palpated. Reach superiorly and anteriorly and the transverse process can be palpated just lateral to the L4-L5 facet. Cobb elevators then are used to elevate the soft tissue from the ala and transverse process.

Ronguers are then used to remove the muscle from the ala and transverse process and up over the lateral portion of the lamina of L5. Care must be taken not to bite too deeply with a ronguer in the area distal to the transverse process of L5 at its junction with the body of L5. The L5 nerve transverses this area. Meticulous decortication is essential to obtain a fusion. All bone is taken from one of the iliac crests through the same incision, which is undermined over to the crest. Care must be taken not to violate the L4-L5 facet unless the fusion is to be more than one level. Closure is routine over hemovac tubes. A subcuticular skin closure is used for comesis.

Fusion rate was 100%. The average time to fusion was 7½ months. Hospital stay averaged 17 days. The most common length of stay was 11 days, and most patients were ambulated between 2 to 5 days. Another 30 days were spent at home in bed except for meals and bathroom privileges.

The fusion was determined to be solid when bending films showed no motion. All surgeries were performed in a kneeling position using either a Hasting or an Andrews frame with the patient in a kneeling position. Both of these frames permit the abdomen to be free. Blood loss was usually about 2 units, and time of surgery was about 3 hours. Complications were minimal: one wound hematoma that resolved with aspiration, and four transient increases in neurologic symptoms that quickly resolved.

One objection to in situ fusion for high-grade spondylolisthesis in the young is that despite fusion, the slip will continue to progress; thus reduction is necessary for cosmesis. I would like to address this objection based on my experience with the previously mentioned patients. A progression of slip is determined on the comparison of preoperative and postoperative radiographs. I have found that there can be a great difference preoperatively in percentage of slip between standing lateral films and those taken in the horizontal position. All fusions will occur in the position that is shown on standing films. Therefore a comparison of preoperative films taken horizontally and postoperative films taken after fusion will likely have a great deal of difference in percentage of slip. Thus the slip will appear to have progressed. Rather, the fusion occurred at the preoperative standing position; when it has fused, even when the patient is lying down, the slip can no longer return to the position it formerly had. Also, most in situ fusions are performed from the midline approach. Most patients who have high-grade spondylolisthesis also have a spina bifida of L5 or S1. The fact that there is a much higher incident of spina bifida in high-grade spondylolisthesis would indicate the midline in these patients is weak and predisposes these patients to slip. Midline approaches for these fusions or midline approaches with laminectomy certainly weaken an already weakened structure. The paraspinal approach that I have described carefully preserves the midline structure. I believe that this is important in obtaining a 100% fusion rate. I think that this is why there is no progression, although no cast is used and the patients are allowed to be up. Even the patient who was followed the longest, 15 years, and had a spondylolisthesis that necessitated the only L3 to S1 fusion showed no evidence of slip progression once the fusion had occurred.

Cosmetic results are often cited as one of the indications for reduction. I did not include that in my questions to patients, but there were no complaints related to the deformity. In fact, as I saw these patients, it was quite apparent that the major components of the abnormal physical appearance had disappeared. The sharp crease in the abdomen and the flat bottom were not present on any of the patients. They were slightly short-waisted but did not appear deformed. One young woman had been a model in New York and Paris. Another young lady is a ballerina in a major ballet company at age 18. Johnson and Kirwan[1a] noted that in 17 patients who had spondylolisthesis, over 50% treated by in situ fusion through the paraspinal approach, "only two patients were conscious of their cosmetic appearance."

I agree with Hensinger's observation that hamstring tightness is not neural in origin.[1] Rather, it is an attempt by the hamstrings to control an unstable area at L5-S1. I found that the average time to fusion was 7½ months, and the average time to resolution of hamstring tightness was 7½ months. I do not believe this to be a coincidence; once fusion occurs there is no longer any necessity for hamstring tightness, since the L5-S1 junction becomes stable.

In short, I have found that in type II high-grade spondylolisthesis in the young in situ fusion through a paraspinal approach will consistently achieve a fusion, giving excellent functional and cosmetic results. Neurologic deficits, hamstrong tightness, and major cosmetic deformities resolve once a fusion occurs. The surgical procedure is not excessively complex and has minimal complications. Postoperative care requires no cast, 2 weeks' hospitalization, and 1 month bed rest at home before the young patient can begin to resume activities on a limited basis. Fusion occurs at 7½ months, and the patients can then resume full activity. At fifteen-year follow-up there is no deterioration of the results and the first mobile segment above the fusion does not deteriorate. I would recommend this same procedure for type II spondylolisthesis regardless of age, symptoms, or degree of anterior displacement.

The adult with type II spondylolisthesis has posed a dilemma. How is it possible to adequately stabilize and yet adequately decompress the neuroelements? With a decompression of the L5 nerve root so much bone is removed that even with a paraspinal approach only the opposite side can be fused. Then to adequately stabilize this patient at 10 days a second procedure is necessary at L5-S1, namely, an anterior fusion by a transperitoneal approach. A body cast and 3 months of bed rest follow this procedure. I was encouraged by the results in my young high-grade spondylolisthesis patients, the oldest being 23 years of age.

Over the past 3 years I have fused 10 adults, age 26 to 66, whose major complaints were related to the legs. Three of these patients had grade III spondylolisthesis. All 10 patients have had complete resolution of their leg pain. Two patients are currently 6 months postoperative and have not yet achieved a solid fusion, but they have total relief of their leg pain. These two patients still have some persistent back pain. Seven of the patients are rated excellent. One patient had 3/5 extensor hallucis longus (EHL) and now has 5 EHL and no functional disability in this extremity and normal sensation. Two of the male patients are involved in extremely heavy work. One is a carpet layer who carries 300-pound rolls of carpet; his fusion became solid at 7 months. The other is a submarine electronics expert, doing heavy work in cramped quarters.

Two females, both with grade III spondylolisthesis, also have done heavy work. One has been an ICU nurse, and the other does geriatric care, including lifting a comatose patient off the floor unassisted. What makes this more amazing is that this patient had the EHL that was 0/5 before fusion. A third female patient, also grade III, is a general practitioner who assists at surgery and does obstetric deliveries without difficulty. I followed the same postoperative care for the adult as I did for the younger patient with high-grade spondylolisthesis with the same good results.

DEGENERATIVE SPONDYLOLISTHESIS

Degenerative spondylolisthesis is a degenerative form of spinal disorder with forward slipping of one vertebra over the other. The typical case would involve a patient over 50 years of age with L4 slipped anterior to L5. This is true in 95% of cases. The L4 vertebral body will be above the level of the pelvis. Statistically, only 25% of the normal population would have an L4 vertebra above the level of the pelvis. I have evaluated 21 patients who were surgically treated for this problem. None had prior back surgery or any compensation or litigation claims. The age range was 49 to 78 years, with a mean of 62 years and the mode of 66 years. Of these, 18 patients had slippage at the L4-L5 levels, one had slippage at the L3-L4 level, and one patient had slippage at L4-L5 and L5-S1. Of the 21 patients, 15 complained mainly of sciatica and 6 patients had symptoms of claudication. The preoperative slip averaged 6.7 mm with a range of 2 to 13 mm and a mode of 4 mm. Electromyography results were abnormal in 41% of the patients tested. Of those that were abnormal, 80% involved the nerve root below the level of the slip, that is, an L4-L5 slip with an L5 nerve root involved. At surgery in such cases it was found that the L4 inferior articular process would compress the L5 nerve root against the body of L5.

Surgical treatment was divided into three groups. The first six patients had articular process resection, and 10 patients had a midline laminectomy at L4-L5 with resection of the medial one third of the articular process and a foraminotomy. Care was taken to preserve the pars. The remaining five patients had, in addition to the previously described procedure, a transverse process fusion at the level of the slip. The follow-up involved the patients' rating of their results. "Excellent" was no pain and no limitation of activity. "Good" was occasional pain, managed by aspirin and/or slight limitation of activity. The patients with articular process resections initially did well, but the results quickly deteriorated. Of the six patients in the group, only two or 33% rated themselves "good" or "excellent." The group with midline decompression had a 78% "good" or "excellent" result. This included those with midline decompression, as well as those with midline decompression and fusion.

More recently, Lombardi and coworkers[2] evaluated a much larger series of patients who had midline decompression and fusion. Of this group, 90% had good or excellent results. No immobilization is necessary postoperatively, although a few patients prefer to have a lumbosacral corset. Patients in general did better if they also had a fusion at the level of the slip.

SUMMARY

For type I, or congenital spondylolisthesis, I recommend the in situ transverse process fusion through a midline skin incision and a paraspinal approach. If there is significant pain in one leg, or the patient cannot stand normally on one leg, then in addition to the fusion through the same paraspinal approach a partial laminectomy should be performed on the side with the involved extremity. It is only necessary to remove the inferior articular process and a small part of the lamina on the involved side. For type II, or isthmic spondylolisthesis, I recommend the in situ transverse process fusion through a midline skin incision and paraspinal approach. I recommend this whether the disorder is grade I or grade IV, even with severe neurologic deficits, and whether it is in the young or adult patient. Decompression is not necessary, no matter how severe the neurologic findings. They will all resolve.

In the type III, or degenerative spondylolisthesis, I recommend a midline approach and a laminectomy, preserving the pars but resecting the medial one-third of the facet, as well as performing a foraminotomy. I also recommend a transverse process fusion at the level of the slip.

REFERENCES

1. Hensinger, R.N.: Spondylolysis and spondylolisthesis in children. In Evarts, C.M., editor: Instructional course lectures: American Academy of Orthopaedic Surgeons, vol. 32, St. Louis, 1983, The C.V. Mosby Co.
1a. Johnson, J.R, and Kirwan, E.: The long-term results of fusion in situ for severe spondylolisthesis, J. Bone Joint Surg. **65B**:43, 1983.
2. Lombardi, J.S., et al.: Treatment of degenerative spondylolisthesis, Spine **10**:821, 1985.
3. Wiltse, L.L.: The paraspinal sacrospinalis-splitting approach to the lumbar spine, Clin. Orthop. **91**:48, 1973.
4. Wiltse, L.L., and Winters, R.B.: Terminology and measurement of lumbar spondylolisthesis, J. Bone Joint Surg. **65A**(6):768, 1983.
5. Wiltse, L.L., et al.: Classification of spondylolysis and spondylolisthesis, Clin. Orthop. **117**: 23, 1976.

EDITORIAL COMMENTARY

There is a question concerning the requirement to reduce the slip of spondylolisthesis concurrent with fusion. Clearly, the methods of reducing the slip seem to be easily applied. Cloward has argued that with posterior lumbar interbody fusion and certain instrumental manipulations of the two interposed vertebral bodies, he can significantly reduce the slip in most cases. Posterior plate and screw techniques may also accomplish this end. However, because there is a poor correlation between the degree of slip and the extent of painful disability, there is no clear relationship between clinical results and degree of resultant correction of the slip. Long-standing, posttraumatic spondylolyses with spondylolisthesis will normally have remarkable compensatory hyperplasia, and hypertrophy of associated ligaments. Subsequently, with the development of even a small degree of end-plate eburnation, these ligaments often lead to complex entrapment of the ganglion and spinal nerve (seldom the root, except as it may traverse a slipped segment, to emerge at the next lower space).

Perhaps the most difficult (and certainly the most often underestimated) part of the procedure for decompression and stabilization lies in dealing with ligamentous entrapment. The surgeon may find it valuable to impact (drive inward, into the underlying vertebral body) the bony course of the nerve after it has been freed of entrapping ligaments (see Chapter 23). One should also remember that the true lateral extent of potential nerve entrapment may lie as far out as the beginning of the ventral surface of the ala; very far lateral, indeed.

Charles D. Ray

EDITORIAL COMMENTARY

Dr. Wiltse has more experience in spondylolisthesis in children than anyone else. It is hard to refute his experience. Spondylolisthesis may be quite different in young adults. I have had to operate on young adults who had fusions for spondylolisthesis without decompressions. My routine surgery for spondylolisthesis in adults is a complete decompression, visualizing the L5 nerve root in its entirety, and then attempting to obtain a fusion. I agree with Dr. Reynolds that it is a large gap to cover once the nerve root has been totally decompressed. There is also the danger of bone growing back over the exposed nerve root. By taking a large piece of free bone from the iliac crest, one can bridge the gap with a single piece of bone, which then acts as a buttress to keep other bone from falling in over the nerve root, or growing in over it. I put the cortical surface of the bone anteriorly.

With the advent of internal fixation, we have been better able to hold an unstable spondylolisthesis while a fusion occurred and therefore have had a greatly increased fusion rate. The early internal fixation with Knodt rods and Harrington rods tended to cause an increase in the spondylolisthesis by the distraction. Now, with the pedicle screws and plates, we are able to reduce unstable spondylolisthesis and hold it rigidly while a fusion occurs nearly 100% of the time. This is a much more formidable surgery than is described by Dr. Reynolds, and exposes the patient to more complications of the internal fixation and scar tissue and potential root damage. When one sees how severely entrapped some of these nerve roots become, it is hard to conceive of them being pain-free with simply a fusion.

Arthur H. White

CHAPTER 29

POSTERIOR LUMBAR INTERBODY FUSION

James Walter Simmons

Change is not made without inconvenience, even from worse to better.
Richard Hooker

Medical writings warn against statements of priority, that is, do not claim to be the first or second to accomplish an achievement.[23] Crock[8] states that the operation of spinal fusion was introduced first by Albee in 1911 for the treatment of spinal tuberculosis. According to Keim,[20] the actual technique of spinal fusion was first performed by Hibbs in 1911 at the old New York Orthopaedic Hospital. Originally, Hibbs's surgery was performed for tuberculosis, but as the years went by it was extended to include many other pathologic conditions in the cervical, thoracic, and lumbar spine. The use of spinal fusions was then extended by the application to anterior interbody fusion methods by Hodgson in Hong Kong and described by Hodgson and Stock[15] in 1956.

The interlaminar fusion of the lumbar spine originally described by Hibbs and Albee[14] in 1911 became the standard fusion technique. In 1936 Mercer[27] was apparently the first to suggest that "the ideal operation for fusing the spine would be an interbody fusion, but the surgical difficulties encountered in performing such a feat would make the operation technically impossible." Posterior interbody fusion after lumbar disc removal was first reported by Jaslow[17] in 1946. However, the honor of being the father of posterior lumbar interbody fusion certainly should fall to Ralph Cloward of Honolulu. In 1945 Cloward[4] devised "The treatment of ruptured lumbar disc by intervertebral fusion—report of 100 cases" and first reported it at the Harvey Cushing Society meeting at Hot Springs, Virginia, in November 1947. With the exception of Cloward's own publications,[5] there has been little enthusiasm for posterior lumbar interbody fusion (PLIF).

PLIF is more popular outside the United States. Crock,[8] of Australia, indicated that theoretically the ideal operation for isolated lumbar disc resorption (localized spondylosis) is the PLIF, allowing bilateral nerve root canal decompression. James and Nisbet[16] of New Zealand used intervertebral fusion in patients with spondylolisthesis, as well as in those with prolapsed discs. They reported the use of tibial grafts for body-to-body fusion, stating that "posterior intervertebral body-to-body fusion is a neater operation." LeVay[22] reported that the PLIF is favored by neurosurgeons in England. In Germany Junghanns and Schmorl[19] are advocates of Cloward's concept of the PLIF. Junghanns[18] believes that the unstable lumbar segments should not only be fused, but should also effect an operative unfolding (distraction) of the disc space: "In the lumbar spine this only could be achieved posteriorly by removing disc tissue, eliminating the cartilaginous plate, unfolding (distraction) of the disc space, and positioning of the osseous packs." Wiltberger[34,35] also favors PLIF, inserting the dowel grafts through the facet without prior dissection or isolation of the nerve root. Christoferson[3] reports 92% good results in 465 consecutive cases done by placing a portion of the lamina, removed during exposure of the intervertebral lumbar disc, in the intervertebral disc space after discectomy. Lin[23] modified Cloward's technique. His continuing interest and success culminated in the formation of the first Posterior Lumbar Interbody Fusion Workshop and Symposium, April 4 and 5, 1981, in Philadelphia.[25]

INDICATIONS

Junghanns and Schmorl[19] were the first to describe the lumbar intervertebral disc as only a part of the motor segment or perhaps better translated as the motion segment *(bewegungssegment)*. The motion segment consists of the intervertebral disc, the intervertebral foramina, the facets, the interlaminal space, the ligamentun flavum, the spinous processes, and the adjoining ligaments. Junghann's concept is that with a change in the disc space, there is also an associated change in all of the motion segments. When a lumbar disc is degenerative or if the disc is removed surgically, the intervertebral disc space will settle and the narrowing is followed with sequential changes of the motion segment as a whole. In addition to disc herniation, there would be posterior spur formation of the vertebral body, facet overriding, spur formation of the facets, and internal envagination of the ligamentum flavum. The size of the intervertebral foramen is further narrowed by the coverage of ligamentum flavum extending laterally as it covers the facet joint to its lateral limit. Various combinations result in neural compression at various sections of the spinal segment. Spinal stenosis, both of the intervertebral foramen and of the spinal canal, often follows simple discectomy with subsequent disc space settling after surgery. These phenomena are also described by Kirkaldy-Willis,[21] Farfan,[11] Crock,[8] Finnison,[13] and Cauthen.[1]

The bottom line of the PLIF procedure is low back pain secondary to abnormalities of the "motion segment"[29] or "functional spinal unit"[33] with or without sciatica. There are many causes of low backpain; although this statement may seem redundant, when determining which of these many causes of low back pain—with or without sciatica—require surgical intervention, a very unique situation is established. Are PLIF indications simply a matter of diagnosing a chronically symptomatic and degenerated disc[5] or does it extend to the disruption of the annulus fibrosus causing disabling pain without "objective" signs, diagnosed on the basis of clinical findings and experience as described by O'Brien.[28]

Some researchers propose definitive indications for PLIF. In recommending the procedure for the chronic, symptomatic, and degenerated disc, Collis[7] describes the indications as:

1. Lumbar pain with or without sciatica

2. A degenerated disc with or without a protrusion
3. A midline disc protrusion
4. A postlumbar laminectomy–discectomy syndrome
5. A recurrent soft tissue protrusion
6. Spondylolisthesis, grade I or grade II
7. Reverse spondylolisthesis
8. Any combination of the preceding seven conditions

Keim[20] listed 10 indications for lumbar spine fusions:

1. Unstable joint complex associated with a long history of low back pain
2. Spondylolisthesis with or without spondylolysis
3. Congenital anomaly, transitional transverse process, or spondylolysis without spondylolisthesis
4. Localized lateral spinal stenosis or degenerative spondylosis at one level
5. Facet resection from previous surgery
6. Heavy labor or sports activity associated with simple disc herniation with or without degenerative change
7. Bilateral disc herniation or massive midline herniation
8. Previous disc surgery at that level
9. Reconstruction for failed back surgery syndrome (FBSS), including pseudarthroses from lateral fusion
10. Obese patients with bilaterally extruded discs, preventing rapid postoperative settling of the disc space

Lin[26] presents a similar list of indications, and Crock[8] lists "absolute indications for operations":

1. Major neurologic deficits may exist. Cases of acute cauda equina compressions due to massive disc tissue in an abnormally small lumbar spinal canal (spinal canal stenosis) may call for spinal canal decompression involving, if necessary, transdural excision of disc fragments.
2. Persistent or recurrent pain, with or without abnormal physical signs, may occur in the legs. This is the most common indication for surgery after an adequate trial of conservative treatment.
3. Progressive neurologic deficit, such as paraparesis or foot drop, may strengthen indications for operative intervention.
4. Persistent spinal deformity, such as lumbar scoliosis or marked lumbar flexion deformity, may be found in certain cases of lumbar disc prolapse or spinal tumor.

Cloward's indications[4] have not changed after 45 years of experience; that is, "the treatment of low back-pain with or without sciatica due to lumbar disc disease."

Our indications have been a combination of pathophysiology, musculoskeletal function, and significantly impaired life-style requirements.

1. Spinal stenosis not responding to nonsurgical measures
2. Discogenic disease not responding to nonsurgical measures or intradiscal enzyme therapy
3. Spinal instability not responding to job or activity modifications

The guidelines given by Collis,[7] Keim,[20] Lin,[26] Crock,[8] and Cloward,[6] who have used and studied PLIF, convey many years of experience in diagnostic and surgical technique. It would therefore be advantageous for the less experienced to evaluate the various indications and combine them with their own training and experience before embarking on any surgical intervention for problems related to the lumbar spine.

BIOMECHANICAL ADVANTAGES

The human spine is an aggregate of superimposed segments, each segment being a self-contained functional unit, with the sum total of all units forming the vertebral column. The functional unit of the spine is composed of two segments, each engineered for a specific job. The anterior segment (Fig. 29-1) contains two vertebral bodies, one superincumbent on the other, separated by a disc, (Fig. 29-2). The posterior segment (Fig. 29-3) contains the two facet articulations. The anterior segment is a supporting, weight-bearing, shock-absorbing structure. The posterior segment is a non-weight-bearing structure, primarily providing directional guidance and movement.

Chronologic studies of the intervertebral disc were first anatomic, later biomechanical, and finally biochemical. The intervertebral disc was first described by Versalius[31] in 1555. The morbid anatomy or pathologic studies of disc disease and degeneration were first reported by Virchow,[32] and later by Schmorl.[19] The lower discs are only a part of the entire low back anatomic complex and must be considered in conjunction with muscles, longitudinal ligaments, facet joints, and the vertebral bodies above and below.

The disc consists of four parts (see Fig. 29-2): the nucleus pulposus, the annulus fibrosus, and two cartilaginous endplates fused to the vertebral bodies above and below.

From a biomechanical point of view the disc is a self-contained fluid system that absorbs shock, permits transient compression, and, due to the fluid displacement with an elastic container, allows some movement. A constant internal disc pressure separates the two endplates and keeps the fibroelastic annulus taut. Resistance to stress by the vertebral column is further augmented by the vertebral ligaments (Fig. 29-4). Ligaments run longitudinally along the vertebral column, and by their attachment restrict excessive movement of the unit in any direction and prevent significant shearing action.

By their position and attachments longitudinal ligaments reinforce the annulus anteriorly and posteriorly. The annulus is bounded posterolaterally by the bony pedicles of the vertebral arch. Of functional and potential pathologic significance, the posterior longitudinal liga-

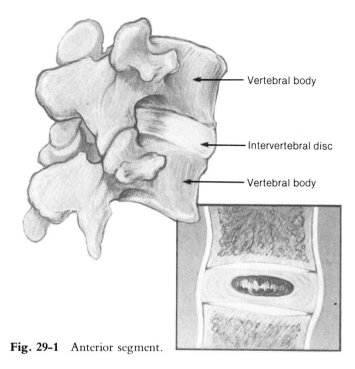

Fig. 29-1 Anterior segment.

290 *Surgical Procedures*

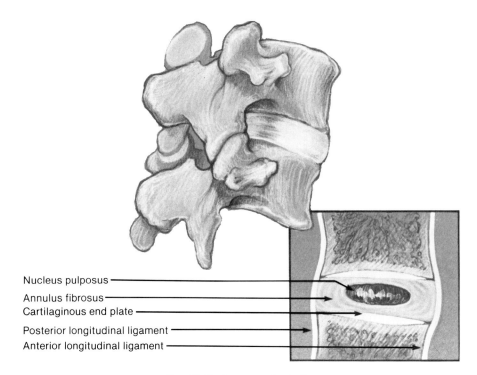

Fig. 29-2 Intervertebral disc.

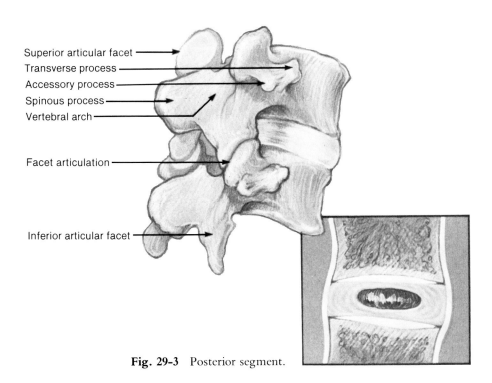

Fig. 29-3 Posterior segment.

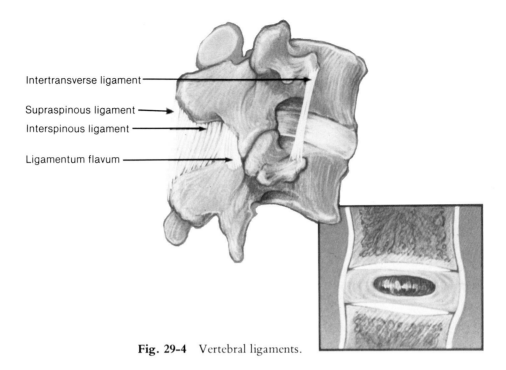

Fig. 29-4 Vertebral ligaments.

ment narrows progressively over the lumbar segments so that, descending to the L5 level, it has retained only one half of its original width. Narrowing of the ligament at these levels provides an inherent structural weakness at the very levels with the greatest static stress and the greatest kinetic strain on the lumbar discs.

The posterior segment (see Fig. 29-3) of the functional unit consists anatomically of two vertebral arches, two transverse processes, a central posterior spinous process, and paired inferior and superior articular facets (apophyseal joints). All but the facets have muscular attachment.

Biomechanical studies have demonstrated that posture brings about marked variation in intradiscal pressure. Reclining, the intradiscal pressure is approximately 7 kg per cm; standing, this rises to 10 kg per cm^2; sitting raises the intradiscal pressure to 15 kg per cm^2.[9]

The nucleus pulposus is a coloidal gel consisting of chondromucopolysaccharide, a protein with strong water-binding property. In this fluid water-loaded state, the nucleus pulposus is incompressible, and by Pasteral's first law exerts strenuous forces equally in all directions against the annulus fibrosus and plates.

Mechanical analysis of the lumbar disc indicates that 80% of weight bearing occurs across the disc.[9] With vertical orientation of the spine, summation of loading is greatest at the lowest lumbar segments. The anatomy, as described previously, can support vertical stress, as well as the forces in rotation and flexion of the spine. Evans[9] describes the motion and the support of that motion.

1. Flexion/extension (sagittal plane): anterior/posterior longitudinal ligaments, facet capsules, and intertransverse, interspinous, and supraspinous ligaments
2. Flexion (coronal plane): facets and capsules, intertransverse ligaments, and possibly the outer annulus

3. Rotation (axial twisting): facet joints and outer annulus
4. Translation (in transverse planes): facet joints, outer annulus, and interspinous ligament

The apophyseal joints and ligamentous structure appear to be passive and are most frequently tested as such. However, there are indications that the ligamentous system is acted on by muscle through the thoracolumbodorsal fascia.[12] The abdominal muscles also can provide an extensional moment when contracted.[10]

Therefore it is apparent that when these normal supportive mechanical structures become dysfunctional, the pathophysiologic responses occur; these responses are well described by Kirkaldy-Willis,[21] Farfan,[11] Crock,[8] Junghanns,[19] and Schmorle.[19] The instability and tropism, which inadvertently occur with dysfunction of the intervertebral "joint,"[11] commands a combination of decompression and stabilization.

Decompression is necessary to relieve the tension placed on the radicals from narrowing of the spinal canal, the lateral spinal recesses, and foraminal stenosis. Because of the instability created with failure of the joint, stabilization of the motion segment is necessary.

CLINICAL ADVANTAGES

Lin[26] lists six clinical advantages of PLIF.

1. PLIF restores the normal anatomic relationship between the motion segment and the neural structures. The narrow disc space and the motion segment are restored to normal anatomic alignment.
2. Further degenerative processes of the fused motion segment are arrested with successful PLIF. However, this increases the range of motion of the adjoining vertebral disc spaces, possibly enhancing their degenerative processes.
3. Recurrent lumbar disc herniation is prevented at the level where the total discoidectomy was needed for PLIF.
4. The lack of motion after a successful PLIF prevents mechanical pulling of the nerve root by the surrounding scar tissue. Thus PLIF prevents painful nerve root irritation from postoperative perineural adhesions.
5. All neural compression from structures other than the disc is relieved by wide laminotomy in PLIF, especially in cases of lateral spinal stenosis.
6. Stress and motion from an abnormal motion segment results in tropism of the facets. The motion is arrested by stabilization; thus PLIF prevents recurrence of tropism or lateral spinal stenosis.

The following reasons are from Cauthen.[1]

1. PLIF reconstitutes the normal anatomic relationship between the motion segment and the neural structures. The narrow disc space and the motion segment are restored to normal anatomic alignment.
2. Successful PLIF arrests further degenerative processes of the fused motion segment. However, because of an increased range of motion of the adjoining vertebral disc spaces, their degenerative processes can be enhanced by PLIF.
3. Total discectomy needed for PLIF prevents recurrent lumbar disc herniation at that level.
4. PLIF prevents painful nerve irritation from postoperative perineural adhesions. Lack of motion after a successful PLIF prevents mechanical pulling of the nerve by the surrounding scar tissue.
5. Wide laminotomy in PLIF relieves all neural compression, especially in cases of lateral spinal stenosis.
6. PLIF restores a constant relationship between all the components of

a motion segment. It also prevents tropism of the facet.

The following are advantages according to Cautilli.[2]
1. It has a wide area of bone surface.
2. It has an adequate blood supply through the cancellous portion of the vertebral body once the cortical plate has been removed.
3. It is proximate to the center of motion and compression forces.
4. It allows complete visualization of the area of nerve root compression.
5. It allows for complete access for removal of the areas of compression centrally (anteriorly and posteriorly), as well as laterally, at the foraminal trough.
6. It preserves interbody distance so there will be no ensuing disc space collapse and possible lateral stenosis as a sequelae of disc excision.

The greatest single advantage of PLIF is that it dynamically decompresses the entire nerve root by holding the vertebral bodies apart. It is a demanding surgical technique that requires a meticulous surgeon with a thorough knowledge of spinal anatomy, causes of nerve root compression, and the basic principles of fusion.

Other important advantages for consideration include visualization and decreased morbidity allowed by the wide decompression. With decompression being carried out to the pedicle, a complete discectomy can be performed, the epidural veins can be cauterized with less risk, and the neural elements are more easily identified. Also, morbidity from the iliac graft is not present when using allograft bone blocks. The operative time is somewhat decreased with the use of allograft bone and good hemostasis. The fear of causing impotency when doing a body-to-body fusion anteriorly is not present. Because of the stability acquired with PLIF, the patient is ambulatory much faster with decreased discomfort and less external support.

SUMMARY

PLIF appears to accomplish all the objectives regarding decompression and stabilization, as well as decreasing the postoperative morbidity associated with spinal fusions in general, particularly when using allograft bones.

REFERENCES

1. Cauthen, J.C.: Lumbar spine surgery indications, techniques, failures and alternatives, Baltimore, 1983, Williams & Wilkins.
2. Cautilli, R.A.: Theoretical superiority of PLIF. In Lin, P.M., editor: Posterior lumbar interbody fusion, Springfield, Ill., 1982, Charles C Thomas, Publisher.
3. Christoferson, L.A., and Selland, B.: Intervertebral bone implants following excision of protruded lumbar discs, J. Neurosurg. **42**:401, 1975.
4. Cloward, R.B.: The treatment of ruptured intervertebral disc by vertebral body fusion: indications, operative technique, after care, J. Neurosurg. **10**:154, 1953.
5. Cloward, R.B.: Lesions of the intervertebral discs and their treatment by interbody fusion methods, Clin. Orthop. **27**:51, 1963.
6. Cloward, R.B.: Posterior lumbar interbody fusion updated, Clin. Orthop. **193**:16, 1985.
7. Collis, J.S.: Total disreplacement: a modified posterior lumbar antibiotic fusion, Clin. Orthop. **193**:64, 1985.
8. Crock, H.V.: Practice of spinal surgery, Vienna, 1983, Springer-Verlag.
9. Evans, J.H.: Biomechanics of lumbar fusion, Clin. Orthop. **193**:38, 1985.
10. Fairbanks, J.C.T., and O'Brien, J.P.: Engineering aspects of the spine, Eng. Med. **7**:135, 1980.
11. Farfan, H.F.: Mechanical disorders of the low back, Philadelphia, 1973, Lea & Febiger.
12. Farfan, H.F.: Muscular mechanism of the lumbar spine and the position of power and efficiency, Orthop, Clin. North Am. **6**:135, 1975.
13. Finnison, B.E.: Low back pain, Philadelphia, 1973, J.B. Lippincott Co.
14. Hibbs, R.A., and Albee, F.H.: An operation for progressive spinal deformities, New York State J. Med. **93**:1013, 1911.
15. Hodgson, A.R., and Stock, F.E.: Anterior spinal fusion: a preliminary communication of the radical treatment of Pott's disease and Pott's paraplegia, Br. J. Surg. **44**:266, 1956.

16. James, A., and Nisbet, N.W.: Posterior intervertebral fusion of lumbar spine: preliminary report of a new operation, J. Bone Joint Surg. **35B**(2):181, 1953.
17. Jaslow, I.A.: Intercorporal bone graft in spinal fusion after disc removal, Surg. Gynecol. Obstet. **82:**215, 1946.
18. Junghanns, H.: Spondylolisthesis Ohne Spalt im Zwischengelenkstueck (pseudospondylolisthesis), Arch. Ortho. Unfallchirurgie **29:** 118, 1931.
19. Junghanns, H., and Schmorl, G.: The human spine in health and disease, ed. 2, New York, 1971, Grune & Stratton, Inc.
20. Keim, H.A.: Indications for spinal fusion and techniques, Clin. Neurosurg. **25:**266, 1977.
21. Kirkaldy-Willis, W.H.: Managing low back pain, New York, 1983, Churchill Livingstone, Inc.
22. LeVay, D.: A survey of surgical management of lumbar disc prolapse in the United Kingdom and Eire, Lancet **1:**1211, 1967.
23. Lin, P.M.: A technical modification of Cloward's posterior lumbar interbody fusion, Neurosurgery **1**(2):124, 1977.
24. Lin, P.M.: Current techniques in operative neurosurgery, New York, 1977, Grune & Stratton, Inc.
25. Lin, P.M.: First Temple PLIF Workshop, Nazareth Hospital, Philadelphia, April 4 and 5, 1981.
26. Lin, P.M.: Introduction of PLIF, biomechanical principals and indications, Springfield, Ill., 1982, Charles C Thomas, publisher.
27. Mercer, W.: Spondylolesthesis with a description of a new method of operative treatment and notes of ten cases, Edinburgh Med. J. N.S. **43:**545, 1936.
28. O'Brien, J.P.: Anterior spinal tenderness in low back pain syndrome, Spine **4**(I):85, 1979.
29. Rolander, S.D.: Motion of the lumbar spine with special reference to the stabilizing effect of posterior fusion, Gothenburg, Sweden, 1966, Tryckeri.
30. Schuerman, H.: Roentgenologic studies of the origin and development of juvenile kyphosis, together with some investigations concerning the vertebral epiphyses in man and in animals, Acta Orthop. Scand. **5:**161, 1934.
31. Vesalius, A.: De Humani Corporis, Fabrica Libri Septem, ed. 1, Basilea [Ex officina Ionnis, Opirini], 1543.
32. Virchow, R.L.: Cellular pathology as based upon physiological and pathological histology, New York, 1860, Dewitt. (Translated from ed. 2 of the original by Frank Chance.)
33. White, A.A., and Panjabi, M.: Clinical biomechanics of the spine, Philadelphia, 1978, J.B. Lippincott Co.
34. Wiltberger, B.R.: The dowel intervertebral-body fusion as used in lumbar-disc surgery, J. Bone Joint Surg. **39A**(2):284, 1957.
35. Wiltberger, B.R.: Intervertebral body fusion by the use of posterior bone dowel, Clin. Orthop. **35:**69, 1964.

EDITORIAL COMMENTARY

Posterior lumbar interbody fusion is the least popular of all of the surgical procedures with the greatest number of authors experiencing complications. Most authors find the procedure of some benefit and a few find it of great benefit. Richard Rothman does not use the procedure at all.

The complications with posterior interbody fusions are well delineated in the chapter. Kirkaldy-Willis states that "most surgeons, myself amongst them, regard it with some trepidation, because the technique is difficult, there is danger of injury to nerves and blood vessels, there is a risk of displacement of the bone grafts, there is a considerable risk of epidural and perineural fibrosis, and the fusion rate is uncertain. I would not embark on this procedure myself."

Vert Mooney states "the posterior interbody fusion has offered the least appealing approach from my standpoint."

Leon Wiltse did his first posterior interbody fusion in 1953. He finds that "theoretically, the posterior interbody fusion fulfills all three criteria for ideal spondylitic surgery. It decompresses the neural component, it distracts the disc space, and it stabilizes the motion segment." However, he says that "I have never used it extensively. I find the indications relatively rare." He finds the fusion rate to be low and the complication rate to be fairly high.

Lumbar laminectomy and disc excision without fusion have been reported to be as successful as any fusion series reported. In my own experience with a controlled series of fusions vs. nonfusions for disc surgery over the past 10 years, there was no greater success by adding a fusion.

There are some theoretic advantages to doing a fusion after disc excision. These are only theoretic and have not been proved by any controlled series. If we are going to add a fusion to our laminectomy and discectomy on theoretic grounds, it would seem reasonable to select a fusion with the least number of complications. The posterior lateral fusion series mentioned in this chapter had very few complications, none of which were serious. Most of the posterior interbody fusion series have complications that are serious.

The extensive neurologic retraction required to place the interbody fusion is a definite potential hazard, and the placement of the bone graft between neurologic structures presents an additional hazard. The extrusion of bone grafts anteriorly or posteriorly can be catastrophic. None of these hazards are present when adding a posterior lateral bone graft.

There are times when posterior interbody fusion is strongly indicated and may be worth the potential hazards. For example, if after disc excision major instability is a highly potential source of future pain, some form of stabilization and fusion is indicated. If there are inadequate posterior elements or small transverse processes, the interbody location for positioning of bone graft seems quite attractive. In such a case I would use bone graft both in the interbody space and intertransverse area and use some form of stabilization with internal fixation, probably including pedicle screws.

Another situation in which I find posterior interbody fusion appealing is after bilaterally removing a disc from a large interspace with very mobile nerves and copious space between the neurologic structures. In anticipation of the settling process, future potential stenosis with the highly available exposure, I will use a posterior interbody technique in place of or in addition to internal fixation. I will not, however, "fight for exposure" or attempt to do the procedure if more neurologic retraction is required than was necessary for the disc removal. If there is any question about the absolute stability of the bone grafts within the interspace, I will use some form of internal fixation to maintain stability and compression of the grafts within the interspace.

The bone grafts or plugs in the interspace usually feel very secure and stable after posterior interbody surgeries. I am always surprised when I find them to shift visibly on x-ray or when I see a case that extrudes. There are many factors responsible for this loosening that we do not understand and are not controlling with conventional posterior or anterior interbody technique. Now that spine surgeons have so many excellent forms of internal fixation that can be applied rapidly, it seems somewhat frivolous not to use internal fixation. The complication of graft extrusion is certainly more potentially severe than complications of most forms of internal fixation.

We do not have a reproducible series of posterior interbody fusions with the use of bone bank allografts in the form of dowels. This technique, with successively sized holes cutters, generally allows only two grafts to be placed. There is a question whether this technique is going to give solid fusion in a significant number of patients. However, as an adjunct to intertransverse fusion or with the additional use of posterior internal fixation, we may find that this very rapid and safe technique will be used more frequently.

Arthur H. White

CHAPTER

30

FAILED POSTERIOR LUMBAR INTERBODY FUSION

James F. Zucherman   David Selby   W. Bradford DeLong

Posterior lumbar interbody fusion (PLIF) has been—and remains—quite controversial. Its proponents have been especially enthusiastic, while many other spine surgeons have been critical of the technical difficulties inherent in the procedure. Theoretically, the PLIF has many advantages, including:

1. Posterior exposure for complete visualization of the neural elements
2. Distraction or disc space restoration maintaining lateral canal patency
3. Fusion stops progressive deterioration of the diseased motion segment
4. Interbody fusion near the center of motion of the motion segment under compression
5. Potential for early stability facilitating rapid postoperative comfort and mobility
6. No necessity for hardware and its unique complications

On the other hand, we believe there are some real disadvantages present, including the following:

1. In its classic form, a high degree of technical difficulty exists requiring more operative time per level than most other fusion techniques.
2. The procedure tends to involve more neural element manipulation than other procedures.
3. Unique complications relating to demands of interdiscal bone graft placement through a limited (posterior) approach are present, including:
   a. Posterior and posterior lateral displacement of bone graft material, which may result in neural element damage or irritation (Fig. 30-1)

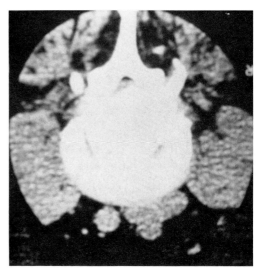

Fig. 30-1 Posterior migration of graft.

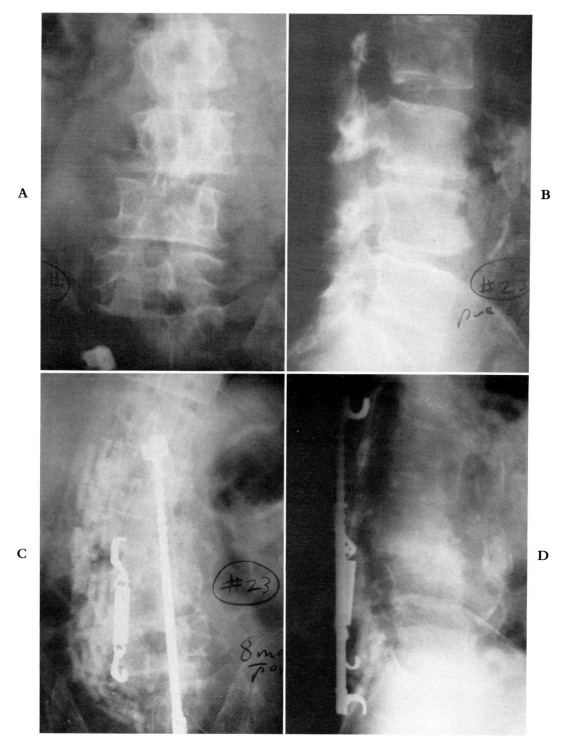

Fig. 30-2 **A** and **B,** Graft collapse with lateral subluxation and instability. **C** and **D,** Refusion with instrumentation.

b. Damage to neural elements while trying to position grafts in the interspace
c. Collapse of vertebral body sometimes resulting in destabilization of the fusion complex (Fig. 30-2)

CLINICAL SERIES

There have been many substantial series on the PLIF, especially in recent years. Variations in techniques are present in each series that make it difficult to accurately judge the procedure in general. Cloward's ingenuity and technical skill in development and refinement of this operation cannot be overemphasized. In 1953 he first published a series[2] of 321 patients with a 1- to 8-year follow-up and reported an 85% cure rate. There were six cases of graft absorption and failure of fusion; four of these required refusion and there was one case of graft dislodgment reported. Homograft was used for the intervertebral space. In 1963 Cloward reported a series of "100 unselected cases"[3] with 84% being completely asymptomatic and 12% good with occasional minor symptoms. Bone grafts had resorbed with questionable fusion in seven out of 100. Four out of these seven were asymptomatic.

In 1964 Wiltberger[16,17] described a series of 192 patients with 2- to 9-year follow-up. A dowel technique was used in 153 of these. There were no or minimal symptoms in 65%. The postoperative regimen included 8 months in a brace preceded by 3 weeks in bed. He reported 21% nonunion in the two-level cases and 13% nonunion in the one-level cases. There were five wound infections, two graft extrusions, and three patients with permanent foot drop.

Blume,[1] using a unilateral dowel technique, reported 216 cases in 1981 with 95% good and excellent results. Of these cases, 10% showed shifting of the interbody autologous dowels. There was one case with dislodgment, which required reoperation. There was one case of anterior extrusion compressing the common iliac vein, which did not require surgery. There were three cases of postoperative lateral stenosis requiring surgery, as well as two infections and a traumatic neuroma.

Lin,[9] a neurosurgeon, in 1982 presented 50 consecutive cases evaluated by two orthopaedists. His technique utilized autologous posterior iliac graft and homograft with retention of the spinous process interspinous ligament complex. In 45 of 50 patients that were examined an 82% fusion rate was present. Good and excellent results overall were found in 69% of the cases. In Lin's series,[10] 500 cases reported in 1983, complications included 5% neurologic deficits, 5% thrombophlebitis, and two cases of urinary incontinence. There were four cases that required immediate reoperation because of graft displacement, and approximately 3% required reoperation for pseudarthrosis.

In 1982 Cloward[9] reported another series of 100 patients evaluated by two orthropaedists. This series had 90% good and excellent results with 60% of the patients being followed greater than 10 years. Of 34 worker's compensation cases, 28 returned to their previous jobs after 6 months. Five patients required reoperation; however, 73% had solid fusions. There were 10 definite pseudarthroses, six of which were asymptomatic.

In 1983 Ma[11] reported 100 consecutive cases with 74% good and excellent results despite a high percentage of patients having secondary gain. Ma has developed mortising chisels and other specialized instruments to shape the interspace and facilitate the procedure; as does Cloward,

Ma uses cadaveric bone graft. In this series, 70% returned to their original jobs. Complications included a 6% graft extrusion rate and a 15% pseudarthrosis rate.

In 1983 Hutter[7] reported his series of 500 cases with an average follow-up of greater than 5 years. There was a 90% fusion rate with 82% excellent and good results. Autologous iliac crest grafts were used. There were technical difficulties in 5%. The series included five infections, five venous thromboses, 18 cases of residual paresis in the affected nerve and three displaced bone grafts. In 88 of the cases that were revisions, there were 64% good and excellent results.

In 1985 Collis[5] reported 950 posterior interbody fusion levels in 750 patients; 50 patients were studied. Of these, 25 patients had previous surgery and 25 had not. The results of 25 cases without prior surgery were all satisfactory. In the 25 patients with prior surgery 84% had satisfactory results. The results with four patients in the group who had previous surgery were considered failures. In addition, 47 patients obtained bony fusion. Three patients with fibrous unions had good clinical results. Out of his series of 750 cases there were four dural tears, four cases of graft extrusion requiring surgery, and three minimal graft displacements that did not require surgery. There were six cases of nerve deficit, all of which were temporary.

In our combined series 120 consecutive cases were performed with a minimum of 9-month follow-up. Of these, 17% had previous chemonucleolysis or surgery. Approximately 33% were performed using bilateral posterior dowel autologous graft from the iliac crest or allograft with instrumentation designed by Dr. H. Crock; 40% were performed using bone blocks in the manner of Cloward. In 20% posterior instrumentation with Luque segmental wiring or interlaminar wiring was added to the PLIF. Autologous chip grafts were used in 10%. About 50% of the cases used autologous bone, and one half used allograft. There was no significant difference in results according to the variation in techniques or the type of bone graft used. Zucherman reviewed the patient results of all three authors of this chapter. The patients' results were categorized into excellent, good, fair, and poor. Excellent was defined as asymptomatic, taking no medicines, and returning to full activities; good was defined as much improved from preoperative state, returning to work with minimal or no limitations with the need for occasional non-narcotic medication; fair was defined as significantly improved from preoperative state but with significant functional limitations and feeling the need to take medications several times a week; poor was defined as the same or worse from the preoperative state with marked functional limitations and the need for pain control measures and medications. Approximately 50% had good and excellent results with 40 patients considered excellent and 21 considered good. There were fair or poor results in 57 patients, 29 fair and 28 poor.

One patient died from apparently unrelated causes 1 month after the procedure. In one case the technique was abandoned because of technical difficulties during the procedure. There was a 17% (20 patients) reoperation rate. In 16 cases these were revisions resulting from graft retropulsion or vertebral subluxation with graft collapse (Figs. 30-3 through 30-5). In three patients hardware was removed only. One patient had a reoperation to remove a drain tip. There was no significant difference in the rate of graft dislodgment by surgeon or by technique.

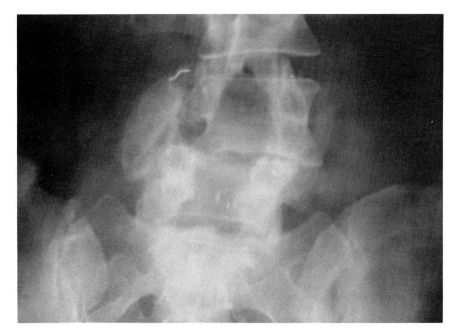

Fig. 30-3 Lateral subluxation after PLIF treated by posterior lateral fusion.

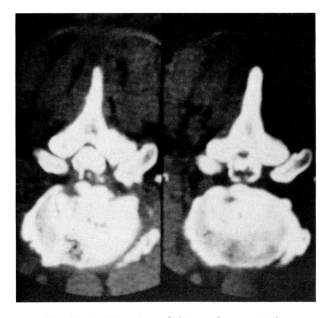

Fig. 30-4 Migration of chip grafts posteriorly.

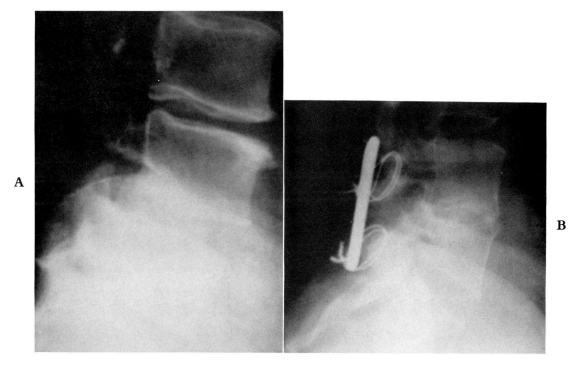

Fig. 30-5 **A,** Posterior migration of PLIF. **B,** Revision with instrumentation.

TECHNICAL ASPECTS

Graft extrusion is one of the principal unique PLIF complications. As Hutter[7] points out, the positioning of the patient is the key factor. If one uses one of the knee-chest frames to free the abdomen from pressure, an increase of lumbar lordosis is also created, which will tend to result in shaping the vertebral space in such a way as to encourage posterior migration of the grafts (Fig. 30-6, *A*); the lumbar lordosis should be reduced (Fig. 30-6, *B*).

When grafts are inserted into the disc space, the upper exiting nerve root traverses the interspace often just out of direct view in the remaining undecompressed lateral recess (Fig. 30-7, *A*). Great care must be taken by both the surgeon and the assistant that the superior lateral corner of the bone graft being inserted does not damage the upper traversing nerve (Fig. 30-7, *B*). Depending on the individual anatomy, it may be difficult or impossible to insert bone grafts without undue traction on neural elements, such as in the case of a conjoined nerve root covering the posterior lateral portion of the disc.

It is essential to be able to slide the grafts across the disc space if bone graft blocks are used. The most inaccessible part of the disc that may block graft positioning is in the midline under the posterior longitudinal ligament (Fig. 30-8, *A*). This is most easily removed with a down-pushing curette or by totally excising the posterior annulus and ligament (Fig. 30-8, *B*).

Although extremely rare, anterior vessel damage by penetrating the annulus is an ever-present danger. A lateral x-ray film with an instrument in the disc space is helpful to gauge its depth. Chisels and curettes can be permanently marked so that their exact depth in the disc space can be gauged readily at any time during the procedure.

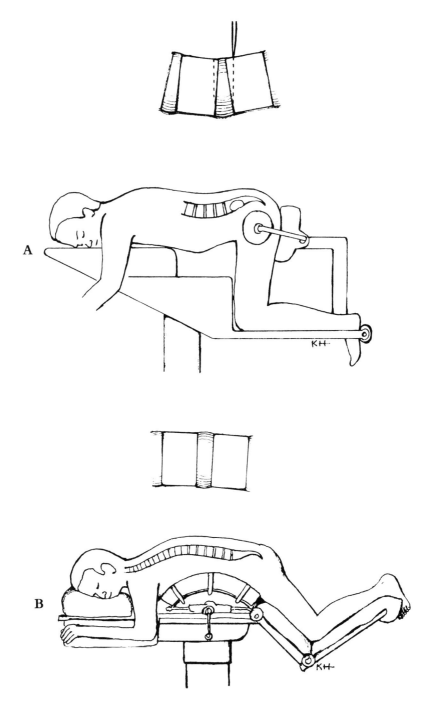

Fig. 30-6 A, Operation with the patient in increased lordosis encourages posterior graft migration. **B,** Appropriate positioning.

Failed Posterior Lumbar Interbody Fusion 303

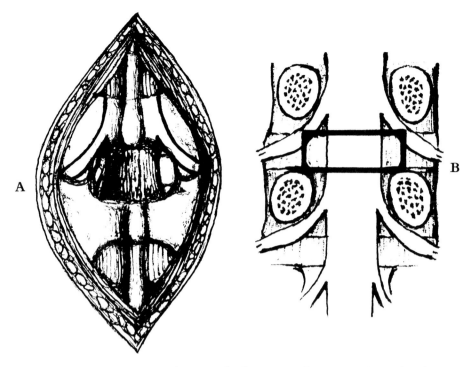

Fig. 30-7 **A,** Exiting roots just out of view under facet joints. **B,** Roots in jeopardy when grafts are inserted.

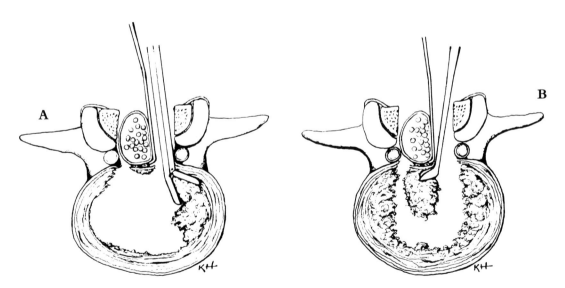

Fig. 30-8 **A,** Removal of lateral most disc. **B,** Midline disc is easily overlooked.

Excellent visualization and exposure is mandatory in this procedure. Hypotensive anesthesia is extremely useful in minimizing bleeding. Epidural veins are controlled with bipolar coagulation and tamponade with Gelfoam or Surgicel. A head lamp is the most effective technique for illumination in our experience.

Although we saw no difference in results using bone-bank bone or autologous bone, there was definitely diminished operative time and technical difficulty using bone-bank bone. In the case of the dowel procedures, using precut dowels seems to significantly reduce the technical difficulties of the procedure.

Osteoporotic patients present a greater technical challenge. Chances of vertebral body collapse with resulting destabilization and bone graft migration are increased. If autogenous bone is used, the variable of bone graft of inadequate strength to support the interspace is introduced. It seems preferable to correct osteoporosis as much as possible before the procedure.

Although some surgeons believe that postoperative epidural fibrosis is minimized because of immediate stabilization, we think that this has been a definite problem with the procedure because of wide posterior decompression and increased manipulation of the neural elements. We have seen great amounts of epidural fibrosis, both in our own cases and in other cases performed by expert PLIF surgeons. The use of fat grafts or Gelfoam around the neural structures appears to help somewhat in reducing scar, perhaps by minimizing postoperative bleeding and dead space.

Although Cloward[4] has reported excellent results in spondylolisthesis, the technical problems are certainly magnified in this situation. It would seem prudent to become very experienced in this technique before attempting it in these cases.

From the series reviewed it is clear that the PLIF can be an effective surgical treatment in some experienced hands. A question that must be answered is what real advantage does it have over other fusion techniques. Another issue is the "learning curve" in perfecting the technique.

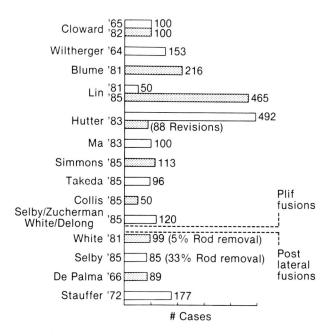

Fig. 30-9 Clinical series of posterior interbody fusion and posterior lateral fusion.

In DePalma's series[6] of 89 patients with 173 levels fused posterior laterally, 76% good and excellent results were reported. Stauffer and Coventry[13] report 81% of 177 patients returning to their original job, with 356 levels posterior laterally fused. Selby and White[12,15] have reported 85% and 70% satisfactory results respectively using posterior lateral fusion with Knodt rods. These results appear to fall within the range of the results reported by various PLIF surgeons (Fig. 30-9).

Our experience and that of other spine surgeons who have recently begun doing PLIFs is of occasional technical complications resulting in poor clinical outcomes. These difficulties are unique to PLIF and are not present in the posterior lateral fusion techniques. Results in worker's compensation cases for the state of Washington have been so dismal that posterior interbody fusions are no longer authorized by the Department of Labor and Industries, based on results in 117 cases.[8]

SUMMARY

PLIF can be effective in the most experienced hands but may not be the easiest or most effective way to accomplish fusion with posterior visualization and decompression. The learning curve in this operation is longer than in others that may accomplish the same goals. Theoretic appeal and the "neatness" of an operation should certainly be secondary consideration to clinical efficacy. We believe that the classic PLIF should be considered only in an ideal setting; that is, performed by very experienced spine surgeons who have had training from an expert in PLIF surgery with an equally qualified assistant. The specialized instrumentation specifically designed for this procedure is mandatory before it should be attempted. Availability of hypotensive anesthesia and a bone bank to diminish technical difficulties is recommended.

REFERENCES

1. Blume, H.G., and Rojas, C.H.: Unilateral lumbar interbody fusion (posterior approach) utilizing dowel grafts, J. Neurol. Orthop. Surg. 2(3):171, 1981.
2. Cloward, R.B.: The treatment of ruptured lumbar intervertebral discs by vertebral body fusion: indication, operative technique, after care, J. Neurosurg. 10:154, 1953.
3. Cloward, R.B.: Lesion of the interbody disks and their treatment by interbody fusion methods (The painful disk), Clin. Orthop. 27:51, 1963.
4. Cloward, R.B.: Spondylolisthesis: treatment by laminectomy and posterior interbody fusion, 1981, pp. 74-8 Clin. Orthop. 154:74, 1981.
5. Collis, J.S.: Total disc replacement: a modified posterior interbody fusion, Clin. Orthop. 193:64, 1985.
6. DePalma, A., et al.: Posterior bilateral fusion of the lumbosacral spine, Clin. Orthop. 47:165, 1966.
7. Hutter, C.G.: Posterior intervertebral body fusion, Clin. Orthop. 179:86, 1983.
8. Johnson, D.A., (Medical Consultant, Department of Labor and Industries, Olympia, Wash.): Personal communication, Nov. 6, 1984.
9. Lin, P.M.: Posterior lumbar interbody fusion, Springfield, Ill., 1982, Charles C Thomas, Publisher.
10. Lin, P.M., et al.: Posterior lumbar interbody fusion, Clin. Orthop. 180:154, 1983.
11. Ma, G.W.: Posterior lumbar interbody fusion with specialized instruments, Clin. Orthop. 193:57, 1985.
12. Selby, D.: Personal communication, March 1985.
13. Stauffer, R.N., and Loventry, M.B.: Posterolateral lumbar spine fusion, J. Bone Joint Surg. 54A:1195, 1972.
14. Takeda, M.: Experience in posterior lumbar interbody fusion: unicortical versus bicortical autologous graft, Clin. Orthop. 193:120, 1985.
15. White, A.H., et al.: Knodt rod distraction lumbar fusion, Spine 8(4):434, 1983.
16. Wiltberger, B.R.: The prefit dowel intervertebral body fusion as used in lumbar disc therapy, Am. J. Surg. 86:723, 1953.
17. Wiltberger, B.R.: Intervertebral body fusion by the use of posterior bone dowel, Clin. Orthop. 35:69, 1964.

CHAPTER

31

LUMBAR FUSION WITH DISTRACTION RODS

Arthur H. White

Internal fixation in spinal fusions has some distinct theoretic advantages. These include the ability to distract, enlarging intervertebral foramina, maintaining disc height, holding vertebra in a stable position while fusions occur, and correcting abnormal curvatures. There are, however, potentially significant complications with internal fixation, including a higher rate of infection, dislodgment of the internal fixation, irritation of neurologic structures, longer operating times, and greater blood loss. One must weigh the risks against the advantages. Overzealous use of internal fixation can lead to unnecessary complications. The desired result may be accomplished by simpler means. With the use of body casts, longer periods of bed rest, more extensive decompressions, and strategic placement of bone grafts such as interbody fusions, very adequate and successful surgeries can be accomplished.

Internal fixation becomes absolutely necessary when stability and distraction cannot be maintained by any other means. In such situations spine surgeons long ago found that conventional techniques did not work. Highly unstable spines in patients who cannot wear body casts and cannot be confined to bed rest may require internal fixation. This is particularly true if there is osteoporosis, scoliosis, spondylolisthesis, and obesity. Any form of surgery in these complex patients is fraught with complications and should not be taken lightly, with or without internal fixation. These cases are usually best treated by a multidisciplinary approach in a spine center that has a team of spine specialists who are equipped to deal with a multiplicity of factors, including metabolic bone disease, pain control, and problems specifically related to the specialties of psychiatry, neurosurgery, orthopedics, internal medicine, and rehabilitation.

Herbert Knodt developed his distraction rods in the 1960s. His rods were frequently used without laminectomy. Knodt rod–fusion success may have been due to the distraction of the intervertebral foramen, which prevented spinal stenosis while a fusion was being accomplished. Fusion alone without internal fixation can leave underlying spinal stenosis potentially symptomatic. Many surgeons

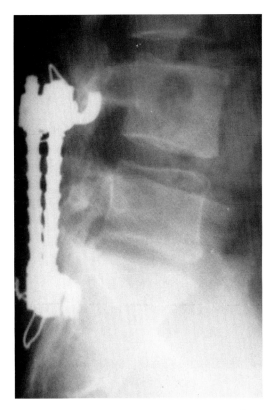 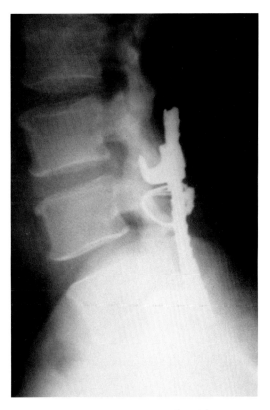

Fig. 31-1 Harrington rods; loss of lordosis from L4 to S1.

Fig. 31-2 Bent Harrington rods with intersegmental wire to maintain same lordosis.

began using Knodt rods after performing a laminectomy to maintain the decompression that had been accomplished.

There have been several reports in the literature on Knodt rods.[1-4] We reported the results of our first 100 Knodt rod fusions in difficult spinal cases in 1983.[4] We found that our success rate with the use of Knodt rods in patients who had over 5 years of low back pain without classical herniated disc was 20% greater than without the use of Knodt rods. We believe the distraction and stabilizing effects of the Knodt rods allowed greater fusion rates and maintenance of disc heights and foramen heights before fusion. These cases were before the CT scan era and our present knowledge of spinal stenosis. We were preventing and correcting spinal stenosis that otherwise could have been overlooked.

With Knodt rods working so well for one- and two-level laminectomies, we began using Harrington rods for three-, four-, and five-level fusions. The Harrington rods had been used for years in scoliosis to correct and maintain alignment. When greater distraction forces became necessary over multiple levels of the spine, the Harrington rods seemed most appropriate. The loss of lumbar lordosis had long been known to be a problem with the use of distraction rods (Fig. 31-1). However, with the advent of intersegmental wiring we found that we were able to retain one or two laminas with which to wire the rods for a three-point fixation and maintain some of the lumbar lordosis (Fig. 31-2). The intersegmental wires also virtually eliminated the other major complication of rod displacement.

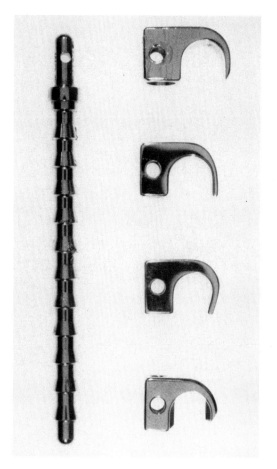

Fig. 31-3 Top three hooks are Harrington hooks of variable size and contour. Bottom hook is a Knodt hook.

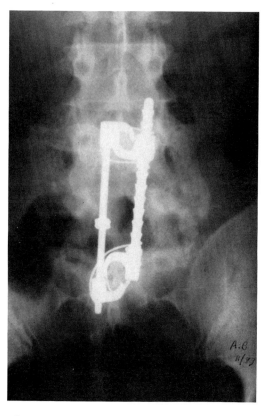

Fig. 31-4 Distraction and compression rods attached to spinous processes.

Sacral fixation has been a problem. There is frequently inadequate space under the S1 lamina to place Knodt rod hooks or Harrington rod hooks. I have used smaller and contoured Harrington rod hooks, which decrease complications but still can cause S1 or S2 root irritation (Fig. 31-3). With three-, four-, and five-level fusions it is relatively easy and safer to use alar hooks. They too can cause nerve irritation at the L5 root, which passes close to the conventional location of an alar hook. I have had to remove several alar hooks for this complication. Contouring and fitting of the rods and hooks of three-level fusions from ala to L3 is time-consuming and complex. Lumbar lordosis, however, can be built into the contour rod, and if the L4 lamina is maintained for intersegmental wiring one can get a very satisfactory alignment and fusion. At times the spinous processes are stout enough to be used for various forms of distraction or compression (Fig. 31-4).

Because of the problem with the sacral and alar hooks I began using screws into the lateral masses of S1 and placing Harrington rods into the open hole in the screws (Figs. 31-5 through 31-7). Some of these screws have worked loose and some have broken, but for the most part this practice provides a safe and effective method of sacral fixation. Dr. Charles Edwards has developed a specialized sacral screw and Harrington rod modular

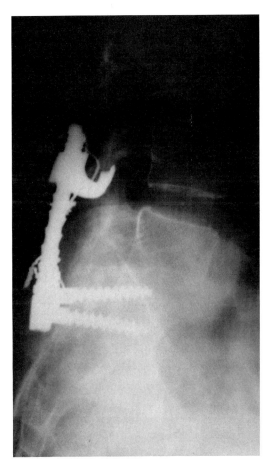

Fig. 31-5 Harrington rods attached to pedicle screws at S1 pedicle, lateral view.

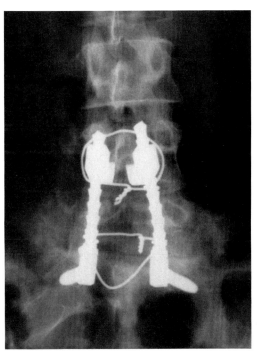

Fig. 31-6 Harrington rods attached to pedicle screws at S1 pedicle, AP view.

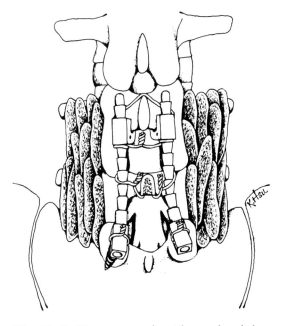

Fig. 31-7 Harrington rods with sacral pedicle screw fixation and intersegmental wiring.

system with hooks to eliminate many problems.* Both distraction and compression systems have been developed. The design of the screw-hook junction at the sacrum maintains the lumbosacral angle and therefore lordosis at that segment. The screw is designed to penetrate both cortices of the sacrum; thus loosening is much less frequent. It remains to be seen how much activity these screws will allow the patient before they fracture. At this point most cases have been kept in a pantaloon-type spica immobilization of one leg for several months. The screws that have fractured in my cases have had either no immobilization or only a light

---

*Zimmer USA, Inc., Warsaw, Ind.

corset. The anatomical hook provided by the Zimmer company also greatly decreases the likelihood of vertebral canal compromise at the proximal end of the lumbosacral fusion. This system also provides pedicle screws and pedicle connectors for multilevel fixation to the rods. Rod sleeves help maintain lordosis.

The Luque system of rods and intersegmental wires does not provide significant distraction, but it can maintain the vertebrae in position after decompression. This system can prevent collapse of the disc space and intervertebral foramen. It may assure stability and a greater fusion rate. Many surgeons are using Luque rectangles to stabilize after interbody fusions or other decompressions. It is sometimes difficult to find a place for an intersegmental wire after a broad multilevel decompression. The surgery has to be planned to preserve the lamina. An adequate decompression and foramenotomy can be performed in most cases while leaving enough lamina for an intersegmental wire (see Fig. 31-7). With far lateral stenosis, however, it is sometimes necessary to remove the complete inferior facet and much of the superior facet to get to the lateral disc and narrowed intervertebral foramen. This type of decompression is hard to perform with the lamina left in place. With the distraction rods and intersegmental wiring these far lateral syndromes are partially corrected by the distraction forces.

Osteoporosis makes segmental wiring less appealing because of inadequate bone support. Intersegmental wires can be placed through intervertebral foramen and around the remaining superior facets (Figs. 31-8 and 31-9). This technique carries with it the obvious possibilities of spinal nerve irritation and facet fracture. Sometimes the transverse processes are large enough to pass a wire intersegmentally to fix a Luque rod. Segmental wiring to the sacrum can be done. A hole is made between the S1 and S2 lamina, and a wire is passed under the lamina.

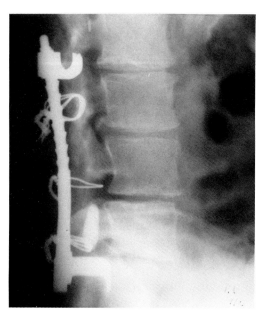

Fig. 31-8 Harrington rod distraction with alar hooks and intersegmental wires passed through intervertebral foramen, lateral view.

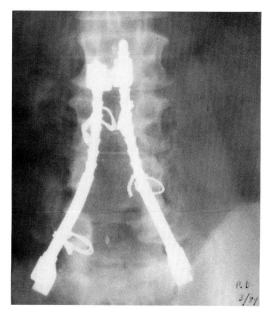

Fig. 31-9 Harrington rod distraction with alar hooks and intersegmental wires passed through intervertebral foramen, AP view.

Alternatively, the rods can be passed into the ilium laterally, crossing the sacroiliac joint with several potential complications.

In my practice I choose the internal fixation to fit the particular needs of the individual case. Knodt rods are used when major distraction forces are not necessary, but some maintenance of disc and foramen height is desired. If larger distraction forces are needed, I use the Harrington rod system. If there is ample room under the lamina of the sacrum I use sacral hooks, and if longer fusions are being done with Harrington rods I use the alar hook. Now with the availability of the sacral screws it is very appealing to use them routinely. Intersegmental wires assure that the rods and hooks do not displace and maintain a more normal lumbar lordosis.

TECHNIQUE

A midline incision is made over the length of the spine to be decompressed and fused. The full lamina and transverse processes are exposed at each level. A liberal and extensive laminectomy is performed bilaterally at the levels with severe stenosis and where discs are to be removed. If possible I retain enough lamina for an intersegmental wire. Each disc is evaluated and excised bilaterally if indicated. Each nerve root is traced thoroughly through its foramen. Foramenotomy is performed until there is free passage of a liberal-sized probe (6 mm in diameter).

The internal fixation to be used is selected. I will describe the most common three-level Harrington rod procedure (Fig. 31-10). The proximal Harrington rod hooks are fashioned as they would be for a scoliosis procedure. If there is adequate room in the facet joint, it is used because the superior facet offers a degree of protection from nerve damage by the hook. After the placement of the hook it is important to evaluate the intervertebral foramen and nerve root at the next most proximal level. If these hooks buckle the ligamentum flavum or protrude into the central canal, they can compress a nerve root or the dura.

The ala of the sacrum is identified, and the space between the ala and the fifth transverse process is exposed. With blunt dissection the free superior surface of the ala is exposed. Care is taken not to injure the L5 nerve root in the depth of this dissection. The alar hook then is slid along the ala with the blade of the hook in contact with the ala at all times so it does not entrap any soft tissue or L5 nerve root in its placement. The hook then is impacted into place, and the L5 nerve root is inspected for free passage.

An appropriately sized Harrington rod is selected and, with a rod bender, contoured with both a lordosis and lateral curvature to pass without excess force from the alar hook to the proximal hook (see Fig. 31-10). Square-ended distal hooks and rods are used because the complexity of the contour of the rod creates

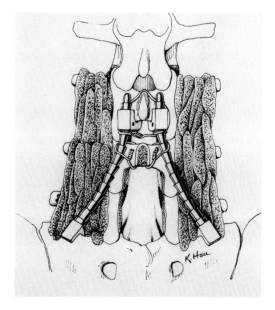

Fig. 31-10 Three-level Harrington rod fusion with contoured rods, intersegmental wiring, alar hooks, and proximal wire serving as C washer.

rotational forces. The rod is placed and distracted. If an L4 lamina has been preserved, a double 18-gauge wire is placed around the lamina and the rod and secured tightly wih a wire twister before full distraction of the rod. After both rods are placed, another 18-gauge wire is passed around the remainder of the L3 spinous process and around both upper hooks and rods, functioning as a C washer (see Fig. 31-10). The ala of the sacrum, all transverse processes, and superior facets to be fused are decorticated, and bone grafts placed over the decorticated area. The bone graft is taken in a routine fashion from the iliac crest through the same skin incision.

If a sacral screw is to be used, it is placed at the base of the superior facet of S1 (see Fig. 31-7). It is angled 30 degrees distally and laterally. One should practice placing this screw on spine models or cadavers, because drilling past the anterior cortex can produce injury to the structures in the pelvis. A depth gauge is used, and an appropriately sized screw is selected to pass both cortices. Some screws have a blunt tip to decrease the danger of damage to pelvic structures. An x-ray film should be taken to verify the position of the screw. If a simple cancellous screw is used, I select rods with a hole drilled in the end to place a wire so the rod does not disconnect from the screw (see Fig. 31-7).

RESULTS

There have been several reports of the results of lumbar spine fixation with rods. The selection of patients and the type of rods used is quite variable. In France Dubuc[2] found Knodt rods to be virtually useless and discovered that most of them had to be removed. In the United States success rates vary from 70% to 90% in relieving low back pain and neurologic symptoms.[1,3,4] Although I have used some form of internal fixation on almost all of my fusions for the past 10 years, I have no quarrel with those who do simple intertransverse fusions or interbody fusions after an adequate one-level decompression and disc excision. The pseudarthrosis rate in two-level or greater lumbar fusions can be high without the use of internal fixation.

I strongly recommend distraction-rod fixation with intersegmental wires in very complex cases with combinations of osteoporosis, spinal stenosis, obesity, deconditioning, and herniated discs. In these difficult kinds of cases surgeons have long ago given up attempting corrective spine surgery. Simple intertransverse fusions were not enough. These patients were relegated to nursing homes and wheelchair existences. I reported on 30 of these cases in 1982 at the International Society of the Lumbar Spine in Cambridge. Since then I have continued to have success on a regular basis with this procedure. Objective and subjective measures indicate a 60% success rate in improving patient's abilities to return to normal activities.

French and German spine surgeons have been using pedicle screws in various forms of spinal fixation for many years. In addition, American surgeons have performed several forms of pedicle screw fixation in the past few years. They have generally been attempting to accomplish the same end—immediate solid fixation and anatomic position by the use of pedicle screws in each involved level without violating any other levels and without undue complications.

Arthur Steffee presented his procedure for plate fixation with pedicle screws to the North American Spine Association in June 1984 and 1986 (Fig. 31-11). His technique is presented in Chapter 33. The advantages were a very strong solid plate with special instruments for ease of insertion of pedicle screws. A major disadvantage was the inability to make a straight

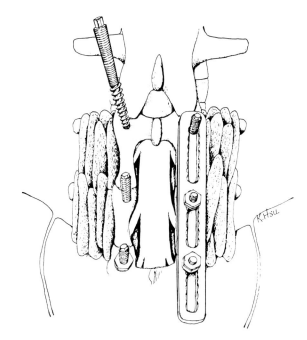

Fig. 31-11 Steffee plate and pedicle screws.

plate conform to pedicle screws that could not be placed in a straight line. Another disadvantage was that the plate protruded above the upper screw far enough to violate the next most proximal facet joint. Dr. Steffee has developed many alterations of his technique; there are now outrigger types of screws that can enter the pedicle at variable angles and still attach to the plate. The most proximal screw can be placed into a pedicle and still attach to the plate without violating the next most proximal facet joint.

The Frymoyer-Vermont internal fixation device was designed mainly for fixation between two segments. It has a single straight rod between the two fixation pedicle screws that can be bent to conform to the location of the pedicle screws. Whether multiple pedicle screws can be placed and this solid rod can be bent to conform to multiple levels remains to be seen. This device was presented to the International Society for the Study of the Lumbar Spine in Australia in April 1985.

Leon Wiltse has developed a similar type of internal fixation pedicle screw device, which attaches two rods to each pedicle screw. The rods are adjustable to almost any configuration of the pedicle screws. His technique does not violate the next most proximal facet joint because the screws can enter the pedicle at various directions. Dr. Wiltse and his colleagues presented his internal fixation apparatus to the North American Spine Society at Laguna Niguel in June 1985.

Charles Edwards, with the assistance of the Zimmer company, has developed a modular internal fixation apparatus, which most closely resembles the Harrington rod internal fixation technique. An anatomic hook has been devised that more closely adheres to the configuration of the spinal canal. Special screws, which adapt to the anatomic Harrington hook, have been developed to enter the pedicle of S1. There is both a distraction and compression means of attaching Harrington rods to these hooks and pedicle screws. The means of attachment of the distal hook to the sacral screw maintains the normal lumbosacral angle. The lumbar lordosis of the higher levels is accomplished by the use of polyethylene elliptical sleeves that are slipped over the rods and exert pressure against the posterior elements. Dr. Edwards presented his fixation device to the American Academy of Orthopaedic Surgeons in Las Vegas in January 1985 and to the North American Society in 1986. There will undoubtedly be more devices to expeditiously fix the lumbar spine in any position that the surgeon finds necessary. The race is on for the "perfect" internal fixation device. The ideal fusion will probably eventually be accomplished percutaneously with any degree of solidity that is biomechanically applicable. Totally solid fusions may not be the best answer. Decreasing stress proportional with the condition of the spine may be quite satisfactory. Available fusions and available internal fixation devices may be better than immediate, totally rigid fixation, which transfers all of the stresses to other levels, resulting in rapid degenerative changes.

The spine surgeon should be familiar with all of the possibilities to accomplish any given surgical task. There is no single surgical procedure that is best for all lumbar spinal surgical conditions. There is no one internal fixation device that will work best for all occasions. Internal fixation is not necessary in the majority of spinal surgery, and the complications of internal fixation—especially in unexperienced hands—far outweigh its value for most lumbar spine surgery at this time.

REFERENCES

1. Beattie, F.C.: Distraction rod fusion, Clin. Orthop. **62**:1969.
2. Dubuc, F.: Knodt rod grafting, Orthop. Clin. North Am. **6**:1975.
3. Knodt, H., and Larrick, R.B.: Distraction fusion of the spine, Ohio State Med. J. **60**(12), 1964.
4. White, A.H., et. al.: Knodt rod distraction lumbar fusion, Spine **8**(4), 1983.

CHAPTER 32

THE KNODT ROD: SPARE THE ROD AND SPOIL THE FUSION

David Selby

The literature on the spine is filled with series of papers that do not equate solid fusion with pain relief. However, one cannot identify the reason for fusion in many of the series. In fact, the normal reason for spinal fusion was only that a disc was removed. No attempt at actual identification of instability with correction of that instability is apparent in these papers.[3] It would seem reasonable that failed fusion in a patient who is inherently stable would give a good result as long as nerve tissue is not compromised by the fusion mass.[4] In contrast, solid fusion of the type that will affix the painful source as identified is necessary for clinical pain relief in the unstable spinal segment.

If you agree, then solid fusion is your goal.

It has always been a conundrum that fractures require fixation—or at least reasonable immobilization—for healing. Yet we expect multiple joint union by placing bone chips along the side of the joint. Afterward the patient may or may not be placed in a brace that offers little or no immobilization of the motion segments. Bed rest may also be ordered, but again it is difficult to identify that this truly immobilizes the motion segments of the spine. It was the hope for rigid internal fixation that led to the use of metallic fixation devices in the lumbar spine.[1,2,5-7]

I started using Knodt rods in the early 1970s. The initial concept, similar to fracture work, was the hope that a form of internal immobilization would promote the healing rate. This was thought to be particularly true in the lumbar spine, where immobilization externally is virtually impossible except perhaps with a spica cast.

The secondary yield with internal fixation was instant ambulation of the patient and reduction of problems associated with bed rest, for example, thrombophlebitis, pneumonia, cystitis, and ileus. Because of the instant rigidity afforded by the rods, these patients were found to have better pain relief after the procedure. A peculiarity of this type of posterior fixation is a fusion in flexion with wide opening of the foramen. This adds to the room afforded to the nerve roots and their exit from the dura, which in itself affects a certain amount of decompression of the nerve roots.

INDICATIONS

Knodt rods are indicated in one- or two-level fusions of the lumbar spine. The rods are most adaptable to transverse process fusions and are particularly easy to use in a two-level fusion where total laminectomy has been done. They will reduce a retrolisthesis but may tend to exaggerate a spondylolisthesis because of the flexion attitude promoted by the fixation. This increase in spondylolisthesis has not been a contraindication. Knodt rods also are used for rotational instability, because they place fixation on both sides of the axis of rotation.

CONTRAINDICATIONS

Knodt rods are contraindicated in any situation where the rod may compromise or damage neural tissue. The patient who has a congenitally small canal may not have room for the hooks without dural crowding. Spina bifida occulta is an absolute contraindication, because the distal bone stock is never sufficient as a good anchor for the distal hooks. Resist the temptation to seat the hooks on the side of the spina bifida, because they will usually migrate medially and dislocate with a concomitant dural tear or nerve-root destruction. Unfortunately, these are usually lower sacral roots and may result in bowel and bladder loss.

The alternative to distal fixation when facing a problem such as spina bifida can be insertion of the distal hooks directly into the space behind the superior articular facet of S1, if wide dissection has been done of the L5 lamina.

TECHNIQUE

Laminectomy is done along with discectomy or any posterior decompression that is necessary to solve the problems of neural encroachment (Fig. 32-1). After the neural tissue is free, begin the insertion of the Knodt rods. Areas for insertion of the hooks are determined with a fitting tool (Fig. 32-2). If the lamina is too thick to accommodate the hooks, slicing thinly from the undersurface of the lamina, thus thinning it gives added room for the dura. This technique is safer than taking off the outer portion of the bone because of the added room for the dura. When all four sites are made for insertion of the hooks, then it is possible to determine the size of the rods to be used (Fig. 32-3). The hooks are inserted into the previously prepared sites, and, by using finger pressure on the turnbuckle, the system is tightened until the hook is engaged and the rod is stable in between the two laminas. A wrench is then used to tighten the turnbuckle, thus effectively putting pressure across the

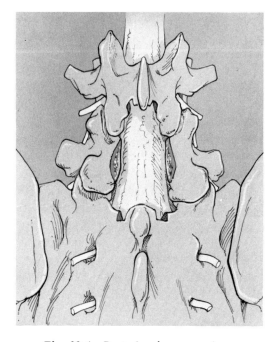

Fig. 32-1 Posterior decompression.

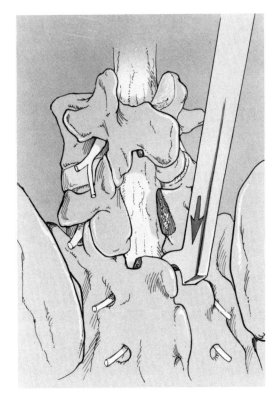

Fig. 32-2 Determining the area for insertion of the hooks with hook fitting tool.

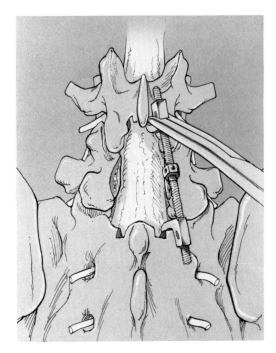

Fig. 32-3 Insertion of Knodt rod.

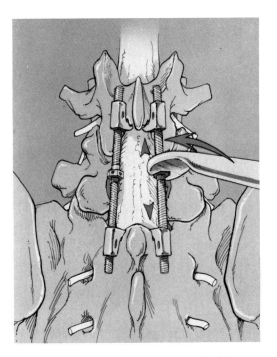

Fig. 32-4 Tightening the turnbuckle.

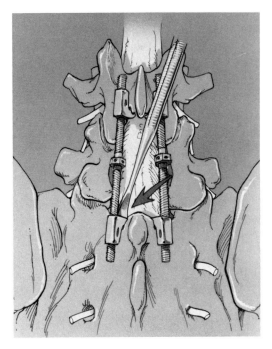

Fig. 32-5 Careful appraisal to assure no impingement on the dura from the hooks.

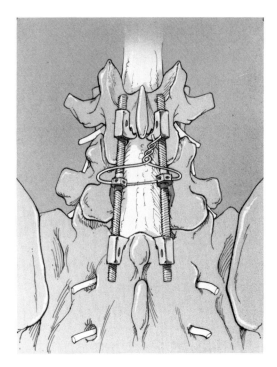

Fig. 32-6 Wires placed between the turnbuckles to prevent loosening motion.

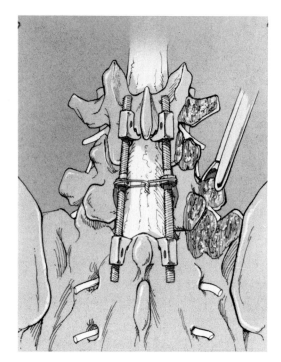

Fig. 32-7 Transverse process decortication is done.

hooks (Fig. 32-4). This tightening procedure is started on one of the rods until there is either some slight bowing of the rod or maxmal flexion has been reached. Next, the other rod is tightened until the first rod is slightly loosened; then they are both tightened. After insertion of the rods, the hooks are carefully checked to be sure there is no dural impingement (Fig. 32-5). An 18-gauge wire is placed in the holes of the nuts to prevent backout (Fig. 32-6). Under direct vision the transverse processes and lateral mass of the pedicles are denuded (Fig. 32-7). Bone graft is placed on the area previously denuded.

POSTOPERATIVE MANAGEMENT

As a general principle rehabilitation is started at the time of initial decision making for surgery. The decision for type of surgery should be effected by ease of rehabilitation. Therefore the postoperative course is set by the preoperative techniques. As in all treatment, I hope to give the responsibility of control to the patient. This requires education concerning (1) the operation, (2) pain and drugs, (3) activities, and (4) wound care.

The Operation

It is impossible for patients to respond intelligently to any kind of postoperative request if they do not understand what has occurred at surgery. They need the confidence that their spine is technically controlled to the point where they are not going to "fall apart." Without this, the fear of the unknown may prevent the patient from going through any type of rehabilitation program. Perhaps the person most able to explain these types of circumstances to the patient is a paramedic. The use of models and visual aids greatly enhances the patient's understanding.

Pain and Drugs

The patient must also understand the trade-off between endorphins and opiates. A preoperative discussion of endorphins and their diminution with different types of drugs give the patient that understanding. We have found a "patient-controlled analgesia" pump that fits into the IV line and allows the patient to control postoperative pain medications very effectively. Most patients are off the intravenous medications within 36 to 48 hours. During that time they have been able to start activity without being obtunded by the opiates, and they are still comfortable. A policy of not discharging patients until they are off narcotics sounds difficult, but in most circumstances it is relatively easy. If the patients are educated in that direction and have some other pain relieving techniques, such as distraction or deep breathing, they frequently will be off narcotic pain medications in 4 to 5 days—even after such operations as spinal fusion. They then can use aspirin, acetaminophen, or antiinflammatories for pain relief. If the physician will examine the medical practice and talk to patients carefully, he or she will find that after the first week narcotics are used essentially in two circumstances, both of them poor. First, the patients wish to increase activity without pain and therefore use a pain pill so that more can be done during the day; and second, patients use narcotics because they feel better from a general standpoint compared to actual pain control. Both of these attitudes are, of course, to be discouraged. This whole concept is radical to the patient and takes considerable education and energy on the part of the surgical team. However, the rewards are great.

Activities

Postoperative activities must be explained and practiced by the patient before surgery so that they are facilitated after surgery. A physical therapist works with the patient on such things as getting out of bed and using walking aids for the first several days. Techniques to log roll and splint the back are taught so that the patient can tolerate increased activity without irritating his or her back. All of these activities should be practiced by the patient before the actual surgery. Teaching these things to the patient after surgery adds to the difficulty of the postoperative course.

Wound Care

Patients and their families are frequently frightened by the care of the wound. Thus the spouse should be involved in all of the preoperative education processes, particularly wound care. The possibility of spontaneous drainage of seromas and other danger signals are warned against. When patients live long distances away, we frequently will teach the family to take out staples and apply Steristrips to the wounds, allowing the patient to prevent prolonged postoperative trips.

It is possible to encourage comparatively high levels of activity after surgery with Knodt rod fixation. Because the limiting factor is usually the bone graft, patients are normally very cooperative. There is no recommendation to restrict activity; the guiding phrase is "if it doesn't hurt, it is okay."

COMPLICATIONS

Loosening of the rod, which most commonly occurs 3 or 4 months after surgery, is by far the most prevalent complication. Patients may experience constant or intermittent sciatica. The pain is frequently relieved by flexion. If there is sacral crowding, the pain may be referred more to the coccyx than a true sciatica. When the rods are removed, the patient usually experiences immediate relief. I have told patients that, like with any

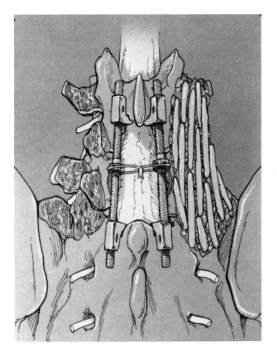

Fig. 32-8 Knodt rods with fusion.

other metal objects, the rods will frequently be removed. My removal rate is approximately one third.

Rod breakage or dislocation is not common and generally occurs in the first 6 weeks. The longer the rod, the higher the chances are of fracture of the metal. I use 6 to 7 cm rods, although they are available up to 10 cm. If an area of fusion is great enough to require a 10 cm rod, it is better to go to a Harrington rod instead of the Knodt. It is not an uncommon experience to identify breakage or dislocation of the rods on an x-ray film in an asymptomatic patient. Under these circumstances I encourage the patient not to have the rods removed unless they become symptomatic.

Dural compromise is reflected in a patient as coccygeal pain that can be identified shortly after the time of surgery. This is caused by the pressure of the Knodt rods as they crowd the nerve roots in the lower sacral segments. If there is no neurologic change, an attempt is made to carry these patients through the first 3 to 4 months until early fusion is seen. Then the rods are removed. If dural compromise is great enough to occur with either bowel or bladder weakness, it is mandatory that the rods be removed immediately.

Dural tear with possible pseudomeningocele can occur with contact of the dura and hooks. This usually represents the dura being pinched between the hook and the lamina and almost always occurs at the caudal anchoring point of the rods. These anchoring points should be carefully checked at the time of insertion of the rods. Dural tears are frequently asymptomatic and are not recognized until the rod is removed for some other reason.

RESULTS

A total of 92 consecutive fusions performed between January 1980 and January 1982 were reviewed. The minimum follow-up period was 1 year, and the maximum follow-up period was 4 years. Of these, 86 patients, or 93%, went on to solid union; 28 patients, or 33%, required removal of the rods; 51 patients were workman's compensation patients and 41 were private patients. Of all of the patients, 85% returned to work. There was repeat surgery, other than removal of the rods, on two of the patients in the series.

SUMMARY

Knodt rods effectively promote fusion in lumbar spine surgery. The chief disadvantage is a removal rate of almost one third. The advantages include a 93% fusion rate and instant mobilization of the patient. I believe that this is a reasonable trade-off.

REFERENCES

1. Beattie, F.C.: Distraction rod fusion, Clin. Orthop. **62:**1969.
2. Dubuc, F.: Knodt rod grafting, Orthop. Clin. North Am. **6:**1975.
3. Frymoyer, J.W., et al.: Disc excision and spine fusion in the management of lumbar disc disease, Spine **3**(1):1978.
4. Goldner, J.L.: The role of spine fusion (symposium), Spine **6**(3):293, 1981.
5. Knodt, H.: Distraction fusion of lumbar spine using Knodt distraction rods, Warsaw, Ind., 1971, Zimmer USA, Inc.
6. Knodt, H., and Larrick, R.B.: Distraction fusion of the spine, Ohio State Med. J. **60**(12):1964.
7. White, A.H., et al.: Knodt rod distraction lumbar fusion, Spine **8**(4):1983.

EDITORIAL COMMENTARY

I have used Knodt rods for internal fixaton since 1969. I reported on my first 100 cases in 1978, and my experience after those cases has continued to be similar. I have had to remove only 5% of the rods inserted. If one avoids using the rods in any case where there is a question about adequate size of the vertebral canal or compromising the spinal nerve, it is rarely necessary to remove the rods. One should be able to pass a dural dissector or freer past the tip of both hooks at the sacral level.

It is also possible to prevent dislodgment by using a segmental wire, both proximally and distally, around the lamina.

A major complication of Knodt rods is overdistraction, which eliminates the normal lordosis and can give postural problems. I have not used epidural fat graft, as has Dr. Selby. My results have been quite good without the fat graft. My fusion rate, however, has not been as great as Dr. Selby's. I have had an 18% pseudarthrosis rate, as indicated by flexion/extension views in my first 100 cases; however, I was using only cancellous bone graft for those cases.

I believe the major advantage to distraction rods is the maintenance of patent intervertebral foramina. The rods do not maintain rotational stability or prevent flexion. They do prevent excessive lumbar extension and resultant narrowing of the intervertebral foramen when the patient stands or attempts to go into lumbar extension.

Arthur H. White

CHAPTER

33

INTERNAL FIXATION WITH PEDICLE SCREWS

**Ken Hsu   James F. Zucherman
Arthur H. White   Gar Wynne**

There is a wide variety of internal fixation devices available for spinal disorders in which significant instability is present and fusion is indicated. So far, all systems have resulted in significant problems and complications; the spine plate and segmental pedicle screws were developed because of these problems. Currently there is a growing number of surgeons who are using the spine plate and pedicle screw system worldwide.

In this chapter, we are presenting our experience with the Variable Spine Plate (VSP) System developed by Dr. Arthur Steffee of Cleveland, Ohio.

Spine plates have been used for many years. Wilson plates[44] and Meurig-Williams plates were designed to be attached to the spinous processes. Reimers[28] also used similar spinous process plates in Europe. Sicard[36] devised plates of synthetic material that were screwed to the posterior aspect of the sacrum and pinned to the spinous processes. Obviously, spine plates cannot be used when wide decompression of the spine is necessary; in general, they do not provide enough holding strength for reduction, realignment, or sagittal contouring of the spine.

Humphries, Hawk, and Berndt[12] reported the use of slotted plates designed to fix and apply compression in anterior lumbar interbody fusion. Noncancellous bone screws are used to gain purchase in the cancellous bone of the vertebral bodies.

PEDICLE SCREWS

Boucher[3] first described passing long screws through the lamina and pedicle into the vertebral body, and Pennel and coworkers[27] reported satisfactory results using Boucher's method of screw fixation. In addition, Harrington and Dickson,[10] McPhee and O'Brien,[26] Sijbrandij,[37] and Vidal and associates[41] have all used screws through the pedicles along with Harrington instrumentation or its modification to achieve reduction and stabilization of spondylolisthesis.

SPINE PLATES AND PEDICLE SCREWS

Schöllner[35] reported a technique of reducing spondylolisthesis using two pedi-

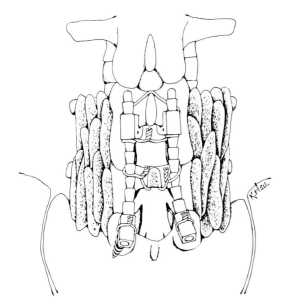

Fig. 33-1 Lumbosacral fusion using Harrington rods, pedicle screw, and wires.

cle screws with dual threads—the cancellous threads for fixation in the vertebra body and the smaller threads to serve the reduction procedure. Reduction is performed against slotted sacral plates anchored in the S2 foramina.

Roy-Camille[33] and Judet of France have developed a system of plates and pedicle screws for stabilization of the spine.[31-34] Louis[19,20] reported 266 cases of plate screw posterior lumbosacral fixation from 1972 to 1982. Rodegerdts[29] of Germany has been reducing spondylolisthesis and achieving excellent fixation using sacral plates with pedicle screws. He recently reported his personal experience of 46 cases over 11 years.

Yamamoto and Yamashita[45] of Japan developed a technique of reduction and stabilization of spondylolisthesis using plates and pedicle screws. The procedure included complete laminectomy of the slipped vertebra, total excision of the disc, reduction and fixation with the spine plate and pedicle screws, and posterior interbody fusion through the window of the plate.

Some published reports on other fixation systems are among the following.
A. Pedicle screws and rods
  1. Harrington and Dickson[10]
  2. Kostuik, Errico, Gleason[14]
  3. Long Beach system (Field, Wiltse, Zindrick, Widell, Thomas)[8]
  4. San Francisco System (White, Zucherman, Hsu)[42] (Fig. 33-1)
  5. Vermont system (Krag, Beynnon, Pope, Frymoyer)[16,17]
  6. Posterior Zielke instrumentation with transpedicular fixation
B. Pedicle screws, wires, and rods
  1. Luque[21] (also developing a spine plate and pedicle screw system)
  2. White and associates
C. External fixation with pedicle threaded pins
  1. Magerl[22-25] (clinically used since 1977, consisting of two pairs of Schanz screws and an adjustable external fixation device, suitable for treatment of unstable spinal injuries and spinal osteomyelitis)

Zindrick and coworkers performed a biomechanical study of different pedicle screws currently available.[46] The screws were inserted into the pedicles of fresh lumbosacral specimens; tension loads were then applied to the screws to the point of failure. Their conclusions included the following.
1. Screws with variable thread patterns gained better purchase if the large threaded areas are kept in the cortical bone of the pedicle. This point applied to the Steffee and the A-O cancellous screws.
2. Larger thread diameters showed the best holding capabilities.
3. A modified awl making starting holes in the superior facet area allowed for more accurate pedicle entry than did drilling.

4. No significant difference was noted with tapping before screw insertion.
5. The second sacral (S2) pedicle provided the weakest fixation.
6. Force required to produce screw failure was inversely proportional to the degree of osteoporosis. Filling the pedicle with larger threads afforded better purchase, especially in osteoporotic specimens. Tapping was not beneficial in very osteoporotic specimens.
7. Methylmethacrylate cement significantly improved the holding power of all screws and was related to the amount and insertion technique used. The methylmethacrylate may leak into the neural canal through defects in the pedicle produced by the screw or tap threads.

VARIABLE SPINE PLATE/PEDICLE SCREW SYSTEM[33-40]

Steffee developed titanium plates with screw slots containing "nests" to allow both adjustment and rigid fixation of vertebra. The plates can be contoured to control the sagittal curve of the spine. The pedicle screws are made with two types of threads: cancellous bone threads and machine threads on the shank to accept tapered nuts.

The variable spine plate (VSP) system allows alignment and stabilization of the spine while fusion takes place. In unstable spondylolisthesis, anatomic reduction is facilitated. After wide decompression and exposure of fusion bed, pedicles are accurately located, reamed, and tapped, and two screws are inserted into each vertebral body. The plates are contoured and placed over the screws. The tapered nuts are tightened down to correct sagittal alignment. Bone graft is placed in the lateral gutter over the transverse processes. In osteoporotic bone, methylmethacrylate cement is injected into the vertebral body through the pedicle to anchor the screws. Steffee is developing a molly bolt to allow good fixation without using cement. Some advantages of the VSP system include:

1. Segmental rigid fixation
2. Good sacral fixation
3. Good control of sagittal curve
4. Allows reduction of spondylolisthesis or retrolisthesis
5. Avoids spinal canal (in contrast to lamina wires and hooks, which are within the canal)
6. Applicable in osteoporotic spine
7. Allows early mobilization and eliminates postoperative bracing
8. Ease of nursing care

Some disadvantages are:

1. Technically difficult
2. Increased bulk of metal implant
3. Implant prominence
4. Implant irritation
5. Implant failure
6. Weakening of facet joints of the lowest unfused segment
7. Increased operative time
8. Increased infection risk

POSTEROLATERAL FUSION USING SPINE PLATES AND PEDICLE SCREWS
Preferred Technique

The patient is placed prone in a knee-chest position on the Andrews frame with the abdomen free. A midline incision is made, and the paraspinal musculature is elevated off the spinous processes and laminas. A point is made to preserve the interspinous ligament and facet joints at the level above. The identification of the appropriate level should be made by morphology or x-ray film.

Laminectomy and decompression are carried out. The dura and the nerve roots are carefully protected from injury. Extensive decompression, including discectomies, foraminotomies, and facetectomies, is performed as indicated.

The dura and nerve roots are then thoroughly inspected. The nerve root canals are gently examined in their entire length and width, using a smooth probe of adequate length. (A "hockey stick" or "foraminal probe" may serve this purpose.) Each nerve root should be followed out past its foramen, to be sure that it is free from lateral compression or impingement.

PREPARATION FOR POSTEROLATERAL BONE GRAFT BED

The facets and transverse processes are exposed. The Wiltse retractors are placed on the tips of the transverse processes. At L5, we prefer to preserve the attachment of the iliolumbar ligament and use a Meyerding or Taylor retractor on the posterior iliac crest for exposure. Soft tissue is removed from the posterior aspect of the transverse processes only. The intertransverse membrane is left intact. The vessels in the caudal axilla of the transverse process lateral to the pars may be cauterized before dissecting in this area.

A small curved curette is used to make a groove in each transverse process longitudinally to its axis. Perpendicular strokes are then made cephalad and caudal to complete the decortication; ¼ inch chisels are used to decorticate the lateral faces of the superior facets, the pars, and the sacral ala. A large flap of bone is taken from the sacral ala and folded over toward the L5 transverse process. (Fig. 33-2.)

PEDICLE SCREW INSERTION

To locate the pedicle several landmarks may be used.
1. The transverse process generally corresponds to the level of the pedicle in the lumbar spine.
2. The caudal tip of the inferior facet.
3. The ridge or junction of the facet, transverse process, and lamina. (Fig. 33-3.)

The pedicle may be palpated with a probe or visualized directly if the exposure is adequate. We have devised pedicle guides to facilitate accurate screw placement (Figs. 33-4 through 33-7). A ¼ inch burr is used to penetrate the posterior cortex, and a pedicle probe or ganglion knife is used to advance the burr hole into the pedicle and the vertebral body. The probe should follow a path of least resistance into the cancellous bone (Figs. 33-8 through 33-10).

A pedicle sounder probe or a depth gauge is used to palpate the hole to be sure it is surrounded 360 degrees by bone (Figs. 33-11 and 33-12). Common errors are breaking through lateral vertebral body cortex, pedicle comminution, entering the spinal canal, or entering the lateral canal.

The hole is then partially tapped with a cancellous bone tap. Using the screw wrench, the pedicle screw is inserted until the large cancellous threads are completely within the vertebral body and pedicle. The screw should be directed slightly medially into the cancellous bone of the vertebral body. If the bone stock is poor, methylmethacrylate cement may be injected into the screw hole before screw placement.

Screw placement is begun at the most

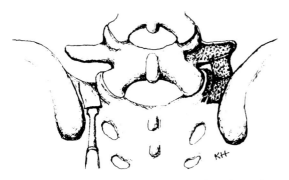

Fig. 33-2 Large flap of bone is taken from the sacral ala and folded over toward L5 transverse process to achieve successful L5-S1 fusion.

326 Surgical Procedures

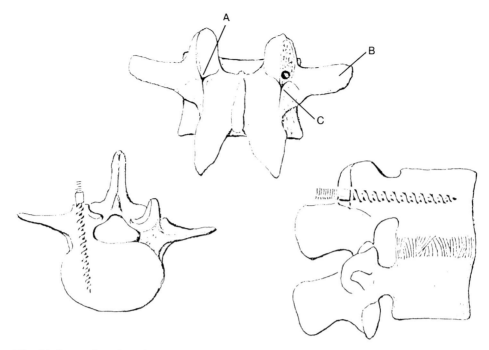

Fig. 33-3 Landmarks to locate pedicle. *A*, Transverse process corresponds to the level of the pedicle. *B*, Caudal tip of the inferior facet. *C*, Junction of facet, transverse process, and lamina.

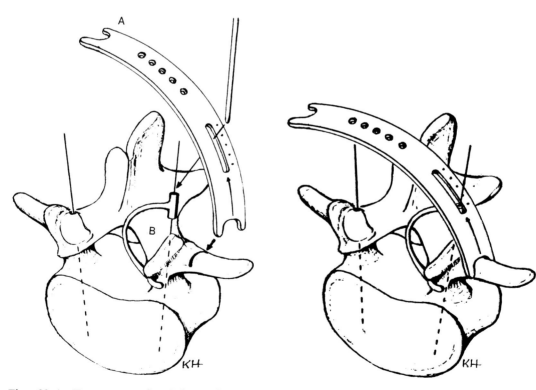

Fig. 33-4 Two types of pedicle guides. *A*, Curved plate and *B*, pedicle aiming device with probe sleeve.

Fig. 33-5 Using the two types of pedicle guides to improve accuracy.

Internal Fixation with Pedicle Screws 327

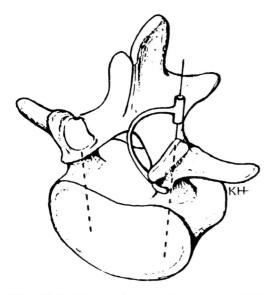

Fig. 33-6 Aiming device with probe or drill sleeve to locate pedicle.

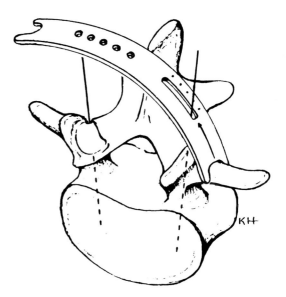

Fig. 33-7 Curved plate with guide slots and holes to direct probe or drill to pedicle.

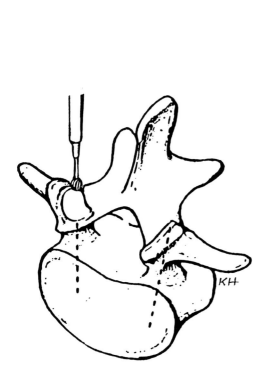

Fig. 33-8 Burr is used to penetrate posterior cortex.

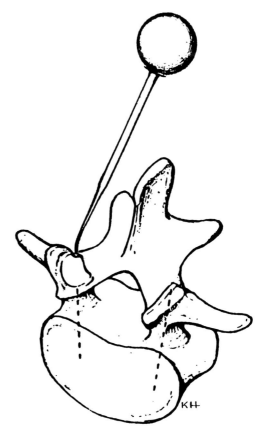

Fig. 33-9 Pedicle probe or ganglion knife is used to advance burr hole into pedicle.

328 *Surgical Procedures*

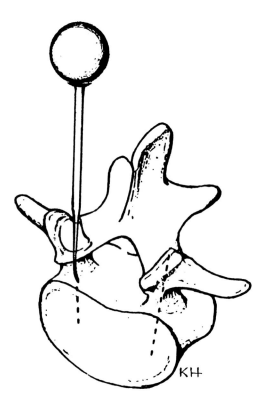

Fig. 33-10 Pedicle probe is advancing through pedicle into vertebral body.

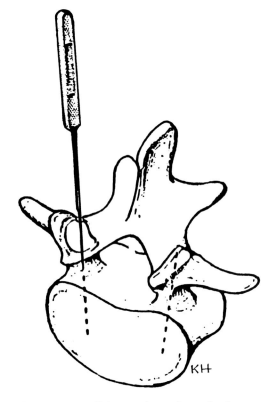

Fig. 33-11 Pedicle sounder probe or depth gauge is inserted into pedicle.

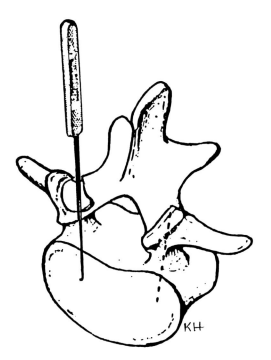

Fig. 33-12 Hole in pedicle is probed with depth gauge to be sure that it is surrounded by bone 360 degrees.

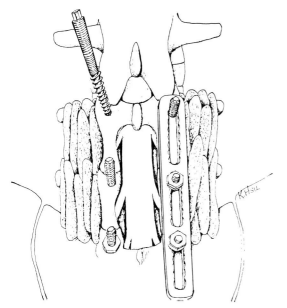

Fig. 33-13 Pedicle screw is inserted until the large cancellous threads are within the bone. (Shown from left upper to left lower levels.) Plate is then placed over the screws with nuts applied anteriorly and posteriorly to lock plate in place. (Shown on right side.)

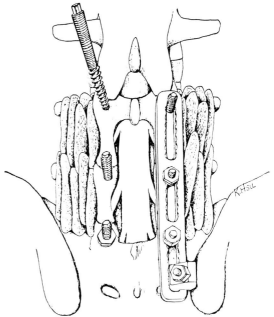

Fig. 33-14 Sacral buttress clamp and additional screw may be used to reinforce sacral fixation (right lower level).

accessible pedicle, but sacral screws are placed last. The screws should be inserted perpendicular to the longitudinal axis of the spine at each level to prevent subsequent screw bending or increased screw torque movement.

A properly placed initial screw can serve as a guide for the remaining screws. The sacral screw is inserted last because there is more suitable bone stock, allowing more variable screw placement. Great care is taken to keep the screws linearly arranged for plate placement (Fig. 33-13).

A tapered nut is advanced with the flat surface up until the round surface is in contact with bone. A malleable template (aluminum) of the same length as the plate is placed against the flat surfaces of the nuts. The template serves as a guide to contour the plate using a plate bender. (We have been using an A-O plate bender with good results.)

The plate is then placed over the screws. It should slide easily over the screws onto the nuts. It is important not to strip the threads by forcing the plate down.

Desired distraction may be applied using screw alignment rods on adjacent screws, screw alignment bar or T-handle nut wrenches. Overdistraction can cause pedicle fracture and screw loosening caused by uneven pedicle pressure. We also suspect this may cause gradual erosion of screw threads through the pedicle in some cases, and cause radicular symptoms. Currently, we do not distract unless there is a specific indication to do so. The upper tapered nuts then are applied to tighten and lock the plate in place. When indicated, sacral buttress clamps and additional screws may be used to reinforce sacral fixation (Fig. 33-14).

Bone graft is positioned over the decorticated surfaces in the lateral gutter (using a Russian forcep or a teaspoon), either before or after the plate is in place. The lateral neural canals are explored to assure patency and that there is no encroachment from bone graft chips.

The opposite-side screws are next applied in a similar manner. The template is again used to contour the plate, because the contour often varies on the right and left sides.

A lateral x-ray film is taken to assure intrapedicle placement of the screw and depth of sacral penetration by the S1 screws. It is desirable to have slight penetration of the S1 screw to ensure that the anterior sacral cortex is engaged.

The portion of the screw above the upper nut is then removed with a bolt cutter. Gelfoam or fat grafts are applied over the exposed dura or nerve roots if desired.

Ambulation is begun on the first postoperative day with the patient in a lumbosacral corset; the corset is worn for a minimum of 3 months. Patients are instructed to limit their activities to less than 1 mile of walking per day and minimize sitting for 3 to 4 months.

Some patients who have been very active appear to have loosened the screw-bone interface and have developed back, hip, and leg pain. This usually resolves with fusion solidity.

Experiences in Spine Plating with Pedicle Screws

Between August 1984 and October 1985, 76 lumbar spine fusions, using Steffee's VSP spine plate and pedicle screw system, were performed at St. Mary's Hospital in San Francisco. Follow-up ranged from 10 to 24 months, with a mean of 15.4 months. Age of the patients ranged from 24 to 76 years, with a mean of 47 years. There were 46 males and 30 females.

The diagnoses for these cases included:

Disc herniation and instability	43%
Spinal stenosis with instability	24%
Segmental instability	11%
Spondylolisthesis with instability	7%
Pseudarthrosis	7%
Herniated disc and stenosis	7%
Spine fracture dislocation	4%
Herniated disc, instability, and poliomyelitis	1%

The numbers of levels ranged from one to five, with an average of 2.5.

Of the 76 patients, 49 (64.4%) had had previous procedures in the area operated. In three cases only chemonucleolysis was performed. In addition, 38 of the 76 patients (50%) were involved in worker's compensation or litigation.

Operative time ranged from 2.5 to 6 hours, with an average of 3 hours 45 minutes. Plate size ranged from 2 to 5 slots bilaterally with a mean of 2.7. The number of pedicle screws used ranged from 4 to 12, with a mean of 6.4. There were two spine surgeons present during each of the procedures, and all procedures were performed by the four authors of this chapter.

We rated our results as follows:

Excellent	No symptoms
Good	Marked improvement
	Occasional pain
	Occasional use of pain medications
	No functional limitations
Fair	Some improvement
	Need for pain medications
	Significant functional restriction
Poor	No change in symptoms or worse

Overall results according to the above criteria follow:

Total	76 cases (10 to 24 months of follow-up)	
Excellent	33%	(25)
Good	29%	(22)
Fair	28%	(21)
Poor	10%	(8)

In those patients without worker's compensation or litigation, the following results were noted:

Excellent	41%	(16)
Good	39%	(15)
Fair	17%	(6)
Poor	3%	(1)

When patients were grouped according to those with worker's compensation or litigation, the results were:

Excellent	24%	(9)
Good	19%	(7)
Fair	38%	(15)
Poor	19%	(7)

In patients without previous surgical procedures, the results were:

Excellent	50%	(14)
Good	39%	(10)
Fair	7%	(2)
Poor	4%	(1)

In 49 patients who had previous procedures, the following results were noted:

Excellent	24%	(12)
Good	23%	(11)
Fair	37%	(18)
Poor	16%	(8)

PROBLEMS AND COMPLICATIONS

There were four cases of deep wound infection as of October 1985; two were diagnosed within 2 weeks of surgery and were treated with early incisions and drainage. In one the metal implants were removed, and in the other the wound was allowed to heal by secondary intensions over the retained metal fixations because of marked preoperative spinal instability. Both had good ultimate results.

Two other infections were found within 2 months after surgery. Both were indolent anaerobic pathogens. Initially, they were treated unsuccessfully with 6 weeks of intravenous antibiotics. Both required removal of the metal implants and delayed wound closure. The infection resolved after implant removal and delayed wound closure.

The infection rate using this metal fixation has been higher than other fusion techniques in our hands. This would appear to be due to increased operative time, the larger volume and surface area of the implant, and high percentage of revision cases in this series. We recommend such infection-minimizing measures as laminar airflow, sterile hoods, frequent irrigation, and IV antibiotics for total joint arthroplasty.

There were 16 patients with one or more broken screws. Three patients were involved in moderate trauma. All three were doing well before the traumatic episodes. Two of the three were improved after removal of metal implants. So far, seven patients with broken screws required reoperation. Screw failure occurred mostly in our younger patients and is probably related to increased activity level and firmer grip at the bone screw interface in younger, less osteoporotic patients. The screws failed at either end of the plate; 70% were at the sacral end.

The incidence of screw breakage was unacceptably high in our series. Recent changes in screw configurations already have been instituted; we expect that this will minimize the complication.

The height of the nuts has also been reduced recently. The resultant lower profile for the hardware should obviate the occasional complaints we have had of hardware being painfully prominent (three out of 76 patients).

Eight of our first 30 patients developed leg pain 1 to 2 months after surgery. This was presumably due to nerve-root irritation and was relieved by selective nerve-root blocks, epidural blocks, or with application of a corset or brace.

This problem occurred in the first portion of our series, when we locked the instrumented vertebrae in distraction. We suspect that distraction places a constant unidirectional torque on the screw against one wall of the pedicle, as shown in the diagram (Fig. 33-15), possibly resulting in erosion, migration of the screw or pedicle fracture (Fig. 33-16). Pedicle fracture was visualized during surgery in one osteoporotic patient. It is important to remember that distraction at one segment causes contraction of adjacent segments that are instrumented.

Distraction

Narrowing
Stenosis } above and below
Screw bending
Pedicle fracture

This mechanism is illustrated in Fig. 33-17; as distraction is applied at one segment the adjacent segment is compressed, causing disc narrowing and foraminal stenosis.

Appropriate contouring of the plate and proper screw alignment should produce a screw plate angle of 90 degrees. Screw plate angle may be an important factor in generating eccentric torque stress against the pedicle. The greater the deviation from the perpendicular, the greater the torque generated when the plate is locked to the flat surface of the nuts, as illustrated in Fig. 33-18.

In similar situations, especially over the sacral curve, the screw bends and becomes weaker as it is locked to the plate (Fig. 33-19). Occasionally, the nuts do

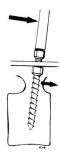

Fig. 33-15 Distraction places a constant unidirectional torque on screw against one wall of pedicle.

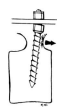

Fig. 33-16 Pedicle fracture or erosion may occur when distraction is applied and a constant unidirectional torque created on the screw against one wall of the pedicle.

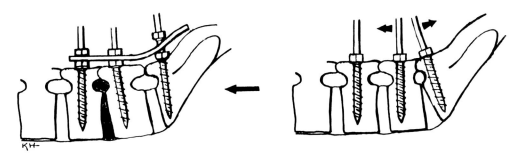

Fig. 33-17 When excessive distraction is applied at one segment, the adjacent segment may become compressed, causing disc narrowing and/or foraminal stenosis.

not lock until the screw finds a stable position, especially over a sharply curved plate. Foraminal stenosis may be produced by this mechanism (Fig. 33-20).

It is important that the nerve root foramina are examined and gently probed after the instrumentation placement to be sure that no stenosis is produced and that bone graft has not been squeezed into the lateral neural canal by the plate.

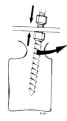

Fig. 33-18 Angular forces are created as nuts are locked eccentrically to plate.

PROBLEM OF STRESS TRANSFER TO ADJACENT LEVELS

We are seeing some patients with problems at the level adjacent to the fusion in the forms of disc degeneration, facet syndrome, and hypermobility. The latter is commonly seen on bending films, although frequently it is asymptomatic. To insert the screw accurately, the normal facet at the first unfused segment is often violated. The capsule and the inferior one fourth of the inferior facet are usually removed, presumably weakening the posterior column of the level above (Fig. 33-21). The frequency and extent that this will weaken the adjacent motion segment are unclear with the short follow-up now available. Increased rigidity of the fixation is also expected to increase stress risers in the adjacent segments. We currently place the plates and screws lateral to the facets to avoid weakening the unfused levels.

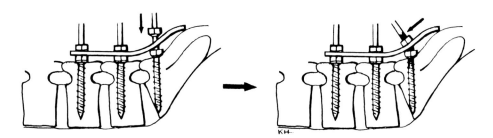

Fig. 33-19 A sharply curved plate, especially over the sacrum, may cause screw to bend and become weaker as nuts are locked to plate.

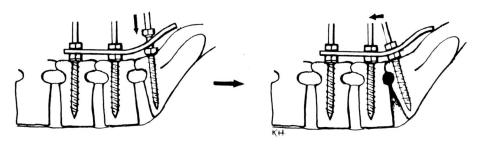

Fig. 33-20 Nuts do not lock until screw finds a stable position over a sharply curved plate. Foraminal stenosis may be produced by this mechanism.

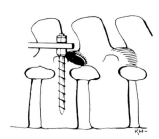

Fig. 33-21 To insert screw into pedicle, the adjacent facet is violated.

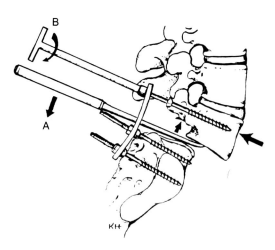

Fig. 33-22 Reduction of spondylolisthesis. L5 vertebral body is levered in position with spinal elevator, *A*, as L5 pedicle screw is tightened toward plate with T-handle wrench, *B*.

We have found it seemingly useful and logical to perform discograms and saline acceptance tests of adjacent levels before all fusions to prevent ending a fusion adjacent to a degenerated, potentially painful segment. This concept is conjectural at this time. However, we are documenting not infrequent radiologic and clinical deterioration in these adjacent segments.

SUMMARY

In spite of the problems we have encountered, the VSP System provides the following.

1. Adequate fixation, even when the posterior elements are totally removed, occurs.

2. It allows good control of sagittal curve and excellent three-dimensional realignment. Most other instrumentations result in flattening of the lumbar lordosis and resultant hyperextension of the upper segments. We believe it is important to place the vertebra above the fusion in the "anatomic angle" of the spine.

3. Superior sacral fixation exists.

4. It allows good reduction of spondylolisthesis when it is necessary (Figs. 33-22 to 33-26).

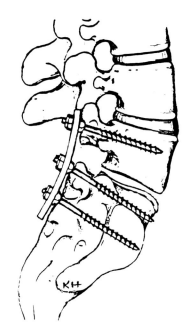

Fig. 33-23 Reduction and stability are maintained with plates and screws as internal fixation.

Internal Fixation with Pedicle Screws 335

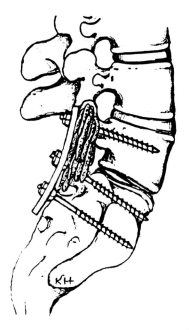

Fig. 33-24 Posterolateral fusion is performed after reduction and fixation.

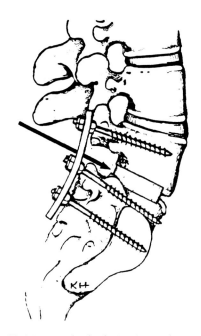

Fig. 33-25 Interbody fusion is another option.

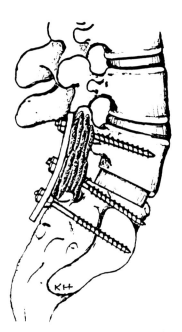

Fig. 33-26 Interbody fusion may be combined with posterolateral fusion.

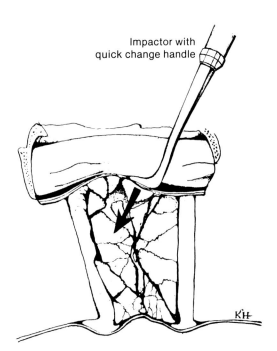

Fig. 33-27 Reduction of retropulsed vertebral fracture fragments using an impactor carefully positioned anterior to dura.

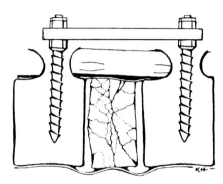

Fig. 33-28 Reduced vertebra is stabilized one level above and below using short plates and pedicle screws.

5. It provides excellent internal fixation for unstable fracture dislocation without sacrificing additional normal levels (Figs. 33-27 and 33-28).

6. It permits early mobilization and ease of postoperative nursing care.

7. We expect fusion rate to be improved because of the rigid fixation.

Younger patients seemed to have slightly less favorable outcome, presumably due to harder bone and increased activity level resulting in more hardware problems, that is, breakage.

The procedure is time-consuming and technically difficult, with significant hardware problems. The latter will hopefully be reduced by advances in design. One should definitely have thorough training in the technique before performing the procedure. An equally qualified assistant is also important.

In general, after this brief experience, we believe that the VSP System has a useful role in spine surgery when used selectively. *Editorial comments on p. 338.*

REFERENCES

1. Allen, B.L., and Ferguson, R.L.: Basic considerations in pelvic fixation cases. In Lugue, E.R., editor: Segmental spinal instrumentation, Thorofare, N.J., 1984, Slack, Inc.
2. Ansel, R., and Scales, J.: A study of some factors which affect the strength of screws and their insertion and holding in bone, J. Biomech. **1**:279, 1968.
3. Boucher, H.H.: A method of spinal fusion, J. Bone Joint Surg. **41B**:248, 1959.
4. Cameron, H., et al.: Use of polymethylmethacrylate to enhance screw fixation in bone, J. Bone Joint Surg. **57A**:655, 1975.
5. Cobey, M.C.: The value of the wilson plate in spinal fusion, Clin. Orthop. **76**:138, 1971.
6. Dickson, J.H., et al.: Results of reduction and stabilization of the severely fractured thoracic and lumbar spine, J. Bone Joint Surg. **60A**:799, 1978.
7. Edwards, C.C.: Sacral fixation device: design and preliminary results, Proc. Scoliosis Res. Soc. 1984.
8. Field, B.T., et al.: The Long Beach spinal fixation system, Proceedings of the second annual meeting of the North American Lumbar Spine Association, Laguna Niguel, Calif., July 1985.
9. Graham, C.: Lumbosacral fusion using internal fixation with a spinous process for the graft, a review of 50 patients with a five-year maximum follow up, Clin. Orthop. **140**:72, 1979.
10. Harrington, P.R., and Dickson, J.H.: Spinal instrumentation in the treatment of severe progressive spondylolisthesis, Clin. Orthop. **117**:157, 1976.
11. Herrmann, H.D.: Transarticular (transpedicular) metal plate fixation for stabilization of the lumbar and thoracic spine, Acta Neurochir. (Wien) **48**(1-2):101, 1979.
12. Humphries, A.W., et al.: Anterior interbody fusion of lumbar vertebrae: a surgical technique, Surg. Clin. North Am. **41**:1685, 1961.
13. King, D.: Internal fixation for lumbosacral spine fusions, J. Bone Joint Surg. **30A**:560, 1948.
14. Kostuik, J.P., et al.: Techniques for internal fixation for degenerative conditions of the spine, Clin. Orthop. **203**:219, 1986.
15. Koranyi, E., et al.: Holding power of orthopaedic screws in bone, Clin. Orthop. **72**:285, 1970.

16. Krag, M.H., et al.: Vermont spinal fixator for posterior thoracic, lumbar, or lumbosacral spinal stabilization: initial mechanical testing and implementation, Proc. Int. Soc. Study Lumbar Spine, 1985.
17. Krag, M.H., et al.: An internal fixator for posterior application to short segments of the thoracic, lumbar, or lumbosacral spine: design and testing, Clin. Orthop. **203**:75, 1986.
18. Lewis, J., and McKibbin, B.: Treatment of unstable fracture-dislocations of the thoracolumbar spine accompanied by paraplegia, J. Bone Joint Surg. **56B**:603, 1974.
19. Louis, R.: Single staged posterior lumbosacral fusion by internal fixation with screw plates, Proc. Int. Study Lumbar Spine, 1985.
20. Louis, R.: Posterior vertebral bone plates, surgical technique, Paris, 1982, Howmedica, CEPRIME Publisher.
21. Luque, E.: Intrapedicular segmental fixation, (In press).
22. Magerl, F.P.: External skeletal fixation of the lower thoracic and the lumbar spine. In Uhthoff, H.K., and Stahl, E., editors: Current concepts of external fixation of fractures, New York, 1982, Springer-Verlag.
23. Magerl, F.P.: Clinical application on the thoracolumbar junction and the lumbar spine. In Mears, D.C., editor: External skeletal fixation, Baltimore, 1983, Williams & Wilkins.
24. Magerl, F.P.: Stabilization of the lower thoracic and lumbar spine with external skeletal fixation, Clin. Orthop. **189**:125, 1984.
25. Magerl, F.P.: External spinal skeletal fixation. In Weber, B.G., and Magerl, F.P.: The external fixator, New York, 1985, Springer-Verlag.
26. McPhee, I.B., and O'Brian, J.P.: Reduction of spondylolisthesis—a preliminary report, Spine **4**:430, 1979.
27. Pennel, G.F., et al.: A method of spinal fusion using internal fixation, Clin. Orthop. **35**:86, 1964.
28. Reimers, C.: Die dorsale Spanverstrebung von Wirbelsäulenabschnitten mittels innerer Schienung, Chirurg. **17**:10, 1956.
29. Rodegerdts, U.: Spondylolisthesis reduction, Proc. Int. Soc. Study Lumbar Spine, 1985.
30. Rosenweig, N.: "The get up and go" treatment of acute unstable injuries of the middle and lower cervical spine, J. Bone Joint Surg. **56B**:392, 1974.
31. Roy-Camille, R., et al.: Vertebral osteosynthesis using metal plates: its different uses, Chirurg. **105**:597, 1979.
32. Roy-Camille, R., et al.: Osteosynthesis of Thoracolumbar Spine Fractures with Metal Plates Screwed Through the Vertebral Pedicles, Reconstr. Surg. Traumatol. **15**:2, 1976.
33. Roy-Camille, R., et al.: Early management of spinal injuries. In McKibbin, B., editor: Recent advances in orthopedics, New York, 1979, Churchill Livingstone, Inc.
34. Roy-Camille, R., et al.: Behandlung von Wirbelfrakturen and luxation am Thorako-Lumbalen Ubergang. Orthopaedic **9**:63, 1980.
35. Schöllner, O.: Ein neues verfahren zur reposition und fixation bei spondylolisthesis, Orthop. Praxis **4**:270, 1975.
36. Sicard, A., and Menegaux, J.: L'abord anterieur de l'articulation sacroiliaque, J. Chir. (Paris) **77**:29, 1959.
37. Sijbrandij, S.: A new technique for the reduction and stabilization of severe spondylolisthesis, J. Bone Joint Surg. **63B**:266, 1981.
38. Steffee, A., et al.: Segmental spine plates with pedicle screw fixation: a new internal fixation device for disorders of the lumbar and thoracico-lumbar spine, Clin. Orthop. **203**:45, 1986.
39. Steffee, A., et al.: Total vertebral body and pedicle arthroplasty, Clin. Orthop. **203**:203, 1986.
40. Steffee, A.: Personal communication, 1985.
41. Vital, J., et al.: Surgical reduction of spondylolisthesis using a posterior approach, Clin. Orthop. **145**:156, 1981.
42. White, A.H., et al.: Lumbosacral fusions with Harrington rods and intersegmental wiring, Clin. Orthop. **203**:185, 1986.
43. Williams, E.W.M.: Traumatic paraplegia. In Matthews, D.N., editor: Recent advances in surgery of trauma, New York, 1963, Churchill Livingstone, Inc.
44. Wilson, P.D., and Straub, L.R.: Lumbosacral fusion with metallic-plate fixation, Instructional Course Lectures: The American Academy of Orthopaedic Surgeons, Vol. 9, St. Louis, 1952, The C.V. Mosby Co.
45. Yamamoto, H., and Yamashita, H.: Pedicular screw and spinal plate for reduction and fusion of spondylolisthesis in aged patients. (Abstracts), Twelfth annual meeting of The International Society for the Study of the Lumbar Spine, 1985.
46. Zindrick, M.R., et al.: A biomechanical study of intrapeduncular screw fixation in the lumbosacral spine. Proc. Int. Soc. Study Lumbar Spine, 1985.

EDITORIAL COMMENTARY

For decades spine surgeons have theorized that the ideal lumbar spine surgery for disc disease would be some form of internal fixation device that would hold the operated segment in anatomic alignment while fusion occurred 100% of the time. Such a fixation device would need to be easy to insert and remove, and would carry no significant complications. We see in this book three devices that seem to meet those criteria.

My experience with over 100 clinical cases of pedicle screw fixation leads me to maintain caution in the use of pedicle screw fixation.

The placement of pedicle screws is not without danger. The pedicle can and does break with insertion or long-range toggle of these screws. New signs and symptoms of nerve-root irritation develop for unknown reasons weeks to months after insertion. Pedicle screws break. New, heavy stresses are placed on the segment adjacent to this immediate rigid fixation device. Adjacent segments can be weakened by the insertion of the device.

Although there is a definite valuable place for these new pedicle screw fixation devices in lumbar spine surgery, I have not found them to be the answer on any routine basis. My clinical success rate was every bit as good with the use of Knodt rods and Harrington rods. The complications with the use of metallic internal fixation probably outweigh the value of increased fusion rates and immediate stability.

The internal fixation devices improved our success rates before we understood spinal stenosis and the need for adequate decompression. The decompression remains the most important aspect of spinal stenosis surgery. A fusion simply decreases the amount of low back pain a patient will experience after a decompression and disc excision. The fusion will prevent postoperative settling and spinal stenosis, which does not have to be a problem with adequate decompression. The fusion may prevent postoperative recurrent herniated discs and recurrent spinal stenosis.

A lumbar decompression and disc excision, when done well, has only a 5% to 10% likelihood of failure and the need for a second operation. To obviate this 10% repeat operation rate, it is probably not worth the risk of a major internal fixation fusion on 100% of lumbar disc surgery patients.

In certain patients such as those with osteoporosis, obesity, spondylolisthesis, multiple failed surgeries, and trauma the failure rate with decompression alone is much greater than 10%. Internal fixation is much more reasonable and, in fact, often necessary for success in some of these patients. One should, however, be very familiar with the device that will be used and take special training in the use of the device before using it surgically.

Arthur H. White

CHAPTER

34

AN INTERNAL FIXATOR FOR POSTERIOR APPLICATION TO SHORT SEGMENTS OF THE THORACIC, LUMBAR, OR LUMBOSACRAL SPINE: DESIGN AND TESTING

**Martin H. Krag   John W. Frymoyer   Bruce D. Beynnon
Malcolm H. Pope**

A new spinal implant has been designed and biomechanical testing completed, intended for application to "short-segment" spinal defects, such as disc degeneration, fracture, spondylolisthesis or tumor. Major improvements over currently available devices include: (1) only two to three vertebrae are spanned, not five to seven as with Harrington rods, (2) true three-dimensional fixation is achieved, preventing such problems as hook or rod dislocation, (3) three-dimensional adjustment is easily accomplished, allowing fracture or spondylolisthesis reduction to be readily performed, (4) attachment to vertebrae is by means of transpedicular screws, eliminating deliberate encroachment into the spinal canal, such as Luque wires or Harrington hooks, (5) no special alignment between screws is needed (such as with holes or slots in a plate), allowing screw placement to fully conform to anatomical structures, and (6) laminectomy sites and lumbosacral junction are readily instrumented.

Background investigations presented here for design of this device include: (1) CT-defined pedicle morphometry showing that screws may be larger than those currently used, (2) effect of pitch, minor diameter and tooth profile on screw pullout strength, (3) mechanical testing of a compact, three-dimensionally adjustable, non-loosening articulating clamp, and (4) establishing of the relationship between depth of penetration and strength of fixation of transpedicular screws.

THE VERMONT SPINAL FIXATOR

Significant improvements remain possible in the design of surgical implants for posterior spinal stabilization, to be used for dealing with single-motion-segment instability in the thoracic, lumbar or lumbo-sacral level (such as fracture, spondylolisthesis, "segmental instability"). This is true, even though major advances have been made in this field in recent years,[13,49,61,116,140] biomechanics has been increasingly applied to spine problems,* and a growing variety of spinal implants have become available.†

Bearing in mind that a single ideal implant is probably undefinable, we have designed a substantially different posterior implant referred to as the Vermont Spinal Fixator (VSF). Presented here is the rationale for its design, new anatomic data related to it, biomechanical testing of it, and initial experience with its cadaver implantation.

Minimum Length of Spinal Involvement

When fusion is indicated for single-level instability, only two vertebrae in principle need to be incorporated in the fusion mass. Even in the case of instability from a severely comminuted fracture, only three vertebrae need be fused. From a mechanical viewpoint, a short fusion is not strengthened by adding to its length (a 1-foot length of chain is as strong as a 3-foot length of chain). From a biologic viewpoint, unnecessary disruption of normal tissue should certainly be avoided.

Despite this, five, six, or even seven vertebrae are typically involved when using Harrington distraction rods, the most commonly used implant for dealing with instability, used either in their standard configuration* or with modifications.† This is related to the history of Harrington rods,[57] which were devised for management of multiple-segment deformities, such as scoliosis, and then subsequently applied to single-level problems (instability, spondylolisthesis, fracture).

However, mechanical characteristics of single-level problems are quite different, thus an implant specifically designed for this application is needed. Placement of Harrington hooks more closely together than five vertebrae fails to achieve adequate stabilization. This same dependency on five or more segments occurs with posterior plates and screws, such as Williams,[156,161] Wilson,[56,84,162] or Roy-Camille.[60,86,124,126,127,147] One method of decreasing the fusion length is the "rod long, fuse short" technique,[4,21,63,64] in which the rods are removed after the graft is solid. Not only does this involve a second operation, but early evidence[68,69] suggests that facet arthrosis may become a problem at the levels temporarily immobilized but not grafted.

Three-Dimensional Fixation

One major purpose of any fixation device is to increase the likelihood of achieving successful bone fusion. There is no data to suggest that motion in any particular direction is better or worse than motion in any other, in terms of achieving fusion. Thus, fully three-di-

---

*References 6, 17, 20, 34, 36, 37, 50, 53, 62, 65, 71, 73, 76, 81-83, 85, 93, 96, 98, 99, 103, 106, 107, 118, 122, 132, 133, 136, 137, 141, 149, 150, 153, 154, 158, 159, 163, 164, 166.
†References 5, 12, 15, 19, 35, 51, 54, 70, 86, 87, 89, 90, 100, 110, 114, 115, 119, 121, 126, 127, 128, 138, 139, 146, 152.

---

*References 1, 4, 8, 21, 22, 30, 32, 33, 43, 44, 55, 58, 66, 77, 94, 97, 111, 130, 135, 143, 156, 160, 165.
†References 11, 16, 18, 31, 34, 38-42, 45, 48, 65, 72, 100, 104, 134, 142, 144, 145, 164.

mensional fixation becomes a logical objective. A second purpose of a fixation device is to limit intervertebral motion so as to prevent nerve root or spinal cord pressure. This may potentially be produced by any one of various displacements (either rotations or translations), so again three-dimensional fixation becomes the objective.

Despite this, most current spinal posterior implants do not produce such three-dimensional fixation. This occurs for one or more of three reasons: (1) absence of a rigid attachment to the vertebra itself, (2) reliance upon soft-tissues to not stretch out or "creep," or (3) absence of rigid attachment between components of the device.

The most commonly used spinal implant, the Harrington rod system, has all three of the above characteristics. The hooks simply push (or pull) against their attachment sites, and they rely on soft tissue resistance,[2,3,8] as well as external trunk support (bracing), to produce sufficient vertebral-motion limitation. As a result, lordosis flattening in the lumbar spine[59,100] or overdistraction at a fracture site[2,3,8] can occur. Once displacement occurs, the hooks may detach from the rod. Modified hooks[11,39,62] or segmental wiring[34,87,144] represent significant improvements, but flexion/extension can still occur by means of the lamina rotating within the hook or wire loop. This lack of three-dimensional fixation at the attachment sites of Harrington hooks (or Luque wires for that matter), is a part of the reason that these implants must span five, six, or even seven vertebrae for adequate stability.

With posterior plates and screws, the screw does provide a rigid grip on the vertebra. However, the screw is not rigidly mechanically linked to the plate. Rather, sufficient compression between plate and underlying bone is needed to prevent "toggle" of the screw in its plate hole[132] or excessive shearing forces on the screw. The occurrence of this toggle is probably related to the falloff in screw tension known to occur in vivo.[10] This issue is one of concern even when these plates are mounted onto broad surfaces such as the femur or tibia.[23] The problem becomes greater yet when the plates are attached to the spine where the bone bed is quite irregular.[60,163] This results in relatively small bone-plate contact areas and thus high contact pressures, increasing the likelihood of bending or shear loads being applied to the screws. These plates, of course, overlay a significant portion of the surface normally used as a graft bed.[163] As with the rods, here also, five vertebrae must be instrumented for adequate control of significant instability.[126,127]

The Magerl external fixator[91,92,133,163] does obtain a rigid grip on each vertebra, it does not rely upon soft tissues, and its components are rigidly linked together in three dimensions. Thus this device represents a major advance in spinal implants. It does have the characteristics of any external fixator in that pin-track infections may occur and the posterior prominence of the device is an inconvenience. The flexibility caused by the unsupported span of the Schanz pins has been conjectured to provide a certain "shock absorbing" quality. However, this same characteristic also requires supplemental internal fixation in more unstable cases, preventing application of this device in a "closed" fashion. In addition, this flexibility often requires the device to be used as either a distractor or a compressor, rather than as a fixator. Thus it relies upon soft tissues being sufficiently intact to prevent excessive creep.

Spinal Canal Avoidance and Safe Implantation

Deliberate encroachment into the spinal canal is a routine part of most device implantations, either with hooks (Harrington, Weiss, Knodt) or wires (Luque) or both. Use of hooks alone has been quite safe, although problems do occur,[52,95] and there is the always-present risk of intra-operative errors when working within the spinal canal. The use of laminar wires has caused some major complications either during their placement[67,123,157] or removal,[9,108] or when used in combination with Harrington hooks.[123,157]

All of these complications are related to deliberate violation of the spinal canal necessary for implantation of these devices. Pedicle screw placement, however, does not require entrance into the canal. Extensive experience with the safety of this method has been gathered, either with plates, external fixators, or facet joint fusions.[14,74,112] The risks of screw placement too far medially or too far anteriorly do exist, but modern image intensifiers allow good intra-operative visualization to guard against both these risks. A further safeguard to keeping the screw within the pedicle is the fact that the medial and inferior pedicle borders may be easily and safely palpated intra-operatively.[89,90,126]

Concerning the issue of anterior cortex engagement by the pedicle screw, it appears that this is unnecessary. Deliberate avoidance of anterior cortex is recommended by Roy-Camille,[126,127] based on his extensive experience in which screw bone interface loosening apparently is not a problem. Supportive evidence exists in the mechanical testing by Lavaste,[82,83] which showed that engagement of the anterior cortex provides only slight additional screw pull-out strengthening. The issue of cortex engagement, as well as a number of other important aspects of pedicle screw placement have been addressed by Zindrick and coworkers,[166] using certain commercially available screw types.

Use of Safest Surgical Approach

The choice between anterior and posterior approach devices depends upon many factors, but certainly there are advantages to avoiding abdominal or thoracic cavity involvement. For cases in which the anterior approach is selected primarily in order to perform spinal canal decompression, a variety of stabilizing devices are becoming available.* These involve only a limited segment of spine and do not require spinal canal encroachment. At least one of them[35] provides a full three-dimensional rigid fixation, although anterior prominence and proximity to the aorta is an issue about which some concern exists.

Device Removal

Although Harrington rods are not routinely removed when accompanied by bone grafting along the entire length of the rod, their upper hooks or cut ends may cause sufficient irritation to require removal. The "rod long, fuse short" technique[4,21,63,64] described above does of course require device removal. The benefit to avoidance of a second operation for device removal is certainly obvious.

Avoidance of Transcutaneous Components

Preliminary experience with an external spinal fixator is growing.[89-92] This device has certain unique and useful advantages, but it does present the risk of pin track infections, which limits the length of time the device can remain in place. Furthermore, the external components appear to be somewhat cumbersome, requiring a special brace and mattress.

In order to simultaneously satisfy all six of the above criterion, our approach has been to devise an "internal fixator"

---

*References 12, 35, 51, 54, 70, 115, 119, 121, 126-128.

which (1) could be adjusted to span as short as a single motion segment, (2) provides rigid three-dimensional fixation by attachment through the pedicle into the vertebral body, (3) does not violate the spinal canal, (4) uses the posterior approach, (5) does not require removal, and (6) is completely internalized.

DESIGN APPROACH

In attempting to satisfy these six criteria, five major design issues were identified for further investigation.

In Vivo Loads

Little data are available concerning the loads that the implant needs to support. Schlaepfer and coworkers[133,163] have presented their results using an external spinal fixator as a load transducer, but the data are not fully three-dimensional and do not allow full separation of the various load components. This important work, however, does suggest that the implant is very largely "shielded" from bending loads by the trunk extensor muscles. Other in vivo measurements have been made using strain gages on Harrington rods in humans[105,120,151] and in sheep,[106] or on Dwyer cables in dogs,[136] but these are difficult to convert into loads acting at the site of instability. "Free-body analysis" estimates of in vivo loads are only as good as the estimates on which they are based, and do not deal at all with load sharing between vertebrae and muscles.

Thus for present purposes the best answer to the question "How strong should the implant be?" comes from the empiric clinical experience that has been accumulated in five areas. First, posterior plates are typically attached[126,127] using 3.5 to 4.5 mm cortical screws. Although ideally these screws are protected from all but pure tensile loads, in practice this seems to be quite unlikely, especially for the screws at the ends of the plates. As noted earlier, these screws are almost surely exposed to some shearing and bending loads. Despite this, screw breakage has not been reported as a significant problem.[124-127] Thus, whatever the in vivo loads actually are, 3.5 to 4.5 mm screws are strong enough to prevent breakage.

Second, in vivo bending of the plates themselves has not been reported to be a problem. Mechanical testing in vitro[82,83] has shown that plastic deformation of the Roy-Camille plates occurs at only 11.3 Nm (8.3 ft. lbs). For comparison, this is even weaker than the bending strength (14.7 Nm or 10.85 ft. lbs) of the 5 mm portion of the Schanz pins used in the external spinal fixator (see following). Thus in vivo bending loads taken by the plate must be less than 11.3 Nm.

Third, Cyron and coworkers[25] have shown in vitro that spondylolysis can be produced with a mean moment of 35 Nm for L5 vertebrae and 28 Nm for L1 vertebrae. These must represent upper limits to in vivo moments, since spondylolysis does not routinely develop after spinal injuries, even with complete paraplegia in which trunk muscle denervation may occur.

Fourth, significant experience has been reported for facet joint fusions with a screw placed obliquely across the facet joint in conjunction with posterior bone grafts for various nontraumatic conditions. Boucher[14] encountered only two broken screws out of a total of 482. Out of 44 L5-S1 fusions, King[74] does not describe any breakages. In the 150 patients of Pennal and coworkers,[112] only one screw broke. In the first two studies, screw diameters were not specified, but were probably approximately ⅛ inch. In the last study, screw minor diameter was specified as ⅛ inch.

Fifth, the external spinal fixator[89,90,132,133] uses 6 mm Schanz pins thinned down to 5 mm along their anterior 6 cm. These pins, of course, are fully exposed to all the loads taken by the fixator. Breakage or bending of these pins has not been reported. This should probably not be surprising, since the bending strength (load needed to produce plastic deformation) of the 5 mm portion of pin is 14.7 Nm per pin or 29.4 Nm per pair. Thus it can be seen empirically that 5 mm certainly seems to be strong enough. If an even larger size could be used, the margin of safety would only increase.

Vertebral Morphometric Constraints

The pedicle seems to be the strongest site accessible posteriorly through which to obtain a three-dimensionally rigid "grip" onto the vertebra. Certainly, no other site with this property seems to have been proposed. The limiting factor to the size of the screw that can be placed from posteriorly through the pedicle into the vertebral body, is the mediolateral width of the pedicle. Saillant[129] has reported certain important data from cadavera, but these data have certain drawbacks. First, only average values were given and not the ranges or standard deviations. Second, bone screw path length was only reported for a purely sagittal screw placement: other screw placement angles may be preferable[89,90] and would alter this length. Third, only the pedicle diameter perpendicular to the pedicle axis was reported: for screws placed at any other direction than along the pedicle axis, an effectively smaller pedicle diameter may be present (Fig. 34-1). Finally, data were obtained from cadavera alone, without any radiographic correlation, the latter being more appropriate to the clinical situation. Thus a morphometric study addressing these issues was undertaken. The major findings are presented below, and full details are reported elsewhere.[80]

Pedicle Screw Design

Bone-screw interface strength is commonly the limiting factor in the overall strength of a stabilizing implant, at least over the first few days or weeks (fatigue of metal or resorption of bone may become a problem later on). Some testing of mechanical characteristics of pedicle screws has been performed. Lavaste[82,83] compared various commerically available screws in pull-out tests. Zindrick and coworkers[166] compared certain commercially available screws, and also the effects of various details of screw placement technique.

Optimizing pedicle screw pull-out strength requires a systematic study in which various screw design features are varied systematically. This has not previously been reported for pedicle screws. Furthermore, despite a fairly large literature characterizing the pull-out strength of various screw designs in limb bones, it does not appear that a systematic study has been done which independently varies the different screw design features such as tooth profile, pitch, and minor diameter. Bechtol[7] compared pull-out strength from dog limb bones of screws with one each of eight different tooth profiles, but the minor diameters were unspecified and various pitches were used in such a way as to not allow the effect of this variable to be isolated. Koranyi and coworkers[75] reported equal pull-out strengths for both "V" toothed Sherman screws and buttress-toothed A-O screws, using dog or cattle femora. However, neither major nor minor diameters were specified although tooth heights were the same. Lyon and associates,[88] Nunamaker and Perren,[109] and Schatzker and coworkers[131] each studied various groups of different commercially available screws, but the individual effects of pitch, major diameter, and minor diameter could not be isolated, since these parameters were not systematically varied.

To design a pedicle screw with optimal bone-metal interface strength, we undertook the study reported here (reported in

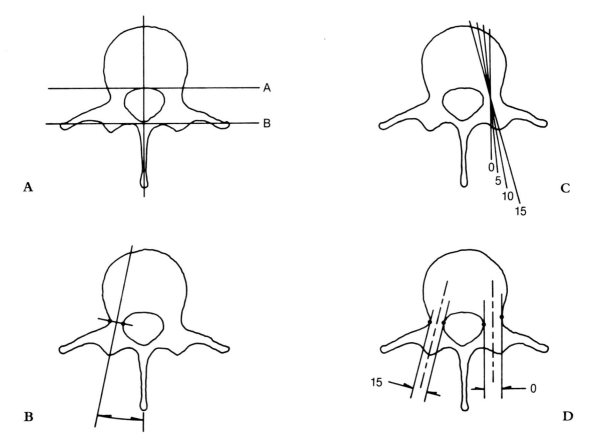

Fig. 34-1 Construction lines used to obtain measurements from vertebral CT scans. **A,** Vertebral body length from anterior cortex to line A, pedicle length from line A to posterior cortex or to line B ("facet corrected"). **B,** Pedicle axis angle measured from sagittal plane (posterolateral positive), pedicle diameter along perpendicular to axis. **C,** Screw path length (or chord length) from anterior to posterior cortex at 0 degrees, 5 degrees, 10 degrees, or 15 degrees posterolaterally from the sagittal plane. **D,** Pedicle diameter at 0 degrees and 15 degrees. Note that bone contact points do not fall along a common perpendicular to the pedicle axis.

more detail elsewhere),[78] using various combinations of pitch, minor diameter, and tooth profile, for each of various major diameters. Pull-out testing was used, since we believed that this load type would be most sensitive to thread design variations. Of course, pure pull-out loads alone are not likely to occur in vivo, since additional kinds of loads (bending, shearing) would usually occur simultaneously.

Articulating Clamp

Some sort of mechanism is needed to rigidly link together the four pedicle screws after they are placed into the vertebra above and the vertebra below the site of instability. The four most important design objectives were felt to be adjustability, strength, compactness and security. Adjustability in all three dimensions was sought, since this would simplify pedicle screw insertion: no special alignment between the screws would need to be maintained during their insertion. Adjustability in three dimensions also allows the reduction (in the case of fractures or spondylolisthesis) to be "unconstrained" and can be performed in a controlled fashion with the fixator already in place (but before tightening the locking mechanism). The strength of this articulating clamp should exceed that of the pedicle screw, so as not to become the limiting factor to overall implant strength. Compactness is obviously important for comfort and for normal muscle function. Finally, "security" means that the likelihood for loosening be extremely low.

To prevent loosening, the threads which the clamp bolt engage inside the rod clamp are of a special pattern known as Spiralock.* This "state-of-the-art" thread is primarily used in aircraft and other critical high-vibration applications. Other advantages of this thread besides security against loosening include (1) it may be repeatedly tightened, loosened and retightened without degradation, (2) it has a much better distribution of loads along the engaged bolt threads compared to standard threads, and (3) a separate locking nut is not needed.

In order to satisfy all four of these criteria, a series of clamping systems were designed and tested by mock-up cadavera implantation. The current design is that shown in Fig. 34-2 and Fig. 34-3. Note

*MicroDot Co., Fullerton, Calif.

that fine stepwise adjustability exists for rotation about the x (transverse) axis, in increments of 6 degrees, since there are 60 radially arranged teeth on the "face gear" on the head of the bone screw. Infinite adjustability exists for longitudinal axis rotation *(Ry)* and longitudinal translation or lengthening *(Ty)*.

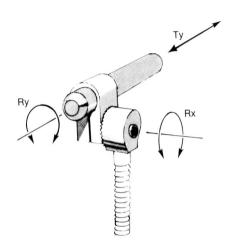

Fig. 34-2 Articulating clamp assembly showing adjustability between components. Flexion/extension (x axis rotation, *Rx*), axial rotation (y axis rotation, *Ry*), intervertebral separation (y axis translation, *Ty*).

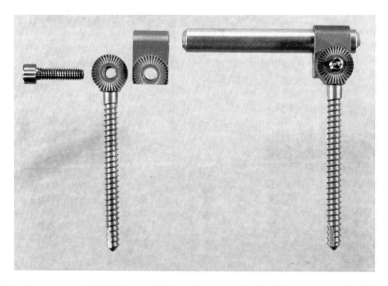

Fig. 34-3 Component of VSF assembled and separated. Pedicle screw, articulating clamp, clamp bolt and connecting rod.

Depth of Screw Penetration into Vertebra

How close to the anterior cortex should the tip of the pedicle screw be placed? The greater the depth of penetration (Fig. 34-4), the more secure the screw "grip" on bone, but the greater the risk of cortical breakthrough and damage to aorta or other structures.

Magerl[89,90] recommends placement of the screw tip just into but not through the anterior cortex. Direct testing of various depths of placement, however, does not appear to have been done. Roy-Camille,[126,127] on the contrary, recommends avoidance of anterior cortex engagement. His clinical reports do not describe in detail the depth of penetration actually used, but illustrative x-rays show penetration of approximately 50% to 60% depth. Screw loosening has not been reported as a significant problem. Mechanical testing in vitro by Lavaste[82,83] suggested that anterior cortex engagement did not add significantly to the pullout strength of the screws. It appears from this experience that even a close approach to the anterior cortex is not necessary.

Because of these conflicting recommendations concerning depth of screw penetration, specific investigation of this issue seemed indicated and is reported here.

METHODS
Vertebral Morphometry

A retrospective review was performed of CT scans of 91 vertebrae from T9 to L5, for evaluation of 41 patients for various spinal conditions (10 single-level fractures, 12 herniated or bulging discs, 3 unspecified cord lesions, 2 bony degenerative changes, and 14 negative studies). Individual vertebrae with positive findings were excluded. The age range was 18 to 75 years (mean of 36 and median of 28 years); there were 14 females and 27 males. The number of specimens at each level were as follows: 7 at T9, 9 at T10, 11 at T11, 12 at T12, 11 at L1, 7 at L2, 12 at L3, 12 at L4, and 10 at L5. A Seimens Somatom-2 third-generation scanner was used, with 4 mm cuts and a 5-second scan time.

The CT image was selected on which the width of both pedicles appeared the largest (thus passing through the midheight of both pedicles). Measurements of the parameters defined in Fig. 34-1 were obtained directly from the film and were corrected to lifesize by the appropriate scale factor of 1.25. Three parameters are of particular interest here. First, pedicle axis angle was measured relative to the sagittal plane, with positive values for anteromedial angulation (see Fig. 34-1, B). Second, pedicle diameter was measured both perpendicular to the pedicle axis (see Fig. 34-1, B), and at the specified approach angles of 0 degrees and 15 degrees (see Fig. 34-1, D). Third, screw path length (chord length) was measured between anterior and posterior cortices along a line passing through the middle of the pedicle and inclined at 0 degrees, 5 degrees, 10 degrees, and 15 degrees (see Fig. 34-1, C). Other measured parameters and further methodological details are reported elsewhere.[80]

To establish the validity of the CT scan

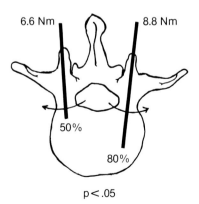

Fig. 34-4 Effect of screw depth of penetration on peak "cut-out" loads (Ry or rotation about long axis); 80% penetration allows 32.5% higher loads than 50% penetration.

Table 34-1 *Test design for pull-out of 6 mm screws*

Screw type	Tooth profile	Minor diameter (mm)	Thread pitch (mm)	Block 1	Block 2	Block 3
1	V	3.8	2	X		X
2	V	3.8	3	X		X
3	V	5.0	2	X		
4	V	5.0	3	X		
5	B	3.8	2		X	X
6	B	3.8	3		X	X
7	B	5.0	2		X	
8	B	5.0	3		X	

Eight experimental screw types resulted from using two values for each of three design variables (tooth, minor diameter, and pitch). In each block, one variable was held constant. In Block 1, only screws with "V" threads were used, allowing the effect of minor diameter and pitch to be studied. Block 2 was similar, but for buttress ("B") screws alone. In Block 3, only screws with a minor diameter of 3.8 mm were used, allowing the effect of tooth profile and pitch to be studied.

measurements, eight cadaver vertebrae (one at T12, three at L2, three at L3, one at L4) had their inferior endplates embedded in polymethylmethacrylate and were attached to a positioning jig for CT scanning using the same method as for patient CT scans. The vertebrae were then sectioned through the midpedicle transverse plane and direct measurements of selected parameters were obtained, which were then correlated to the CT scan measurements.

Screw path length cannot be directly measured from routine lateral x-ray films. Occasionally it may be convenient to predict screw path length when CT scans are not available. For this reason, the ratios between path length and midsagittal AP diameter of vertebral body (which can be measured on lateral x-ray films) were calculated for various approach angles.

Screw Design

The pedicle diameter dictates the maximum major diameter for the screw, but choice remains concerning minor diameter (root diameter), pitch, and tooth profile. Two values for each of these three parameters were selected for study, giving a total of eight possible screw designs. For the 6 mm major diameter screws, the values were: thread profile either "V" or buttress, minor diameter of 3.8 or 5 mm, and pitch of 2 or 3 mm. For the 7 mm major diameter screws, the values were: thread profile buttress only, minor diameter of 5 or 6 mm, and pitch of 2 or 3 mm. Two screw types at a time were directly compared by placement into the right and left pedicles of individual excised cadaveric vertebrae, which had been embedded in base blocks of polymethylmethacrylate. Predrill diameter was 85% of the minor diameter of the screw. Predrilling was done along the pedicle axis and to the same depth as subsequent screw penetration, which was 80% of path length. No pretapping was performed. Thread-cutting flutes were present on the tips of all screws. The polymethylmethacrylate blocks were then attached to an MTS machine for pull-out testing of each screw, one at a time, with the pull-out direction along the long axis of the screw.

A randomized balanced incomplete block experimental design was used (see Table 34-1, and 34-2). This was chosen because (1) there were 3 variables of interest but only 2 pedicles per vertebra and (2) significant variation between vertebral

Table 34-2 *Test design for right-left pedicle pairings of experimental screws for pull-out*

Vertebral group	Block 1 Right	Block 1 Left	Block 2 Right	Block 2 Left	Block 3 Right	Block 3 Left
A	1	2	5	6	1	2
B	1	3	5	7	1	5
C	1	4	5	8	1	6
D	2	3	6	7	2	5
E	2	4	6	8	2	6
F	3	4	7	8	5	6

In Block 1, each of the six possible pairings (A-F) of screw types no. 1, 2, 3 and 4 were placed respectively into the right and left pedicles of individual vertebral specimens. In Block 2, a similar arrangement was used, for screw types no. 5, 6, 7 and 8. In Block 3, screw types no. 1, 2, 5 and 6 were studied. Each vertebral group consisted of two vertebral specimens, giving a total of 36 vertebrae (72 pedicles) tested.

specimens was noted on preliminary experiments. Three blocks were defined, each one consisting of a subgroup of four screw types (Table 34-1). For each subgroup, there were six possible combinations of screw types taken two at a time (Table 34-2). Each combination was studied by placement in the two pedicles of a vertebra; two vertebrae per combination were used to provide duplicate measurements, for a total of 24 pull-outs per block. A direct comparison of 6 mm vs. 7 mm major diameter screws was not performed, since the strengthening effect of major diameter has already been established.[88,109] Further details of the test procedure and data analysis are presented elsewhere.[78]

Articulating Clamp

Three types of static testing were considered important. See Fig. 34-2, which shows the coordinate system used in the testing. Moments about the transverse axis (flexion-extension, Mx) are probably the largest loads to which the device will be exposed. Axial torsional moments (twisting, My) may also be significant. Finally, axial compression forces. (Fy) will be large, but will probably be located anterior to the rod, tending to produce a "jamming" effect of the clamp on the rod. As pointed out previously, the actual in vivo loads to which this device will be exposed are really not known. This is emphasized by the large disparity between the in vivo strain-gauge measurements from the external spinal fixator and typical predictions from free body analysis. The former showed peak bending moments of only 8 Nm,[162] while the latter predicts bending moments of 91 Nm at 40 degrees flexed posture.[101,155]

Depth of Screw Penetration into Vertebra

Vertebral specimens were prepared in a manner identical to that used in the screw design study. In all cases the screws were 6 mm major diameter, 5 mm minor diameter, 2 mm pitch, and buttress tooth. One screw was implanted into each of the right and left pedicles, but using a different depth of penetration on each side (see Fig. 34-4). Some specimens were used to compare 50% vs. 80% penetration, others were used to compare 80% vs. 100% penetration. The results of only the former are presented here. Loading to failure was then performed using a moment about either (1) the transverse or x axis ("cut-up" loading, tending to force

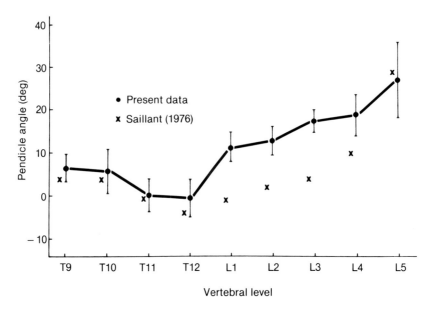

Fig. 34-5 Pedicle axis angle relative to sagittal plane for each vertebral level. Means ± 1 SD are shown, compared to means *(x)* from Saillant.[129]

the screw tip up through the superior end plate), or (2) the longitudinal or y axis ("cut-out" loading, tending to force the screw tip out through the lateral cortex of the vertebral body) as shown in Fig. 34-4. The moments were applied about a point near the center of the pedicle, in such a way as not to constrain subsequent screw motion. Four specimens were used for each load type. These load types were chosen because it was believed that they would be the most sensitive to different depths of penetration, and also that they were at least as realistic as the pull-out loading.

RESULTS
Vertebral Morphometry

Pedicle axis angle data are shown in Fig. 34-5. The minimum angulation is at T12, with a value of −0.6 degrees (that is, very slight anterolateral angulation). The maximum is at L5 with an angulation of +27.2 degrees. In rough terms, the axis angle is 0-10 degrees in the lower thoracic spine, and gradually increases caudally throughout the lumbar region.

Standard deviations are fairly small (typically 3 to 5 degrees). The data of Saillant[129] are shown for comparison: good agreement exists except for L1 to L4, where our data show substantially larger pedicle axis angles.

Pedicle diameter data are shown in Fig. 34-6 and Table 34-3. The former shows the results of all three different methods for measuring pedicle diameter. It may be seen that (1) pedicle diameter is almost constant from T9 to L1, with a means at each level of approximately 7 mm, (2) a gradual increase in diameter occurs from L1 to L5, (3) very similar results are obtained from the three different measures of pedicle diameter, (4) the standard deviations at each vertebral level are quite small (most are less than 2 mm), and (5) quite good agreement exists with the data of Saillant,[129] although our values tend to be a little lower.

Table 34-3 shows for each vertebral level the distribution by size of pedicle diameter (measured perpendicular to the pedicle axis). Note that (1) pedicles smaller than 5 mm were never encoun-

An Internal Fixator for Posterior Application to Short Segments of the Spine 351

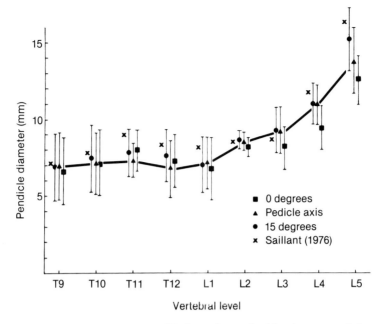

Fig. 34-6 Pedicle diameter means ± 1 SD for each vertebral level, measured three different ways (see Fig. 1, *B* and *D*) and compared to means *(x)* from Saillant.[129]

Table 34-3 *Pedicle diameter and distribution by size*

Level	Mean	SD	No.	3-3.9 mm	4-4.9 mm	5-5.9 mm	6-6.9 mm	7-7.9 mm	8-19.4 mm
T9	6.88	2.23	14	14%	7%	14%	21%	7%	35%
T10	7.47	2.24	18	11		11	39		39
T11	7.83	1.56	22			14	18	14	55
T12	7.63	1.79	24			21	21	12	46
L1	7.01	1.84	22	9		18	18	14	41
L2	8.67	0.64	14					7	92
L3	9.30	1.51	24				8	12	79
L4	11.03	1.36	24						100
L5	15.15	1.97	20						100

Pedicle diameter and distribution by size. Diameter was measured perpendicular to pedicle axis (Fig. 34-1, *B*). Means (±1 SD) are graphed in Fig. 34-6. Note large number of pedicles 8 mm or larger, especially at lower vertebral levels.

tered below T10, with the exception of L1, and elsewhere they were infrequent, (2) pedicles 8 mm or larger were encountered in significant numbers at all levels, from 35% at T9 up to 100% at L5.

Screw path length (chord length) data are shown in Fig. 34-7 for both the 0 degrees and the 15 degrees approach angles. Major features of these results include (1) a slightly longer path length always results from the more steeply inclined approach (15 degrees), (2) path length is almost constant over the vertebral levels studied, with a small decrease occurring caudally (45.1 mm at T9, 36.4 mm at L5), (3) standard deviations are relatively small, and (4) good agreement is present with the data of Saillant.[129]

The accuracy of our CT scan measurements is illustrated in Fig. 34-8. The various measurements obtained by CT scanning of cadaver vertebrae are plotted

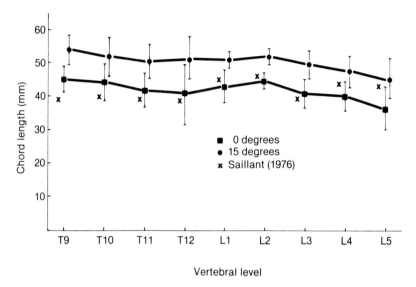

Fig. 34-7 Screw path length (chord length) measured along line at 0 degrees and 15 degrees relative to sagittal plane (see Fig. 1, C), and compared to means *(x)* from Saillant.[129]

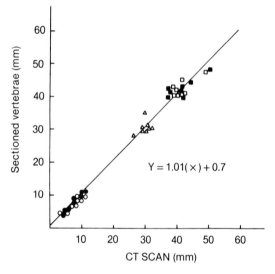

Fig. 34-8 Correlation between caliper measures and CT scan measurements on cadaver vertebrae.

Table 34-4 *Significance of screw design variables on pull-out strength of 6 mm and 7 mm screws*

Variable	Major diameter (mm)	Block 1 (V tooth subgroup)	Block 2 (B tooth subgroup)	Block 3 (3.8 minor subgroup)
Minor	6	p .05*	p .01†	—
	7	—	ns	—
Pitch	6	ns	p .01‡	ns
	7	—	ns	—
Tooth	6	—	—	ns
	7	—	—	—
Minor and pitch	6	ns	ns	—
	7	—	ns	—
Pitch and tooth	6	—	—	ns
	7	—	—	—

*1093 N vs. 864 N adjusted mean pull-out of 3.8 mm and 5.0 mm minor diameter screws respectively.
†1408 N vs. 1181 N adjusted mean pull-out of 3.8 mm and 5.0 mm minor diameter screws respectively.
‡1416 N vs. 1174 N adjusted mean pull-out of 2 mm and 3 mm pitch screws respectively.
The significance level is noted for each design variable and certain combinations of variables, for each of the Blocks (1, 2, and 3) and for each of the 6 mm and 7 mm diameter sizes; n.s., nonsignificance, (p = .05); variables the significance of which were not testable.

against the same measurement obtained by calipers. All these data are seen to fall very close to the y = x line, with an acceptably low correlation coefficient.

The ratio between screw path length and AP diameter of vertebral body was calculated for both the 0 degrees and the 15 degrees approach angle. The mean (±1 SD) at 0 degrees was 1.32 ± .12, and at 15 degrees was 1.60 ± 0.9. In other words, the path length is approximately one third longer than the AP body diameter for a 0 degree approach angle, and two thirds longer for a 15 degree approach angle.

Screw Design

Table 34-4 shows the significance of each screw design variable. Minor diameter is significant for 6 mm screws, both for the V tooth and B tooth subgroups. In each case, the smaller minor diameter (3.8 mm vs. 5 mm) is somewhat stronger: 26% for the V tooth (1093 N vs. 864 N adjusted mean strengths) and 19% for the B tooth (1408 N vs. 1181 N adjusted mean strengths). However, for 7 mm screws with B teeth, minor diameter was not significant.

Pitch was significant only for 6 mm B threads: 2 mm pitch screws were 21% stronger than 3 mm pitch (1416 N vs. 1174 N adjusted mean strengths). This effect was not seen for 6 mm V threads or 7 mm B threads.

Tooth pattern (V vs. B) was not significant for the one subgroup tested, which was the 6 mm major, 3.8 mm minor screws. Finally, the interaction between variables (minor and pitch, pitch and tooth) can also be seen to be not significant (n.s.) in the areas tested.

Table 34-5 shows the mean pull-out strengths of the various screw types studied, with no adjustment for vertebral specimen bone density, size, or donor age, and with no consideration given to the right-left pedicle pairing used in the analysis to produce Table 34-4. Because of this, direct comparison between means is not appropriate. Nonetheless, it is valid to note that the screw type with lowest mean value is still substantial at 715 N (161 lbs.), that many of the means are

Table 34-5 *Mean pull-out strengths of various experimental screw types*

Screw type	Tooth profile	Major diameter (mm)	Minor diameter (mm)	Thread pitch (mm)	Pull-out (N) Mean	SD	Range	No.
1	V	6	3.8	2	1326	692	818-2942	13
2	V	6	3.8	3	1645	944	625-3592	13
3	V	6	5.0	2	976	330	630-1580	6
4	V	6	5.0	3	715	253	395-1101	6
5	B	6	3.8	2	1978	868	700-3494	12
6	B	6	3.8	3	1435	624	700-2747	12
7	B	6	5.0	2	1132	600	550-2063	6
8	B	6	5.0	3	1248	440	600-1840	6
1	B	7	5.0	2	1675	41	1120-2014	6
2	B	7	5.0	3	1410	464	825-2000	6
3	B	7	6.0	2	1288	456	743-1839	6
4	B	7	6.0	3	1387	213	1123-1645	6

The mean pull-out strength of each experimental screw type is presented, as well as the standard deviation (SD), range, and number of screw pull-outs performed (No.). No adjustment has been made for vertebral specimen age, size, or bone density. All screws were placed along the pedicle axis to a depth of penetration equal to 80% of the vertebral path length.

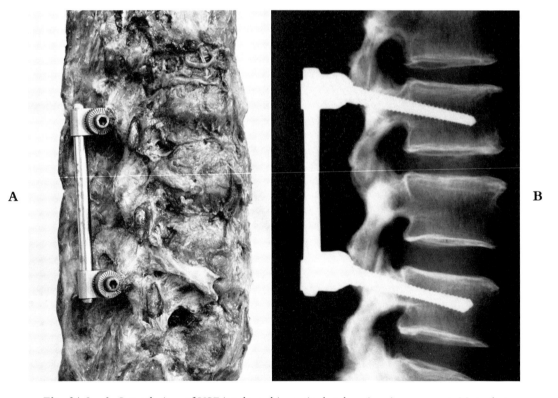

Fig. 34-9 A, Lateral view of VSF implanted in excised cadaveric spine segment. Note that graft bed is unobstructed and that prominence of implant is less than that of spinous process. **B,** Corresponding lateral x-ray film. Note pedicle screws may be aligned to conform to anatomic constraints and do not extend to anterior cortex.

over 1000 N, and that the highest mean is 1978 N (440 lbs.).

Articulating Clamp

Static testing has been performed for each of three different types of loading, as shown in Fig. 34-2. To produce rotation of the bone screw relative to the articulating clamp about the clamp bolt (x axis rotation, or flexion/extension), moments must exceed 149 Nm (110 ft. lbs). For rotation of the connecting rod within the articulating clamp (y axis rotation, or axial twisting), moments of 27.5 Nm (20.3 ft lbs) may be sustained. Finally, sliding of the rod within the clamp (y axis translation or axial collapse) requires loads of at least 4878 N (1095 lbs) for 6 mm diameter rods, and at least 10690 N (2400 lbs) for 8 mm diameter rods.

Depth of Screw Penetration

Fig. 34-4 illustrates the results of the moments about the y axis ("cut-out" or twisting loads). The screws placed at 50% depth failed at an average of 6.58 Nm (4.84 ft. lbs) while those at 80% depth failed at an average of 8.72 Nm (6.41 ft. lbs). This 32.5% strength improvement is significant ($p = .05$). For the x axis moments ("cut-up" or extension loads), corresponding data were 6.50 Nm (4.79 ft. lbs) and 8.41 Nm (6.12 ft. lbs), for an improvement of 29.3%, which is also significant ($p = .05$).

Current Design

Based on these studies, a prototype design has been completed and cadaver implantations performed as shown in Figs. 34-9 and 34-10. The individual device

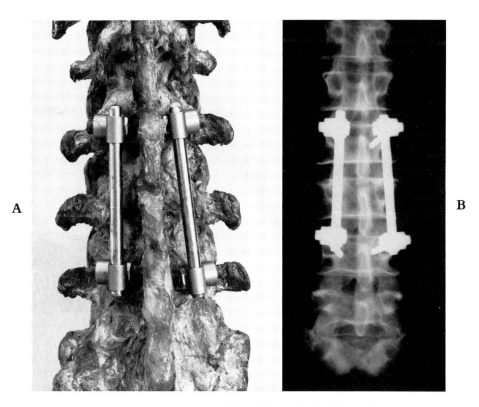

Fig. 34-10 A, Posterior view of VSF implanted in excised cadaver spine segment, corresponding to Fig. 9. Note that connecting rods do not obstruct graft bed and are placed medial to the pedicle screws to allow extensor muscle approximation to midline. **B,** Corresponding posterior x-ray film. Note convergence of right and left pedicle screws, producing "toe-nailing" effect for increased strength of fixation.

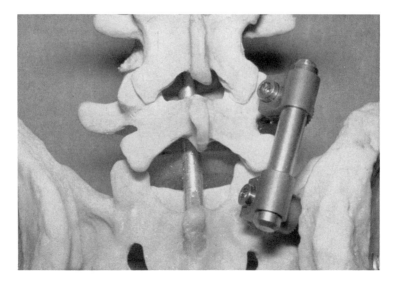

Fig. 34-11 Posterior view of VSF at L5 to S1 junction. Attachment to sacrum presents no particular difficulties, as it does with certain other stabilization devices. Note that ilium protrudes even more posteriorly than does VSF.

components are shown in Fig. 34-3. Placement is readily accommodated, not only in the thoracolumbar or lumbar area, but also the lumbosacral junction as shown in Fig. 34-11. The simplicity, short length, adjustability, and compactness may be noted.

DISCUSSION

An important principle that relates to surgical management of single-motion-segment instability (for example, fracture, spondylolisthesis, "segmental instability") is that normal tissue should not be disrupted; both the implant and the bone graft should involve only the abnormal motion segment. A second principle is that the implant should be a fixator, rather than either a distractor or a compressor, in order to provide mechanical stabilization, and to do so without reliance upon intact soft tissues. Since instability can involve motion in any direction,[46,47,117] the fixation produced should be three-dimensional. Finally, the safety of the implantation process should be maximized.

Placement of screws through the pedicle is considered by some to be particularly dangerous. To the contrary, this procedure has certain aspects which render it particularly safe. First, this method completely avoids the need for violation of the spinal canal, such as passage of circum-laminar wires or placement of Harrington hooks with the potentially associated neurologic complications.[67,123,157] Second, device removal (either for intraoperative repositioning or as a separate procedure) is even safer than device placement, quite in contrast to the situation with circum-laminar wires.[9,108] Also related to safety is the issue of screw depth of penetration. Recommendations concerning this issue are in disagreement, as already mentioned. Our data (see Fig. 34-4) do show that 80% depth of penetration produces an approximately 30% stronger "grip" for the pedicle screw, compared to only 50% depth of penetration. This is statistically significant, but whether it is functionally significant remains to be established; in vivo comparison of screw depths or measurement of implant loads will be needed to fully answer this question. An additional commentary on the safety of the pedicle route is that (1) there has been extensive clinical experience with screw fixation into the pedicle,* (2) biopsies of the vertebral body are commonly done through the pedicle[24] for the thoracolumbar and lumbar spine, and (3) the pedicle has been used as a surgical route either for placement of vertebral body bone grafts[26,27] or for "shelling out" of cancellous bone from the vertebral body for management of scoliosis.

A final observation concerning pedicle screw placement safety is that even if the pedicle cortex is disrupted, neurological damage does not necessarily follow. In a retrospective x-ray film study of patients with Roy-Camille plates and pedicle screws, Saillant[129] noted that 10% of 375 screws in 56 patients were outside the pedicle cortex, and yet there were only two CSF leaks (which spontaneously resolved), and there were no neurologic deficits produced. Adding further to this benign experience, it should be noted that correct screw placement is much easier with the VSF, since there is no plate with fixed-position screw holes to "force" the screws into anatomically undesirable positions. Intraoperative use of an x-ray image intensifier also provides substantial additional safety.

The issue of anterior vs. posterior surgical approach is of course a complex one. Significant advances have been made in the design of anterior spinal implants. However, these devices are really only appropriate (1) in cases which require spinal canal decompression and (2) in cases for which the anterior surgical approach is selected, instead of a posterior or posterolateral approach. In all other cases, however, a posterior device is probably preferable.

---

*References 38, 60, 86, 89, 90, 119, 126, 127, 138, 146.

Vertebral Morphometry

The new data presented here extend significantly the dimensional information previously available,[129] relative to spinal fixation devices. CT scanning has been shown to be highly accurate (not surprisingly) compared to direct measurements, allowing preoperative measurements to be depended upon.

The pedicle axis (see Fig. 34-5) is almost always anteromedially directed, and gradually increases to substantial levels between L1 (11.5 degrees) and L5 (27.2 degrees), a finding differing somewhat from Saillant.[129] Our data tend to support the recommendation of Magerl[89,90] that pedicle screws be angulated anteromedially, following the axis of the pedicle. One benefit of this angulated placement is that right and left pedicle screws are not parallel, producing a "toenailing" effect which should substantially increase pull-out strength of the fully assembled fixator.

The size of screws previously reported for pedicle attachment vary from 3.2 mm minor diameter[112] up to 5.0 mm major diameter.[89,90] Our data (see Fig. 34-6 and 34-3) show that substantially larger screws may be safely accommodated by the pedicle at many vertebral levels. Whether it is mechanically beneficial to use a diameter larger than 5 mm remains to be established. Future experience with various sized screws, or alternatively measurement of the loads acting upon the fixator in vivo will be needed to resolve this issue.

Pedicle diameter is not influenced very much by screw approach angle. This is helpful for intraoperative safety in screw placement, since an exact screw placement angle is not necessary.

The fairly constant screw path length (see Fig. 34-7) found from T9 to L5 also benefits safety of screw placement, by preventing the need for a large range of screw sizes. Fine increments of screw lengths probably are also not needed, since exact placement of the screw tip just deep to the anterior cortex of the vertebral body appears to be unnecessary.[82,83] Intraoperative safety in screw placement is further aided by the observation that screw path length is consistently longer for more anteromedial screw angulation: this knowledge should help in preventing anterior cortex penetration.

Pedicle Screw Design

The pedicle screw design experiments reported here were undertaken because certain major questions remained unanswered by the fairly extensive literature on bone screws. Our data (see Tables 34-4 and 34-5) certainly do not provide the complete answers, but we believe that the test approach used here is a valuable one, since for the first time it allows the effect of various individual screw-design variables to be analyzed independently.

The issue of minor diameter is particularly interesting in applications such as ours in which the screw is subjected to bending and shear loads, as well as pull-out loads. A larger minor diameter increases the screw's resistance to bending, but its effect on pull-out strength has apparently not been previously tested, even though recommendations for a deep thread have been made[28,113] for cancellous screws. We predicted that changing the minor diameter should have no effect on pull-out, for the following reason. Screw pull-out causes shear failure of a cylinder of bone, equal to or somewhat greater than the major diameter of the screw.[75] The force need for pull-out is related to the surface area of this cylinder, which is determined only by the diameter and depth of penetration of the screw. Note that the minor diameter is unimportant: a smaller minor diameter (thus a deeper thread) does not change the area of bone which must be sheared off, and thus does not affect pull-out strength. A smaller diameter does produce a larger volume of bone interposed between the metal threads, but this is not the important parameter.

Thus we predicted that minor diameter would be a non-significant variable. Our results do not provide a clear-cut answer: minor diameter is significant for the 6 mm major diameter screws, but is not significant for the 7 mm screws. The explanation for this difference is not yet clear. One factor that may be important is the range of minor diameters used in our experiments. For the 7 mm major diameter screws the range was only 1 mm, whereas for the 6 mm major diameter screws the range was slightly larger, namely 1.2 mm. Perhaps this was just enough to produce the insignificance of minor diameter seen in the 7 mm screws. A larger sample size may also help resolve this issue.

From these data the obvious choice to maximize pull-out strength would be the 3.8 mm minor diameter for the 6 mm screws. However, this would produce a screw with substantially reduced resistance to bending loads (theoretically only 58% compared to a 5 mm minor diameter). The proper balancing between these two effects fundamentally requires knowing the in vivo loads acting on the fixator. In the absence of such data we have selected a minor diameter of 5 mm for the 6 mm major diameter screws, for two reasons. First, the actual pull-out strength of even the 5 mm minor screw is quite strong (1132-1248 N, or 514-567 pounds, for the buttress threads). Second, our estimate is that relatively higher demands will be made on the implant in vivo will arise from loads tending to produce screw bending, than from loads tending to produce screw pull-out. Bending resistance is improved by a larger minor diameter.

We predicted that pitch would also be a variable that does not have a significant effect on pull-out strength. The surface area of the cylinder of bone which must be sheared off during screw pull-out (as discussed above), is not affected by the pitch; for the smaller pitch, each tooth of bone is smaller, but the larger number of them exactly counterbalances this. This argument is particularly true for metal screws in bone, since the relatively high stiffness of metal produces a fairly uniform load distribution along the entire length of the screw.

Our data fairly strongly support this prediction. Pitch is insignificant in three out of the four areas in which it was tested (6 mm V tooth subgroup, 6 mm 3.8 minor diameter subgroup, and 7 mm B tooth subgroup). Pitch was significant only in the 6 mm B tooth subgroup. Surprisingly, it was the smaller pitch that was stronger (21%). This is in contrast to the view that widely separated threads (that is, a large pitch) provide greater resistance to pull-out,[113,148] a view that apparently has not been supported by biomechanical testing. Why pitch is a significant variable for the 6 mm major and not the 7 mm major B tooth subgroup (subexperiment 2) is not clear. Furthermore, why it should occur for the 6 mm major B tooth subgroup but not the V tooth subgroup is also not clear. Further testing will be needed for a resolution of this issue.

For current purposes we are using a pitch of 2 mm for the 6 mm major diameter screws. The reasons are (1) we have chosen the B (buttress) tooth pattern as discussed below, and it is for this subgroup that the lower pitch appears to be stronger, and (2) only minimal increased effort is involved in fabrication or implantation of the lower pitched screw. For the 7 mm major diameter screws, we have also chosen 2 mm pitch, for similarity to the 6 mm screws.

Concerning tooth profile, it seems to have been widely accepted that buttress (B) threads are superior to more traditional V threads. The essential features of the buttress thread are (1) the trailing edge is perpendicular (or very nearly so) to the long axis of the screw while the leading edge is inclined, and (2) the space between adjacent teeth is significantly greater than the space occupied by the teeth themselves.

It is not at all clear that the buttress thread is mechanically superior. The only directly applicable experimental work which seems to have been reported is that by Koranyi and coworkers.[75] Comparison was made of V and B threads of identical tooth height, but major diameters were not stated; one can only presume that they were the same. No rationale for use of buttress threads is mentioned by Muller[102] or Perren.[113] This latter work cites the extensive, pioneering experience of Danis.[28,29] However, neither of these monographs contains or cites experimental work related to this issue. The stated rationale for the asymmetric tooth profile is only that this thread pattern is used in the screws for attaching railway rails to the wooden ties.[29] The slope of the leading edge of each tooth was later steepened enough that the interspace between teeth was six times larger than the space occupied by the teeth themselves, the reason given being that bone is only one sixth as strong as metal.[28] Apart from the apparent absence of experimental support for this design, even on theoretical grounds this latter reason is not clearly valid: increasing the space between teeth does not alter the surface area of the cylinder of bone that must be sheared off to produce pull-out (as discussed above regarding pitch), and thus should not affect pull-out strength.

Our data (see Fig. 34-3) fail to show any significant difference between V and B threads, for any of the subgroups tested. This confirms our initial hypothesis. Faced with equivalent pull-out strengths, we have chosen to use a buttress thread simply for the reasons that (1) they may be slightly easier to implant, because a smaller volume of bone is crushed by the less-voluminous teeth and (2) many surgeons seem accustomed to using buttress threads.

Articulating Clamp

The three dimensional adjustability of the articulating clamp (see Figs. 34-2 and 34-3) provides a number of benefits: (1) safer pedicle screw placement, since correct anatomical placement is unconstrained by the VSF design, (2) easier pedicle screw placement since no special alignment between screws is required, (3) easy adjustment of fracture or spondylolisthesis reduction, even with the VSF fully implanted, and (4) accommodation to unusual anatomical configurations or only partially reducible fractures.

Based on cadaver implantation, as well as subjective comparison to existing implants, we believe that the compactness of this device is more than adequate. This is particularly true when one considers the substantially decreased length of this device compared to many currently used implants.

Although the in vivo loads to which this device will be exposed are not known for sure, the articular clamp component of the VSF certainly is not the "weak link" in the overall system. A pedicle screw placed at 80% depth of penetration can tolerate up to 8.72 Nm (6.41 ft. lbs) of "cut-out" or y-axis moment. The connecting rod, however, requires moments of 27.5 Nm (20.3 ft. lbs) before slippage occurs. This is a safety factor of more than 3. An even greater safety factor exists for "cut-up" or x-axis (extension) moments. The pedicle screw can tolerate 8.41 Nm (6.12 ft. lbs) while the articulating clamp attached to the head of the pedicle screw can tolerate 149 Nm, a safety factor of 18.

How strong does a spinal implant really need to be? Although significant research has been done concerning forces on the normal spine, only limited and partial information is known[*] concerning forces acting at the site of injury or other types of instability. Major unresolved issues include (1) to what extent does muscle activity alter the loads to which the implant is exposed, (2) to what extent can the unstable motion segment safety bear loads, and (3) what is the time-course of healing and return to normal load-bearing capacity.

It is only after such in vivo forces are known that optimal design of a spinal fixator can be completed.[79] The morphometric data that we present here define the upper limits on what the screw diameter and length could be, but the question remains of what the dimensions actually should be. To answer this question, we need to know the forces. We have shown the relative strengths of various pedicle screw designs, but a final selection among these designs requires knowledge of the forces. The static strength of the articulating clamp in our current prototype has been measured, but to what extent it may be "over-designed" depends upon the in vivo loads. Finally, we have measured the strengthening effect of a depth of pedicle screw penetration, but how much strength do we need? Again the knowledge of the in vivo loads is required.

SUMMARY

Presented here is a new type of posterior spinal implant for dealing with various types of destabilizing conditions (fractures, spondylolisthesis, degenerative "instability"). The major characteristics of this device, referred to as the Vermont Spinal Fixator (VSF) are (1) only two to three vertebrae need to be

---

[*]References 105, 106, 120, 132, 133, 136, 151, 163.

used; (2) it is a fixator and not a distractor or a compressor; (3) fixation is fully three-dimensional and is obained directly at the site of instability rather than two or three vertebrae away from it; (4) no reliance is placed upon intact soft tissues to achieve stabilization; (5) attachment is by means of specially designed screws into the vertebral body through the pedicles; (6) no violation of the spinal canal is required, such as with hooks or circumlaminar wires; (7) the VSF is fully internalized, with no pins transfixing skin and muscle; and (8) a three dimensionally adjustable articulating clamp mechanism allows safe and easy pedicle screw placement (no special alignments between screws is needed), as well as full adjustability of fracture or spondylolisthesis reduction even after VSF implantation.

New experimental data are reported concerning pertinent vertebral dimensions. These data show that the pedicle can safely accommodate a vertebral screw of ample diameter in almost all cases. Safety is further enhanced by (1) the near constancy in screw path length at different vertebral levels, (2) the dependable orientation and diameter of the pedicles, and (3) the knowledge that path length is longer with anteromedial angulation of the screw.

Mechanical testing was performed on a variety of experimental pedicle screw designs, using various combinations of minor diameter, pitch and tooth pattern. A special experimental design allowed the effect of each variable to be isolated. Minor diameter appears to be a significant variable for 6 mm but not 7 mm screws. Pitch is insignificant in three out of four areas tested, and tooth pattern is insignificant in all areas tested.

The strength of the articulating clamp has been determined for static loading. This device can readily accommodate loads that are high compared to pedicle screw attachment strength, which in turn has been shown by extensive clinical experience to be adequately secure.

Mechanical testing of various pedicle screw depths of penetration has been performed, addressing the conflicting recommendations in the literature concerning this issue. Our data show that an approximately 30% gain in screw-placement strength occurs by increasing depth of penetration from 50% to 80%. Whether this is functionally significant will require knowledge concerning in vivo implant loads.

Cadaver implantation has demonstrated the ease with which the VSF may be implanted. Fatigue testing is currently under way to document the security of the articulating clamp against loosening. Clinical implantations are planned in the near future. Postoperative monitoring of residual motion at the site of instability will be used to assess the in vivo mechanical performance of the VSF.

REFERENCES

1. Akbarnia, B.A., et al.: Contoured Harrington instrumentation in the treatment of unstable spinal fractures: the effect of supplementary sublaminar wires, Clin. Orthop. **189:**186, 1984.
2. Amis, J., and Herring, J.A.: Iatrogenic kyphosis: a complication of Harrington instrumentation in Marfan's syndrome: a case report, J. Bone Joint Surg. **66A:**460, 1984.
3. Anden, U., et al.: The role of the anterior longitudinal ligament in Harrington rod fixation of unstable thoracolumbar spinal fractures, Spine **5:**23, 1980.
4. Armstrong, G.W.D.: Harrington instrumentation for spinal fractures, Proc. Scoli. Res. Soc. 1976.
5. Attenborough, C.O., and Reynolds, M.T.: Lumbo-sacral fusion with spring fixation, J. Bone Joint Surg. **57B:**282, 1975.
6. Barrack, R.L., et al.: Retrieval and analysis of failed Harrington rods, Proc. Ortho. Res. Soc. 1983.
7. Bechtol, C.O.: Internal fixation with plates and screws. In Bechtol, C.O., et al.: Metals and engineering in bone and joint surgery Baltimore, 1959, Williams & Wilkins.

8. Benner, B., et al.: Instrumentation of the spine for fracture dislocations in children, Child's Brain 3(4):249, 1977.
9. Blackman, R., and Toton, J.: The sublaminal pathway of wires removed in SSI, Proc. Scoli. Res. Soc. 1984.
10. Blumlein, H., et al.: Longterm measurements of axial tension in bone screws in vivo (German), Zeitschr. Orthop. 115:603, 1977.
11. Bobechko, W.P.: The instant Harrington, Proc. Scoli. Res. Soc. 1981.
12. Bohler, J.L.: Operative treatment of fractures of the dorsal and lumbar spine, J. Trauma 10:1119, 1970.
13. Bohlman, H.H.: Current concepts review. Treatment of fractures and dislocations of the thoracic and lumbar spine, J. Bone Joint Surg. 67A:165, 1985.
14. Boucher, H.H.: A method of spinal fusion, J. Bone Joint Surg. 41B:248, 1959.
15. Bridwell, K.H.: The treatment of flexion/distraction spinal fractures with SSI and Luque rectangles, Proc. Scoli. Res. Soc. 1984.
16. Brown, C.W., Donaldson, D.H., Odom, J.A., Jr.: A new approach to low lumbar fractures, Proc. Scoli. Res. Soc. 1984.
17. Brunski, J.B., and Hill, D.C.: Stresses in a Harrington distraction rod: their origin and relationship to fatigue fractures in vivo, Proc. Orthop. Res. Soc., Anaheim, Calif., 1983.
18. Bryant, C.E., and Sullivan, J.A.: Management of thoracic and lumbar spine fractures with Harrington distraction rods supplemented with segmental wiring, Spine 8:532, 1983.
19. Cabot, J.R., et al.: La panarthrodese lombosacree avec la plaque crabe, Acta Orthop. Belg. 47(4-5):657, 1981.
20. Casey, M.P., and Jacobs, R.R.: Internal fixation of the lumbosacral spine: a biomechanical evaluation, Proc. Int. Soc. Study Lumbar Spine, 1984.
21. Casey, M.P., et al.: The rod long-fuse short technique in the treatment of thoracolumbar and lumbar spine fractures, Proc. Scoli. Res. Soc. 1984.
22. Convery, F.R., et al.: Fracture-dislocation of the dorsal-lumbar spine: acute operative stabilization by Harrington instrumentation, Spine 3:160, 1978.
23. Cordey, J., and Perren, S.M.: Limits of plate on bone friction in internal fixation of fractures, Proc. Orthop. Res. Soc. 1985.
24. Craig, F.S.: Vertebral-body biopsy, J. Bone Joint Surg. 38A:93-97, 1956.
25. Cyron, B.M., et al.: Spondylolytic fractures, J. Bone Joint Surg. 58B:462, 1976.
26. Daniaux, H.: Technik und Ergebnisse der transpedikularen Spongiosaplastik bei Bruchen in thorakolumbalen Ubergangs und Lendenwirbelsaulebereich, Hefte Unfallheilkunde 165:182, 1983.
27. Daniaux, H.: Technik und erste Ergebnisse der transpedikularen Spongiosaplastik bei kompressions Bruchen in Lenden-wirbelsaulebereich, Acta Chir. Aust. (Suppl.) 43: 79, 1982.
28. Danis, R.: Theorie et pratique de l'osteosynthese, Paris, 1949, Masson Publishers.
29. Danis, R.: Technique de l'osteosynthese: Etude de quelque procedes, Paris, 1932, Masson Publishers.
30. Denis, F., et al.: Acute thoracolumbar burst fractures in the absence of neurologic deficit: a comparison between operative and nonoperative treatment, Clin. Orthop. 189:142, 1984.
31. Denis, F., et al.: Comparison between square-ended distraction rods and standard round-ended distraction rods in the treatment of thoracolumbar spinal injuries: a statistical analysis, Clin. Orthop. 189:162, 1984.
32. Dewald, R.L.: Burst fractures of the thoracic and lumbar spine, Clin. Orthop. 189:150, 1984.
33. Dickson, J.H., et al.: Results of reduction and stabilization of the severely fractured thoracic and lumbar spine, J. Bone Joint Surg. 60A:799, 1978.
34. Drummond, D., et al.: Interspinous segmental spinal instrumentation for unstable fractures, Proc. Scoli. Res. Soc. 1984.
35. Dunn, H.K.: Anterior stabilization of thoracolumbar injuries, Clin. Orthop. 189:116, 1984.
36. Dunn, H.K., et al.: A comparison of spinal bending stability with posterior and anterior fixation devices, Proc. Scoli. Res. Soc. 1979.
37. Dunn, H.K., and Bolstad, K.E.: Fixation of Dwyer screws for the treatment of scoliosis, J. Bone Joint Surg. 59A:54, 1977.
38. Edwards, C.C.: Sacral fixation device: design and preliminary results, Proc. Scoli. Res. Soc. 1984.
39. Edwards, C.C., et al.: A new spinal hook: rationale and clinical trials, Proc. Scoli. Res. Soc. 1984.
40. Edwards, C.C., et al.: Determinants of hook dislodgement: rigidity of fixation, rod clearance, and hook design, Proc. Int. Soc. Study Lumbar Spine, Montreal, 1984.

41. Edwards, C.C., et al.: Early clinical results using the spinal rod sleeve method for treating thoracic and lumbar injuries, Proc. Am. Acad. Orthop. Surg. 1982.
42. Edwards, C.C.: The spinal rod sleeve. Its rationale and use in thoracic and lumbar injuries, Proc. Orthop. Res. Soc. 1981.
43. Erwin, W.D., et al.: Clinical review of patients with broken Harrington rods, J. Bone Joint Surg. **62A:**1302, 1980.
44. Flesch, J.R., et al.: Harrington instrumentation and spine fusion for unstable fractures and fracture-dislocations on the thoracic and lumbar spine, J. Bone Joint Surg. **59A:**143, 1977.
45. Floman, Y., et al.: The simultaneous application of a compressive wire and Harrington distraction rods in the treatment of fracture dislocation of the thoracolumbar spine, Proc. Israel Ortho. Soc. 1980.
46. Frymoyer, J.W., and Krag, M.H.: Spinal stability and instability: general concepts. In Schmidek, H., and Frymoyer, J.W.: The unstable thoracic and lumbosacral spine, New York, 1985, Grune & Stratton, Inc.
47. Frymoyer, J.W., and Selby, D.: Segmental instability: rationale for treatment, Spine **10:**280, 1985.
48. Gaines, R.W., et al.: Stabilization of thoracic and thoracolumbar fracture-dislocations with Harrington rods and sublaminar wires, Clin. Orthop. **189:**195, 1984.
49. Gaines, R.W., and Humphreys, W.G.: A plea for judgment in management of thoracolumbar fractures and fracture-dislocations: a reassessment of surgical indications, Clin. Orthop. **189:**36, 1984.
50. Gaines, R.W., et al.: Harrington distraction rods supplemented with sublaminar wires for thoracolumbar fracture dislocation: experimental and clinical investigation, Proc. Scoli. Res. Soc. 1982.
51. Gardner, A.D.H.: Four years' experience with an anterior spinal distraction device for the correction of kyphotic deformities, and its use as a permanent implant. Proc. Scoli. Res. Soc. 1982.
52. Gertzbien, S.D., et al.: Harrington instrumentation as a method of fixation in fractures of the spine: a critical analysis of deficiencies, J. Bone Joint Surg. **64B:**526, 1982.
53. Goel, V.K., et al.: Biomechanics of the Harrington instrumentation for injuries in the thoraco-lumbar spine, Proc. Internat. Soc. Biomech. 1983.
54. Hall, J.E.: Dwyer instrumentation in anterior fusion of the spine: current concepts review, J. Bone Joint Surg. **63A:**1188, 1981.
55. Hannon, K.M.: Harrington instrumentation in fractures and dislocations of the thoracic and lumbar spine, South Med. J. **69:**1269, 1976.
56. Hardy, A.G.: Treatment of paraplegia due to fracture-dislocation of the dorsolumbar spine, Paraplegia **3:**112, 1965.
57. Harrington, P.R.: History and development of Harrington instrumentation, Clin. Orthop. **93:**110, 1973.
58. Harrington, P.R.: Instrumentation in spine stability other than scoliosis, S. Afr. J. Surg. **5:**7, 1967.
59. Hasday, C., et al.: Gait abnormalities arising from iatrogenic loss of lumbar lordosis secondary to Harrington instrumentation in lumbar fractures, Proc. Scoli. Res. Soc. 1982.
60. Hermann, H.D.: Transarticular (transpedicular) metal plate fixation for stabilization of the lumbar and thoracic spine, Acta Neurochir. (Wien) **48**(1-2):101, 1979.
61. Jacobs, R.R., and Casey, M.P.: Surgical management of thoracolumbar spinal injuries. General principles and controversial considerations, Clin. Orthop. **189:**22, 1984.
62. Jacobs, R.R., et al.: A locking hook spinal rod system for stabilization of fracture-dislocations and correction of deformities of the dorsolumbar spine: a biomechanic evaluation, Clin. Orthop. **189:**168, 1984.
63. Jacobs, R.R., et al.: A locking hook-spinal rod: current status of development, Paraplegia **21:**197, 1983.
64. Jacobs, R.R., et al.: A locking hook-spinal rod: a preliminary clinical report on its use in thirty thoracolumbar spinal injuries, Proc. Int. Soc. Study Lumbar Spine, 1982.
65. Jacobs, R.R., et al.: Reduction, stability, and strength provided by internal fixation systems for thoracolumbar spinal injuries, Clin. Orthop. **171:**300, 1982.
66. Jacobs, R.R., et al.: Thoracolumbar spinal injuries: a comparative study of recumbent and operative treatment in 100 patients, Spine **5:**463, 1980.
67. Johnston, C.E, II, et al.: Delayed paraplegia following segmental spinal instrumentation, Proc. Scoli. Res. Soc. 1984.
68. Kahanovitz, N., et al.: The effects of internal fixation on the articular cartilage of unfused canine facet joint cartilage, Spine **9:**268, 1984.
69. Kahanovitz, N., et al.: The effect of internal fixation without arthrodesis on human facet joint cartilage, Clin. Orthop. **189:**204, 1984.

70. Kaneda, K., et al.: Burst fractures with neurologic deficits of the thoracolumbar-lumbar spine: results of anterior decompression and stabilization with anterior instrumentation, Spine 9(8):788, 1984.
71. Kaneda, K., et al.: Biomechanical study of the anterior spinal fixation device in pig spine, Proc. Scoli. Res. Soc. 1984.
72. Keene, J.S., et al.: Mechanical performance of the Wisconsin compression system, Proc. Orth. Res. Soc. 1980.
73. Kempf, I., et al.: Osteosynthesis of dorsolumbar spinal fractures. Biomechanical approach and comparative study: reversed Harrington pins and hooks. Roy-Camille bone plates (French), Rev. Chirurg. Orthop. 65(11):43, 1979.
74. King, D.: Internal fixation for lumbosacral spine fusions, J. Bone Joint Surg. 30A:560, 1948.
75. Koranyi, E., et al.: Holding power of orthopaedic screws in bone, Clin. Orthop. 72:283, 1970.
76. Kostuik, J.P., et al.: Comparison of spinal fracture fixation devices under dynamic cyclical loading of calf spines, Proc. Scoli. Res. Soc. 1984.
77. Kostuik, J.P., et al.: Posterior segmental spinal instrumentation in adults, Proc. Scoli. Res. Soc. 1984.
78. Krag, M.H., et al.: Effect of minor diameter, pitch, and tooth profile on pull-out strength of transpedicular vertebral screws: application to surgical spinal fixation (submitted for publication), 1985.
79. Krag, M.H., et al.: Mechanisms of spine trauma and features of spinal fixation methods. In Ghista, D.N., ed. Mechanisms of injury, Springfield, Ill., 1986, Charles C Thomas, Publisher.
80. Krag, M.H., and Weaver, D.L.: Morphometry of the thoracic and lumbar spine related to transpedicular screw placement for surgical spinal fixation (Submitted for publication), 1985.
81. LaBorde, J.M., et al.: Comparison of fixation of spinal fractures, Clin. Orthop. 152:303, 1980.
82. Lavaste, F.: Biomechanical experimental study on the thoracic and lumbar spine (French), Thesis "Ingeneur," Ecole Nationale des Ars et Metiers a Paris, 1979.
83. Lavaste, F.: Biomechanique du rachis dorsolombaire. Deuxieme Journees d'Orthop. de la Pitie, Paris, 1980, Masson Publishers.
84. Lewis, J., and McKibbin, B.: Treatment of unstable fracture-dislocations of the thoracolumbar spine accompanied by paraplegia, J. Bone Joint Surg. 56B:603, 1974.
85. Liu, Y.K., et al.: Torsional fatigue of the lumbar intervertebral joint, Spine 10:894, 1985.
86. Louis, R.: Single-staged posterior lumbosacral fusion by internal fixation with screw-plates, Proc. Int. Soc. Study Lumbar Spine, 1985.
87. Luque, E.R., et al.: Segmental spinal instrumentation in the treatment of fractures of the thoracolumbar spine, Spine, Spine 7:312,
88. Lyon, W.F., et al.: Actual holding power of various screws in bone, Ann. Surg. 114:376, 1941.
89. Magerl, F.P.: External spinal skeletal fixation. In Weber, B.G., and Magerl, F.P.: The external fixator, New York, 1985, Springer-Verlag.
90. Magerl, F.P.: Stabilization of the lower thoracic and lumbar spine with external skeletal fixation, Clin. Orthop. 189:125, 1984.
91. Magerl, F.P.: Clinical application on the thoracolumbar junction and the lumbar spine. In Mears, D.C., editor: External skeletal fixation, Baltimore, 1983, Williams & Wilkins.
92. Magerl, F.P.: External skeletal fixation of the lower thoracic and the lumbar spine. In Uhthoff, H.K., and Stahl, E.: Current concepts of external fixation of fractures, New York, 1982, Springer-Verlag.
93. McAfee, P.C., et al.: A biomechanical analysis of spinal instrumentation systems in thoracolumbar fractures: comparison of traditional Harrington distraction instrumentation with segmental spinal instrumentation, Spine 10(3):204, 1985.
94. McAfee, P.C., et al.: Anterior decompression of traumatic thoracolumbar fractures with incomplete neurological deficit using a retroperitoneal approach, J. Bone Joint Surg. 67A:89, 1985.
95. McAfee, P.C., and Bohlman, H.H.: Complications of Harrington instrumentation in thoracolumbar fractures: ten year experience, Proc. Scoli. Res. Soc. 1984.
96. McAfee, P.C., et al.: A biomechanical analysis of spinal instrumentation systems in thoracolumbar fractures: comparison of traditional Harrington distraction instrumentation with segmental spinal instrumentation, Proc. Scoli. Res. Soc. 1984.

97. McAfee, P.C., et al.: The unstable burst fracture, Spine **7**:365, 1982.
98. Miller, F., et al.: Biomechanical analysis of segmental spine fixation in a fracture model, Proc. Ortho. Res. Soc. 1982.
99. Mino, D.E., et al.: Torsional loading of Harrington distraction rod instrumentation compared to segmental sublaminar and spinous process supplementation, Proc. Scoli. Res. Soc. 1984.
100. Moe, J.H., and Denis, F.: The iatrogenic loss of lumbar lordosis, Proc. Scoli. Res. Soc. 1976.
101. Morris, J.M., et al.: Role of the trunk in stability of the spine, J. Bone Joint Surg. **43A**:327, 1961.
102. Muller, M.E., et al.: Manual of internal fixation, ed. 2, New York, 1979, Springer-Verlag.
103. Munson, G., et al.: Experimental evaluation of Harrington rod fixation supplemented with sublaminar wires in stabilizing thoracolumbar fracture-dislocations, Clin. Orthop. **189**:97, 1984.
104. Murphy, M.J., et al.: Treatment of the unstable thoracolumbar spine with comparison Harrington distraction and compression rods, Proc. Scoli. Res. Soc. 1981.
105. Nachemson, A., and Efstrom, G.: Intravital wireless telemetry of axial forces in Harrington distraction rods in patients with idiopathic scoliosis, J. Bone Joint Surg. **53A**:445, 1971.
106. Nagel, D.A., et al.: In vivo measurement of load on Harrington distraction rods in sheep spines with and without fusion, Proc. Ortho. Res. Soc. 1984.
107. Nagel, D.A., et al.: Stability of the upper lumbar spine following progressive disruptions and the application of individual internal and external fixation devices, J. Bone Joint Surg. **63A**:62, 1981.
108. Nicastro, J.F., et al.: Intraspinal pathways of sublaminar wires during surgical removal, Proc. Scoli. Res. Soc. 1984.
109. Nunamaker, D.M., and Perren, S.M.: Force measurements in screw fixation, J. Biomech. **9**:669, 1976.
110. Ogilvie, J.W., and Bradford, D.S.: Lumbar and lumbosacral fusion with segmental fixation, Proc. Scoli. Res. Soc. 1984.
111. Osebold, W.R., et al.: Thoracolumbar spine fractures: results of treatment, Spine **6**:13, 1981.
112. Pennal, G.F., et al.: Method of spinal fusion using internal fixation, Clin. Orthop. **35**:86, 1964.
113. Perren, S.M.: Physical and biological aspects of fracture healing with special reference to internal fixation, Clin. Orthop. **138**:175, 1979.
114. Pietruszka, I.: Early rehabilitation after fracture fixation using Daab's serrate plate and cancellous autotransplants (Polish), Chir. Narzadow Ruch, Ortop. Pol. **45**(6):507, 1980.
115. Pinto, W.C., et al.: An anterior distractor for the intraoperative correction of angular kyphosis, Spine **3**:309, 1978.
116. Pope, M.H., et al.: Fixation methods. In Ghista, D.N., editor: Mechanisms of spine trauma and features of spinal fixation methods. II. Springfield, Ill., 1986, Charles C Thomas, Publisher.
117. Pope, M.H., and Panjabi, M.: Biomechanical definitions of spinal stability, Spine **10**(3):255, 1985.
118. Purcell, G.A., et al.: Twelfth thoracic-first lumbar vertebral mechanical stability of fractures after Harrington rod instrumentation, J. Bone Joint Surg. **63A**:71, 1981.
119. Puschel, J., and Zielke, K.: Transpedicular vertebral instrumentation using VDS instruments in ankylosing spondylitis, Proc. Scoli. Res. Soc. 1984.
120. Quintin, J., et al.: Mesure de la deformation des implant in vivo, Acta Orthop. Belg. **48**(4):688, 1982.
121. Rezaian, S.M., et al.: Spinal fixator for the management of spinal injury (the mechanical rationale), Engin. in Med. **12**:95, 1983.
122. Roaf, R.: A study of the mechanics of spinal injuries, J. Bone Joint Surg. **43B**:810, 1960.
123. Rossier, A.B., and Cochran, T.P.: The treatment of spinal fractures with Harrington compression rods and segmental sublaminar wiring: a dangerous combination, Spine **9**(8):796, 1984.
124. Roy-Camille, R., et al.: Behandlung von Wirbelfrakturen und -luxation am thorakolumbalen Ubergang, Orthopaedie **9**:63, 1980.
125. Roy-Camille, R., et al.: Vertebral osteosynthesis using metal plates: Its different uses (French), Chirurg. **105**(7):597, 1979.
126. Roy-Camille, R., et al.: Early management of spinal injuries. In McKibbin, B., editor: Recent advances in Orthop. New York, 1979, Churchill-Livingstone, Inc.
127. Roy-Camille, R., et al.: Osteosynthesis of thoracolumbar spine fractures with metal plates screwed through the vertebral pedicles, Reconstr. Surg. Traumatol. **15**:2, 1976.

128. Ryan, M.D., et al.: New instrumentation for anterior lumbar and thoracolumbar interbody spinal fusion, Proc. Scoli. Res. Soc. 1981.
129. Saillant, G.: Anatomical study of vertebral pedicles: surgical application (French), Rev. Chirurg. Orthop. **62**(2):157, 1976.
130. Savastano, A.A., et al.: Experiences with Harrington instrumentation for unstable fractures of the truncal spine, Rhode Island Med. J. **62**(8):325, 1979.
131. Schatzker, J., et al.: The holding power of orthopaedic screws in vivo, Clin. Orthop. **108**:115, 1975.
132. Schlaepfer, F., et al.: Stabilization of the lower thoracic and lumbar spine: comparative in vitro investigation of an external skeletal and various internal fixation devices. In Uhthoff, H.K., and Stahl, E., editors: Current concepts of external fixation of fractures, New York, 1982, Springer-Verlag.
133. Schlaepfer, F., et al.: In vivo measurements of loads on an external fixation device for human lumbar spine fractures, Inst. of Mech. Eng. **C131/80**:59, 1980.
134. Schlicke, L., and Schulak, J.: The simultaneous use of Harrington compression and distraction rods in a thoracolumbar fracture-dislocation, J. Trauma **20**:177, 1980.
135. Schmidek, H.H., et al.: Management of acute instable thoracolumbar (T11-L1) fractures with and without neurological deficit, Neurosurgery **7**:30, 1980.
136. Shapiro, F.D., et al.: Telemetric monitoring of cable tensions following Dwyer spinal instrumentation in dogs, Spine **3**:213, 1978.
137. Shen, G., et al.: Biomechanical aspects of Harrington spinal instrumentation, Proc. Scoli. Res. Soc. 1978.
138. Sijbrandij, S.: A new technique for the reduction and stabilization of severe spondylolisthesis, J. Bone Joint Surg. **63B**:266, 1981.
139. Slot, G.H.: A new distraction system for the correction of kyphosis using the anterior approach, Proc. Scoli. Res. Soc. 1981.
140. Stauffer, E.S.: Current concepts review: internal fixation of thoracolumbar spine fractures, J. Bone Joint Surg. **66A**:1136, 1984.
141. Stauffer, E.S., and Neil, Y.L.: Biomechanical analysis of structural stability of internal fixation in fractures of the thoracolumbar spine, Clin. Orthop. **112**:159, 1975.
142. Sullivan, J.A.: Sublaminar wiring of Harrington distraction rods for unstable thoracolumbar spine fractures, Clin. Orthop. **189**:178, 1984.
143. Taylor, T.K.F., and Cummine, J.: Harrington instrumentation for fractures and dislocations of the thoracolumbar spine, J. Bone Joint Surg. **60B**:289, 1978.
144. Tello, C.A.: Early results with a variation of spinal instrumentation, Proc. Scoli. Res. Soc. 1984.
145. Trias, A., et al.: Modified Harrington rod, Proc. Scoli. Res. Soc. Denver, Colo., 1982.
146. Vercauteren, M., et al.: Reduction of spondylolisthesis with severe slipping, Acta Orthop. Belg. **47**(4-5):502, 1981.
147. Vlahovitch, B., and Fuentes, J.M.: Recent fractures of the dorsolumbar spine. Reduction of the double shroud technique (French), Nouv. Presse Med. **6**:3107, 1977.
148. Wagner, H.: Die einbetting von Metalschrauben im Knochen und die Heilungsforgange des unter dem einflus der stabilen Osteosynthese, Langenbeck Arch. Klin. Chir. **305**:28, 1963.
149. Ward, J.J., et al.: Cyclic torsional testing of Harrington and Luque spinal implants, Proc. Scoli. Res. Soc. 1984.
150. Ward, J.J., et al.: Biomechanical evaluation of the neural arch, Proc. Scoli. Res. Soc. 1984.
151. Waugh, T.R.: Intravital measurements during instrumental correction of idiopathic scoliosis, Acta Orthop. Scand. Suppl. **93**:1, 1966.
152. Weiss, M.: Dynamic spine alloplasty (spring-loading corrective devices) after fracture and spinal cord injury, Clin. Orthop. **112**:150, 1975.
153. Wenger, D.R., et al.: Laboratory testing of segmental spinal instrumentation versus traditional Harrington instrumentation for scoliosis treatment, Spine **7**:265, 1982.
154. Wenger, D., et al.: Evaluation of fixation sites for segmental instrumentation of the human vertebra, Proc. Scoli. Res. Soc. 1981.
155. White, A.H., et al.: Knodt rod distraction lumbar fusion, Spine **8**:434, 1983.
156. Whitesides, T.E., Jr., and Shaw, S.G.A.: On the management of unstable fractures of the thoracolumbar spine: rationale for use of anterior decompression and fusion and posterior stabilization, Spine **1**:99, 1976.
157. Wilber, R.G., et al.: Postoperative neural deficits in segmental instrumentation: a study using spinal cord monitoring, J. Bone Joint Surg. **66A**:1178, 1984.
158. Wilder, D.G., et al.: Cyclic loading of the intervertebral motion segment, Proc. Northeast Bioeng. Conf., Hanover, New Hampshire, 1982.

159. Willen, J., et al.: Thoracolumbar crush fracture: an experimental study on instant axial dynamic loading: the resulting fracture type and its stability, Spine **9:**624, 1984.
160. Willen, J., et al.: Unstable thoracolumbar fractures: a study by CT and conventional roentgenology of the reduction effect of Harrington instrumentation, Spine **9:**214, 1984.
161. Williams, E.W.M.: Traumatic paraplegia. In Mathews, D.N., editor: Recent advances in surgery of trauma, New York, 1963, Churchill-Livingstone, Inc.
162. Wilson, P.D., and Straub, L.R.: Lumbosacral fusion with metallic-plate fixation, Instructional course lectures: The American Academy of Orthopaedic Surgeons, St. Louis, 1952, The C.V. Mosby Co.
163. Worsdorfer, O.: Operative stabilization of thoracolumbar and lumbar vertebrae: comparative biomechanical investigation of the stability and stiffness of various dorsal fixation systems (German). Thesis (Habilitationsschrift), Clinical-Medical Faculty, University of Ulm, Sweden, 1981.
164. Yamagata, M.: Biomechanical study of posterior spinal instrumentation for scoliosis, J. Jpn. Orthop. Assoc. **58:**523, 1984.
165. Yosipovitch, Z., et al.: Open reduction of instable thoracolumbar spinal injuries and fixation with Harrington rods, J. Bone Joint Surg. **59A:**1003, 1977.
166. Zindrick, M.R., et al.: A biomechanical study of intrapedicular screw fixation in the lumbosacral spine, Proc. Int. Soc. Study Lumbar Spine, 1985.

CHAPTER

35

ANTERIOR LUMBAR INTERBODY FUSION: STEP-BY-STEP PROCEDURE AND PITFALLS

Bryan Barber

Anterior lumbar interbody fusion (ALIF) has been proved in several large series to be a valuable and effective means of obtaining arthrodesis in the lumbar (and thoracic) spine. Its advantages are many and the disadvantages few for those surgeons who have adequately prepared themselves to perform this procedure. The complications, on the other hand, can be substantial for the uninitiated, that is, the surgeon who does not take the opportunity to watch the procedure being performed by one who is experienced in the procedure or the surgeon who is not familiar with the anatomy of the abdominal cavity and the retroperitoneal space. The prepared and meticulous surgeon, however, will find the ALIF a tremendous aid in the stabilization of one or more motion segments.

HISTORY

The ALIF is not a new procedure. Burns[1] was the first to report its use in a young man with spondylolisthesis in 1933. Since then, there have been numerous reports by many surgeons concerning its effectiveness.[2,4-6,9-17,19-22]

ADVANTAGES

The interbody fusion is biomechanically the most stable of all fusions, if one compares it to any other single kind of fusion (see Chapter 6). Other advantages are:

1. The ALIF avoids violation of the spinal canal and its nerve roots, thereby reducing the formation of scar tissue and its proclivity for causing chronic pain.
2. The ALIF has been demonstrated pragmatically to significantly reduce sciatica in the patient who has had a previous unsuccessful discectomy.[10]
3. It offers some degree of immediate stabilization of the motion segment(s).
4. It has an acceptable fusion rate, if not superior to other kinds of bone stabilization procedures.

5. It can decompress the bulging or herniated disc.

6. The ALIF can restore the vertical height of a disc to a large degree (dramatic restoration of the vertical height is not advised in those patients suspected of having arachnoiditis, since such restoration may increase painful tethering of nerve roots).

DISADVANTAGES

The disadvantages can be considerable in the hands of the uninitiated. The trained, meticulous surgeon, however, can avoid almost all of these disadvantages. The disadvantages are as follows in order of severity.

1. Damage to nerve roots of the cauda equina resulting from instrument violation of the spinal canal
2. Laceration of the inferior vena cava or iliac veins (very fragile structures that are difficult to repair) or the abdominal aorta and iliac arteries (less fragile, more resistant to injury, and easier to repair)
3. Damage to the superior hypogastric plexus with resultant retrograde ejaculation (actual incidence of this complication is quite low, 0.42%)[7]
4. Rare pulmonary embolism, minimized with aspirin after surgery
5. Excessive blood loss during surgery (can be markedly reduced by proper technique as discussed later)
6. Abdominal wall hernia (can be avoided with proper technique)
7. Not substantially useful in retrieving a sequestered disc or lysing adhesions in the spinal canal

TECHNIQUE
Preparation of the Patient

With the patient supine on the operating table and under general endotracheal anesthesia, a nasogastric (NG) tube and Foley catheter are inserted. The NG tube decompresses the stomach throughout the procedure and thus makes for better exposure of the spine. The NG tube also shortens the time of postoperative ileus that usually occurs (it is usually 2 to 3 days before the patient can take fluids or food by mouth). The Foley catheter deflates the bladder, because a full bladder can cause some obstruction when fusing the L5-S1 space.

Intravenously, 1 g of Ancef is given by push and 1 g Ancef is placed in the IV system (1000 ml Ringer's lactate). After surgery, the patient receives Ancef 500 mg intravenously every 6 hours for 24 hours.

Retroperitoneal Exposure

Exposure of the anterior lumbar spine can be accomplished by more than one approach. One can use a subcostal oblique approach or an abdominal approach, the latter by a midline or paramedian incision. I use the left paramedian incision, which is made and carried down through the subcutaneous tissue to the fascia of the rectus abdominis, electrocoagulating all bleeders encountered (Fig. 35-1). Self-retaining retractors are placed in the wound, and the anterior rectus sheath is incised the length of the wound. Kochers and then applied to the medial edge of the anterior rectus sheath, and the sheath is lifted to expose the attachment of the tendinous intersections to the linea alba (Fig. 35-2). These attachments are defined, clamped, transected and tied with 2-0 polyglycolic sutures. Any branches of the superior or inferior epigastric vessels (beneath the rectus abdominis muscle) that interfere with lateral retraction of the rectus abdominis are similarly ligated.

Next, the rectus abdominis muscle is retracted laterally, and the arcuate line is identified (Fig. 35-3). The arcuate line is actually the distal end of the posterior rectus sheath (the sheath is quite thick). The visceral peritoneum is loosely ad-

370 *Surgical Procedures*

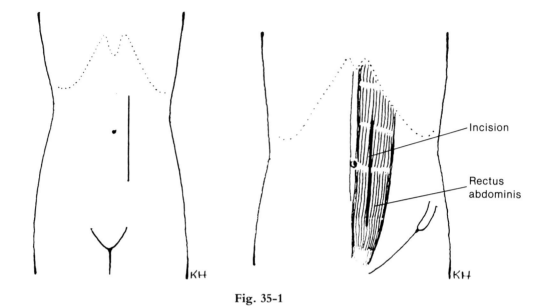

Fig. 35-1

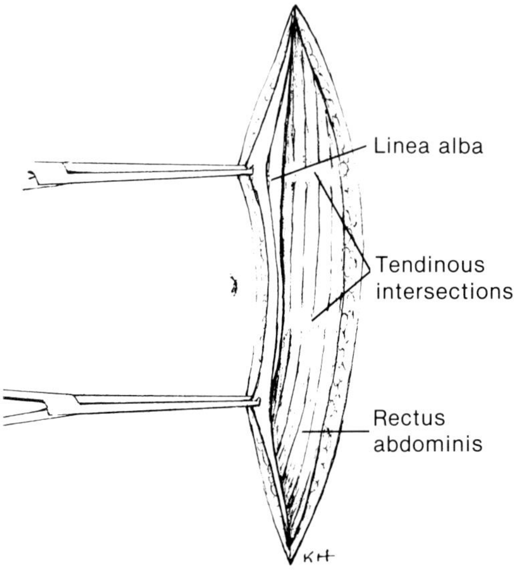

Fig. 35-2

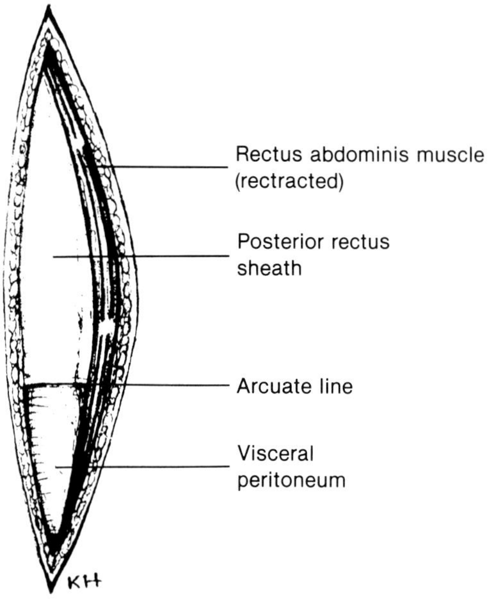

Fig. 35-3

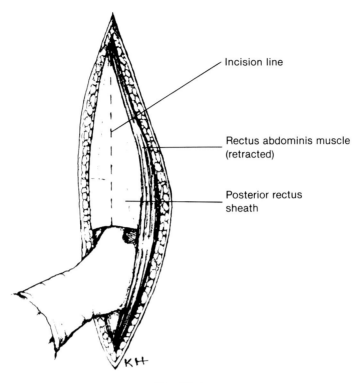

Fig. 35-4

hered to the undersurface of the posterior rectus sheath. At the arcuate line, the visceral peritoneum can be seen to progress distally toward the pubis, ultimately blending with the transversalis fascia (see Fig. 35-3). The visceral peritoneum must be separated from its attachment from the undersurface of the posterior rectus sheath. This can usually be accomplished by blunt finger dissection (Fig. 35-4). Occasionally, it is necessary to use Kittners (peanuts) at the arcuate line to develop this plane.

Another way to separate the visceral peritoneum from the posterior rectus sheath is to separate the visceral peritoneum distal and lateral to the arcuate line from its attachment to the parietal peritoneum laterally by blunt finger dissection (see Fig. 35-4). In this way the surgeon can sneak up to the lateral edge of the arcuate line through the distal retroperitoneal space, which is the space the surgeon is attempting to enter. Once the visceral peritoneum has been separated from the posterior rectus sheath, the sheath is incised in its midline as far proximal as possible with scissors (see Fig. 35-4).

Next, the abdominal contents are swept to the patient's right and cephalad by means of blunt finger dissection between the visceral and parietal peritoneum, that is, the abdominal contents are taken to the patient's right and cephalad, thus exposing the lumbar spine (beneath the great vessels) (Fig. 35-5). At this point one can appreciate the left ureter to have traveled along with the visceral peritoneum and its contents. Any rents in the visceral peritoneum are closed at this time with 2-0 chromic catgut.

Next, the very thin parietal peritoneum overlying the great vessels is incised with the Metzenbaum scissors to expose those disc spaces that are to be arthodesed (see Fig. 35-5). If the parietal

372 *Surgical Procedures*

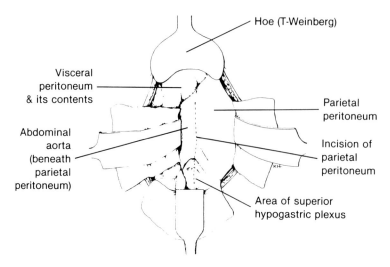

Fig. 35-5

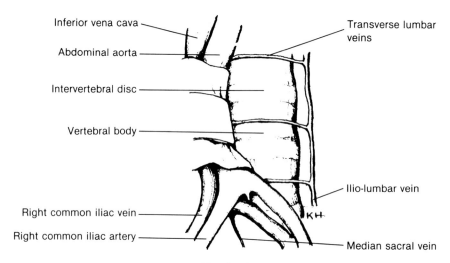

Fig. 35-6

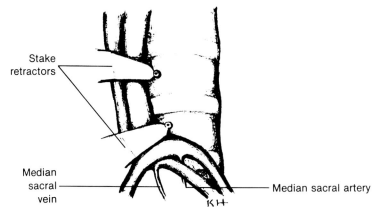

Fig. 35-7

peritoneum is not readily identifiable as to its thickness, one can inject some saline beneath it, thereby elevating it from its underlying loose attachment to the great vessels. I have never found this to be necessary, however.

Next, ligate and transect all lumbar veins or arteries that interfere with retracting the inferior vena cava and abdominal aorta (to the patient's right). These tributaries are usually venous and almost in all instances traverse transversely across the midportion of the vertebral bodies, except at the L5-S1 level, where the median sacral artery and vein pass directly and vertically across the L5-S1 disc (Figs. 35-6 and 35-7). Depending on the level or levels to be fused, these tributaries are identified, divested of thin overlying connective tissue with Kittners, clamped, ligated with 2-0 silk sutures, and transected.

Rarely, it will be necessary to ligate and transect the left iliolumbar vein. This vein takes off from the superior aspect of the left common iliac vein, and on occasion interferes with retraction of the great vessels (to the patient's right) at the L4-L5 level (see Fig. 35-6). The L4-L5 disc is almost always the most difficult disc to fuse because the abdominal aorta and inferior vena cava usually bifurcate at this level.

PITFALLS

If any tear occurs in the veins, whether the inferior vena cava, the common iliacs, the internal iliacs, or any of the tributaries (these should have been ligated firmly), complete attention is mandatory to repairing the tears (or runaway tributaries that have escaped their ligatures). Until all bleeding or significant oozing is under control, any further surgery should not be entertained. The presence of a qualified vascular surgeon can be much appreciated under these conditions, although with some experience the orthopedic surgeon will become adept at using various vascular clamps and repairing tears in veins with 6-0 vascular sutures.

Care must be taken to avoid damaging the superior hypogastric plexus. This plexus is located beneath the parietal peritoneum and overlies the L5-S1 level, just distal to the bifurcation of the abdominal aorta and over the sacral promontory (see Fig. 35-5). The plexus is usually shifted more to the patient's left side. Its fine, interconnecting, weblike filaments can be seen if one looks closely while *pushing* the loosely adherent tissue away from the L5-S1 disc with Kittners. Electrocoagulation should be avoided in this area, especially if there is a "pool" of blood. To repeat, damage to the hypogastric plexus can easily be avoided by gently *pushing* the nerve filaments to the right and left with Kittners.

The superior hypogastric plexus feeds the inferior hypogastric plexus. The latter plexus innervates the bladder sphincter, seminal vesicles, prostatic urethra, ejaculatory ducts, corpora cavernosa.[23] When the superior hypogastric plexus is sufficiently damaged, the bladder sphincter contracts during ejaculation. The seminal fluid, therefore, is blocked from its normal urethral pathway and ends up in the bladder. Retroejaculation obviously renders the patient incapable of normal conception.

The potential complications of retroejaculation should be discussed with the patient before surgery. With proper technique the incidence is extremely low.[7]

TRANSPERITONEAL EXPOSURE

If the patient has had previous abdominal surgery, it will not be possible to develop the retroperitoneal space, since the visceral and parietal peritoneum are densely adhered. In these cases, one simply incises the posterior rectus sheath and the visceral peritoneum to enter the abdominal cavity.[8] The omentum and intestines are retracted to the patient's right, and the visceral and parietal peritoneum overlying the great vessels (and the spine) are incised.

After the fusion, the peritoneum will have to be closed (the deep visceral and parietal peritoneum together in one layer; the superficial visceral peritoneum separately except where it is firmly adhered to the undersurface of the posterior rectus sheath). Actually, the transperitoneal approach is easier than the retroperitoneal approach. This is because the retroperitoneal approach requires more time to develop the retroperitoneal space by blunt finger and hand dissection.

PITFALLS

The left ureter must be identified with the transperitoneal approach, since it will remain in its normal anatomic position in the left retroperitoneal space and thus more exposed to injury when the surgeon transects the deep visceral and parietal peritoneum.

ABDOMINAL RETRACTION

Up to this point an assistant has been retracting the abdominal contents (enclosed within the visceral peritoneum) with deavers and hoes. To reduce the risk of tearing the great vessels and to maintain adequate exposure during arthrodesis, I use Stake retractors (Raney retractors) (Fig. 35-8) and the Thompson retractor (Fig. 35-9). These are crucial instruments, and I will not undertake an ALIF without them. These self-retaining retractors not only allow for consistent exposure (with reduced risk of iatrogenic injury to the vessels), they also allow for more maneuverability on the part of the assistant on the other side of the operating table. With these retractors the ALIF can be performed with one surgeon and one assistant.

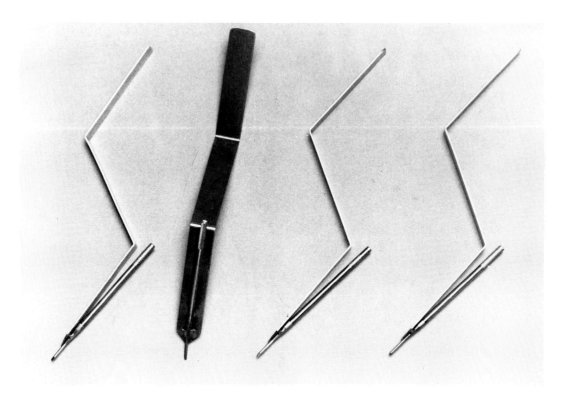

Fig. 35-8 Stake retractors. (Courtesy Thomson & Shelton Instrumentation Co., Dallas, Tex.)

The Stake retractors are gently impacted into the vertebral bodies to hold the great vessels away from the disc to be fused (see Fig. 35-7). They are placed far enough from the disc space so as not to interfere with the removal of the disc contents and preparation of the disc space for grafting. If they are too close to the disc space or angled too severely, the spike of the Stake retractor will penetrate the end-plate of the disc and interfere with disc evacuation and scarification of the end-plates.

The rectangular frame of the Thompson retractor is affixed to the operating table. Various size retractors are then attached to this frame in whatever position gives the best exposure. I suggest the large Hoe (T-Weinberg) for the most cephalad position (see Fig. 35-5).

PITFALLS

Obviously, the surgeon should avoid driving the Stake retractors through vessels, the latter of which are held well out of the way with Deavers by an assistant until the Stake retractors can be impacted into proper position.

The intestinal contents, within the visceral peritoneum, usually sneaks out beneath the various retractor blades of the Thompson retractor. This can be avoided

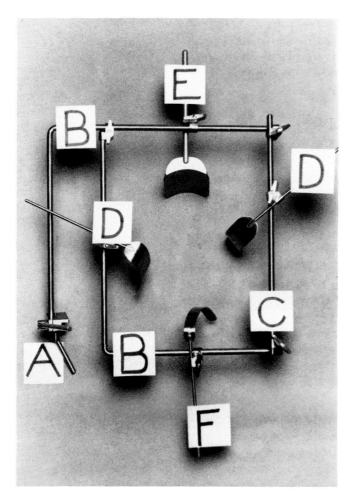

Fig. 35-9 Thompson retractor (*A*, rail clamp; *B*, 90-degree rods; *C*, straight rod; *D*, 2-inch Crile blades; *E*, T-Weinberg; *F*, 1-inch Crile blade. (Courtesy Thompson Surgical Instruments, Inc., Barrington, Ill.)

by first covering the visceral "sack" with damp lap sponges and then putting the retractor blades into position.

THE FUSION

The disc space to be fused is first divested of its contents. The annulus fibrosus (along with the anterior longitudinal ligament) is incised with a no. 10 scalpel (long handle) in a rectangular fashion (Fig. 35-10), the plane developed between the disc contents and the subchondrol bone of the vertebral end-plates with curved osteotomes (Fig. 35-11), the disc contents grasped with a Kocher, and a large portion of the disc contents removed in bulk with the no. 10 scalpel (Fig. 35-12). Pituitaries will remove what remains in the disc space as deep as the posterior longitudinal ligament (actually, the disc is concave and one is protected to *some* degree from violating the spinal canal by these concave end-plates deep in the disc space).

Next, the end-plates are scarified to bleeding subchondral bone with osteotomes and ring curettes (Fig. 35-13). A trough or excavation is then fashioned into the midportion of the motion segment for seating of the slot graft (Fig. 35-14).

It has been my experience that the slot graft is important in stabilizing the motion segment (it prevents torque or torsion). When the slot graft is trapezoid in shape, it will be locked in (will not displace anteriorly out of the disc space) and thus prevents translational and torsional motion. With the slot graft preventing torsional and translational motion, the other onlay tricortical grafts tend not to displace. Dr. Leonard J. Goldner, however, feels that perservation of the subchondral boney end-plates is important and that the fusion rate is significantly higher if only onlay tricortical grafts are used.[11] There have been no studies to date comparing the ALIF with and without

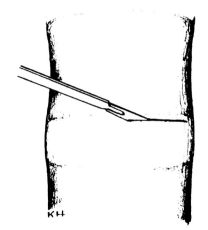

Fig. 35-10

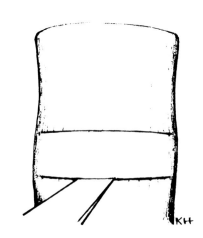

Fig. 35-11

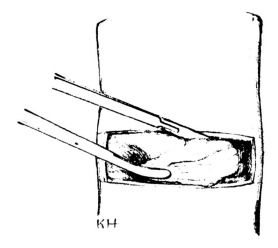

Fig. 35-12

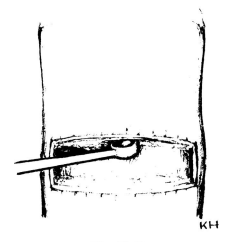

Fig. 35-13

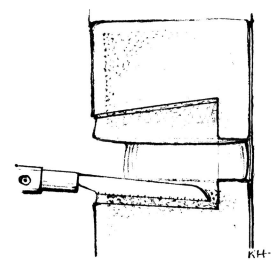

Fig. 35-14

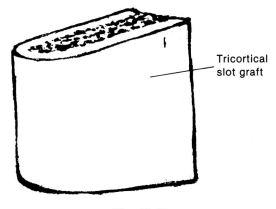

Fig. 35-15

slot grafts. I suggest that the individual surgeon rely on personal experience. One recent failure of fusion at three levels in the same patient has caused me to seriously wonder if the benefits of the slot graft outweigh the risk of nonunion.

The trough for the slot graft is fashioned by cutting into the end-plates with a reciprocating saw (under direct vision) and then making the transverse cut with an osteotome (see Fig. 35-14). The transverse cut should be slightly diagonal, not straight down, so that the trough is trapezoid in shape for fitting of the trapezoid-shaped slot graft (Fig. 35-15). The block of bone thus outlined with the reciprocating saw and osteotome can be pried out with an osteotome to complete the excavation.

The disc space is now ready for placement of the grafts. The raw, bleeding surfaces in the disc space can be packed with Thrombin-soaked Gelfoam and one small sponge and attention given to obtaining the grafts.

PITFALLS

Excavation of the disc space must be meticulous so that no instruments inadvertently violate the spinal canal. Resting the forearm on the patient's abdomen can prevent sudden, unexpected lunging forward of the surgeon's hand, which is holding, for example, an osteotome or reciprocating saw.

HARVESTING THE GRAFT

I always use autogenous bone for the slot graft. If only one space is to be fused, the onlay grafts are also autogenous. When two or more spaces are fused, full thickness allografts are used for the onlay grafts. The allografts are prepared and gas sterilized as outlined by Cloward.[3]

The graft is taken from the anterior lateral aspect of the left iliac crest with particular attention given to leaving the anterior superior iliac spine intact. After the routine exposure full thickness grafts are obtained. The graft site is not closed until after the disc space(s) have been grafted (in case more graft is needed). The raw bleeding surfaces of the graft site, however, are covered with Thrombin-soaked Gelfoam held firmly against the bleeding surfaces with small sponges or lap sponges. When the graft site is closed, the gap remaining in the iliac crest is replaced with methylmethacrylate.[18] In my experience large gaps of this type can be an ongoing source of discomfort for the patient, especially since this is the area on which rests the patient's belt.

FUSION

The slot graft is seated first. The height of the graft is determined by holding it up against the trough and thus obtaining a direct measurement. The graft is then cut with a reciprocating saw, taking care to cut the graft into a trapezoid shape. The depth of the slot graft, its length, is determined by measuring the depth of the disc space. The slot graft is then impacted into the trough using Cloward impactors (Fig. 35-16). Because the slot graft is trapezoid in shape, it is usually not possible to seat it unless the disc space is opened up. Opening up the disc space can be accomplished by breaking the operating table or prying the disc space open with Cloward's Puka chisels (see Fig. 35-16). If the table is broken, it must be returned to a straight position after seating of the slot graft.

On each side of the slot graft a full thickness onlay graft is seated (after being tailored in height and length) (Fig. 35-17). Usually there is no room for any more grafts. However, if there is a small space or crevice unfilled, these areas can be packed with cortical-cancellous pieces of autogenous graft. Cloward's Puka chisels are very helpful if one wishes to

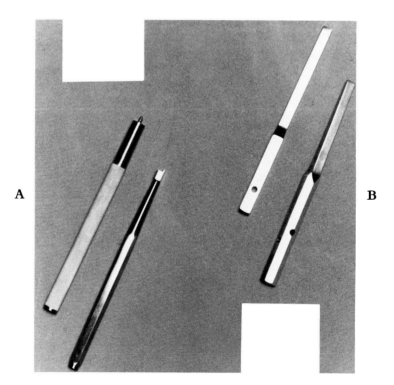

Fig. 35-16 Cloward impactors **(A)** and Puka chisels **(B)**. (Courtesy Codman & Shurtleff, Inc., Randolph, Mass.)

walk a graft one way or the other to create space for more graft material.

If there is any doubt about any of the grafts backing out, that is, displacing anteriorly, they can be shimmed with a piece of cortical bone (Fig. 35-18). When in doubt, *shim*.

When all graft material is in place, the disc is covered with Thrombin-soaked Gelfoam (cut to size) and the latter is pressed firmly against the disc space with a folded "sponge on a stick." This Gelfoam is left in situ.

When the Stake retractors are removed, there can be brisk oozing of blood from the vertebral body. This can be controlled by pressing and holding a small piece of Thrombin-soaked Gelfoam against the puncture site with the index or long finger. When the stake retractors are removed, the retroperitoneal space is observed for 5 minutes for excessive oozing or bleeding.

CLOSURE OF THE ABDOMINAL WOUND

Once the surgeon is convinced that hemostasis is adequate, the Thompson retractor blades are removed, the abdominal contents allowed to fall back into their proper place, the visceral peritoneum examined for any tears, and the wound closed.

First, the edges (at the arcuate line) of the previously cut posterior rectus sheath are grasped with Kochers and the sheath approximated from proximal to distal with a running no. 1 polyglycolic (Dexon) or polyglacetin (Vicryl) suture (Fig. 35-19), the anterior rectus sheath with a running no. 1 polyglycolic suture reinforced with several interrupted sutures of the same material, the subcuta-

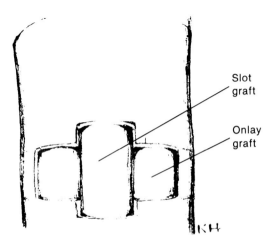

Fig. 35-17

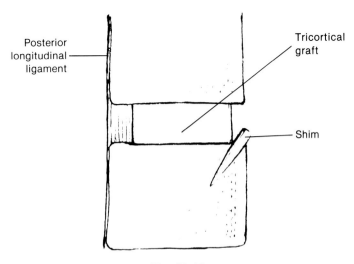

Fig. 35-18

380 *Surgical Procedures*

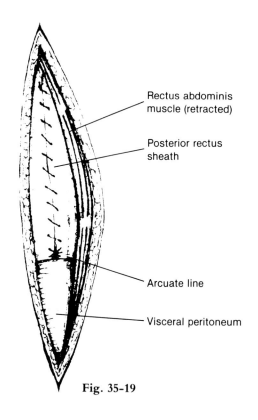

Fig. 35-19

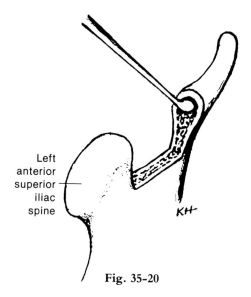

Fig. 35-20

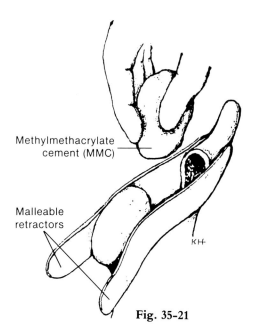

Fig. 35-21

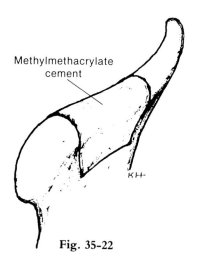

Fig. 35-22

neous tissue with no. 2 polyglycolic suture (very close to the dermis), and the skin with a running no. 3 polyglycolic intradermal suture, topped with betadine solution, Telfa and dry sterile dressing.

CLOSURE OF THE GRAFT SITE

The ilium is prepared for the methylmethacrylate (MMC) by fashioning anchoring holes in the exposed cancellous graft site areas with curved osteotomes or curettes (Fig. 35-20). The raw, bleeding cancellous areas are then covered with Thrombin-soaked Gelfoam (apply sponge pressure). A malleable retractor is then placed on each side of the gap and held in position with Kochers or bone clamps; the Gelfoam is removed, and the gap is filled with MMC (Fig. 35-21). The MMC is molded to conform to the brim of the ilium (Fig. 35-22). The rest of the soft tissue closure is accomplished in the routine fashion.

PITFALLS

Run your fingers along the malleable retractors, especially deep, to be certain that no MMC has escaped in globs and to ensure that the iliac crest has been restored as closely as possible to its previous configuration.

AFTER SURGERY

Intravenous Ancef is discontinued in 24 hours. The hematocrit and hemoglobin results are observed until adequate and stable. If confident that hemostasis is very secure, aspirin suppository (1200 mg) is given in the recovery room and continued twice daily until the patient can take aspirin by mouth (600 mg twice daily). Aspirin is discontinued when the patient is up and about. The NG tube is removed when bowel sounds are present. The Foley catheter is usually removed the first day the patient is allowed out of bed.

The patient wears a lumbosacral corset with metal stays when out of bed for approximately 3 months. The patient is prohibited from bending at the waist but may sit, stand, or walk as comfort will allow.

X-ray films are taken every 6 to 8 weeks. If x-ray films or the clinical picture suggest a nonunion at 9 months or more after surgery, lateral stress x-ray films are performed (with the patient extending and flexing as far as possible while in the standing position). If these stress x-ray films demonstrate no motion at the suspected site of nonunion, they are repeated with the patient in the lateral decubitus position on the x-ray table, but this time the patient is stressed into extension and flexion with aid from the surgeon. This latter type of stress x-ray film, in my experience, is more helpful in determining a nonunion than the CT scan or magnetic resonance imaging.

If stress x-ray films demonstrate an unequivocal nonunion, *and* if the nonunion is judged to be the source of ongoing, intractable pain, an intertransverse fusion of the level in question can be performed. An intertransverse fusion was necessary at one level in three of my patients (out of a total of 44). The intertransverse fusion became solid in all three patients. I believe that an intertransverse fusion in patients with a failed interbody fusion probably has a very high incidence of "take" by virtue of the interbody grafts, which may not have fused to one end-plate (or two), but which by their presence reduce movement in the motion segment.

REFERENCES

1. Burns, B.H.: Operation for spondylolesthesis, Lancet **1**:1283, 1983.
2. Chow, S.P., et al.: Anterior spinal fusion for deranged lumbar intervertebral discs, Spine **5**: 452, 1980.
3. Cloward, R.B.: Gas-sterilized cadaver bone grafts for spinal fusion operations: a simplified bone bank, Spine **5**:4, 1980.
4. Crock, H.V.: Anterior lumbar interbody fusion: indications for its use and notes on surgical technique, Clin. Orthop. **165**:157, 1982.

5. Crock, H.V.: Observations on the management of failed spinal operations, **58B**:193, 1976.
6. Crock, H.V.: Practice of spinal surgery: with a contribution on the management of spinal injuries by Sir George Bedbrook, New York, 1983, Springer-Verlag.
7. Flynn, J.C., and Price, C.T.: Sexual complications of anterior fusion of the lumbar spine, Spine **9**:489, 1984.
8. Freebody, D., et al.: Anterior transperitoneal lumbar fusion, J. Bone Joint Surg. **53B**:617, 1971.
9. Fujimaki, A., et al.: The results of 150 anterior lumbar interbody fusion operations performed by two surgeons in Australia, Clin. Orthop. **165**:164, 1982.
10. Goldner, J.L., et al.: Anterior disc excision and interbody spinal fusion for chronic low back pain, Orthop. Clin. North Am **2**:543, 1971.
11. Goldner, J.L.: Personal communication, Oct. 24, 1986.
12. Harmon, P.H.: Lumbar disc excision and vertebral body fusion: application to complicated and recurrent multi-level degenerations, Am. J. Surg. **97**:649, 1959.
13. Harmon, P.H.: Operative technique and some ten year end results from abdominal disc excision and vertebral body fusions in the lumbar spine, J. Bone Joint Surg. **41A**:1355, 1959.
14. Harmon, P.H.: Anterior lumbar disc excision and fusion. I. Study of the long term results, various grafting materials, Clin. Orthop. **18**:169, 1960.
15. Harmon, P.H.: Anterior lumbar disc excision and fusion. II. Operative technique including observation upon variations in the left common iliac veins, Clin. Orthop. **18**:185, 1960.
16. Harmon, P.H.: Anterior excision and vertebral body fusion operation for intervertebral disc syndromes of the lower lumbar spine: three to five year results in 244 cases, Clin. Orthop. **26**:107, 1963.
17. Harmon, P.H.: Anterior disc excision and fusion of the lumbar vertebral bodies: a review of diagnostic level testing with operative results in more than 700 cases, J. Internat. Coll. Surgeons **40**:572, 1963.
18. Lubicky, J.P., and DeWald, R.L.: Methylmethacrylate reconstruction of large iliac crest bone graft donor sites, Clin. Orthop. **164**:252, 1982.
19. Kirkaldy-Willis, W.H., et al.: Surgical approaches to the anterior elements of the spine: indications and techniques, Can. J. Surg. **9**:294, 1966.
20. Raney, F.L., and Adams, J.E.: Anterior lumbar disc excision and interbody fusion used as a salvage procedure, Proc. West. Orthop. Assoc. J. Bone Joint Surg. **45A**:667, 1963.
21. Raney, F.L.: Spinal disorders, diagnosis and treatment, Philadelphia, 1977, Lea & Febiger.
22. Sacks, S.: Anterior interbody fusion of the lumbar spine, J. Bone Joint Surg. **47B**:211, 1965.
23. Warick, R., and Williams, P.L.: Gray's Anatomy, ed. 35 (British), Philadelphia, 1973, W.B. Saunders Co.

CHAPTER 36

ANTERIOR LUMBAR FUSION

David K. Selby   Robert J. Henderson
Scott Blumenthal   Drew Dossett

The technique of anterior fusion is well established in fracture treatment and in tuberculosis.[8] However, in degenerative disease it has been and remains highly controversial. The various reports in the literature virtually contradict each other in such reported items as fusion rate and complications.* Suffice it to say, we believe that anterior fusion has reasonable risks and reasonable results.

INDICATIONS

The traditional indication for anterior fusion in degenerative disease has been as a salvage operation when all other procedures fail.[6] This "surgery by desperation" tends to be a poor application; it is hoped that more precise indications will be followed.

Perhaps the present most common use of anterior fusion is for a posterior nonunion. This has the advantage of giving an approach to the spine without the vicissitudes of going through the previous posteriorly operated area. It further allows bony fusion in an area that is not already infiltrated with fibrosis and cartilaginous change. The success rate of this type of procedure is relatively high because there is usually partial immobilization from the fibrous union posteriorly, and this allows even better healing anteriorly.

The most proper use of any interbody fusion is when it can be proved that pain is coming directly from the intervertebral disc space. In most circumstances this can only be done by an anterior arthrogram of the three-joint complex. This enters the realm of the controversial discogram. It is not within the scope of this article to discuss the arguments concerning discography. However, discography is the only direct method of ascertaining integrity of the anterior joint of the three-joint complex. The reproduction of the patient's symptoms, combined with architectural change, represents a significant diagnostic event. With the specificity of the diagnosis of anterior column pain it is seemingly more logical to have the thrust of the immobilization at the painful site. Posterior types of fusions do not specifically immobilize the vertebral inter-

---

*References 3, 5, 6, 7, 10, 12, 14, 15.

space itself because the elasticity of bone allows motion through the pedicles, therefore affording motion of the intervertebral space. This is probably the mechanism of failure of pain relief from well-healed posterior fusions.

The diagnosis of disc disruption syndrome can be made only by discography. Specific treatment for this requires interbody fusion, and the anterior approach is recommended. Any practitioner of spine surgery who is not aware of the diagnosis of disc disruption syndrome is encouraged to read the noted articles as this is an important reason for undiagnosed back pain.[1,4,11]

Anterior fusions are contraindicated when the pathologic process is posterior to the pedicles. Again, the principle of directing the surgical procedure at the source of pathology applies. Previous anterior surgery may create a situation where adhesions make it very difficult to get to the anterior aspect of the spine and may be a relative contraindication. Obesity is another relative contraindication, because the grossly obese person may present a situation where the surgical procedure itself becomes dangerous. Working at the end of the instruments close to major vessels is an uncomfortable circumstance for the surgeon and the patient. The presence of well-developed arteriosclerosis in the older patient may be a relative contraindication for anterior fusion. In our series there have been two incidences of plaque emboli that have required embolectomy at the femoral artery.

THE TEAM AND EQUIPMENT

It is advantageous for the orthopedic surgeon to be working with a vascular surgeon who has specific interest in this. The vascular surgeon is familiar with the area of exposure, and is also familiar with the complications that occur and is easily able to treat them. The ability of the vascular surgeon to handle the left common iliac vein can frequently speed procedural time and save on potential complications. We have found it best for the vascular surgeon and orthopedic surgeon to be present throughout the procedure and to approach it as a team effort. This is in contradistinction to the philosophy of the vascular surgeon opening the abdomen and gaining exposure. After that, the orthopedic team moves in and does the procedure and then somebody closes. Constant teamwork adds greatly to the flow.

It is also advantageous to have an extra light source and magnification for precise delineation of structures, particularly in the posterior aspect of the disc area.

All of our instruments have been designed by Dr. Crock.[3,4] There have been some modifications to simplify the instrumentation. This is an attempt to make the procedure easier for us surgeons without Dr. Crock's surgical dexterity. Full instrumentation is important.

APPROACH TO THE LUMBAR SPINE

Exposure to the anterior lumbar spine is important in effecting the ease, efficiency, and effectiveness of the spinal fusion procedure itself and in many cases the end result.[5,8,9,13] Therefore due deliberation must be given to the type of exposure to be attempted and the appropriate level on the skin to initiate the approach. It is important to delineate the anatomic relationship between the highest interspace to be fused with the superior iliac crest. This is done by evaluating the anterior-posterior lumbar x-ray films. Generally we find the transverse incision overlying the left rectus muscle will be just below the umbilicus when exposing for the L4-L5, or L4-L5 and L5-S1, and approximately halfway between the umbilicus and symphysis pubis when exposing the L5-S1 (Figs. 36-1 and 36-2). Those individuals requiring more than two sequential levels to be

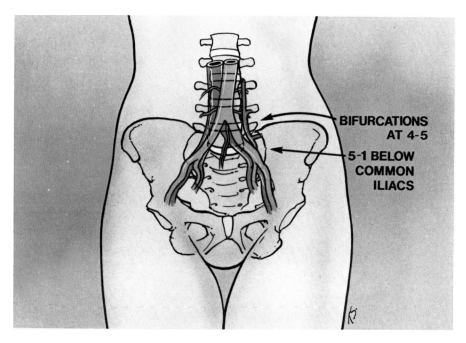

Fig. 36-1 Anatomic relationships.

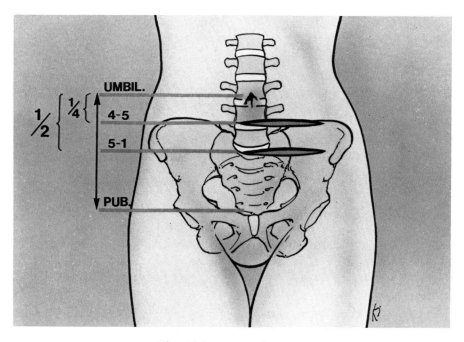

Fig. 36-2 Incision location.

fused, who are more than moderately obese, or who require a fusion above the L3-L4 level need to be approached by a paramedian vertical incision.

Exposure is carried down to the rectus sheath, which is then incised transversely (Fig. 36-3). It is extended caudally on the medial side and cephalad on the lateral side (Fig. 36-4). The rectus muscle is then freed hemostatically with electrocautery from the anterior rectus sheath (Fig. 36-5) and mobilized medially, exposing the neurovascular bundles, one or two, that need to be sacrificed in most cases to facilitate exposure (Fig. 36-6). The posterior rectus sheath is then incised on a vertical plane down to the peritoneal sac (Fig. 36-7). Blunt finger dissection is then

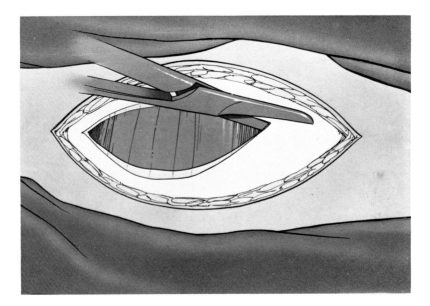

Fig. 36-3 Incise rectus sheath.

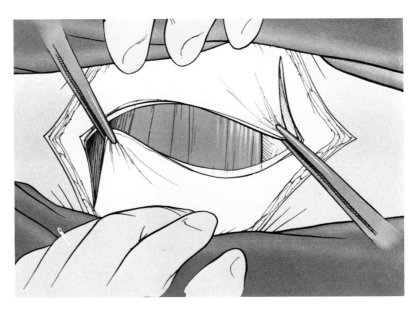

Fig. 36-4 Extend rectus sheath incision.

used to mobilize the left hemiperitoneal sac from its attachments (Fig. 36-8). It is important not to dissect behind the psoas muscles and not to disturb the genital, femoral, and ilioinguinal nerves. As the iliac vessels are exposed, they are left in-situ, but the left ureter is mobilized with the peritoneal sac (Figs. 36-9, A and B). Please note in Fig. 36-9, B, the use of the distinct right-angle retractors, modified hip retractor is available in 4-, 6-, 8- and 10-inch lengths. These allow maximal exposure in the depths of the approach, therefore obviating the need for additional soft tissue destruction.

With the kidney rest extended, hyperextending the interspaces, manual palpation identifies the appropriate interspaces

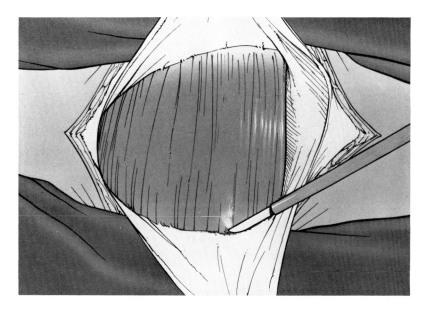

Fig. 36-5 Free rectus muscle.

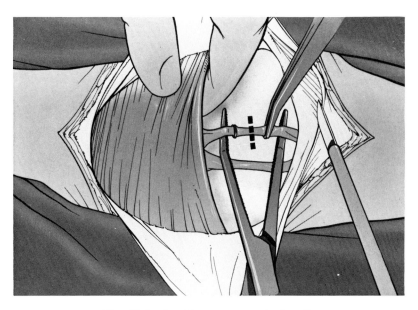

Fig. 36-6 Sacrifice neurovascular bundle.

388 Surgical Procedures

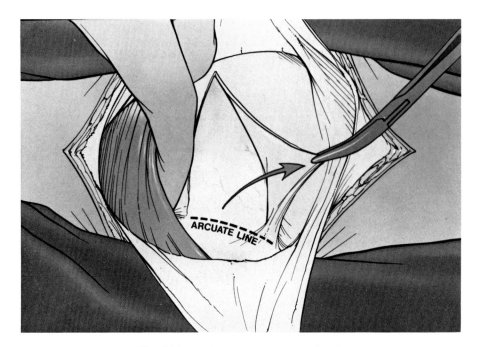

Fig. 36-7 Incise posterior rectus sheath.

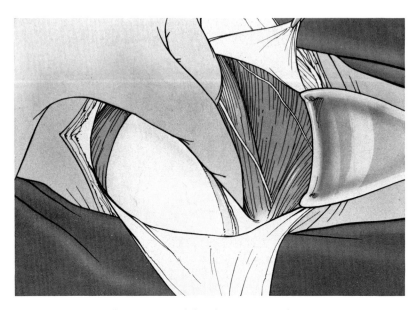

Fig. 36-8 Mobilize hemiperitoneal sac.

Anterior Lumbar Fusion 389

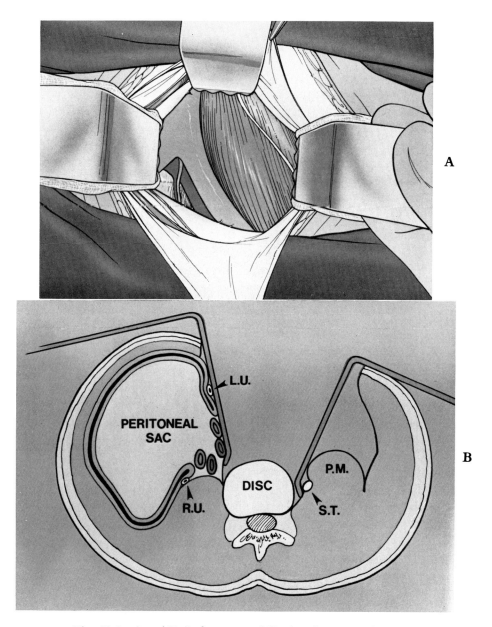

Fig. 36-9 **A** and **B,** Left ureter mobilized with peritoneal sac.

counting up from the sacral prominence. If there is a question of the interspace, x-ray verification should be done. When exposing the L5-S1, the iliac vessels are mobilized cephalad and laterally, carefully dividing the presacral veins, in many cases for additional exposure; it is important to use only blunt dissection in this area to avoid inadvertently injuring the branches of the sympathetic nerve plexus (Fig. 36-10).

Exposure of L4-L5 is also done by blunt dissection, mobilizing the distal aorta and the left common iliac vessels to the right (Fig. 36-10, *B*). The sympathetic trunk is usually intact at this level and can easily be moved to the left as shown. It is sometimes necessary to divide small branches off of the left common iliac vessels to augment satisfactory exposure. Occasionally the ascending lumbar vein, the first major branch off of the common iliac vein, will need to be transected after first securing it with double ligatures on each side. Additional exposure can also be obtained by taking

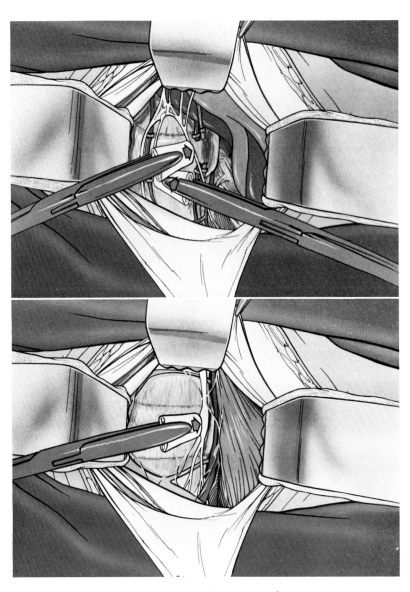

Fig. 36-10 Sympathetic nerve plexus.

the paravertebral transverse vessels usually crossing the midportion of the vertebral bodies beginning with L4 (Fig. 36-11).

After obtaining satisfactory exposure, it is important to maintain exposure in such a way as to protect the major vessels from accidental injury from the instruments being used with the fusion, as well as protecting the vessels from the instruments maintaining exposure.

Closure of this approach is anatomic, posterior rectus sheath (Fig. 36-12), anterior rectus sheath (Figs. 36-13 and 36-14), Scarpa's (Fig. 36-15), and skin.

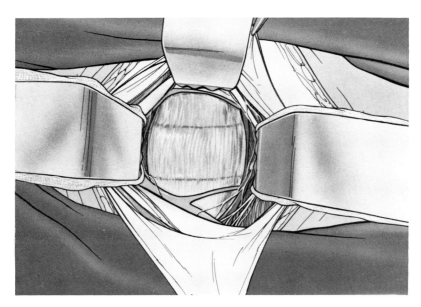

Fig. 36-11 Paravertebral transverse vessels.

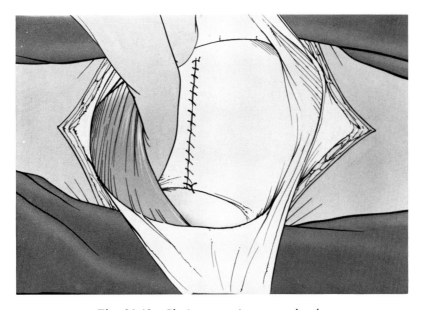

Fig. 36-12 Closing posterior rectus sheath.

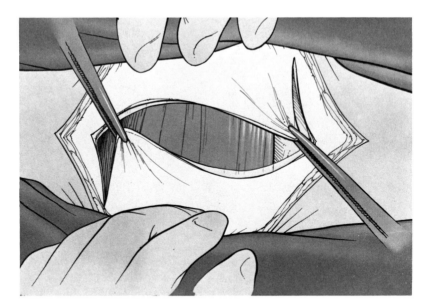

Fig. 36-13 Closing anterior rectus sheath.

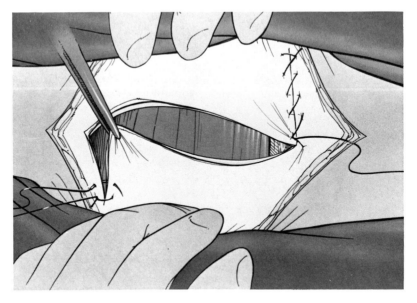

Fig. 36-14 Closing anterior rectus sheath.

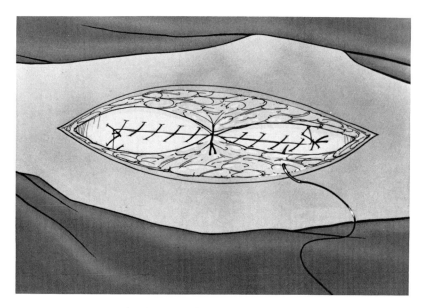

Fig. 36-15 Closing Scarpa's sheath.

ORTHOPEDIC TECHNIQUE

The orthopedic portion of the procedure begins after adequate exposure of the disc space. The orthopedic surgeon must be acutely aware of the structures surrounding the relatively small working space. It is the joint responsibility of both the vascular surgeon and orthopedic surgeon to protect the vasculature and sympathetic trunk. Instruments, particularly the curettes, should be manipulated away from the fragile structures.

To begin, identify the gray line that denotes the end-plates. Be aware of the lateral extension of the sympathetic trunk and the left iliac vein (see Fig. 36-11). Subperiosteal exposure of the end-plate is demonstrated in Fig. 36-16. The Bovie is used to cut through the anterior longitudinal ligament because it reduces bleeding from the edges of the incision. After this, a small cuff of the periosteum of the vertebra is turned back to better mark the vertebral edge (Fig. 36-17). Anterior spur should be taken down to the plane of vertebral surface. The end-plate then can be separated from the subchondral bone by the periosteal elevator (Fig. 36-18). Caution should be exercised in determining the depth of the instrument during the period of separation. This step gives immediate exposure of subchondral bone after excision of the disc and facilitates and speeds complete discectomy.

Loosened disc material is removed with a large pituitary ronguer with a Kocher on the disc material where further separation is done with the periosteal elevator (Fig. 36-19). The remaining disc material is removed by curettage. Shown here is the large curette developed by Dr. John O'Brien in Oswestry (Fig. 36-20). Fig. 36-21 demonstrates the use of Dr. Harry Crock's curette, which is more precise for removal of the most posterior disc material.

After complete discectomy and curettage, including all disc material and end-plate and down to subchondral bone, the depth of the vertebra is determined and compared to the marking lines on the dowel cutter (Fig. 36-22). A circular chisel is used to make a starting cut to seat the teeth of the reamer (Fig. 36-23). It is

Text continued on p. 398.

394 *Surgical Procedures*

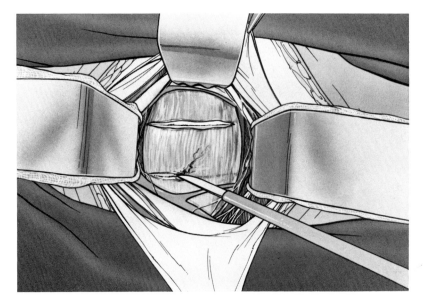

Fig. 36-16 Subperiosteal exposure.

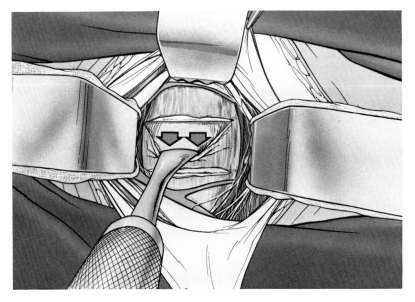

Fig. 36-17 Reflect periosteum to visualize vertebral edge.

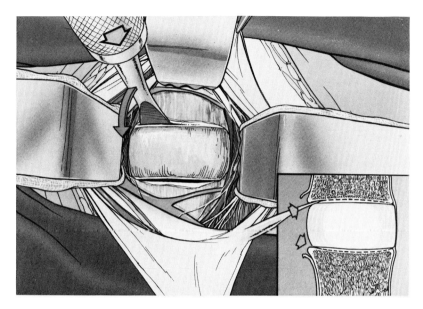

Fig. 36-18 Separate end-plate from subchondral bone.

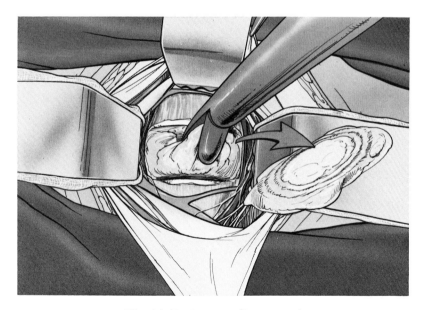

Fig. 36-19 Remove disc material.

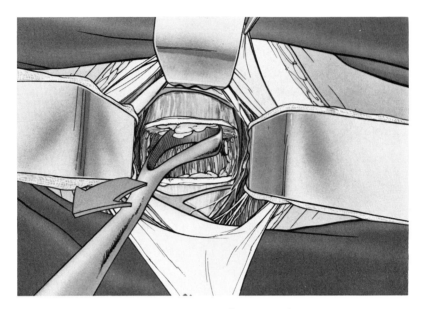

Fig. 36-20 Curette disc material.

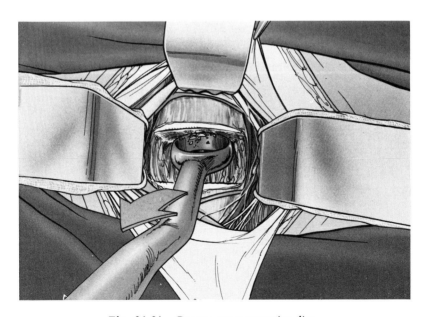

Fig. 36-21 Curette most posterior disc.

Anterior Lumbar Fusion 397

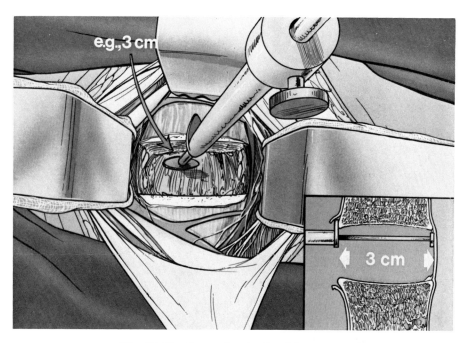

Fig. 36-22 Determine depth of disc space.

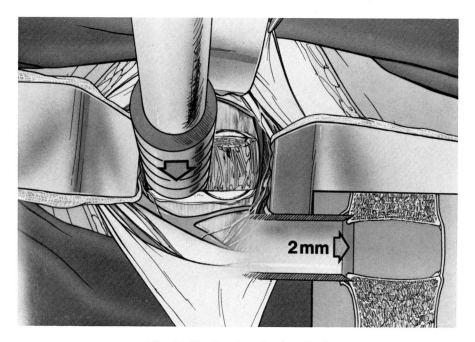

Fig. 36-23 Starting circular chisel.

important that this is done with sufficient depth to prevent the reamer from "jumping" and causing damage to nerve or vein. The circular chisels come in sizes equivalent to the dowel cutters and are used to measure which cutter may be used in the intervertebral space, 0 to 3. It is advantageous to use the smallest size that will still give distinct cuts on both sides of the interspace. Be sure to compensate for the concavity of the disc surfaces.

The dowel cutter is used to ream out a circular cut across the intervertebral space (Fig. 36-24). The cutting end should be under the direct vision of the surgeon at all times. A headlamp and loops are helpful in this regard. If visual supervision becomes difficult, palpation of the dowel cutter within the vertebral bodies can be done with the Penfield no. 4 and can give the surgeon preception as to the depth. This dowel cutter can be on a Hudson brace, on a T-ratchett handle, or on an airpowered drill.

The core evacuation gouge is helpful in removing the bone fragments (Fig. 36-25). The AP view in Fig. 36-25 properly demonstrates a shoulder of bone in the distal aspect of the dowel cut. This acts as a buttress for seating the grafts and preventing protrusion through the nerve tissue. The lateral view would indicate a full cut across the intervertebral space without the protecting buttress and is to be avoided.

Fig. 36-26 demonstrates the site prepared for seating of the grafts. Again, note that there is bleeding bone both proximally and distally at the cuts, the interspace is well cleaned out, and there is a buttress of bone between the graft and the dura. The grafts are inserted and tapped home (Fig. 36-27). The kidney rest is up until this part of the procedure. It is then let down and the grafts are impacted into the intervertebral space. Occasionally, an edge may protrude, which may possibly compromise vascular tissue. If this is the case, removal with a double-action ronguer will quickly give a smooth surface.

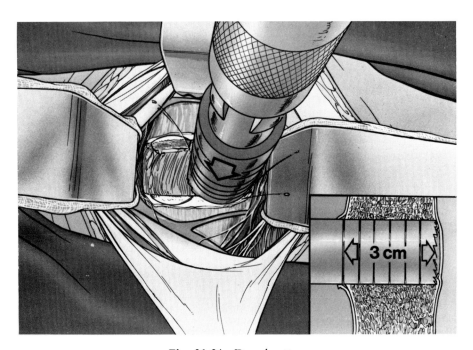

Fig. 36-24 Dowel cutter.

Anterior Lumbar Fusion 399

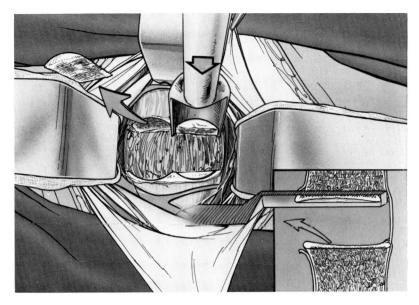

Fig. 36-25 Core evacuation gauge.

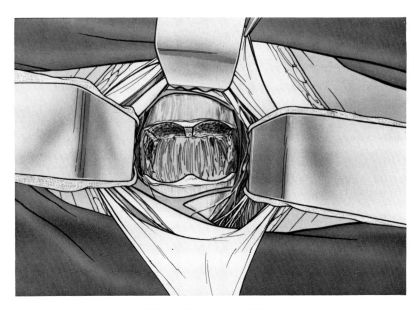

Fig. 36-26 Site prepared for graft.

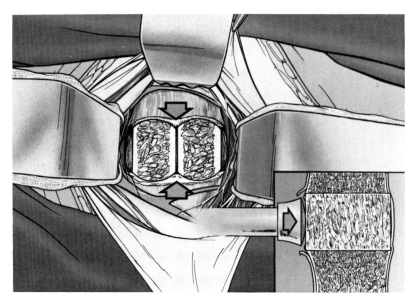

Fig. 36-27 Grafts inserted.

FURTHER COMMENTS ON TECHNIQUE
Kidney Rest

The kidney rest we are referring to is a movable portion of the operating table that has the capacity of extending up from the table. With proper positioning the patient can be placed into hyperextension. As noted earlier, we start the procedures with the kidney rest down. When exposure of the disc space is effected, the kidney rest is cranked up. This places the spine much closer to the surface and enhances the procedure to a very large extent. When the kidney rest is initially extended, the anesthesiologist takes it all the way up and then down two revolutions. This allows the dowel cuts to be made without the patient fully extended. When the grafts are inserted, the patient is fully extended, and this makes the grafts easier to place. The kidney rest is then let down, impacting the grafts in the intervertebral space.

Bone Grafts

The use of donor bone grafts taken with the Crock dowels is advantageous because it avoids the postoperative difficulty associated with the bone graft site. Our rate of fusion has been equal using homogenous vs. autogenous bone. If bank bone is not available, we follow Crock's[4] technique of taking bone off of the anterior iliac crest. Usually a separate counter-incision is made over the crest, and a tricortical graft is taken with the dowel cutter one size larger than that used to ream the intervertebral space.

Dowel Cutters

The dowel cutters are numbered 0 to 4 and progress upward so that the higher number is always used to take the graft for the number below it. Consequently, the 0 dowel cutter is only used for intervertebral cuts and the no. 4 dowel cutter is only used to take the graft. Most commonly, we have used the no. 1 cutter with the no. 2 grafts. The reader is encouraged to read Crock's description of this procedure.[4]

POSTOPERATIVE CARE

The grafts offer immediate stabilization, and immobilization of the patient is unnecessary. In over 2000 grafts only two have backed out. Therefore postoperative care can be directed at rapid rehabilitation from the surgical procedure. Immediate ambulation is encouraged. Nasogastric tubes are not used, and most patients will be on clear fluids for 36 to 48 hours and then progressed to a general diet as they prove bowel motility. Urinary bladder catheters are seldom used and are inserted only on an individual basis.

The use of a patient controlled analgesic pump tends to decrease narcotic dosage and increase comfort levels in patients. Most patients go on to oral medications on the second or third day and are discharged from the hospital in approximately 1 week.

At home patients are encouraged to start a walking program and are reassured about any activity requiring straight flexion-extension. However, the grafts are peculiarly unstable to rotational stress. This is most commonly demonstrated by twisting and moving in bed with logrolling. Patients may continue to have some pain at night when they rotationally stress their back 8 or 9 months after surgery. Bracing is not used, but many physicians doing anterior fusions do recommend bracing for a 3-month period.

COMPLICATIONS

The most common complication is a change in sympathetic response because of trauma from retractors or other instruments on the left sympathetic trunk. This is demonstrated objectively by a temperature change in the legs, the left side being warmer. Subjectively, it is frequently reflected by the patient complaining of coldness in the right foot. This normally reverses itself between 3 and 6 months, and no long-term problems have been identified in our group of patients. The severe problem with the sympathetic change is retrograde ejaculation. In a large series of patients this has been seen four times on a temporary basis, reverting back to normal in a 3- to 6-month period. In a special circumstance where a patient had three anterior procedures because of complications at the L5-S1 area, retrograde ejaculation was permanent. Obviously, multiple procedures at the L5-S1 interspace should be avoided.

Plaque emboli to the femoral artery are possible in older patients with artheriosclerosis. This can be prevented by careful control over the retractor, particularly that on the right side. This may very well be a contraindication for patient selection. This condition is normally recognized when the drapes are removed and a cold, pale leg is evident. It should respond to immediate embolectomy and have minimal, if any, long-term sequelae.

Graft impingement of neural tissue is possible if the graft extrudes posteriorly because of technical error. Patients who have the onset of severe radicular symptoms after anterior fusion have an immediate CT scan; if graft impingement is demonstrated, then a posterior decompression is probably the procedure of choice.

SUMMARY

Anterior fusion is an efficacious method of treatment in those patients who have anterior column disease. A single-level fusion rate of 86% and a two-level fusion rate of 70% is acceptable. Those patients with nonunions normally under posterolateral fusion and with the completion of the posterior fusion will then go on to anterior fusion. The complication rate has been low and patient satisfaction high.

The ability to treat the anterior joint of the three-joint complex without disturbing neurologic tissue is believed to be the major advantage of this method.

REFERENCES

1. Crock, H.V.: Traumatic disc injury. In Vinken and Bruyn, editors: Handbook of clinical neurology, Amsterdam, 1976, North-Holland Publishing Co.
2. Crock, H.V.: Observations on the management of failed spinal operations, J. Bone Joint Surg. **58B:**193, 1976.
3. Crock, H.V.: Anterior lumbar interbody fusion, indications for its use and notes on surgical technique, Clin. Orthop. **165:**1981.
4. Crock, H.V.: Practice of spinal surgery. New York, 1983, Springer-Verlag.
5. Freebody, D.: Anterior transperitoneal lumbar fusion, J. Bone Joint Surg. **53B:**617, 1971.
6. Goldner, J.L., et al.: Anterior disc escision and interbody spinal fusion for chronic low back pain, Orthop. Clin. North Am. **2:**543, 1971.
7. Harmon, P.H.: Anterior excision and vertebral body fusion operation for intervertebral disk syndromes of the lower lumbar spine: three to five-year results in 244 cases, Clin. Orthop. **26:**107, 1963.
8. Hodgson, A.R., and Stock, F.E.: Anterior spinal fusion: the operative approach and pathological findings in 412 patients with Pott's disease of the spine, Br. J. Surg. **48:**172, 1960.
9. Hodgson, A.R., and Wong, S.K.: A description of a technic and evaluation of results in anterior spinal fusion for deranged intervertebral disc and spondylolisthesis, Clin. Orthop. **56:**133, 1968.
10. Humphries, A.W., et al.: Anterior interbody fusion of lumbar vertebrae: a surgical technique, Surg. Clin. North Am. **41:**1685, 1961.
11. Johnson, P.M.: Interal disc disruption. J. Arkansas Med. Assoc. **81:**425, 1985.
12. Kirkaldy-Willis, W.H., et al.: Surgical approaches to the anterior elements of the spine: indications and techniques, Can. J. Surg. **9:**294, 1966.
13. Lane, J.E., Jr., and Moore, E.S., Jr.: Transperitoneal approach to the intervertebral disc in the lumbar area, Ann. Surg. **127:**537, 1948.
14. Sacks, S.: Anterior interbody fusion of the lumbar spine: indications and results in 200 cases, Clin. Orthop. **44:**136, 1966.
15. Stauffer, R.N., and Coventry, M.B.: Anterior interbody lumbar spine fusion, J. Bone Joint Surg. **54A:**756, 1972.

CHAPTER

37

THE RANEY TECHNIQUE OF ANTERIOR INTERBODY FUSION

†Frank L. Raney, Jr.

The Raney technique of anterior interbody fusion involves the use of both iliac crest and fibular bone grafts to provide a continuing support throughout the course of the healing phase of the fusion. This technique has been highly consistent in repairing posterior pseudoarthroses. It is quite useful after failed laminectomy and disc excision in that it does restore the disc space to its original height. It has been used successfully as a primary procedure, especially in large frame males and in patients with three level disc disease, especially if the L3 to L4 disc is very symptomatic.

TECHNIQUE

The technique of the Raney anterior interbody fusion is as follows. Preoperative, intraoperative, and postoperative antibiotics are given. The patient is positioned on his/her back with an x-ray film under the back between the mattress and the sheet. The right iliac crest is elevated with a sandbag under the right buttocks. The kidney rest is placed directly at the anterior iliac spine level so that when the kidney rest is elevated the lower three disc spaces will be elevated to their maximum height. An indwelling catheter is placed. The arms are wrapped to protect the ulnar nerve. The draw sheet is placed over the arm and under the patient so that the sandbag and x-ray film can be removed during the procedure without disturbing the arm position. A pneumatic tourniquet is placed on the right thigh. Bone grafts are then obtained from the anterior iliac crest and from the fibula (Fig. 37-1).

The iliac crest graft is obtained by starting an incision at the level of the anterior iliac spine just below the crest and developing along the crest for approximately 5 inches. The incision is developed through the skin's subcutaneous tissue and directly down to the top of the ilium. The conjoined tendon of the abdomen is detached from the top of the crest, the iliacus from the inside of the crest, and the

†Deceased.

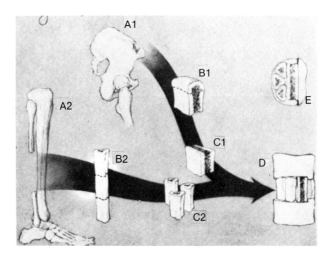

Fig. 37-1

tensor fascia femorus from the outside of the crest. Care is taken to locate and protect the branch of the iliohypogastric nerve so that the patient will not have thigh numbness after surgery. The full thickness of the crest is exposed to a depth of approximately 2 cm. Rectangular blocks of crest are then obtained by making saw cuts with an operating saw to a depth of approximately 1.5 cm and with the cuts approximately 3 cm apart to give a block of bone that is 3 cm in length in its long axis and about 1.5 cm in depth. This is amputated at its base then to give a full thickness graft of the ilium, which will have two cortices with cancellous bone sandwiched between them. One such graft will be obtained for each space that is being fused. The graft thus obtained is further trimmed by removing the rounded cortical top surface to give a completely rectangular block of full thickness iliac bone. The corners are trimmed from this so they will not project out into the intervertebral foramen. The graft finally will be trimmed to fit exactly into the prepared disc space with the disc space elevated to its maximal height.

The donor site is then trimmed to make it smooth and the cancellous surface covered with bone wax. The iliacus is fastened back to the tensor fascia femorus over the remaining iliac crest. The conjoined tendon of the abdominal wall is plicated over the tensor fascia so that there will be no slack and therefore no sagging of the lower abdominal wall. The remainder of the wound is then closed in layers.

Next, the fibular graft is obtained. To avoid producing ankle instability, it is important that the distal 4 inches of the fibula be left in place and that there be no tearing of the distal tibiofibular syndesmosis ligament by levering on the distal fragment. The incision over the fibula is started 4 inches proximal to the tip of the lateral malleolus and is carried proximally for 6 to 7 inches directly in line with the posterior margin of the fibula. It is developed through skin, subcutaneous tissue, and deep fascia and down to the fibula in the interval between the peroneus longus and soleus. The distal portion of the exposure is completed first, and then exposure is carried proximally in a subperiosteal fashion. The needed length of

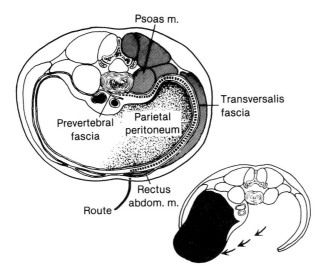

Fig. 37-2

fibula is exposed and the fibula is then transsected with an oscillating saw first distally and then proximally. The removed full thickness fibular graft is almost always relatively triangular shaped. The lateral upper end of the distal fibular fragment is trimmed, and the medullary canal of both fragments remaining are plugged with bone wax. The deep part of the wound is then inspected for any venous bleeding.

The deep fascia is then closed from each end to within 2 inches of the middle and the tourniquet is then deflated. Any bleeding present is controlled, and the deep fascial closure is then completed; the rest of the wound is closed in layers, and a sterile compression dressing is applied within the sterile field. The iliac crest and fibular grafts are protected by placing them in a locked bone box until they are finally prepared for insertion into the prepared disc space.

The abdominal approach to the anterior aspect of the lumbar spine is then carried out through an oscillating left paramedian incision. This extends through both the anterior and posterior rectus sheaths and extends from the level of the pubis to approximately 2 inches above the umbilicus. The dissection is carried between the peritoneum and the transversalis fascia, across the left psoas, and over to the vertebral body (Fig. 37-2). The lumbosacral space is exposed in the bifurcation and the L3-L4 and L4-L5 spaces are exposed along the left side of the great vessels with the great vessels being displaced to the right (Fig. 37-3).

Once the vessels have been adequately displaced, self-retaining retractors are driven into the vertebral bodies to maintain the exposure. The disc spaces are then prepared, usually starting with the top one that is to be included. Initially, an annular flap is formed at either L3-L4 or L4-L5. The flap is reflected to the right to help hold the great vessels over to the right. The intervertebral disc material is then excised back to the posterior annulus, using a combination of ring and spoon curettes and a pituitary rongeur. It can be determined when the back of the disc space has been reached in that the direction of the annular fibers changes. The disc end-plate is normally quite concave, and when the vertebral bodies are observed to start to approach each other

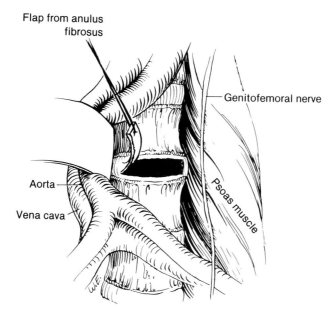

Fig. 37-3

at the back of the disc one will see this change occur.

Once the disc material has been removed, the cortical plates are excised within 1 cm of the posterior margin of the disc space to produce a posterior ledge that will prevent any bone graft from being driven into the neural canal. At each level the opposing end-plates are removed in this manner. The kidney rest is elevated on the operating table. This first hyperextends the lumbar spine, which tightens the disc annulus, and then as the elevation is continued, all of the ligaments are stretched tight and the disc space is elevated to its original maximal height. To secure blocking of the space in this position, a tightly fitting combination of cancellous and cortical bone grafts (iliac crest and fibula) is then placed into the space. By having the combination, the cortical bone maintains disc space height while the cancellous bone is incorporated, and the incorporated cancellous bone then continues to support while the cortical graft is softened during its incorporation. This results in continuous support throughout the healing stage of the fusion.

Once the disc space has been appropriately prepared, both the iliac crest and fibular grafts are measured to fit the elevated disc space with it at its maximal height. The iliac crest graft is placed with the cortical plates oriented vertically and with the long axis of the graft transverse; the graft is then driven back against the previously formed ledge. When this graft is in place, the cortices are vertical and the cancellous bone of the graft is in contact with the cancellous bone of the vertebral body above and below and the bodies are kept the maximal distance apart by the vertical position of the cortices of the graft.

The fibular grafts are then measured and cut with an oscillating saw. An attempt is made to place three such fibular grafts, two with their triangular bases facing posteriorly, and the third with its base facing anteriorly to act as a keystone graft. The triangular shape of the fibular strut is made use of in this manner. All of the fibular struts are placed entirely within the disc space so that they are inside the anterior cortices of the vertebral body. The annular flap that was formed is then closed back over the front of the space and sutured in place. This is used to hold strips of Surgicel in place to establish hemastasis. Pressure is held against the annular flap and Surgicel until bleeding has stopped. Bacitracin solution (1000 units per ml) is placed into the disc space around the graft and also into the retroperitoneal space. Each level to be fused is then dealt with in the same manner, with the exception that at L5-S1 the procedure is done in the great vessel bifurcation and the annular flap is tipped to the left rather than to the right. When all levels to be fused have been completed, closure of the abdominal wall is then carried out in layers, sterile dressings are applied to the abdominal and iliac crest wounds, and an elastic abdominal binder is applied over this; the patient then is transferred onto a guerney and to the recovery room.

POSTOPERATIVE CARE

After surgery, blood loss is replaced until preoperative hematocrit and hemoglobin levels are restored. The patient is fed orally as soon as peristalsis has been reestablished. Ambulation and weight-bearing (within tolerance of pain), with an elastic binder on is permitted on the first or second postoperative day. Initially, this activity usually consists of just standing at the bedside, to be increased gradually to walking as the pain in the donor sites and abdominal wound will allow.

As soon as tenderness of the abdominal wound subsides, the patient is placed in a previously prepared plastic bivalved, removable and adjustable lumbar spinal jacket. The patient wears this jacket all of the time when he or she is ambulatory except when bathing. Ambulation is encouraged only to the point of fulfilling daily needs; the patient otherwise is encouraged to remain lying down with the lumbar spine flexed either in the contour position or on a side in bed. Hyperextension of the lumbar spine is carefully avoided at all times until the grafts have become fully incorporated. The jacket is continued until there is radiologic evidence of incorporation of the bone grafts, at which time a weaning process is carried out and patient is started on an appropriate rehabilitation program to reestablish muscle power and endurance.

CHAPTER 38

RESULTS OF ANTERIOR INTERBODY FUSION

Robert G. Watkins

There are numerous problems in evaluating fusion studies in general, particularly, anterior lumbar fusion studies. Numerous methods have been used for spinal fusion. The anterior lumbar fusion appears to be, theoretically, an ideal method of stopping motion in any neuromotion segment. Because of significant complication rates and technical difficulties, the popularity of the operation has never matched similar operations such as the anterior cervical fusion. In the past, studies of the results of anterior lumbar fusions have varied from very high fusion rates to low fusion rates, from very high clinical success rates to low clinical success rates.

There are several problems in evaluating these papers, as well as those of other fusion methods. Prospective studies comparing fusion to nonfusion patients is quite difficult. Most studies making this comparison use patients who are being decompressed for radicular symptoms and where outcome depends primarily on the adequacy of the decompression, not the fusion. A better comparison would probably be between fusion patients and patients not treated, or treated nonsurgically.

PROPER REVIEW OF RESULTS

Several measures can be used in a proper review of the results of a specific operation without double blind prospective comparisons:
1. Proper assessment of the preoperative morbidity
2. Establishing a diagnosis
3. Standardization of operative technique
4. Proper assessment of a postoperative morbidity
5. Determination of structural result such as fusion

Clinical morbidity should be determined by a scale encompassing function, pain, and occupation. In a modern society with a high unemployment rate return to prior occupation after back surgery is hardly the sole criteria for improvement of human pain and suffering.

The functional activities of the patients, their ability to become an active community ambulator as opposed to bedridden patients, the ability to avoid narcotic medications, and a change from constant pain to intermittent pain may be more than enough justification for a specific operation. It is very important to know how sick these patients who are proposed for fusion are. Patients who have had a mild problem for a short period of time will often get well with no treatment, good nonoperative treatment, or with a safer operation. Fusion permanently changes spinal biomechanics. There is added stress and strain at adjacent levels. An unfused healed disc is better than a fused one. It is important that fusion patients have significant morbidity to warrant the operation.

The best way to consistently judge this is to use a standardized evaluation of morbidity. A proper morbidity scale should be evaluated preoperatively and at proper postoperative intervals. Documentation should be made in a standard—preferably numerical—form of the patient's pain, function, and occupational status. Subjective evaluation by the surgeon and sometimes by the patient is notoriously inaccurate. Too often these evaluations are more a reflection of their expectations of clinical results rather than the true clinical result.

Finally, an independent reviewer is preferred when reviewing a surgeon's work.[9,10] A truly independent review is difficult to obtain. Anyone reviewing clinical material with sufficient knowledge to understand the material present may have some inherent biases with regard to its results.

PROPER DIAGNOSTIC STUDIES

Proper diagnostic studies are at the heart of any review of surgical results. Without understanding the diagnosis for which the operation was performed, very little future information can be determined from the results of the operation. Most fusion studies have used a great variety of methods for determining which levels to fuse: the presence of spondylolisthesis, hypermobility on motion films, hypomobility on motion films, and the presence of radiographic changes on plain x-ray films, myelograms, discograms, EMG, clinical examination, CT scanning, and different combinations of these tests. To compare one fusion study that uses myelographic changes as its indication for fusion to one that uses motion studies for its indication for fusion is quite difficult. There must be a consistent diagnosis and consistent diagnostic testing criteria to compare clinical results.

As for anterior interbody fusion, it is imperative that the surgical approach be standardized and done by the most skilled hands available for this type of surgery. There are certain inherent complications in an anterior approach to the spine, and every effort should be made to standardize the technique in the approach to keep these complications to a minimum.[32] In addition to the approach, grafting technique is a consideration. There are a number of grafting techniques available, from the dowel method[4,5,10] to fibular grafts, to tricorticate iliac crest grafts,[17,19] and bank bone to autogenous bone. For evaluation of a series of cases it is best to have the same grafting technique in all the cases. Having a great mixture of grafting techniques and bone graft used will introduce many factors into the clinical study.

Different reviewers often have a marked difference in opinion concerning what constitutes a fusion.[6] Plain radiographic evaluation of possible postoperative fusion is difficult indeed. CT scanning techniques have improved this method and may be a future source of determination of fusion. Bone scanning techniques offer a very gross evaluation of the activity of a fusion. Motion studies are probably the best method of determining stability but fall short of defining what type of tissue is present in the fusion area. Evaluation of fusion results should be a combination of radiographic appearance, as well as motion studies. Specifically, vigorous flexion/extension films with documentation of the amount of motion at a prior fusion level should be the test to use. The margin for error in doing this measurement is not well defined.

INDICATIONS FOR ANTERIOR LUMBAR SURGERY

Any fusion operation should proceed with the basic understanding that abnormal motion is present in the area of the spine to be fused. The spine is a multiunit, biomechanical structure in which each disc and its two facet joints combine with adjacent levels to produce a combined motion. The disc and its two facet joints, the nerves innervating that area, and the muscles and ligaments attached to that area are considered one neuromotion segment. The mechanical forces present in a neuromotion segment are a complex variety of coupled motions, for example, flexion, extension, rotation, shear, compression, and tension. A neuromotion segment is a living viscoelastic structure that responds with creep, hysteresis, stress, strain, injury, and permanent deformity. The biomechanical changes in a neuromotion segment are continually evolving in response to prior stimuli. The neuromotion segment is richly innervated with sensory fibers and can respond to noxious stimuli with intense pain. Disc herniations, disc space infections, acute annular tears, fractures, and other pathologic conditions can totally immobilize the patient. It is most difficult to determine how much motion is abnormal, what type of motion is abnormal, and how much stress is needed to produce pain through an abnormal motion.

In making the decision to stop motion surgically in a neuromotion segment, one must be concerned with documenting abnormal motion and pain production from that neuromotion segment. Motion x-ray films in flexion/extension films can be of benefit, but they are hindered by the fact that the abnormal motion present may in no way be reflected as hypermobility. Very often the most inflamed, painful disc is splinted and will be moving less than an adjacent, normal disc whose hypermobility is a reflection of the pathology at the abnormal level. Flexion/extension films reflect only certain aspects of the motion present in a neuromotion segment. The best use of flexion/extension films is probably in degenerative spondylolisthesis. The operative care of degenerative spondylolisthesis is usually conducted for radicular disease and involves a decompression. The flexion/extension film is an indicator of future radicular disease that is due to progressive olisthesis. Flexion/extension films are a less reliable indicator of fusion for back pain in degenerative spondylolisthesis. In cervical spine disease fusing either the stiff or the hypermobile segment for neck pain is fraught with error.

The fact that the cases in which union was achieved often does not match the cases in which the greatest clinical successes were achieved has led investigators to the skeptical opinion that fusion was not the causative factor in the patient's clinical outcome and therefore should not be a worthy therapeutic modality. An anterior lumbar fusion operation may not produce a total ablation of all motion at the neuromotion segment. A pseudoarthrosis may produce a sufficient ablation of the noxious motion at that neuromotion segment and thereby produce an excellent clinical result. A pseudoarthrosis may have eliminated all of the shear forces through an intervertebral disc but not eliminated 3 to 5 degrees of flexion on a vigorous flexion/extension film. Despite this possibility, any fusion operation should be designed and conducted to achieve solid bony union with no motion present in the neuromotion segment. Consistent inability to obtain solid union requires that the surgical technique and procedures be reevaluated.

A prerequisite for anterior lumbar fusion is that the pathologic condition can be affected by an operation on the anterior column of the spine. As a general rule, spinal column pain, discogenic pain, axial pain are more likely to respond to anterior interbody fusion than posterior column pain, radicular pain, or leg pain. The latter is treated commonly by a decompressive operation of the posterior column. An ideal would be one procedure for both anterior and posterior disease. One example is anterior cervical fusion, which is indicated and has the best results in cervical radiculopathy. Another is the posterior lumbar interbody fusion. Anterior lumbar fusions have been shown to produce a significant improvement in radicular symptoms. Stopping motion in a neuromotion segment does decrease nerve-root irritation from a lesion adjacent to the nerve root, but it is important to choose the most efficient and effective method of dealing with a specific pathologic situation. A large primary space-occupying lesion, such as disc herniation or free fragment, is best removed posteriorly whereas a nerve root scarred to a disc that is moving abnormally may best be handled with an anterior interbody fusion. Anterior lumbar fusion may or may not be the most effective method of dealing with radicular pain, depending on the cause of the radicular pain.

Determining the Need for Fusion

The first step in determining the need for an anterior lumbar fusion is to determine the need for fusion. With the acknowledged difficulties in documenting the type of abnormal motion present in a neuromotion segment, clinical decision-making is often on an empirical basis using indirect criteria. Criteria for fusion at the time of an initial disc herniation include a long history of mechanical back pain before the herniation and radiographic signs of abnormal mechanical stress at the disc space, such as hypermobility or traction spurs. The predictive value of the height of the disc space is questioned because the higher the disc space the greater chance for hypermobility and instability. Yet the narrowing of early degeneration in a disc may indicate abnormal mechanical stress on an intervertebral disc and result in severe back pain but less overall motion. Relative indications for primary fusion include a massive central herniation in which the annulus is totally insufficient for any hope of normal biomechanics in that disc in the near future.

Disc herniation with spondylolysis or spondylolisthesis is an indication for fusion. Reherniation in cases other than a reextruded fragment within the first 6 weeks is a reasonable indication that the disc has undergone sufficient damage that prophylactic fusion will improve the overall clinical result.

Age is an important consideration. Young patients are more likely to have instability from an injury or disc herniation but are more likely to heal. Fusions in young people are more likely to produce degenerative change at adjacent levels because they are under higher activity loads for longer periods of time. The young to midportion of life is the most economically productive time; thus people are less able to endure a long disability. Immediate fusion that insures stability, although it may be prophylactic in nature, is often preferred against two potential periods of disability and convalescence. As patients near retirement they are usually less willing to undergo a procedure with a high complication rate just because the procedure offers hope of total perfection when successful. Physiologically, the older the patient, the less likely a fusion is needed. Neuromotion segments stiffen naturally. If symptoms are the result of spinal stenosis, the segment is usually stable. The prime time for fusion for disc disease appears to be age 35 to 55. A clinician must be very selective in using these relative criteria for the choice of fusion in any specific patient.

The Importance of Accurate Diagnosis

Diagnostic accuracy is a key to successful surgical results in most medical conditions and spinal fusions are no exception. Obviously, if the wrong level is fused a poor clinical result can be expected. Motion studies are limited by a lack of understanding of abnormal motion in a neuromotion segment. Static studies of the spinal column are limited by our knowledge of which structural abnormalities cause pain under what biomechanical conditions. Myelographic and CT scan changes may not be the source of a patient's pain. Discography is a test commonly used to determine patients for fusion.[11,21] Discography offers the ability to evaluate the structural integrity of the intervertebral disc through the morphologic changes seen on the discogram. Also, it allows a symptomologic reproduction of pain. The discogram reproduces the patient's pain by introducing noxious stimuli into an inflamed, irritated, or injured area. The injection of the needle, the pressure of the fluid introduced, or the chemical irritation of the fluid introduced will usually reproduce pain from an injured, symptomatic intervertebral disc. This allows the clinician to return another time and block the disc with local anesthetic, hopefully relieving the patient's pain complex.

There are difficulties encountered in interpreting discography, just as there are with other diagnostic tests. Some patients are too emotionally distraught to participate in pain reproduction studies.

Their tests will be inaccurate. Often patients with a long pain history are too suggestible and subjectively involved in their pain to accurately report pain reproduction. When conducted accurately, discography offers the potential for identifying which neuromotion segment is responsible for the patient's pain. Further evidence can be achieved by ablation of that pain with local anesthetic. It improves the chances of an operation designed to stop motion in that neuromotion segment, relieving the patients pain. Multilevel discography has the additional benefit of allowing evalaution of levels adjacent to that proposed for fusion. Patients with multilevel symptomatic degenerative disc disease are less likely to improve from an isolated level fusion. Multilevel positive discography is a relative contraindication to an isolated level interbody fusion. Multilevel discography has demonstrated cases in which the most obviously degenerated spondylolisthetic level was not the source of the patient's pain while an adjacent, normal appearing radiographic level was. There will be cases in which symptomatic discs on discography may not be the source of the patient's pain either.

THE PREOPERATIVE EVALUATION

A preoperative evaluation of a patient with back pain must include some method to eliminate intrathecal tumors and high lumbar disc herniations as a source of the pain. Myelograms, contrast CT scans and/or nuclear magnetic resonance imaging (MRI) are important in this area.

Discography is a test for discogenic disease.[21] Myelograms and CT scans are a better test for radicular disease. Often the two disease processes may be present in the same patient, but they may not be. Discography should not be the diagnostic procedure of choice for a predominantly radicular clinical problem. An evaluation of potential fusion patients should pinpoint as accurately as possible the neuromotion segment or segments responsible for a patient's pain. Diagnostic accuracy is imperative in anterior fusions, and discography should be an integral part of the diagnostic workup. Very little information can be confirmed at surgery, therefore complete reliance is on preoperative tests.

The discograms are performed under direct fluoroscopic guidance in the radiology department. The discogram need not be a terrifying ordeal for the patient. In a cooperative patient a three-level discogram could be completed in approximately 30 minutes.

Procedure for Discography

The patient is first premedicated before coming to radiology, but not sedated too much to respond. A modified lateral approach is used rather than a midline approach. First and most important, the dural sac is avoided. This reduces the incidence of headaches and other side effects so frequently encountered during myelography. Second, any epidural extravasation would imply annular and ligamentous disruption and must not be confused with potential leakage of contrast through the needle tract. In patients with clinical radicular pain, the approach used is the side opposite to their leg pain, to avoid any confusion that might occur if the lumbar nerve is encountered with the needle. The patients are placed in the prone semi-oblique position with a bolster under the abdomen in an effort to open up the disc spaces. After sterile preparation, local anesthesia is employed so the patient is awake and can relate any pain response upon disc injection. Using fluoroscopy, exact measurements on needle placement are not needed. The procedure can be performed in the surgical suites with a mobile C-arm fluoroscopic unit. The patient is in an oblique position so that the "Scotty dog" appearance of the posterior arch is visible. After local anesthesia with Xylocaine, an 18-gauge spinal needle is inserted down to the midpoint of the disc until contact with the annulus fibrosus is achieved. At certain levels it is necessary to angle the C-arm or fluoroscopic x-ray tube so that the disc space is seen in profile. If a nerve is accidentally encountered by the needle, the patient relates this to the radiologist, who subsequently repositions the needle.

There are a variety of discogram needles ranging from 3- and ¾-inch spinal needles to 8-inch needles for obese patients. A skinny 22- or 23-gauge Chiba needle (20 cm in length) is passed through the 18-gauge needle after the stylet has been removed. The patient may feel some discomfort as the annulus is punctured. The 22-gauge needle can be manipulated by forming a curve 2 to 3 cm from its tip. This is usually necessary for the L5-S1 level, but it is generally not required for other levels. By turning the beveled needle in either direction, the needle tip can be deflected in the direction away from the bevel. Using such maneuvers the Chiba needle is advanced until its tip is within the center of the disc space. This is confirmed with the patient either turning onto the side or stomach or by rotating the C-arm so that the disc and needle are visualized in two planes. Once the position of the needle is centrally located within the disc, contrast material is carefully injected while monitoring the flow of contrast and the patient's pain response.

With a normal disc, between 0.5 and 1 ml can be injected, whereupon there is resistance to further injection. Herniated or degenerated discs may accomodate up to 4 or 5 ml with little or no resistance. Injection should be stopped with either increased resistance to injection, frank annular rupture with extravasation of contrast, or reproduction of the patient's clinical pain. Finally, before the removal of the needle intradiscal Xylocaine or

Marcaine was injected for symptomatic relief and to avoid confusing pain responses at different levels.

With this technique, there is little morbidity and discomfort to the patient. The complication rate is quite low and has been limited in my practice to one case of disc space infection.

MORBIDITY CRITERIA

Patients proposed for anterior lumbar fusion should have sufficient morbidity to justify an operation with a significant complication rate that produces a spine with abnormal biomechanics. The complication rate with anterior lumbar fusion in most reviews is approximately 20%. The inherent risk of vascular complications is not present in posterior approaches. Careful assessment of the patient's morbidity may determine that the potential hope of success with the operation warrants the potential complications. The more disabled patients are before surgery, the more they will notice the improvement and the more tolerant they will be of complications and a failure to improve. Combining morbidity ratings with time of pain and disability offers a reasonable indication of severity of the symptoms. Not only can one establish criteria for fusion in the clinician's own patient, but one can also have an objective assessment of clinical results.

To fuse a disc—especially in the midportion of the lumbar spine—produces abnormal biomechanics. This abnormal situation may be an improvement to the painful abnormalities present before surgery, but any realistic expectations after anterior interbody fusions would realize that mechanics are different. There are increased stresses at adjacent levels. Patients who have suffered an injury to an intervertebral disc at one level are more likely to suffer an injury at another level. Even with normal discography at adjacent levels degenerative changes are more likely to occur in people who have had other degenerated levels, although the chance of suffering a second totally incapacitating disabling injury will be much less. Pain from degenerative disc disease and disc injury is a ubiquitous problem. Only a minute fraction of patients suffering this type of pain should ever require spinal fusion.

An additional indication for fusion is a failure of nonsurgical treatment. Properly conducted nonsurgical treatment results in a very high success rate in treating patients with discogenic problems. Only after exhausting all nonsurgical treatment methods will one have an accurate assessment of the true role of the operation in the patient's improvement. The clinician will also significantly increase the overall patient success rate by conducting these aggressive nonsurgical treatment methods.

If it is accepted that abnormal motion is present and a fusion is indicated, the method of the fusion is considered immediately. The posterior approach to the spine offers a great variety of surgical procedures. There is the ability to decompress the neurologic structures and achieve stabilization after that decompression. Methods include a posterior and posterolateral fusion; decompression, laminectomy, and foraminotomy with a lateral fusion; decompression, lateral fusion, and internal fixation; and posterior lumbar interbody fusion. Each of these posterior methods has been conducted with good results by numerous clinicians. A brief review of specifics and difficulties with these procedures includes:

1. *Posterior and posterolateral fusion.*[30] Success with posterior and posterolateral fusion for relieving back pain alone has not been accepted as sufficient to warrant the procedure except in cases of spondylolisthesis. The amount of residual motion in the disc space after a solid posterior and posterolateral fusion may be sufficient to allow continued annular pain

because of flexibility of the posterior fusion mass. The paraspinous approach does offer good exposure of the area to be fused and the ability to avoid the scarred midline area.

2. *Decompression with posterolateral fusion.* The procedure allows a maximum decompression and attempts to compensate for instability by fusing the remaining posterior elements. Decompression removes a significant portion of bone available for fusion. This may compromise the union rate and produce a greater chance of instability. There is a greater chance of pain due to motion under a solid fusion because it decreases the bulk of the fusion mass.

3. *Decompression, posterolateral fusion, and internal fixation.* Internal fixation may or may not improve fusion rates, probably depending on the method of internal fixation. The techniques of internal fixation of the lumbar spine are varied and continually under revision and, hopefully, improvement. Multilevel fixation and pedicle screw fixation have great promise but will follow the same evolution of successes and failures as internal fixation in other orthopedic conditions. A successful interbody fusion offers a good chance of complete immobilization of a neuromotion segment. At least it should have a greater chance of having a profound effect on the motion of a neuromotion segment than a posterior fusion.

4. *Posterior lumbar interbody fusions* offer the opportunity for total decompression in addition to fusion.[3,20] This operation is technically demanding. The usual indication for the posterior lumbar interbody fusion is a postlaminectomy syndrome patient with back and radicular pain. Postlaminectomy patients are the most difficult to perform additional back surgery on because of the dural scarring; they will have the highest neurologic complication rate. Posterior lumbar interbody exposure of articular surfaces to be fused is not as good as the anterior exposure. The carpentry is less precise compared to the anterior exposure. The exposure itself causes intense scarring, and when fusion is unsuccessful it may contribute to postoperative pain.

5. *Anterior lumbar interbody fusion.* Anterior interbody fusion offers the ability to avoid prior areas of neurologic scarrings as in postlaminectomy cases. Avoid prior posterior column infected areas. It offers excellent disc exposure and the ability to use skill and precision in the carpentry of the fusion technique under direct visualization. Approaching the spine through transperitoneal or retroperitoneal approach is similar to numerous transperitoneal and retroperitoneal operations for other conditions. The disadvantages are that decompression of neurologic structures is usually done in an indirect manner by stopping motion. Although direct removal of tissue from the posterior annulus and spinal canal through the disc space is possible, it is technically very difficult. There is a consistent 10% to 20% complication rate that must be considered with the choice of an anterior lumbar fusion. Anterior lumbar fusion should be considered a one-time operation. Repeat approaches to the anterior lumbar spine have a high vascular complication rate. Biomechanical considerations of the effects of anterior resection of the annulus and anterior longitudinal ligament are unknown.

Several past published reports (Table 38-1) stand out. An overall view of experience with anterior lumbar fusion demonstrates varying success with the procedure. The best results were with one surgeon doing all of the cases.* This allowed an accumulation of experience that improves results. Retrospective reviews of a number of surgeons at one institution doesn't show as good results.[1,7,29] Most of the cases with fewer numbers have less than ideal results.[1,7,28]

---

*References 2, 8, 9, 18, 22, 28.

Table 38-1 *Results of past studies*

	Union %	Clinical success %
Calandruccio[1]	32	56
Chow[2]	63	89
Flynn[7]	67	52
Freebody[8]	85	91
Fujimaki[10]	96	76
Goldner[11]	81	82
Harmon[12]	83,99	
Harmon[14]		100
Harmon[15]	83	95
Harmon[16]	95,85	79
Hodgson[17]	83	96
Hoover[18]	70	70
Humphries[19]	78	70
Nisbet	42	74
Raney[22]	83	63
Raney[23]	81	76
Ragstad[24]	81.6	82.2
Sacks[27]		88
Sacks[25]	72	88
Sijbrandij[28]	61	
Stauffer[29]	56,64	56
Taylor	44	

Using the same grafting technique helps to compare results but there is variance of technique between studies and within studies.[8,12,33]

Among the many contributions in this area, several studies offer specific information. Chow and associates,[2] in relating the Hong Kong experience, reviewed 97 patients, most of whom had back and leg pain from disc disease. Using strict radiographic criteria for union of their corticocancellous autogenous iliac plugs, they showed a marked disparity between one- and two-level fusion rates—85% to 45%. There was a 95% relief of sciatica and a 32% complication rate.

Freebody's work[8,9] was standardized by technique and surgeon and was reviewed independently. The fusion rate was 92.4% with disc lesions of a lower rate with spondylolisthesis of 84.3%. The clinical success was excellent, 90%.

Goldner's review[11] has a wealth of information. Discography was used effectively, and other diagnostic methods were discussed. The diagnostic categories were defined and the technique—iliac corticocancellous plugs—explained. There was 78% relief of back pain and 85% relief of leg pain. There was an 83% overall fusion rate that decreased with multilevels.

Harmon's diagnostic criteria[12,13,14,15,16] is difficult to understand. He uses Pantopaque myelogram and motion studies; 244 out of 650 cases were reviewed, meaning a great number of cases were not included. Those included had a strangely low complication rate of 1%, and great results of a clinical success rate of 90% and union rate of 95%.

Raney[22,23] had an 81% union rate and 76% clinical success rate using a combination of fibula and iliac crest. There is an extensive list of complications and methods to avoid them.

Rangstad[24] showed a lower union rate with spondylolisthesis of 76.9% compared to an overall rate in all cases of 87.0%. There was no correlation between the 82.2% who had good success and age, duration of symptoms, duration of disability, or union.

Sacks[25,26,27] has published extensively on anterior lumbar fusions. Using broad indications, a mixture of autologous and allogenous graft and occasional internal fixation, he had an 88% clinical success.

Stauffer[29] found a low 36% clinical success rate and advised use only when posterior fusion could not be done. The fusion rate was 56% and thought to be increased by a spica cast after surgery. There was no consistent diagnostic criteria nor standard technique among the seven surgeons that tried the procedure over an 8-year period. This study may be a better example of the ineffectiveness of anterior lumbar interbody fusion as an occasional operation rather than an indictment of faulty mechanics resulting

Table 38-2 *Preoperative morbidity review of total cases*

	Pain		Function		Occupation	
Scale 1	0	0%	3	3.5%	9	11%
Scale 2	7	8.5%	16	19.5%	14	17%
Scale 3	16	19.5%	24	29%	16	20%
Scale 4	59	72%	39	48%	43	52%
TOTAL	82		82		82	

from the anterior approach.

Flynn[7] had a union rate of 56% and clinical success of 52%. There was no correlation between union and clinical success. He presented retrograde ejaculation to be a transitory, overated complication.

In a review of severe failed back patients in whom O'Brien[33] performed an anterior lumbar fusion using a single midline strut with cancellous packing, the union rate was 77% and the clinical success rate was 90%.

A composite of papers of this kind shows what type of results can be expected. It allows one to choose some factors responsible for success.

1. Experience
2. Good grafting technique
3. Safe approaches

In a retrospective review of anterior lumbar fusions I reviewed the results of another surgeon.[32] An attempt was made to evaluate all cases done within the certain period of time. There was good clinical chart data on 82 patients; 60 were seen in follow-up.

The preoperative and postoperative morbidity was assessed by comparison of three categories of pain, function, and occupation (see box). The severity of preoperative morbidity is critical in justifying the operation (Table 38-2). The patients had 85 months with preoperative back pain and averaged 32 months of preoperative disability. Using the rating scales (Tables 38-3 to 38-5), the patients showed an average disability of 3.37 with 1 being minimum disability and 4 being the maximum. A 4 rating would be unable to work, bedridden, or on narcotics because of spinal pain. Of all the patients, 53% were work compensation cases and most were laborers or housewifes, 49% had at least one prior laminectomy.

The diagnosis for these patients was segmental instability. To condense the diagnostic criteria the patients had a history of mechanical and/or radicular pain with activity; 80% had positive straight leg raisings. Surgical decisions were

---

Morbidity ratings

Pain
1. No pain to mild pain, minimal discomfort with activity
2. Moderate pain, may take non-narcotic medication
3. Constant low grade or severe intermittent pain, intermittent narcotic use, may interfere with sleep
4. Constant severe pain, regular narcotic use, minimal to no relief of pain

Function
1. No impairment
2. Impairment of function
3. Inaffective community ambulator
4. Inaffective household ambulator

Occupation
1. Full-time
2. Part-time
3. Changed jobs
4. Unemployment

Table 38-3 Preoperative and postoperative pain ratings of patients available for review

Scale	Preoperative		Postoperative	
1	0	0%	26	43%
2	6	10%	25	42%
3	13	22%	3	5%
4	41	68%	6	10%
Total	60		60	

Table 38-4 Preoperative and postoperative function ratings of patients available for review

Scale	Preoperative		Postoperative	
1	3	5%	22	37%
2	12	20%	24	40%
3	19	32%	10	17%
4	26	43%	4	6%
Total	60		60	

Table 38-5 Preoperative and postoperative occupation ratings of patients available for review

Scale	Preoperative		Postoperative	
1	8	13%	22	42%
2	8	13%	6	12%
3	10	17%	9	17%
4	34	57%	15	29%
Total	60		52	

Table 38-6 Clinical improvement

	Number	Percent
Improved	55	91
Same	4	6
Worse	1	3

based predominantly on multilevel discography. All patients had discography and 60% had myelography, an important adjunctive test. Discography showed abnormal configuration, reproduced the patient's symptoms, and usually allowed symptom blocking with local anesthesia at each level to be fused.

The technique was the transperitoneal approach, iliac crest (autogenous and allogenous) tricorticate plugs after disc space distraction and chiseling of the endplate.

The postoperative clinical improvement was dramatic—91% improved, 6% remained the same and 3% worsened (Table 38-6). The morbidity ratings fell from 3.37 to 2.03; 41% improved their occupational rating.

The union rate was determined by flexion-extension films and radiographic appearance; 2 degrees of motion was labeled a nonunion. The union rate was 60%. Although it is significantly low, it had no correlation with clinical improvement. A significant number of fibrous unions and nonunions showed clinical improvement.

Postlaminectomy patients showed improvement equal to primary surgical patients. This may be an indication that anterior lumbar fusion is a reasonable choice for postlaminectomy patients because most other operative methods would have a lower success rate compared to primary surgery. Also, when worker's compensation cases with morbidity ratings of 3 to 4 in every category were reviewed as a separate group, they had an excellent recovery rate, indicating that anterior lumbar fusion has a role as a salvage operation for difficult patients (Table 38-7).

What are the indications for anterior lumbar interbody fusion? The ideal case is a patient who has had multiple operations, who is totally disabled with back and with leg pain. Discography is posi-

Table 38-7 *Postoperative clinical success rate in severely disabled patients (rating 3 and 4)*

	Pain	Function	Occupation
General population			
Asymptomatic	40%	19%	22%
Improved	47%	44%	19%
Same	11%	6%	27%
Worse	2%	0%	2%
Severely disabled worker's compensation cases			
Asymptomatic	22%	20%	9%
Improved	61%	73%	36%
Same	12%	7%	46%
Worse	5%	0%	9%

tive at one level (L4-L5) only, without spondylolisthesis. In discussing indications an assumption is made that the patient has sufficient morbidity and failure to respond to nonsurgical care to warrant an operation. It is best that the problem be confined to one or two levels with normal adjacent levels confirmed by discography. Relative indications include:

1. Primary large central disc herniation
2. Annular tear and segmental instability of an intervertebral disc
3. Primary disc herniation with a long history of disabling back pain
4. Postlaminectomy syndrome resulting from segmental instability
5. In combination with a posterior fusion for severe instability or deformity
6. In combination with anterior instrumentation in lumbar scoliosis

Special circumstances in which anterior lumbar fusion has distinct advantages over other methods include:

1. More back pain than leg pain
2. Dense scar around nerve and posterior elements
3. Posterior pseudoarthrosis
4. Prior posterior infection
5. Disc space infection

When choosing an anterior lumbar fusion as a treatment for a lumbar spine problem, a surgeon should be comfortable with not only the technique of the operation but also the philosophy of the operation. Being well trained and knowledgable concerning anterior lumbar fusions requires a reasonable number of cases to become proficient. Most surgeons performing this operation come in three groupings.

1. The surgeon who rejects entirely interbody fusion as a treatment for disc damage producing back pain regardless of the amount of pain and any concommitant conditions such as sciatica. These surgeons may use anterior lumbar fusion for lumbar scoliosis, disc space infection, and fractures only.
2. The second group of anterior lumbar surgeons consists of those who reserve the operation for the most difficult of lumbar spine disc problems. This includes circumferential fusions for certain types of lumbar instabilities such as spondylolisthesis, posterior pseudoarthrosis, posterior infection, kyphotic deformities, and failed surgery cases with predominantly back pain.
3. The third category of surgeons includes the most frequent users of anterior lumbar fusion. They would use anterior lumbar fusion, in addition to the indications outlined above, for primary disc herniations, postlaminectomy syndrome, an annular tear of the intervertebral disc with back pain only, and degenerative spondylolisthesis. These surgeons believe in the use of discography and anterior lumbar fusion as surgical treatment for incapacitating pain from the annulus of the intervertebral disc. It becomes a primary surgical procedure.

Some parameters of application for anterior lumbar fusion have been presented, but its exact role in the operative care of the lumbar spine may ultimately be an individual clinical-patient decision.

Editorial comments on p. 432.

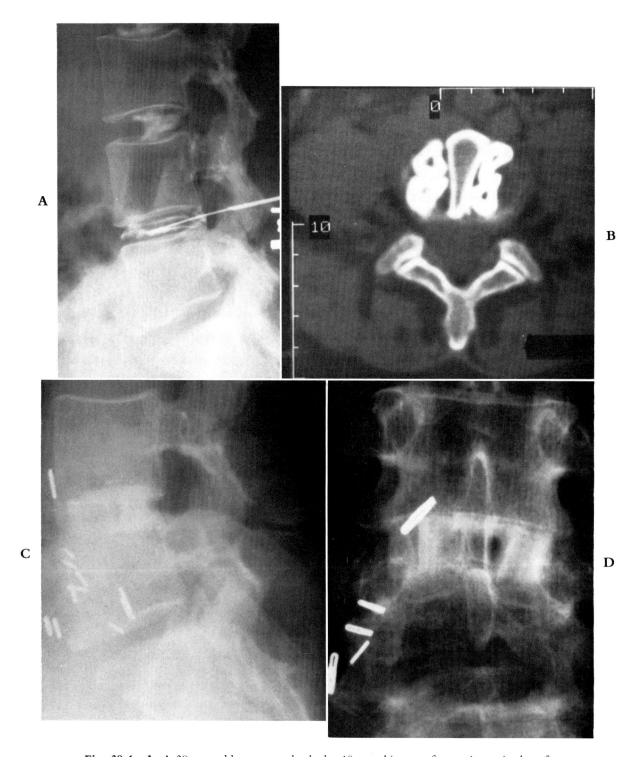

Fig. 38-1 A, A 39-year-old woman who had a 10-year history of recurring episodes of mechanical axial back pain. With childbirth and delivery the patient developed an excruciatingly severe back pain that predominantly confined her to bed rest for 6 months before evaluation. Patient had severe mechanical back pain that increased on coughing, sneezing and straining. There was no radiculitis or radiculopathy. Myelogram and CT scan (not shown) had no evidence of an intracanal lesion. Preoperative discography demonstrated normal levels at L2-L3, L3-L4, L5-S1, and symptomatic abnormal discography at L4-L5. L4-L5 disc was blocked with local anesthetic, producing significant relief in patient's symptoms. **B,** Postoperative CT scan showing a 4 fibula and 1 iliac crest graft. **C** and **D,** At follow-up patient is totally asymptomatic with no motion present in disc space.

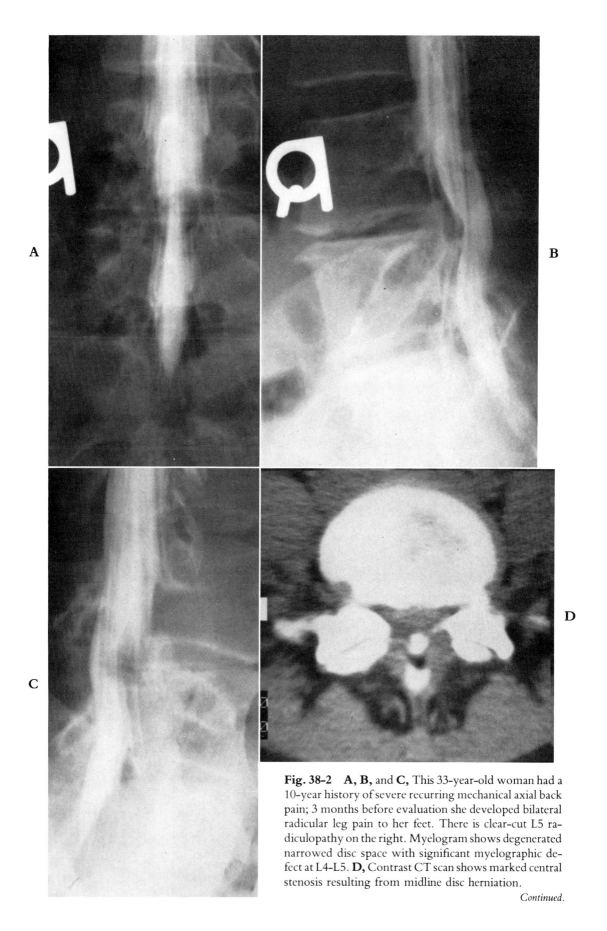

Fig. 38-2 **A, B,** and **C,** This 33-year-old woman had a 10-year history of severe recurring mechanical axial back pain; 3 months before evaluation she developed bilateral radicular leg pain to her feet. There is clear-cut L5 radiculopathy on the right. Myelogram shows degenerated narrowed disc space with significant myelographic defect at L4-L5. **D,** Contrast CT scan shows marked central stenosis resulting from midline disc herniation.

Continued.

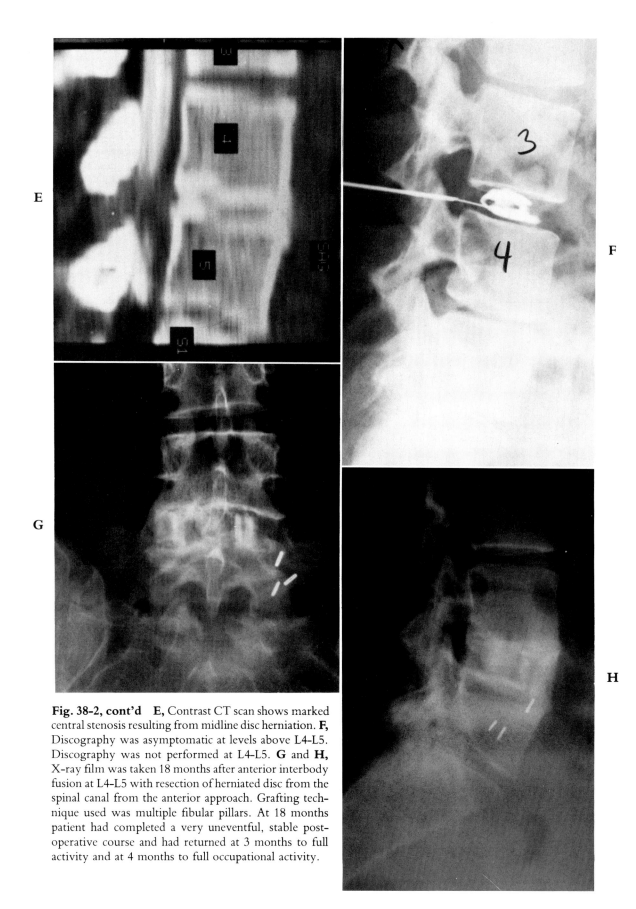

Fig. 38-2, cont'd **E**, Contrast CT scan shows marked central stenosis resulting from midline disc herniation. **F**, Discography was asymptomatic at levels above L4-L5. Discography was not performed at L4-L5. **G** and **H**, X-ray film was taken 18 months after anterior interbody fusion at L4-L5 with resection of herniated disc from the spinal canal from the anterior approach. Grafting technique used was multiple fibular pillars. At 18 months patient had completed a very uneventful, stable postoperative course and had returned at 3 months to full activity and at 4 months to full occupational activity.

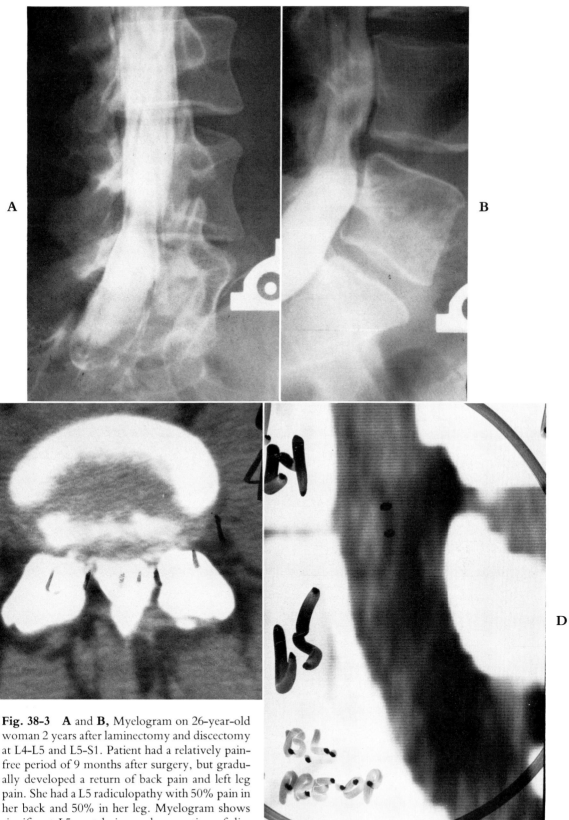

Fig. 38-3 **A** and **B,** Myelogram on 26-year-old woman 2 years after laminectomy and discectomy at L4-L5 and L5-S1. Patient had a relatively pain-free period of 9 months after surgery, but gradually developed a return of back pain and left leg pain. She had a L5 radiculopathy with 50% pain in her back and 50% in her leg. Myelogram shows significant L5 root lesion and suggestion of disc herniation at L4-L5. **C** and **D,** Her CT scan showing scar, stenosis, and recurrent disc herniation at L4-L5. Although laminectomy and disecectomy had also been performed at L5-S1, radiographic changes at that level were not as significant.

Continued.

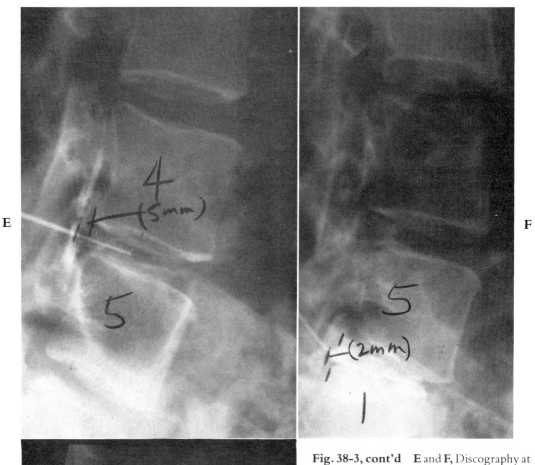

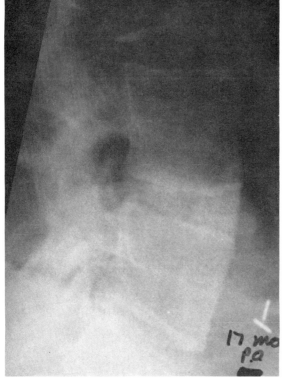

Fig. 38-3, cont'd **E** and **F,** Discography at L2-L3 and L3-L4 were negative. Discography at L4-L5 reproduced patient's pain exactly and allowed for partial ablation of pain with local anesthetic injection. L5-S1 disc was asymptomatic on discography. **G,** X-ray film was done 17 months after anterior interbody fusion using fibular graft. Patient is totally asymptomatic, has returned to work, and is working in body reconditioning program. It was elected not to fuse L5-S1 level because patient had minimal symptoms from that area, had a clear-cut myelographic, CT scan, discographic lesion at L4-L5 that matched her clinical symptoms.

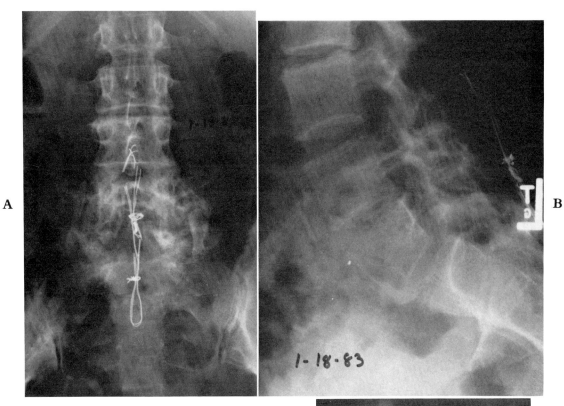

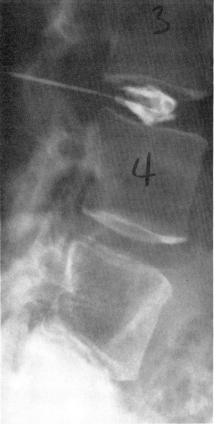

Fig. 38-4 This 41-year-old woman had past history of three prior spine operations, the last a posterior and posterolateral fusion at L4 to S1. She was pain-free approximately 6 months and then developed severe back and radiating leg pain. Her pain was with forward bending and had a reproducible mechanical component. Discography could not be performed because of size of posterior fusion mass, but motion was measured through center of fusion mass, indicating pseudarthrosis. **C,** Discography at level above fusion mass proved to be negative. There is narrowing of the L2-L3 disc space. This was asymptomatic on discography.   *Continued.*

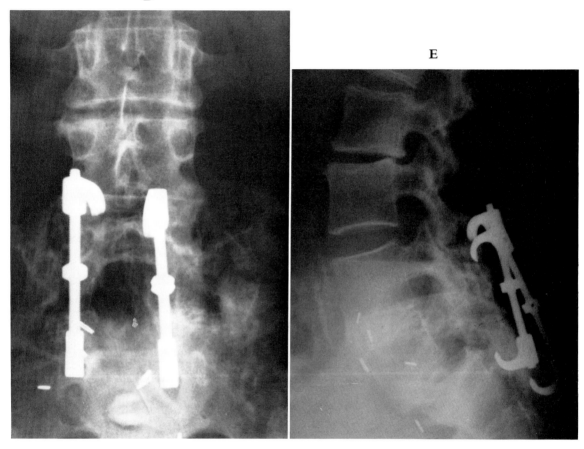

Fig. 38-4, cont'd **D** and **E,** Patient underwent two-stage anterior and posterior fusion, the first stage being a posterior pseudarthrosis resection, regrafting and Knodt rod internal instrumentation. The bony bed posteriorly for regrafting was very poor. Second stage was a 2-level anterior lumbar fusion. Patient has had marked symptomatic improvement but is still unable to work 2 years after surgery. Poor quality of bone posteriorly was believed to be totally inadequate for posterior refusion.

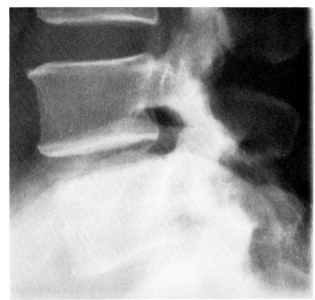

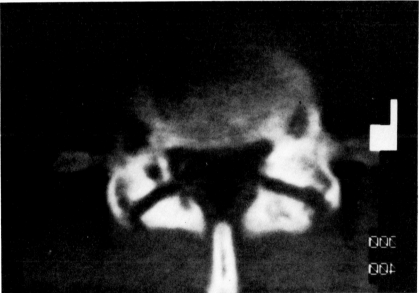

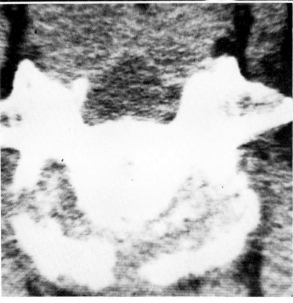

Fig. 38-5 A, This 46-year-old male had a history of 6 months of back and leg pain before an evaluation by an orthopaedic surgeon. Based on positive myelogram and CT scan for disc herniation, patient underwent chemonucleolysis. **B,** CT scan taken 30 days after surgery reveals evidence of infection. Patient had normal sedimentation rate and was afebrile, but he had extreme back pain with a drop foot on the left. Based on this CT scan he underwent a major posterior decompression and debridement. Postoperative cultures were negative, but they showed an intense red granulation tissue. **C,** CT scan done 11 months after laminectomy shows that total facetectomy and laminectomy had been carried out. Patient had return of significant back and leg pain after 3-month pain-free interval. *Continued.*

Fig. 38-5, cont'd **D,** Patient's x-ray film, demonstrating what appears to be an infection; 11 months after surgery the patient had a Craig needle biopsy, revealed no evidence of infection or reactive bone. The cultures were negative. Sedimentation rate was 28. At this point patient has excruciating back pain, is unable to ambulate, and is unrelieved by narcotic medication. **E,** Immediate postsurgical films demonstrate satisfactory disc space distraction and graft in place. Anterior fusion was carried out after anterior debridement revealed no evidence of infection on Gram's stain or frozen section. There was excellent bleeding and clean bone for grafting surface. Autogenous iliac crest was used. **F,** Graft collapse and suggestions of early fusion 8 months after surgery. Patient is asymptomatic.

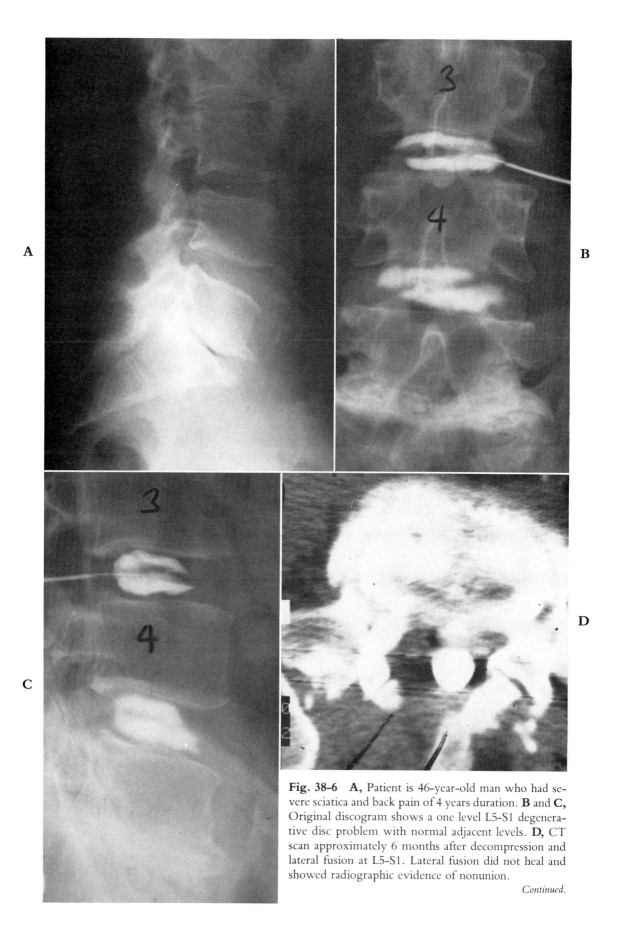

Fig. 38-6 **A,** Patient is 46-year-old man who had severe sciatica and back pain of 4 years duration. **B** and **C,** Original discogram shows a one level L5-S1 degenerative disc problem with normal adjacent levels. **D,** CT scan approximately 6 months after decompression and lateral fusion at L5-S1. Lateral fusion did not heal and showed radiographic evidence of nonunion.

Continued.

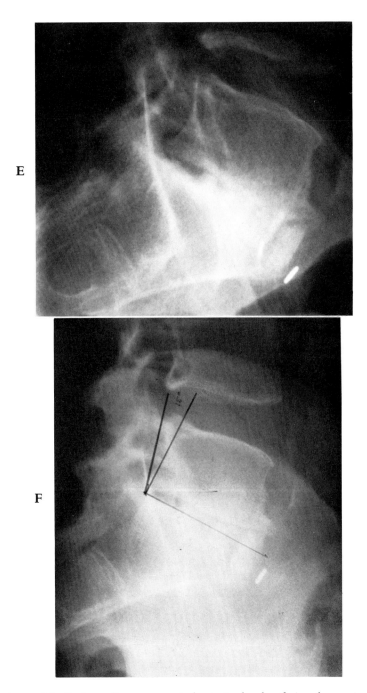

Fig. 38-6, cont'd **E,** Immediate postsurgical anterior lumbar fusion demonstrating distraction of disc space. **F,** Follow-up film showing progression of satisfactory union with no motion on flexion/extension films. There is improvement in symptomatology at 16 months after surgery.

REFERENCES

1. Calandruccio, R.A., and Benton, B.F.: Anterior lumbar fusion, Clin. Orthop. **35**:63, 1964.
2. Chow, S.P., et al.: Anterior spinal fusion for deranged lumbar intervertebral discs, Spine **5**:452, 1980.
3. Cloward, R.B.: Spondylolisthesis: treatment by laminectomy and posterior interbody fusion: review of 100 cases, Clin. Orthop. **154**:74, 1981.
4. Crock, H.V.: Observations on the management of failed spinal operations, J. Bone Joint Surg. **58B**:193, 1976.
5. Crock, H.V.: Anterior lumbar interbody fusion: indications for its use and notes on surgical technique, Clin. Orthop. **165**:157, 1982.
6. DePalma, A.F., and Rothman, R.H.: The nature of pseudoarthrosis, Clin. Orthop. **59**:113, 1968.
7. Flynn, J.C., and Hogue, M.A.: Anterior fusion of the lumbar spine, J. Bone Joint Surg. **61A**:114B, 1979.
8. Freebody, D.: Treatment of spondylolisthesis by anterior fusion via the transperitoneal route, J. Bone Joint Surg. **46B**:788, 1964.
9. Freebody, D., et al.: Anterior transperitoneal lumbar fusion, J. Bone Joint Surg. **53B**:617, 1971.
10. Fujimaki, A., et al.: The results of 150 anterior lumbar interbody fusion operations performed by two surgeons in Australia, Clin. Orthop. **165**:164, 1982.
11. Goldner, J.L., et al.: Anterior disc excision and interbody spinal fusion for chronic low back pain, Orthop. Clin. North Am. **2**:543, 1971.
12. Harmon, P.H.: Experiences with anterior interbody spinal fusion, J. Bone Joint Surg. **41A**:562, 1959.
13. Harmon, P.H.: Operative technique and some ten year end results from abdominal disc excision and vertebral body fusions in the lumbar spine, J. Bone Joint Surg. **41A**:1355, 1959.
14. Harmon, P.H.: Anterior lumbar disc excision and fusion. I. Study of the long term results, various grafting materials. Clin. Orthop. **18**:196, 1960.
15. Harmon, P.H.: Anterior lumbar disc excision and fusion. II. Operative technique including observation upon variations in the left common iliac veins, Clin. Orthop. **18**:185, 1960.
16. Harmon, P.H.: Anterior excision and vertebral body fusion operation for intervertebral disc syndromes of the lower lumbar spine: three to five year results in 244 cases, Clin. Orthop. **26**:107, 1963.
17. Hodgson, A.R., and Wong, S.K.: A description of a technique and evaluation of results in anterior spinal fusion for deranted intervertebral disc and spondylolisthesis, Clin. Orthop. **56**:133, 1968.
18. Hoover, N.W.: Indications for fusion at the time of removal of intervertebral disc, J. Bone Joint Surg. **50A**:189, 1968.
19. Humphries, A.W., et al.: Anterior interbody fusion of the lumbar vertebrae: a surgical technique, Surg. Clin. North Am. **41**:1685, 1961.
20. Hutter, C.G.: General orthopedics: posterior intervertebral body fusion, 25 year study, Clin. Orthop. **179**:86, 1983.
21. Kingston, S., and Watkins, R.G.: Principles and techniques of spine surgery, Baltimore, 1986, Aspen Systems.
22. Raney, F.L. Jr., and Adams, J.E.: Anterior lumbar disc excision and interbody fusion used as a salvage procedure (proceedings of the Western Orthopedic Association), J. Bone Joint Surg. **45A**:667, 1963.
23. Raney, F.L. Jr.: Spinal Disorders, 1977.
24. Ragstad, T.S., et al.: Acta Orthop. Scandia **53**:561, 1982.
25. Sacks, S.: Anterior interbody fusion of the lumbar spine, J. Bone Joint Surg. **47B**:211, 1965.
26. Sacks, S.: Experiences with posterior, anterior and posterolateral spine fusions. J. West. Pacific Orthop. Assoc. **6**(1)187, 1969.
27. Sacks, S.: Anterior spinal surgery in Ballarat (proceedings of the Australian Orthopedic Association) J. Bone Joint Surg. **52B**:392, 1970.
28. Sijbrandij, S.: The value of anterior interbody vertebral fusion in the treatment of lumbosacral insufficiency, with special reference to spondylolisthesis, Arch. Chir. Neelandicum. **14**:37, 1962.
29. Stauffer, R.G., and Coventry, M.D.: Anterior interbody lumbar spine fusion, J. Bone Joint Surg. **54A**(4)756, 1972.
30. Watkins, M.B.: Posterolateral bone grafting for fusion of the lumbar and lumbosacral spine, J. Bone Joint Surg. **41A**:388, 1959.
31. Watkins, R.G.: Surgical approaches to the spine, New York, 1983, Springer-Verlag.
32. Watkins, R.G.: Anterior interbody fusion: a clinical review; presentation, American Academy of Orthopedic Surgeons meeting, Las Vegas, 1985, (Submitted for publication).
33. Watkins, R.G., et al.: Comparisons of preoperative and postoperative MMPI data in chronic back patients treated by anterior lumbar fusion, Spine, 1985, (In press).

EDITORIAL COMMENTARY

The anterior interbody fusion was the fourth most popular surgical procedure among the authors of this text. All find it of some value, and half find it of great value. Six authors have had significant complications with the procedure. Although Vert Mooney and David Selby find that they are able to do anterior interbody fusions rapidly and reliably by the use of Harry Crock's hole cutter and dowel technique, other authors, such as Leon Wiltse, Kirkaldy-Willis and Hugo Keim, find the procedure demanding and with significant potential dangers. Richard Rothman seldom finds this procedure necessary and has experienced no significant complications.

Leon Wiltse points out that the success rate seems to be directly related to the volume used and the accuracy of fitting the bone in the interbody space. He finds that "the rate of failure in anterior interbody fusion has traditionally been distressingly high." His indications for anterior interbody fusions are patients who have had failed surgery posteriorly, after infections that have not fused and for "idiopathic vertebral sclerosis."

In San Francisco we find few indications for the use of anterior interbody fusion. There is usually a condition within the vertebral canal or intervertebral foramen that is a probable source of the patient's pain. Our primary thrust has therefore been to deal with the primary source of pain posteriorly and, if a fusion is necessary, do it posteriorly. We agree with Kirkaldy-Willis who uses "this procedure for the treatment of discogenic pain. The results for mechanical and degenerative lesions are at best equivocal."

Anterior interbody fusion has been popular for cases in which posterior fusion has failed to give a solid fusion. Since the advent of internal fixation many of those previously using anterior interbody fusion now prefer a repeat posterior fusion with the adjunct of Luque rods or pedicle screws.

Discograms on some of our failed posterior fusion cases have revealed painful discs that have not previously been excised under solid posterior fusions. Anterior interbody fusion would, of course, be an excellent choice for such a situation.

Arthur H. White

PART THREE

SPINE SURGERY: AN ANTHOLOGY

CHAPTER 39

BONE GRAFTS AND IMPLANTS IN SPINE SURGERY

Ken Hsu   James F. Zucherman   Arthur H. White

Recent advances in both fusion techniques and instrumentation have markedly facilitated the treatment of spinal disorders. Yet a significant number of patients exist who continue to have pseudarthroses. Despite the surgical advances the essentials of a successful spinal fusion still appear to be the effective application of sound bone grafting principles. These principles, along with the techniques, problems, and complications associated with bone grafting, are reviewed in this chapter.

The loss of bone in the spine often presents serious difficulties not seen in other areas. The most favorable replacement would still be a bone graft that fills the defect and becomes incorporated into the spine. However, the availability of appropriate bone to replace the loss is a significant problem. Alternatives to bone grafts, including a number of implants used to stabilize the spine, are also surveyed.

Bone grafts have often played the roles of scaffolds, bridges, spacers, fillers of defects, and replacements of bone lost. Immobilization of multiple motion segments is frequently necessary in the spine; great demands are made on bone grafts. In the lumbosacral spine, body weight and muscular forces impart loads equal to three or four times body weight.[121] It is not surprising that the highest rate of bone graft failure is seen in the lumbosacral spine. Hence, the following is a discussion of technical problems, biomechanical and physiologic characteristics of bone grafts, and implants.

THE AUTOGRAFT

Autograft, or bone graft transplanted from one site to another in the same individual, is considered to be the most biologically suitable. Its advantages include:
1. Has superior osteogenic capacity
   a. Contributes cells capable of immediate bone formation
   b. Allows for bone induction by recipient bed where nonosseous

tissue is influenced to change its cellular function and become osteogenic
2. Lack of histocompatibility differences or immunologic problems
3. Ease of incorporation
4. No disease transmission

The disadvantages include:
1. Additional incision or wider exposure, prolonged operative time, and increased blood loss
2. Increased postoperative morbidity
3. Sacrifice of normal structure and weakening of donor bone
4. Risks of significant complications
5. Limitations in size, shape, quantity, and quality

For optimal results harvest autogenous cancellous bone in the following manner.
1. In thin strips
   a. Not exceeding 5 mm in thickness[51,106]
   b. To provide maximal exposure of superficial cells
   c. To allow rapid vascularization
2. Graft wrapped in a gauze soaked in patient's blood
   a. To avoid exposure to high intensity lights
   b. Kept in temperature less than 42° C[51]
   c. Not stored in saline or antibiotic solution[3,109]
   d. Without the use of chemical sterilization[109]
3. Transfer the graft to the recipient bed as soon as possible to
   a. Avoid exposure to air for more than 30 minutes[51]
   b. Protect the viability of the surface cells
4. Place the graft
   a. In well-vascularized bone bed
   b. In well-decorticated bone surface (cancellous site is superior)
   c. With healthy soft tissue coverage
5. Minimize surgical trauma because, for example, high speed burring and inadequate irrigation retard healing[1,117]
6. Position the cancellous surface
   a. On opposing cancellous surface
   b. On surrounding soft tissue with good blood supply
   c. So that total mass of graft is not too thick to prevent nutrient diffusion from recipient bed
7. Always avoid
   a. Dead space
   b. Hematoma
   c. Interposition of necrotic tissue
8. To minimize risk, be aware of
   a. Anatomy
   b. Potential complications

The *iliac crest* is the most versatile bone graft reserve. It is relatively subcutaneous and easy to harvest in prone, supine, lateral, or other positions. It is expendable, and it has a large reserve of cortical and cancellous bone. In addition, it allows carpentering of different shapes and sizes.

Anterior Iliac Crest Grafts

Anterior iliac crest bone grafts are used for anterior interbody fusion of the cervical, thoracic, or lumbosacral spine. The subcutaneous anterior superior iliac spine and iliac crest and easily palpable. The iliac tubercle is the widest portion where a large quantity of corticocancellous bone is found. (See Fig. 39-8.)

A skin incision is made parallel to or in line with the iliac crest. It is advantageous to center the incision over the iliac tubercle. The incision is carried down to the bone of the crest, and the muscles are elevated subperiosteally to expose the wing of the ilium.

The tensor fascia latae, gluteus medius, and gluteus minimus originate from the lateral aspect of the ilium. They are innervated by the superior gluteal nerve. The abdominal muscles are also attached to the iliac crest and are segmentally innervated. The incision over the crest is therefore "internervous" and safe.

An appropriate osteotome or chisel may be used to outline a cortical window in the lateral iliac surface from which to procure the bone graft. Longitudinal parallel cuts may be made (Fig. 39-1). Strips of cancellous bone may be removed with a curved gauge. Care must be taken not to violate the inner table of the iliac wing where hernia is a significant potential complication.

Bone graft may be obtained from the inner table of the iliac wing. However, there are risks of peritoneal perforation and significant bleeding with formation of hematoma in the retroperitoneal space.

It is important not to carry the incision to or anterior to the anterior superior iliac spine. Injury to the lateral femoral cutaneous nerve or the inguinal ligament must be avoided. Detachment of the inguinal ligament may result in inguinal hernia. If bicortical bone is taken too close to the anterior superior iliac spine, fracture may occur. (See Fig. 39-6.) Avulsion of the anterior superior iliac spine may occur by the action of the attached muscles, such as the tensor fascia lata or sartorius.

Bone may be removed in the form of block, dowel, strips, and by way of cortical window or "trap door" (Figs. 39-1 to 39-4). The iliac crest contour can be preserved by removing the bone deep to the crest, or by temporarily detaching and repositioning it later (Fig. 39-5). The anterior superior iliac spine should be left intact to maintain normal appearance. The region of the iliac spine should not be weakened by removing bone adjacent to it. Fracture and displacement of the inguinal ligament may result (Fig. 39-6).

The wound should be closed properly. The muscles and fascia must be sutured to their original anatomic positions and the defects closed; an effective drain should be used.

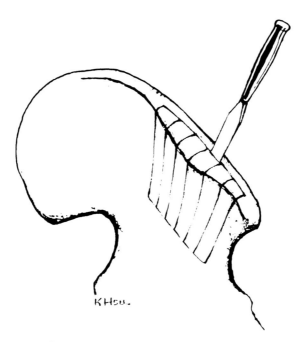

Fig. 39-1 Corticocancellous bone graft is obtained from lateral iliac surface using longitudinal parallel cuts with an osteotome or chisel.

Bone Grafts and Implants in Spine Surgery 437

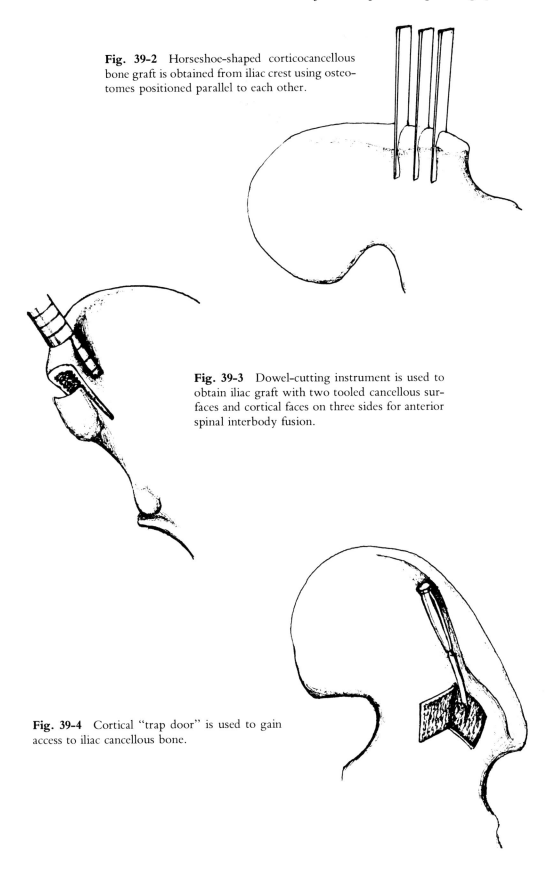

Fig. 39-2 Horseshoe-shaped corticocancellous bone graft is obtained from iliac crest using osteotomes positioned parallel to each other.

Fig. 39-3 Dowel-cutting instrument is used to obtain iliac graft with two tooled cancellous surfaces and cortical faces on three sides for anterior spinal interbody fusion.

Fig. 39-4 Cortical "trap door" is used to gain access to iliac cancellous bone.

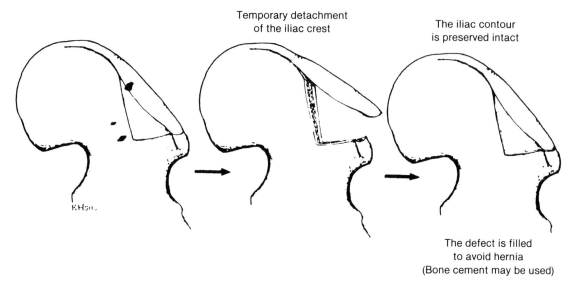

Fig. 39-5 Large iliac graft is obtained with preservation of the iliac contour.

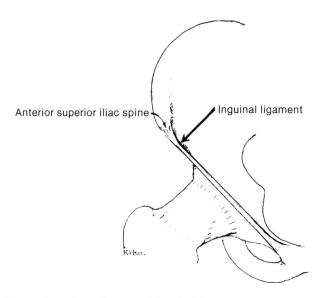

Fig. 39-6 Illustration of attachment of inguinal ligament to anterior superior iliac spine. Detachment of inguinal ligament may lead to inguinal hernia. Injury to lateral femoral cutaneous nerve should also be avoided.

Posterior Iliac Crest Grafts

The posterior iliac crest provides a large quantity of cortical cancellous bone graft. The posterior superior iliac crest is palpable under the skin dimple in the superior medial aspect of the gluteal region. The iliac crest curves cephalad and laterally from the posterior superior iliac spine.

An oblique, curved or vertical incision may be made over the posterior iliac crest or in line with it. The cluneal nerves cross the iliac crest 7 to 12 cm anterolateral to the posterior superior iliac spine (see discussion under Complications) and must be protected (see Fig. 39-13).

A midline spine incision may be extended distally and the posterior iliac crest approached laterally under the skin and subcutaneous fat. This avoids the use of a second skin incision.

The incision is carried down to the bone of the crest, and the muscles are elevated subperiosteally from the posterior lateral surface of the ilium. This approach does not denervate the muscles. The gluteus maximus, medius, and minimus originate from the lateral surface of the ilium. The superior gluteal nerve innervates the gluteus medius and minimus, and the inferior gluteal nerve innervates the gluteus maximus. The paraspinal musculature innervated segmentally originates from the iliac crest.

It is very important to remember the following rules.
1. Stay on bone and work subperiosteally.
2. Avoid the sciatic notch and protect the sciatic nerve.
3. Protect the superior gluteal vessels (see discussion under Complications) and protect the pelvic stability.
4. Avoid the sacroiliac joint.
5. Protect the posterior sacroiliac ligaments.

The removal of bone in the vicinity of the sciatic notch can weaken the thick bone that forms the notch. This can produce instability of the pelvis. It is important to stay cephalad to the sciatic notch and remove bone only from the false pelvis. For a landmark, an imaginary line dropped anteriorly from the posterior superior iliac spine with the patient in the prone position can be used as the caudal limit of bone removal (see Fig. 39-15, *A* and *B*). Care must be taken not to enter the sacroiliac joint, which may become a source of persistent pain and instability when injured.

A sharp surgical instrument (that is, an osteotome or tip of Taylor retractor) may injure the sciatic nerve deep to the sciatic notch. Laceration of the superior gluteal vessels is a significant danger in this region. The vessels leave the pelvis via the sciatic notch. A divided vessel can easily retract into the pelvis and presents a very alarming complication (see discussion under Complications) (see Fig. 39-14).

Nutrient vessels supplying the ilium found in the mid portion of the anterior gluteal line may present troublesome bleeding and should be controlled with Gelfoam, Surgicel, bone wax, or electrocoagulation.

A relatively painless bone graft donor site for lumbar spine fusion is possible by applying the following technique. A separate incision over the iliac crest is *not* made through the skin. The fascia through the wound of the lumbar surgery is grasped with Kochers clamps and pulled medially. The subcutaneous tissue is carefully elevated off the fascia laterally and caudally until the fascia immediately above the posterior iliac crest and posterior superior iliac spine is reached. A Taylor retractor is placed in the subcutaneous tissue lateral to the crest over the ilium posteriorly. The periosteum is not dissected from the ilium except from the superior-most crest. The fascia is incised over the crest, and an elevator is used to scrape the superior crest free of perios-

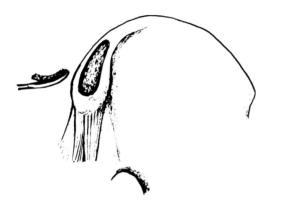

Fig. 39-7 A gouge is used to remove posterior "roof" of ilium and the cancellous bone between cortical layers.

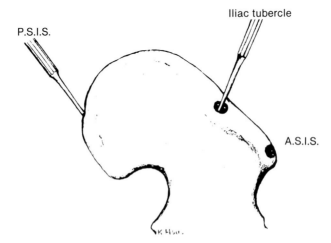

Fig. 39-8 Cancellous bone is removed from iliac tubercle, anterior or posterior iliac spine region through small cortical opening.

teum to bare bone. Gouges are used to remove the "roof" of the ilium and the cancellous bone between the cortical layers, leaving the cortices intact laterally and medially with their soft tissue attachments (Fig. 39-7). This technique minimizes postoperative donor site pain and prevents uncomfortable scar tissue from forming over the ilium, as when the lateral cortices are removed.

When limited quantity of cancellous bone is required, the following methods may be advantageous:

Currettage allows harvest of cancellous graft with least morbidity through a small round cortical window using a sharp curette as shown in Fig. 39-8. Cancellous bone is most abundant in the posterior aspect of the iliac crest, followed by the iliac tubercle and anterior superior iliac spine areas.

A *"trap door"* cut in the anterior or posterior outer table of the ilium and hinged on muscles can be opened to allow access to cancellous bone. The trap door is closed at the end. Postoperative pain appears to be less with this technique. Cosmetic deformity is minimal (see Fig. 39-4).

Wolfe and Kawamoto[125] reported a technique of obtaining full thickness bone graft from the anterior ilium. Incision is made through the iliac crest. The outer ridges of the iliac crest are split obliquely with the muscular and periosteal attachments remaining. All the iliac bone be-

Bone Grafts and Implants in Spine Surgery 441

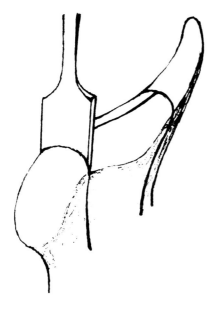

Fig. 39-9 Wolfe and Kawamoto's technique of obtaining full thickness bone graft from the anterior ilium. A sharp osteotome is used to make appropriate cuts shown above and in Fig. 39-10.

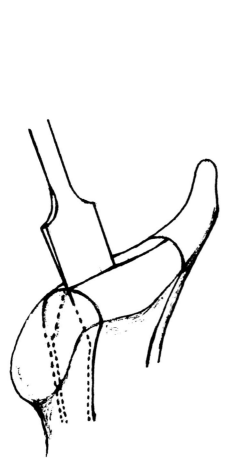

Fig. 39-10 The ridges of the iliac crest are split obliquely with the osteotome. The muscular and periosteal attachments should remain.

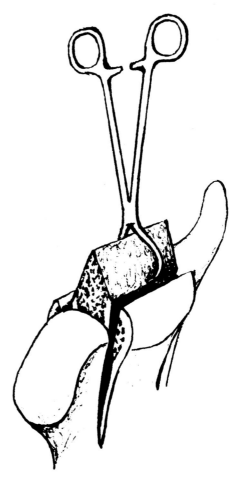

Fig. 39-11 A large full-thickness bone graft can be removed as shown, using Wolfe and Kawamoto's method.

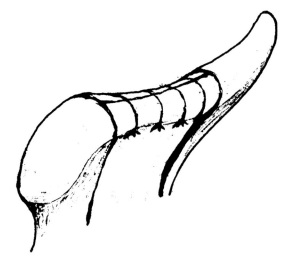

Fig. 39-12 Wolfe and Kawamoto's technique of reapproximating the two fragments of the crest, using wires or sutures. Figure eight wire or suture may be passed through the bone with an awl and fixed to adjacent bone.

neath this can then be removed. The edges of the crest may be reapproximated, thus minimizing cosmetic deformity, hernia, hematoma, and postoperative morbidity (Figs. 39-9 to 39-12).

COMPLICATIONS

Complications involving the iliac bone graft donor site are not uncommon. Although some of these complications may not be serious, they add to the patient's discomfort and prolong the convalescence. The complications that are due to graft removal from the ilium include:
1. Major blood loss
2. Hematoma
3. Nerve injury (neuroma formation)
4. Severe pain (chronic pain)
5. Hernia
6. Cosmetic deformity
7. Fracture
8. Sacroiliac joint injury
9. Pelvic instability
10. Hip subluxation
11. Gait disturbance
12. Peritoneal injury
13. Ureteral injury
14. Heterotopic bone formation
15. Infection

Cockin[24] reviewed 118 cases of iliac crest bone graft procedures and found major complications in 3.4% and minor complaints in 6%. There were two cases of meralgia paresthetica, one of hernia, and one of hip subluxation after extensive removal of the iliac crest. The minor complaints included wound pain, hypersensitivity, and buttock anesthesia.

Nerve Injuries

Possible *nerve injuries* include the following.
1. Lateral femoral cutaneous nerve[24,118]
2. Iliohypogastric (lateral cutaneous branch) nerve
3. Superior cluneal nerve (cutaneous branches of dorsal rami L1, L2, L3)[25,35]
4. Middle cluneal nerve (cutaneous branches of dorsal rami S1, S2, S3)
5. Sciatic nerve
6. Ilio-inguinal nerve[10]
7. Femoral nerve
8. Superior gluteal nerve

Superior cluneal nerves are lateral branches of the posterior primary division of the upper three lumbar nerves that run posteriorly through the lumbosacral fascia at the lateral origin of sacrospinatus

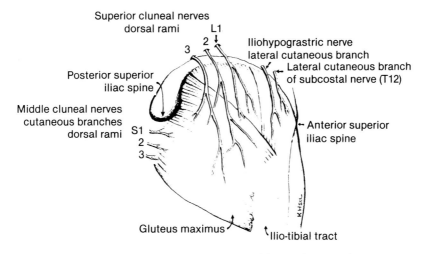

Fig. 39-13 Illustration of the nerves that may be injured during the procedure to remove bone graft from the iliac crest.

muscle. They cross over the dorsal aspect of the posterior iliac crest and provide sensation to the skin of the buttocks. They are found 7 to 12 cm anterolateral to the posterior superior iliac spine in the adult. When incision is made across or parallel to the posterior iliac crest, the cluneal nerves may be injured (Fig. 39-13).

Painful neuritis of the buttocks has been reported.[25,35] That these nerves are a cause of disability can be demonstrated by relief of symptoms after they have been infiltrated with local anesthetics. Permanent relief can be obtained by resection of the nerves with the transected ends allowed to retract into the soft tissue.

The sciatic nerve may be injured when the dissection is extended down to the sciatic notch. A surgical instrument such as an osteotome may be passed deep to the sciatic notch to cause this injury. The bony rim of the notch should be palpated before the dissection is carried to this area. An imaginary plumb line dropped from the posterior superior iliac spine with the patient in the prone position will pass through the bony rim of the sciatic notch. This serious complication can be avoided if you stay cephalad to this line (see Figs. 39-14 and 39-15).

The ilioinguinal nerve may be injured when the abdominal wall is retracted medially from the anterior iliac crest. The nerve may be compressed beneath the retractor on the inner part of the wall of the ilium. It occurs when the inner cortex of the anterior ilium is exposed for removal of bone grafts. Ilioinguinal neurologic injury is characterized by pain radiating from the iliaca toward the inguinal and genital areas. This complication is well discussed by Smith and associates.[101]

The iliohypograstric nerve (lateal cutaneous branch, L1 ventral rami) is found over the midlateral aspect os the iliac crest. It should be protected when working in this region (see Fig. 39-13).

Vascular Injuries

Vascular injuries may include the superior gluteal artery (and vein),[40,57] the deep circumflex iliac artery, the iliolumbar artery, and the fourth lumbar artery.

The superior gluteal artery is a branch of the internal iliac artery that curves around the rim of the sciatic notch as it leaves the pelvis. It may be injured when dissection is carried close to the sciatic notch. An osteotome or the sharp point of a Taylor retractor may enter the notch

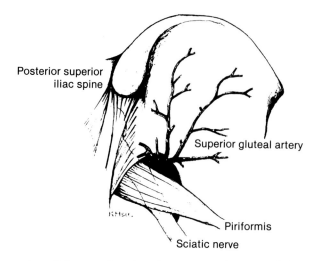

Fig. 39-14 Illustration of the superior gluteal artery, curving around the rim of the sciatic notch as it leaves the pelvis.

and pose similar danger to the artery. This complication can become alarming, since the divided vessel easily retracts into the pelvis (Fig. 39-14).

If the superior gluteal vessel is lacerated, it can be compressed locally and exposed for ligation or clipping. A finger may be used to apply direct pressure to the vessel against the bone. Kahn[57] discussed the use of a Raney-modified Kerrison rongeur to remove the upper margin of the sciatic notch to expose the bleeding vessel. If the bleeding vessel is still not accessible, the patient may be positioned for a retroperitoneal or transperitoneal exposure of the vessel. Arterial occlusion by embolization or using a Fogerty catheter is another option.

Injury to the superior gluteal vessels can be prevented if the surgeon is well aware of the anatomy in this region. The bony origin of the gluteus maximus or the roughened area anterior to the posterior superior iliac spine is a good landmark and can be used as the caudal limit of bone removal (Fig. 39-15, *A* and *B*). An imaginary plumb line dropped from the posterior superior iliac spine with the patient in the prone position will pass through the bony rim of the sciatic notch. It is important to stay cephalad to this line.

Escalas and DeWald[40] reported a case of combined traumatic superior gluteal arteriovenous fistula and ureteral injury complicating removal of bone graft from the posterior ilium. The tip of a Taylor retractor accidentally dislodged and penetrated into the sciatic notch to cause this unusual injury.

The *deep circumflex iliac artery*, the *iliolumbar artery*, or the *fourth lumbar artery* may cause troublesome bleeding when working on the inner table of the ilium. Occasionally, peritoneal perforation accompanies the arterial injury. The anatomic position of the arteries are illustrated in Figs. 39-16 and 39-17. It is very important to stay subperiosteally and carefully elevate the abdominal wall muscles off the crest and the iliacus muscles off the inner table of the ilium (Fig. 39-18).

A *hernia* through the iliac bone graft donor site may occur after the removal of full thickness bone from that site. It may appear as an iliac swelling, sometimes associated with pain or symptoms of bow-

Bone Grafts and Implants in Spine Surgery 445

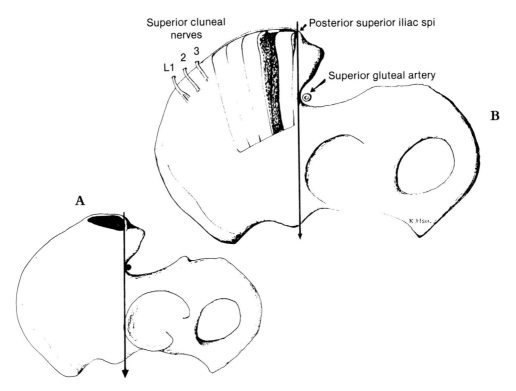

Fig. 39-15 **A,** The bony origin of the gluteus maximus or the roughened area anterior to the posterior superior iliac crest is a good landmark and can be used as the caudal limit of bone removal. An imaginary plumb line dropped from the P.S.I.S. with the patient in the prone position will pass through the bony rim of the sciatic notch. The superior gluteal artery is adjacent to the bony rim. **B,** A large amount of bone graft can be removed safely if the surgeon stays cephalad to the P.S.I.S., the sciatic notch and the imaginary line joining them.

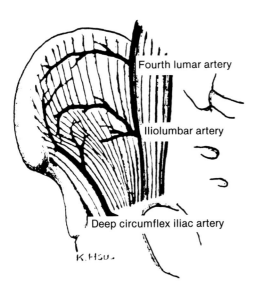

Fig. 39-16 Illustration of the anatomic positions of the arteries that may cause troublesome bleeding when working on the inner table of the ilium.

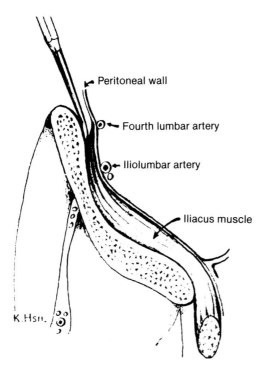

Fig. 39-17 The anatomic locations of the peritoneal wall and the vulnerable arteries are shown relative to the iliacus muscle and the inner wall of the ilium.

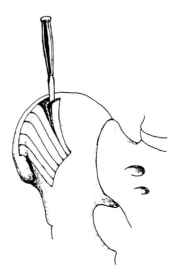

Fig. 39-18 It is very important to stay subperiosteally and carefully elevate the abdominal wall muscles off the crest and the iliacus muscle off the iliac wall before removing the bone from the inner table of the ilium.

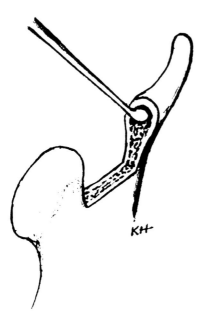

Fig. 39-19 The large defect left in the iliac wall may be repaired and iliac contour restored using bone cement. Anchoring holes are made with a curette before the cement is applied.

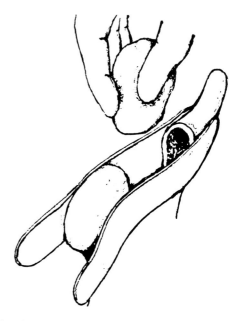

Fig. 39-20 The iliac wing defect is filled with bone cement. Malleable blades are used to repair the iliac wall as shown.

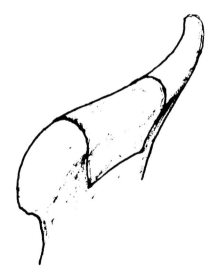

Fig. 39-21 The iliac wall is reconstructed with bone cement.

el obstruction.[45,67,80,88,90] Strangulated hernia and valvulae are very rare occurrences.[21] Symptoms were reported to have occurred from 24 days[21] to 15 years[116] after the formation of the iliac defect.[27]

Treatment requires the reduction of the hernia and repairing the defect by:
1. Using soft tissue[7,21,67,80,91] advancement, imbrication, flaps, or fascial flaps
2. Using a prosthesis[88] (tantalum or Marlex mesh)
3. Using methylmethacrylate cement to reconstruct the iliac wall[68] (Figs. 39-19 to 39-21)
4. The Bosworth technique:[7,27] removing the remaining wings of the ilium on either side of the defect followed by layered soft tissue closure.

Pelvic Instability

Removal of a large quantity of bone graft from the posterior ilium may disrupt the mechanical keystone effect of the sacroiliac joint and the posterior sacroiliac ligament, causing instability. Lichtblou[65] first reported such complications after a bone grafting procedure in which the posterior sacroiliac ligaments were postulated to be interrupted. The ensuing instability transferred the stress forces to the pelvic ring, causing fractures of the superior and inferior pubic rami. Coventry and Tapper[26] reported six cases of pelvic instability following removal of bone graft from the ilium. The patients with such instability often developed symptoms indistinguishable from other spinal disorders. History of clicking or thudding, as well as pain in the thigh and gluteal region, is characteristic.

Sacroiliac stability is maintained by formation of the sacrum as a keystone with interlocking eminences and depressions, plus ligamentous support mostly in the posterior and superior aspect.[10] Multiparous women with lax ligaments and anatomic variations in the sacroiliac joints are more prone to develop such pelvic instability. Radiologic examination of the entire pelvic ring is important. Changes in the sacroiliac joint, the pubic rami, and the symphysis pubis should be looked for.

The Tibia

The *tibia* provides strong full thickness cortical graft and is occasionally used in spine fusion. The subcutaneous anteromedial aspect of the tibia is a convenient donor site. The periosteum should be left intact and sutured over the defect. The condyles also supply cancellous bone. However, there are significant risks to the use of the tibia as a donor site. Biomechanically, it is changed from a closed section to an open one when bone graft is obtained from the tibia. It is markedly weakened and much less able to resist torsional and bending loads.

Frankel and Burstein[42] discussed the effect of cortical graft removal from the tibia. They described the torque and angular deformation to failure of the tibia to be reduced to 30% of normal and energy absorption capacity to 10% of normal. Even when the corners of the cutout are rounded, open section overshadows any reduction in stress concentration gained.

Fatigue fractures are relatively high, and the tibia should be cast immobilized from 6 to 12 months after bone graft is obtained.[37] Thus the disadvantages of autogenous tibial graft far outweigh the benefits.

The Fibula

Although the upper two thirds of the fibula may be removed as bone graft, the middle one third provides the best cylindric cortical bone graft. The fibula graft is strongest in resisting compressive loading and can be depended on for longer periods of structural support in interbody fusion. For large defects in the vertebral bodies, fibula struts may be used to achieve stability. Because of the small amount of cancellous bone in the fibula, iliac cancellous graft should be supplemented to enhance osteogenesis.

Peroneal nerve injuries may occur when obtaining the graft from the proximal one third of the fibula. Valgus deformity of the ankle is a serious risk when the lower one third is violated. Significant donor site pain and compartment syndrome have also been reported.

Ribs have been used for thoracic spine fusion. However, their modest cortex and porous cancellous bone are rarely appropriate for lumbar spine fusion.

Free Vascularized Bone Grafts

Free vascularized bone grafts may be used to circumvent the disadvantage of large cortical grafts, most of which become necrotic.[75,89] Recent progress in microsurgical techniques is making this possible.[107,119] Continuing circulation and increased viability of the bone grafts facilitate the problem to that of fracture healing. Vascularized grafts are less dependent on the recipient bed for survival, and their use is advantageous in poorly vascularized bed after previous surgery, trauma, infection or irradiation. The fibula, rib, and anterior or posterior ilium may be used. However, their application is usually limited by the small size and need for time-consuming highly specialized microvascular techniques. In special circumstances the use of free vascularized bone graft may be advantageous in spine fusion.

Dupuis and coworkers[34] used a free vascularized fibular graft in a case of progressive congenital kyphosis with success, following the work of O'Brien and Ostrup. In a similar situation, an avascular strut graft becomes weaker to the point of mechanical failure as it is replaced by creeping substitution, which may take two or more years to complete.

Muscle-pedicle bone grafting procedures were reported by Hartman and associates for failed lumbosacral spinal fusion.[49] An iliac crest autograft with an intact quadratus lumborum muscle pedicle was used in this case.

ALLOGRAFTS

Allografts are the most frequently used alternatives to autografts in spine surgery. They are bones transplanted from one individual to another and are used to circumvent the problems encountered with autografts.[9,39,79,120]

Allografts are readily available and come in a wide variety of shapes and sizes. They can provide immediate support and minimize the use of stabilization hardware or braces. Bone allografts can replace missing structures and become incorporated into the spine. They provide biologic scaffolding that is gradually replaced with the patient's own bone.

Major problems lead to decreased effectiveness of allografts.[15-17,50] Immunologic rejection of implanted graft,[6,100] delayed union, nonunion, and fracture of the graft have not been uncommon. Incorporation of allografts by the host is slower. Vascular penetration is slower and less dense. There is less perivascular new bone formation when compared to autografts. Transmission of disease from allografts is also a serious concern.

The major weakness of the allograft is that it is *dead* and cannot contribute directly to osteogenesis, as do fresh autografts. Burwell[14] found a way around this problem by combining the osteogenic potential of autogenous marrow with allografts. The use of autogenous marrow to provide superior osteogenic capability in allografts and xenografts, as well as autografts, is finding greater clinical application (see further discussion on xenograft and synthetic implants). The use of bank bone is very advantageous if storage problems, immunologic reactions, and infection could be eliminated.

The allograft must be aseptically obtained soon after death or properly sterilized and processed early to:
1. Minimize its antigenicity
2. Prevent degradation by proteolytic enzymes
3. Maintain the mechanical structure
4. Preserve the osteogenic induction property

Freezing and Freeze-Drying

Freezing and freeze-drying are the most widely used preservation methods that allow storage of bone in a biologically useful (but nonviable) state.*

Freezing of allografts is carried out as soon as possible after procurement. Currently, the length of safe storage for bone is not known. However, based on the knowledge of autolysis retardation by cold, lower temperatures are expected to extend the "shelf life" of allografts.[43] At $-15°$ C to $-30°$ C, using a home type of mechanical freezer, long-term storage of

---
*References 11, 43, 61, 62, 70, 71.

bone is difficult. This form of freezing is not advisable because ice crystals grow rapidly in this temperature range and mechanically destroy the tissue viability.[71] Freezing at $-76°$ C is achieved in dry ice. At $-60°$ C to $-90°$ C using a laboratory type of mechanical deep freezer and at $-150°$ C or colder using a refrigerator with cryogenic gases, more effective preservation of bone is possible. At temperature near $-70°$ C, ice crystal formation is slower.[71] Bones frozen to $-70°$ C have been stored for several years and successfully applied clinically.[43] Freezing in a cryoprotective agent such as glycerol at controlled cooling velocity may be a more effective option.

Freeze-drying is a process in which the bone is first frozen to $-70°$ C and then sublimated in high vacuum. The bone is freeze-dried until the water content is reduced to 5% or less. The freeze-dried bone graft then can be shipped and stored conveniently at room temperature indefinitely in a vacuum container. Since freeze-dried bone is very brittle, it must be reconstituted by immersing in normal saline before use.[72] The reconstitution time depends on the size and shape of the graft. Chips of bone may not require any rehydration, whereas larger cortical bone may require up to 24 hours for reconstitution.[43]

As for their clinical application in spinal fusion, Malinin and Brown[71] reported the union rate of freeze-dried allografts under compression load (interbody or strut grafts) not to be delayed by low grade immunologic response. This is in contrast to a high incidence of resorption with cortical graft placed under tension posteriorly in the spine.

Biomechanical Properties

Biomechanical properties of bone grafts may be changed by the techniques used for preservation, although Sedlin's study showed that freezing and thawing do not significantly change the mechanical properties of bone.[98]

Bright and Burstein,[8] as well as Triantafyllou and coworkers,[108] studied the biomechanical properties of freeze-dried and irradiated bones. Komender[60] found that freezing to $-78°$ C does not alter the mechanical properties of bone. Pelker and associates[86] also concluded that freezing allograft bone to temperature as low as that of liquid nitrogen ($-196°$ C) does not significantly alter the biomechanical properties. They showed that freeze-drying does diminish the torsional and bending strength but not the strength in compression. The data of Pelker and coworkers indicate that frozen bones are better suited than freeze-dried bones when they are subjected to torsional loads.[85,86]

Both frozen and freeze-dried bones are acceptable when compressive forces are the primary concern. It must be remembered that the initial biomechanical properties of the bone graft will change with resorption, incorporation, and remodeling by the host. Surgical technique, internal fixation, and postoperative management must therefore be planned accordingly.

Radiation, Heat, and Chemical Treatment of Allografts and Xenografts

Although most of the aseptically procured cadaver bones do not require sterilization procedures, allografts or xenografts have been sterilized by physical means such as high energy radiation, and heat (boiling, autoclaving); and by chemicals such as merthiolate (Thimerosol), ethylene dioxide, Propiolactone, or using antibiotic solutions. Some of these sterilization methods were used in the past and are discussed for historical interest only.

Radiation of at least 2 megarads is required to kill bacteria; 4 megarads inactivates some viruses.[71] The same dose of radiation (2 to 4 megarads) needed for sterilization or to destroy antigens, also significantly impairs the inductive repair capacity of the bone graft.[12,110,111] Increased solubility of collagen and glycosaminoglycan, destruction of bone matrix fibrillar network[12,18] and discoloration[71] of irradiated bone have been reported. In cobalt-60 irradiated bone Ostrowski[83] reported free radicals of unusual stability to be present, although their effect on the host tissue is unclear.[71]

The effect of radiation on the biomechanical properties of bone is not well defined at this time. The effect seems to be minimal with low level radiation. Radiation doses exceeding 3 megarads are known to destroy bone matrix fibrillar network.[12,18] There appears to be significant drop of breaking strength of bone with more than 3 megarads. This effect is magnified when radiation is combined with freeze-drying. Komender noted 6 megarads of radiation reduced the strength in bending, compression, and torsion.[60] Irradiation of freeze-dried bone with only 3 megarads markedly diminished the bending strength, but not the strength in compression or torsion.

Boiled bones have been used for graft material since the early part of this century.[46] Although some good clinical results have been reported,[66,124] boiled allografts and xenografts have generally produced undesirable consequences. Boiling destroys all inductive capacity.[124] Heat may be intended to destroy transplantation antigen, but it only denatures the antigenic proteins into another unacceptable material.

Autoclaving of contaminated bone may be tempting to use in the operating room, but this produces haversian canal coagulation and denaturation of bone protein,[12,71] which severely retard host incorporation.

Chemical processing of bone graft may

present significant problems such as potential carcinogenesis and difficulty of penetration into bone. Propiolactone (1% solution) has been found to be more bacteriocidal than ethylene dioxide, which is more difficult to use.[71]

Merthiolate-treated grafts have in general produced poor results; 30% of the grafts failed in the study by Reynolds and coworkers.[92] There appears to be three times as many failures as with autografts. Reduced callus formation and osteogenesis have been noted. When the graft fractured, there was minimal healing. When washed before use, no significant host sensitivity to Merthiolate was noted in Merthiolate-treated bone graft.[71]

Benzalkonium chloride completely destroys osteogenic inductive capacity of bone, according to Urist and associates.[111] Antibiotic solutions do not penetrate completely into bone. Their germicidal effect in bone graft is variable. In general, antibiotics appear to inhibit the osteogenic inductive capacity of bone.[3,71]

Bone Morphogenetic Protein

Urist states that allograft bone must be removed from the donor within 4 to 8 hours after death or within the minimal biodegradable time.[111] Radiation sterilization with more than two megarads, heating over 60° C, exposure to chemicals such as hydrogen peroxide, beta-propriolactone, benzalkonium chloride, cryolysis, immediate freeze-drying, and prolonged storage at 0° to 30° must be avoided to preserve the inductive properties of the bone. Urist and coworkers have extensively studied osteogenic induction and discovered a bone morphogenetic protein (BMP) that is capable of inducing the differentiation of host perivascular mesenchymal cells into cartilage and bone.[112] They have separated BMP from demineralized cortical bone and osteosarcomas of man and mouse. BMP is characterized as glycoprotein(s). Its clinical application now is being evaluated in the form of an injectable substance linked to different delivery systems.[114]

AAA bone is a chemosterilized, autodigested, antigen-extracted allograft developed and clinically tested by Urist and coworkers. It is an allogeneic bone of high osteogenetic property and low immunogenicity prepared in five basic steps. Urist believes that BMP is also preserved by these measures.[111,112,115]

1. Lipids and cell membrane lipoproteins are extracted using chloroform-methanol.
2. Endogenous intra- and extracellular transplantation antigens are removed by neutral phosphate buffer autodigestion in the presence of sulfhydral group enzyme inhibitors to preserve BMP.
3. Acid-soluble proteins are extracted and matrix demineralized by 0.6 N hydrochloric acid.
4. The bone is freeze-dried. Residual proteins including BMP are preserved.
5. The processed AAA bone is stored in sterile double plastic envelope and outer vacuum-sealed glass container.

Urist and Dawson[113] reported 40 intertransverse process fusions in 36 cases of degenerative joint and disc disease including spinal stenosis and spondylolisthesis, as well as 4 cases of thorocolumbar fracture dislocation. A composite of AAA cortical bone strips and local autologous bone was used in all cases. There were over 80% excellent and good results with a nonunion rate of 12%.

XENOGRAFTS

Xenografts, or bones transplanted from other species, have been used in spine surgery.[55,73] The application of ivory,[54,69] animal horns,[54] corals,[52,53] and other exotic materials has been explored. Animal horns and ivory are very resistant to incorporation into the host bone.[94] Fresh xenograft bones have been shown to be unacceptable. Invariably, they produce inflammation, fever, sequestration, resorption, or other manifestations of rejection.[12] Fibrous envelopment occurs as over a metal plate. Even when fusion takes place, sequestration of the xenograft is observed. Urist believes that xenografts should not be used in patients.[111]

Bovine bones have been relatively popular because they incorporate and remodel with less difficulty.[94] Different types of preserved bovine bone have been tried since the nineteenth century.

1. Frozen calf bone
2. Freeze-dried calf bone (Boplant)[87] and
3. Decalcified ox bone[47] (as well as decalcified calf and sheep bone) evaluated experimentally and clinically, but found unsatisfactory

Deproteinized xenografts, including "os purim," "anorganic bone," "Oswestry bone," and "Kiel bone,"[73,94-96] have also been tried.

"Kiel bone," partly deproteinized bone from freshly killed calf, sterilized either by ethylene dioxide or by gamma radiation, has been commercially available. Experimental studies showed that it is very weakly antigenic and does not possess active bone-inducing capacity.[95] Since its introduction in 1957, Kiel bone has been used in almost every possible bone graft site, and varying success rates have been reported clinically.[55,73,94]

In spinal fusion, Jackson[55] noted that Kiel bone implant became surrounded by autogenous bone with time. For larger defects he recommended the use of autogenous and Kiel bone composite. McMurray[78] presented clinical, radiologic, and histologic data on the fate of Kiel bone implants in four anterior spinal fusions that failed. Biopsies of the Kiel bone implants showed invasion by fibrous tissue. There was no ossification and no incorporation into the surrounding bone. Such deproteinized bone could be invaded by host new bone when placed in excellent vascular bed with potentially osteogenic cells. When impregnated with autogenous bone marrow cells, it may prove to be an excellent scaffolding with good bone conduction property.[94,95] Salama[94] and Salama and coworkers[95,96] reported good results using autogenous bone marrow-Kiel bone composite grafts in patients. The red marrow can be easily aspirated from the patient's own iliac crest.

SYNTHETIC IMPLANTS

Synthetic implants can be prepared to fit any size or shape, but they have been traditionally considered to be subject to wear and not biologically incorporated into the host bone.[12] A number of implants fashioned from metals have been tried as replacement for bone in the spinal column (see, for example, Steffee's titanium vertebral replacement: "Total Vertebral Body and Pedicle Replacement"[104,105]).

Metal scaffolds with the shape of bone being replaced may be covered by ground autologous bone grafts of small particle size. In animal experiments ingrowth of bone occurred over the total surface area of fiber metal implants and bone penetrated deep into the composite.[2]

Titanium mesh implants have been clinically applied by Leong,[63,64] and coworkers for anterior spinal fusion after discectomy in the lumbar spine. This porous implant allows ingrowth of bone and appears to obviate the use of bone graft. It acts as a spacer and can provide immediate stability, while allowing time for the slow ingrowth of bone and long-term stability.

Experimentally, porous titanium mesh blocks with a 50% void allows rapid ingrowth of bone in canine long bone. A 12-year follow up was possible in two patients who are asymptomatic, and the implants have remained unchanged and undisplaced; 10 patients had more than 5-year follow up. Of these, seven patients were asymptomatic, two had more than 70% symptomatic relief, and one retained a very stiff back. Radiologic analysis showed that disc height was maintained at 5 years with no movement between the adjacent vertebral bodies, often with bony overgrowth anterior to the implant.

Nonmetallic Synthetic Implants

There is a growing number of other synthetic implants being used as bone substitutes. According to Osborn and Nemesley[82] the chemical nature of the implant determines the biodynamics and reaction of the recipient bed in the interaction with living bone. They considered the following materials.[19,82]

1. Bone cement and stainless steel as *biotolerant,* resulting in *distance osteogenesis* with a fibrous layer separating the implant from bone
2. Alumina and carbon materials as *bioinert,* resulting in *contact osteogenesis*
3. Glass ceramic, calcium phosphate ceramics and hydroxyapatite ceramics as *bioactive,* resulting in *bonding osteogenesis*

Bioinert porous ceramics of alumina were noted by Benum and associates[4] to be bound to bone by the ingrowth of bone 3 to 4 mm thick in regions exposed to compressive forces.

Thus far, evidence strongly suggests that porous calcium phosphate ceramics are the most biocompatible synthetic bone substitute with the ability to become chemically bonded by living bone and with a chemical composition devoid of toxicologic liabilities.[56] They are shown to be superior to biodegradable polymers, such as polylactic acid and polyglycolic acid, which have been considered as bone substitutes.[20,56] The implants may be in dense form or porous. The minimum pore size for ingrowth of bone is shown to be 100 μm.[58] Corals provide such porous structures.[19,52]

Holmes and coworkers[53] performed histologic and biomechanical studies in dogs using hydroxyapatite converted from sea coral calcite as bone substitute. The material was incorporated in bone and became almost as strong as the native bone. They also reported encouraging clinical application with fractures in 18 patients.

Another material, Replam Hydroxyapatite-Porites (RHAP), is a ceramic with three-dimensional interconnected porous material of calcium hydroxyapatite from the exoskeleton of porites (coral). It may be carved by the surgeon before implanting. RHAP was approved for evaluation in spinal fusion in several centers under Mooney and associates. (See Chapter 41.)

Bioactive and biodegradable porous ceramics of hydroxyapatite or tricalcium phosphate have been studied. Jarcho[56] stated that they are usually well tolerated and become chemically bonded to bone by natural bone-cementing mechanisms.

Porous hydroxyapatite ceramics have been used in dog experiments for the spine[29] and other skeletal defects. Porous ceramics and autologous marrow composites were studied by Nade and associates.[77] Porous alumina, calcium aluminate, calcium hydroxyapatite, and tricalcium phosphate were placed with bone marrow into intermuscular sites. Bone was found to adhere to the ceramics and to penetrate the interior if the pore size were greater than 100 μm. The marrow cells were shown to play a significant part in new bone formation into the framework. Nade and coworkers believe that the appropriate histocompatible biodegradable ceramic material would act as a scaffold by virtue of its porosity for retention of bone marrow cells, and provide mechanical strength, while bone ingrowth is progressing. This type of bone substitute would also allow a wide selection of sizes and shapes in sterile form.

Porous biodegradable ceramic and BMP composites were evaluated by Urist and coworkers.[114] They reported that an aggregate of B-tricalcium phosphate and bone morphogenetic protein (TCP/BMP) induced the differentiation of cartilage in 8 days and in lamella bone in 21 days. The yield of new bone was more than 12 times greater from the TCP/BMP than from the BMP alone. It is possible that a porous ceramic acts as a slow-release delivery system to distribute BMP more favorably and to potentiate its activity.

Calcium phosphate-coated metallic implants showed superior bone-bonding characteristics according to Ducheyne and associates.[30] Such implants may solve the problem of weak mechanical strength of ceramics, particularly the porous ones. Ceramic implants by themselves are probably unsuitable for restoration that would have to withstand significant impact, or torsional or bending stresses,[56] as in the spinal column.

Calcium phosphate-containing bone cements are also being developed.[55,73] Recently, calcium hydroxyapatite in powder form was used as an expander of a patient's own cancellous bone graft. It has been used in spine fusion, especially in children, when there is insufficient autologous bone graft available.[68a]

METHYLMETHACRYLATE CEMENT

Knight[59] was the first to report the use of acrylic cement to fix the cervical spines with chronic fracture dislocation, atlanto-axial subluxation, and cervical spondylosis. He also stabilized the lumbar spine using the cement in one patient with disc disease. Scoville and coworkers[97] reported the use of acrylic plastic for vertebral replacement or fixation in metastatic tumor destruction of the spine.

In recent years the clinical use of methylmethacrylate cement for spine stabilization has become more popular. Harrington[48] documented the use of methylmethacrylate for vertebral body replacement and anterior stabilization of the spine with metastatic tumor. His series included 14 patients treated by anterior decompression and stabilization using metal and the bone cement.

The strength of methylmethacrylate is about one half that of bone.[123] Attempts have been made to strengthen the cement by adding fibers,[74] but clinical data are still unavailable. After polymerization, methylmethacrylate becomes a rigid and brittle solid that can withstand significant compression. However, it fails under tension or shear forces. It is reasonable to use it in replacement of vertebral body where compression is the predominant force present. It is important to remember that when used alone the outer part of the cement mass is still subject to tension when bending and will fail with time in a clinical setting. The primary indication for application of methylmethacrylate in spinal stabilization is in patients with malignant disease and limited life expectancy.[38,76] It should not be expected to provide long-term support of the spine.[31]

In the spinal column, methylmethacrylate cement should be used with secure metal fixation such as the Dunn,[32,33,41] Harrington, Luque, Steffee,[103,105] or other instrumentation. It may be used as reinforcement for screws and hooks in cancellous bone. The cement does enhance fixation of implants by increasing the contact area, especially in osteoporotic bone.

REFERENCES

1. Albrektsson, T.: The healing of autologous bone grafts after varying degrees of surgical trauma, J. Bone Joint Surg. **62B:**403, 1980.
2. Andersson, G.B.J., et al.: Segmental replacement of the femur in baboons with fiber metal implants and autologous bone grafts of different particle size, Acta Orthop. Scand. **53:**349, 1982.
3. Bassett, C.A.L.: Clinical implications of cell function in bone grafting, Clin. Orthop. **87:**45, 1972.
4. Benum, P., et al.: Porous ceramics as a bone substitute in the medial condyle of the tibia: an experimental study in sheep: long-term observations, Acta Orthop. Scand. **48:**150, 1977.
5. Blakemore, M.E.: Fractures at cancellous bone graft donor sites, Injury **14:**519, 1983.
6. Bonfiglio, M., and Jetter, W.S.: Immunological response to bone, Clin. Orthop. **87:**19, 1972.
7. Bosworth, D.M.: Repair of herniae through iliac crest defects, J. Bone Joint Surg. **37A:**1069, 1955.
8. Bright, R., and Burstein, A.: Material properties of preserved cortical bone. Trans. Orthop. Res. Soc. **3:**210, 1978.
9. Brown, K.L.B., and Cruess, R.L.: Bone and cartilage transplantation in orthopaedic surgery, J. Bone Joint Surg. **64A:**270, 1982.
10. Brown, L.T.: The mechanics of the lumbosacral and sacro-iliac joints, J. Bone Joint Surg. **19:**770, 1937.
11. Brown, M.D., et al.: A roentgenographic evaluation of frozen allografts versus autografts in anterior cervical spine fusions, Clin. Orthop. **119:**231, 1976.
12. Burchardt, H.: The biology of bone graft repair, Clin. Orthop. **174:**28, 1983.
13. Burchardt, H., et al.: Freeze-dried allogenic segmental cortical-bone grafts in dogs, J. Bone Joint Surg. **60A:**1082, 1978.
14. Burwell, R.G.: A study of homologous cancellous bone combined with autologous red marrow after transplantation to a muscular site, J. Anat. **95:**613, 1961.
15. Burwell, R.G.: Studies in the transplantation of bone. V. The capacity of fresh and treated homografts of bone to evoke transplantation immunity, J. Bone Joint Surg. **45B:**386, 1963.
16. Burwell, R.G.: Studies in transplantation of bone. VIII. Treated composite homo-autografts of cancellous bone, J. Bone Joint Surg. **48B:**532, 1966.
17. Burwell, R.G.: The fate of bone grafts. In Apley, A.G., editor: Recent advances in orthopaedics, 1969, Baltimore, Williams & Wilkins.
18. Burwell, G.R.: The fate of freeze-dried bone allografts. Transplant Proc. (Suppl. 1) **8:**95, 1976.
19. Burwell, R.G.: The function of bone marrow in the incorporation of a bone graft, Clin. Orthop. **200:**125, 1985.
20. Cameron, H.U.: Evaluation of a biodegradable ceramic, J. Biomed. Mater. Res. **11:**179, 1977.
21. Challis, J.H., et al.: Strangulated lumbar hernia and volvulus following removal of iliac crest bone graft, Acta Orthop. Scand. **46:**230, 1975.
22. Chalmers, J., and Rush, J.: Observations on the induction of bone in soft tissues, J. Bone Joint Surg. **57B:**36, 1975.
23. Cobey, M.L.: A national bone bank survey, Clin. Orthop. **110:**333, 1975.
24. Cockin, J.: Autologous bone grafting—complications at the donor site, J. Bone Joint Surg. **53B:**153, 1971.
25. Cooper, J.W.: Cluneal nerve injury and chronic post-surgical neuritis, J. Bone Joint Surg. **49A:**199, 1967.
26. Coventry, M.B., and Tapper, E.M.: Pelvic instability: a consequence of removing iliac bone for grafting, J. Bone Joint Surg. **54A:**83, 1972.
27. Cowley, S.P., and Anderson, L.D.: Brief note: hernias through donor sites for iliac-bone grafts, J. Bone Joint Surg. **65A:**1023, 1983.
28. Curtiss, P.H., et al.: Immunological factors in homologous bone transplantation, J. Bone Joint Surg. **41A:**1481, 1959.
29. Dawson, E.: The fate of bone substitution with porous hydroxyapatite implants in the dog spine. Transactions of the 27th Annual Meeting, Orthopaedic Research Society Vol. 6, 1981.
30. Ducheyne, P., et al.: Effect of hydroxyapatite impregnation on skeletal bonding of porous coated implants. J. Biomed. Mater. Res. **14:**225, 1980.
31. Dunn, E.J.: The role of methylmethacrylate in the stabilization and replacement of tumors of the cervical spine, Spine **2:**15, 1977.
32. Dunn, H.K.: Internal fixation of the spine—a new implant system: proceedings of the Scoliosis Research Society. Orthop. Trans. **3:**47, 1979.

33. Dunn, H.K., et al.: Comparative assessment of spine stability achieved with a new anterior spine fixation system, Trans. Orthop. Res. Soc. **5**:192, 1980.
34. Dupuis, P.R., et al.: Anterior free vascular transplant of the fibula for the treatment of kyphosis, J. Bone Joint Surg. **64B**:259, 1982.
35. Drury, B.J.: Clinical evaluation of back and leg pain due to irritation of the superior cluneal nerve, J. Bone Joint Surg. **49A**:199, 1967.
36. Editorial. Bone harvesting and transplantation, Lancet **2**:730, 1981.
37. Edmonson, A.S., et al.: Campbell's operative orthopaedics, ed. 6, St. Louis, 1980, The C.V. Mosby Co.
38. Eftekhar, N.S., and Thurston, C.W.: Effect of irradiation on acrylic cement with special reference to fixation of pathological fractures, J. Biomech. **8**:53, 1975.
39. Enneking, W.F., et al.: Autogenous cortical bone grafts in the reconstruction of segmental skeletal defects, J. Bone Joint Surg. **62A**:1039, 1980.
40. Escalas, F., and Dewald, R.L.: Combined traumatic arteriovenous fistula and ureteral injury: a complication of iliac bone-grafting, a case report, J. Bone Joint Surg. **59A**:270, 1977.
41. Evarts, C.M.: Surgery of the musculoskeletal system, New York, 1983, Churchill Livingstone, Inc.
42. Frankel, V.H., and Burstein, A.H.: Orthopedic Biomechanics, Philadelphia, 1970, Lea & Febiger.
43. Friedlaender, G.E.: Current concepts review—Bone-banking, J. Bone Joint Surg. **64A**:307, 1982.
44. Friedlander, G.: Autigenicity of freeze-dried allografts, Transplant Proc. (Suppl. I) **8**:195, 1976.
45. Froimson, A.I., and Cummings, A.G., Jr.: Iliac hernia following hip arthrodesis, Clin. Orthop. **30**:89, 1971.
46. Gallie, W.E.: The use of boiled bone in operative surgery, Am. J. Orthop. Surg. **16**:373, 1918.
47. Gupta, D., et al.: Bridging large bone defects with a xenograft composited with autologous bone marrow: an experimental study, Int. Orthop. (SICOT) **6**:79, 1982.
48. Harrington, K.D.: The use of methylmethacrylate for vertebral body replacement and anterior stabilization of pathological fracture dislocations of the spine, due to metastatic disease. J. Bone Joint Surg. **63A**:36, 1981.
49. Hartman, J.R., et al.: A pedicle bone grafting procedure for failed lumbosacral spinal fusion, Clin. Orthop. **178**:223, 1983.
50. Heiple, K.G., et al.: A comparative study of the healing process following different types of bone transplantation, J. Bone Joint Surg. **45A**:1593, 1963.
51. Heppenstall, R.B.: Fracture treatment and healing, Philadelphia, 1980, W.B. Saunders Co.
52. Holmes, R.E.: Bone regeneration within a coraline hydroxyapatite implant, Plast. Reconstr. Surg. **63**:626, 1979.
53. Holmes, R., et al.: A coralline hydroxyapatite bone graft substitute: preliminary report, Clin. Orthop. **188**:252, 1984.
54. Hughes, C.W.: Rate of absorption and callus stimulating properties of cow horn, ivory, beef bone and autogenous bone, Surg. Gynecol. Obstet. **76**:665, 1943.
55. Jackson J.W.: Surgical approaches to the anterior aspect of the spinal column, Ann. R. Coll. Surg. Engl. **48**:83, 1971.
56. Jarcho, M.: Calcium phosphate ceramics as hard tissue prosthetics, Clin. Orthop. **157**:259, 1981.
57. Kahn, B.: Superior gluteal artery laceration: a complication of iliac bone graft surgery, Clin. Orthop. **140**:204, 1979.
58. Klawitter, J.J., and Hulbert, S.F.: Application of porous ceramics for the attachment of load bearing orthopaedic applications, J. Biomed. Mater. Res. **2**:161, 1971.
59. Knight, G.: Paraspinal acrylic inlays in the treatment of cervical and lumbar spondylosis and other conditions, Lancet **2**:147, 1959.
60. Komender, A.: Influence of preservation on some mechanical properties of human haversian bone, Mater. Med. Pol. **8**:13, 1976.
61. Kreuz, F.P., et al.: The preservation and clinical use of freeze-dried bone, J. Bone Joint Surg. **33A**:297, 1974.
62. Langer, F., et al.: The immunogenicity of fresh and frozen allogeneic bone, J. Bone Joint Surg. **57A**:216, 1975.
63. Leong, J.C.Y., et al.: The use of porous titanium mesh implant after discectomy in patients with deranged lumbar intervertebral disc—The five-year results of a prospective trial, (abstracts), Twelfth annual meeting of the International Society for the Study of the Lumbar Spine, 1985.
64. Leong, J.C.Y.: University of Hong Kong, Personal communication, 1984.
65. Lichtblau, S.: Dislocation of the sacro-iliac joint: a complication of bone-grafting, J. Bone Joint Surg. **44A**:193, 1962.

66. Lloyd-Roberts, G.C.: Experiences with boiled cadaveric bone, J. Bone Joint Surg. **34B**:428, 1952.
67. Lotem, M., et al.: Lumbar hernia at an iliac bone graft donor site: A case report, Clin. Orthop. **80**:130, 1971.
68. Lubicky, J.P., and Dewald, R.L.: Methylmethacrylate reconstruction of large iliac crest bone defect donor site, Clin. Orthop. **164**:252, 1982.
68a. Luque, E.R.: Personal communication, 1985.
69. Magnusson, P.B.: Holding fractures with absorbable materials—ivory plates and screws, JAMA **61**:1514, 1913.
70. Malinin, T.I.: University of Miami tissue bank: collection of postmortem tissues for clinical use and laboratory investigation, Transplant. Proc. (Suppl.) **8**:53, 1976.
71. Malinin, T.I.: Cadaver bone allografts—bone banks. In Turek, S.L., editor: Orthopaedics, principles and their application, Philadelphia, 1984, J.B. Lippincott Co.
72. Malinin, T.I., and Brown, M.D.: Bone allograft in spinal surgery, Clin. Orthop. **154**:168, 1981.
73. McMurray, G.N.: The evaluation of Kiel bone in spinal fusions, J. Bone Joint Surg. **64B**:100, 1982.
74. Mittelmeier, J.H., et al.: PMMA cement with carbon fiber reinforcement and apatite ingredients: mechanical properties and tissue reaction in animal tests, First World Biomat. Cong., Baden, Austria, 1980.
75. Moore, J.B., et al.: A biomechanical comparison of vascularized and conventional autogenous bone grafts, Plast. Reconstr. Surg. **73**:382, 1984.
76. Murray, J.A., et al.: Irradiation of polymethylmethacrylate: in vitro Gamma Radiation Effect, J. Bone Joint Surg. **56A**:311, 1974.
77. Nade, S., et al.: Osteogenesis and bone marrow transplantation, the ability of ceramic materials to sustain osteogenesis from transplanted bone marrow cells: preliminary studies, Clin. Orthop. **181**:255, 1983.
78. Nade, S., and Burwell, R.G.: Decalcified bone as a substrate for osteogenesis: an appraisal of the inter-relation of bone and marrow in combined grafts, J. Bone Joint Surg. **59B**:189, 1977.
79. Oikarinen, J., and Korhonen, L.K.: The bone inductive capacity of various bone transplanting materials used for treatment of experimental bone defects, Clin. Orthop. **140**:208, 1979.
80. Oldfield, M.D.: Iliac hernia after bone grafting, Lancet **248**:810, 1945.
81. Osborn, J.F., and Newesely, H.: Dynamic aspects of the implant-bone-interface, Dental Implants **111**:123, 1980.
82. Osborn, J.F., and Newesely, H.: The material science of calcium phosphate ceramics, Biomaterials **1**:108, 1980.
83. Ostrowski, K.: Current problems of tissue banking, Transplant. Proc. **1**:126, 1969.
84. Pappas, A.M.: Current methods of freezing and freeze-drying, Cryobiology **4**:358, 1968.
85. Pelker, R.R., et al.: Biomechanical properties of bone allografts, Clin. Orthop. **174**:54, 1983.
86. Pelker, R., et al.: The effects of preservation on allograft strength, Trans. Orthop. Res. Soc. **7**:283, 1982.
87. Pierson, A.P., et al.: Bone grafting with Boplant: results in thirty-three cases, J. Bone Joint Surg. **50B**:364, 1968.
88. Pyrtek, L.J., and Kelly, C.C.: Management of herniation through large iliac bone defects, Ann. Surg. **152**:998, 1960.
89. Ray, R.D.: Vascularization of bone grafts and implants, Clin. Orthop. **87**:43, 1972.
90. Ray, R.D., and Holloway, J.A.: Bone implants, J. Bone Joint Surg. **39A**:1119, 1957.
91. Reid, R.L.: Hernia through an iliac bone-graft donor site: a case report, J. Bone Joint Surg. **50A**:757, 1968.
92. Reynold, C.F., et al.: Clinical evaluation of the merthiolate bone bank and homogenous bone grafts, J. Bone Joint Surg. **33A**:873, 1951.
93. Rhinelander, F.W.: Tibial blood supply in relation to fracture healing, Clin. Orthop. **105**:34, 1974.
94. Salama, R.: Xenogeneic bone grafting in humans, Clin. Orthop. **174**:113, 1983.
95. Salama, R., et al.: Re-combined grafts of bone and marrow, J. Bone Joint Surg. **55B**:402, 1973.
96. Salama, R., and Weissman, S.L.: The clinical use of combined xenografts of bone and autologous red marrow: a preliminary report, J. Bone Joint Surg. **60B**:111, 1978.
97. Scoville, W.B., et al.: The use of acrylic plastic for vertebral replacement or fixation in metastatic disease of the spine, J. Neurosurg. **27**:274, 1967.
98. Sedlin, E.: A rheologic model for cortical bone, Acta Orthop. Scand. (Suppl.) **36**:83, 1965.
99. Seres, J.L.: Fusion in the presence of severe metastatic destruction of the cervical spine (case report), J. Neurosurg. **28**:592, 1968.

100. Smith, R.T.: The mechanism of graft rejection, Clin. Orthop. **87**:15, 1972.
101. Smith, S.E., et al.: Ilioinguinal neuralgia following iliac bone-grafting, J. Bone Joint Surg. **66A**:1306, 1984.
102. Spence, W.T.: Internal plastic splint for stabilization of the spine, Clin. Orthop. **92**:325, 1973.
103. Steffee, A., et al.: Segmental spine plates with pedicle screw fixation: a new internal fixation device for disorders of the lumbar and thoracic spine. (Submitted for publication.)
104. Steffee, A., et al.: Total vertebral body and pedicle replacement. (Submitted for publication.)
105. Steffee, A.: Personal communication, 1985.
106. Stringa G.: Studies on the vascularization of bone grafts, J. Bone Joint Surg. **39B**:395, 1957.
107. Taylor, G.I., et al.: The free vascularized bone graft: a clinical extension of microvascular techniques, Plast. Reconstr. Surg. **64**:745, 1979.
108. Triantafyllou, N., et al.: The mechanical properties of the lyophilized and irradiated bone grafts, Acta Orthop. Belg. **41**:35, 1975.
109. Turek, S.L.: Orthopaedics, principles and their application. Philadelphia, 1984, J.B. Lippincott Co.
110. Urist, M.R.: Surface-decalcified allogenic bone implants, Clin. Orthop. **56**:37, 1968.
111. Urist, M.R.: Practical applications of bone research on bone graft physiology, Instructional course lectures. The American Academy of Orthopaedic Surgeons, vol. 25, St. Louis, 1976, The C.V. Mosby Co.
112. Urist, M.R., et al.: Human bone morphorgenic protein (BMP), Proc. Soc. Exp. Biol. Med. **173**(2):194, 1983.
113. Urist, M.R., and Dawson, E.: Intertransverse process fusion with the aid of chemosterilized autolyzed antigen-extracted allogeneic (AAA) bone, Clin. Orthop. **154**:97, 1981.
114. Urist, M.R., et al.: β-tricalcium phosphate delivery system for bone morphogenetic protein. Clin. Orthop. **187**:277, 1984.
115. Urist, M.R., et al.: A chemosterilized antigen-extracted autodigested allo-implant for bone banks, Arch. Surg. **110**:416, 1975.
116. Verheugen, P., et al.: Hernie illique apres prelevement osseux: subobstruction, Acta Chir. Belg. **1051**:1056, 1965.
117. Watson-Jones, R.: Transplantation of bone. In Fracture and joint injuries, vol. 1, ed. 4, Baltimore, 1955, Williams & Wilkins.
118. Weikel, A.M., and Habal, M.B.: Meralgia paresthetica: a complication of iliac bone procurement, Plast. Reconstr. Surg. **60**:572, 1977.
119. Weiland, A.J.: Current concept review: vascularized free bone transplants, J. Bone Joint Surg. **63A**:166, 1981.
120. Weiland, A.J., Phillips T.W., and Randolph, M.A.: Bone grafts: A radiologic, histologic, and biomechanical model comparing autografts, allografts, and free vascularized bone grafts, Plast. Reconstr. Surg. **74**:368, 1984.
121. White, A.A. III, and Panjabi, M.M.: Clinical biomechanics of the spine, Philadelphia, 1978, J.B. Lippincott Co.
122. White, A.A. III, et al.: Spinal stability: evaluation and treatment, Instructional course lectures, The American Academy of Orthopaedic Surgeons, vol. 30, St. Louis, 1981, The C.V. Mosby Co.
123. Wilde, A.H., and Greenwald, A.S.: Shear strength of self-curing acrylic cement, Clin. Orthop. **106**:126. 1975.
124. Williams, G.: Experiences with boiled cadaveric cancellous bone for fractures of long bones, J. Bone Joint Surg. **46B**:398, 1964.
125. Wolfe, S.A., and Kawamoto, H.K.: Taking the iliac-bone graft: a new technique, J. Bone Joint Surg. **60A**:411, 1978.

CHAPTER
40

BONE BANKING

James Walter Simmons

The art of progress is to preserve order amid change and to preserve change amid order.

Alfred North Whitehead

Bone grafting has become a common procedure in the United States, over 200,000 grafts are performed each year.[19] The desire to replace damaged bone with bone derived from other humans or animals has been demonstrated in ancient works of art, as well as early medical records.[8] The first written record of a bone transplant occurs in Russian church records in 1682, when Meekren successfully used a piece of dog skull to repair a defect in the skull of a soldier.[4] Since that time improved surgical skills and aseptic techniques have enabled modern surgeons to use bone in filling bony defects, spinal fusions, treatment of fracture nonunions, reshaping of craniofacial deformaties, and limb-sparing tumor resections.[3,13,17]

For over 40 years, there has been a concerted effort in the field of bone grafting and bone preservation. In 1942 Inclan demonstrated the viability of human bone by freezing and its use in orthopaedic surgery. Since then numerous accounts of the various preservation techniques, banking methods and procedures, and clinical and laboratory studies in support of the biologic potential of stored grafts have been recorded.[3,4,6,12,15]

Histologically, cancellous and cortical autogenous bone transplants have three differences: (1) cancellous grafts are revascularized more rapidly and completely than cortical grafts; (2) creeping substitution of cancellous bone initially involves an appositional bone formation phase, followed by a resorptive phase, whereas cortical grafts undergo a reverse creeping substitution process; (3) cancellous grafts tend to repair completely with time, whereas cortical grafts remain as admixtures of necrotic and viable bone.

Bone morphogenetic protein (BMP) has been found to stimulate regeneration of bone defects caused by injury, malignancy, infection, and congenital deformity. The quantity of BMP in transplants of bone matrix is very small; however, methods are available to produce quantities sufficient for preliminary clinical applications.[28]

The increased number of procedures requiring bone has led to a concomitant increase in the demand for banked bone. Although fresh autogenous bone is considered to be biologically more effective,[8] banked allograft bone obviates the sacrifice of normal bone tissue and eliminates potential donor-site morbidity.[4,8] Also, the quantity of autogenous bone is limited, whereas banked bone can be ordered by size, shape, and quantity for each surgical procedure.

In response to the demand for allograft tissues, the number of tissue banks in the United States is rapidly increasing. The American Association of Tissue Banks (AATB) was formed in 1976 to establish legal, moral, ethical, and medical guidelines for organs and tissues used in transplantation. In 1984 the AATB published a manual of standards for tissue banking to ensure that tissue banks will follow accepted standards of technical and ethical performance.[1]

DONOR SELECTION

It is the responsibility of each tissue bank to use current banking knowledge to protect the potential graft recipient and provide biologically functional grafts.[9] Part of this responsibility involves careful donor selection. The medical history, physical examination or autopsy, and laboratory testing should be closely scrutinized to provide only healthy tissue for transplantation. It is especially important for bone banks that are not using secondary sterilization to be sure that donors are free from infection to prevent transmission of disease to the recipients.[22]

Because autolysis begins immediately after death, it is advisable to refrigerate the donor until the procurement is begun.

The maximum length of time between death and the time of tissue procurement should be less than 12, but no longer than 24 hours.[8,9,22] Completion of a donor information form (Fig. 40-1) can be a valuable tool to prequalify a potential donor. Medical histories that include the following conditions may eliminate a donor from consideration.[8,9,22]

1. Febrile course in hospital
2. More than 72 hours on respirator
3. An active systemic infection
4. An active infection in tissues to be procured
5. Slow virus disease
6. Malignancy that has the potential of metastasizing to the donated tissue
7. Hepatitis or unexplained jaundice
8. Connective tissue diseases
9. Metabolic bone disease
10. Unknown cause of death
11. Chronic parenteral drug abuse
12. History of radiation treatment to the donated tissue
13. Presence of toxic substances that could be transmitted to the recipient in toxic doses
14. AIDS or known homosexual
15. Long-term steroid use
16. Death from CNS diseases of unknown cause

Permission for the donation should be given by the legal next of kin. A typical form that could be used for this purpose is shown in Fig. 40-2. A policy of informed consent is recommended in the AATB standards by explicitly listing the tissues to be removed. The Uniform Anatomical Gift Act allows a living person to donate tissues to be removed at the time of death. It is legal for tissue banks to remove those tissues without seeking permission from the next of kin. However, unfavorable publicity could result if the family should object strongly. It is therefore advisable to inform the family of the donation and ask for their approval.[1]

It is important to approach the family

```
                        DONOR INFORMATION
    Contacted by_____ of _____
    Contact Phone_____ Date _____ Time _____
    Donor Name_____ Age _____ Sex _____
    Cause of Death_____
    Time of Death_____ Date _____
    Treating Physician_____ Department _____
    Injuries present_____
    Hospital_____
    Location of Donor _____
    Hospital Contact_____ Phone _____
    Medical History:
    Surgery_____
    Disease_____
    Other _____
    Lab Tests:
    Hepatitis _____
    Blood Cultures_____ Other Cultures_____
    Is this a Medical Examiner's Case?_____ County _____
    Medical Examiner Phone _____ Is autopsy planned___
    Date & Time of Autopsy_____ Location _____
    Permission given by_____ Date & Time _____
    Family Information:
    Next of Kin_____ Relationship _____
    Telephone _____ Address _____
    Type of permit _____
    Permit for _____
    Permit obtained by _____
    Date and time of procurement _____
```

Fig. 40-1 Donor information.

with sensitivity to their grief. If more than one transplant organization is seeking permission for the donation of tissue from the same donor, assign one person to represent the group of organizations to prevent the family from being approached several times.

After permission has been obtained, it is necessary to arrange the procurement with any other transplant organizations that may be involved. Eye and skin tissues are normally the first to be retrieved after viable organs have been removed. If the coroner or medical examiner is in charge of the case, it is necessary to obtain their approval before tissues are pro-

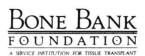

Fig. 40-2 Consent for bone and tissue donation.

cured. In some cases the removal of tissue will be allowed only after an autopsy has been performed.

THE PROCUREMENT

Tissues may be procured in an operating room under aseptic conditions or in a nonsterile environment such as a morgue or funeral home. If a nonsterile method is chosen, the tissue bank must use some means of secondary sterilization during processing.

Sterile procurement is the method of choice when large osteochondral grafts are to be transplanted. Cultures of each tissue removed must be performed to prevent infection in the recipients.[9] If the large bones are to be cut into smaller graft specimens, this must be done under aseptic conditions with additional culturing of the specimens produced.

The nonsterile method of procurement allows the tissue bank to consider more patients as potential donors, since those who have been autopsied or have received severe lacerations usually are not considered for sterile procurement. Tissues removed in the morgue or funeral home are cooled immediately and transported to the bone bank, where they are placed in a freezer that is at least $-70°$ C. Blood from the donor is sent to the laboratory to be tested for Hepatitis B surface antigen, HTLV-III antibody, and RPR for syphillis. None of the tissue is distributed for clinical use until negative laboratory results are received.

Unless notified otherwise, the bone bank should reconstruct the body of the donor to provide a cosmetically acceptable appearance.[1] Wooden dowels may be used to replace the long bones in the arms and legs. If not all of the ribs are removed, the chest will retain its normal contour. If the mandible has been removed, it may be replaced with a plastic facsimile. All incisions should then be sutured with autopsy thread and needles.

PROCESSING OF BONE

Bone that has been procured under nonsterile conditions is processed in a clean but nonsterile facility. Before cutting the bone, all soft tissue is first removed. Various types of saws may be used to cut the bone into the desired sizes and shapes. The cut specimens are then washed to remove blood and bone marrow. Examples of specimens that may be produced from various procured bones to produce the highest yield of transplantable tissues follow.

Procured bone	Specimens produced
Ilium	Tricortical blocks for spinal fusions
	Bicortical blocks for spinal fusions
	Cortical-cancellous strips of various sizes
	Crock dowels for lumbar fusions
	Ilium matchsticks
Femur	Cervical fusion dowels
	Whole femoral heads
	Femoral head cross-sections
	Cancellous chips
	Cortical bone powder
	Crushed cortical bone
	Ground cancellous bone
Tibia	Cervical fusion dowels
	Cancellous chips
	Cancellous blocks
	Cortical struts
	Ground cancellous bone
	Cortical bone powder
	Crushed cortical bone
Fibula	Cross-sections
	Crushed cortical bone
Humerus, radius, ulna, clavicle	Cross-sections
	Crushed cortical bone
	Cortical struts
Ribs	Whole ribs
	Split ribs
	Rib matchsticks
Mandible	Whole mandible
	Hemi-mandible

DEMINERALIZATION

Demineralized or autolysed antigen-extracted allogeneic bone (AAA) consists chiefly of collagen and fiber-entrapped insoluble noncollagenous proteins, including bone morphogenetic protein (BMP); it is stabilized by dehydration and defatting in chloraform-methanol followed by freeze-drying and packaging. The donor bone residue is biologically more compatible with the recipient than septically collected whole bone, either freeze-dried or radiation-sterilized. Though clinical use of AAA bone is limited, preliminary results demonstrate that the organic matrix is more rapidly resorbed with less cell-mediated local immune reaction and more rapid incorporation of the donor tissue in the recipient bed.[27]

Demineralized bone is prepared by extraction with 0.6 ml HCl followed by several washes of distilled water and sequential washes in absolute ethanol and anhydrous ether.[13] Upon rehydration and before implantation the bone is pliable and can be trimmed with scissors to the desired shape. Cancellous bone becomes spongelike in texture and is ideal to use for filling defects. Types of demineralized bone specimens available include crushed cortical (powder), cortical struts, femoral head cross-sections, ribs, fibula cross-sections, and bone chips.

Rapid bone formation has been demonstrated with demineralized implants.[13,14,17,23,24] This process, called *osteoinduction,* is described as the differentiation of migratory mesenchymal cells into osteoprogenitor cells (chondroblasts) with subsequent bone formation.[25] Undemineralized allografts undergo a process termed *osteoconduction,* involving the ingrowth of capillaries, perivascular tissue, and osteoprogenitor cells from the recipient bed, followed by a resorptive phase. Resorption of both the allograft and surrounding living bone takes place to bring about incorporation of the graft.[24]

The clinical advantages or benefits of demineralized bone implants include ease of manipulation and insertion and decreased late resorption—compared to conventional bone grafts—rapid healing of skeletal defects, the ability to induce large quantities of new bone, elimination or avoidance of a surgical procedure to collect donor bone, and the potentially unlimited supply of banked material that increases treatment options.[14] Due to its many advantages, demineralized bone implants will be the favored allotransplant for the future, where fairly immediate return to normalcy of bone structure and stability are desired but where support is not the prerequisite. Nondemineralized allografts will be used clinically where support and weight bearing are essential.

SECONDARY STERILIZATION

Several methods of secondary strilization have been used with varying degrees of success. Urist[25] found that beta-propiolactone and hydrogen peroxide destroy the bone morphogenic protein.[25] Reynolds, Oliver, and Ramsey reported clinical results showing that approximately 30% of Merthiolate- (thimerasol) treated implants failed.[21] Bonfiglio reported that Merthiolate-treated grafts demonstrated poor osteogenic stimulus in host tissues and in fractured grafts, healing of the graft seldom occurred.[2]

Today, most bone banks sterilize with Cobalt gamma radiation or ethylene oxide gas. Bone is usually exposed to 3.5 megarads of cobalt 60 to achieve sterilization. Urist and Hernandez[26] found that this dosage completely eliminated the ability of the graft to initiate a morphogenic response in host tissue. However, if irradiated grafts are in contact with osteogenetically active bone in young patients, it compares favorably with autogenous bone in its osteoconductive function.[25,26]

Ethylene oxide gas has been shown to be an effective sterilant for tissues.[20] Some concern has been expressed regarding the residual levels of ethylene oxide, ethylene glycol, and ethylene chlorohydrin in tissues that have been sterilized with the gas. Prolo[20] conducted an investigation to determine the levels of each residue in bone, dura mater, and fascia that had been sterilized with ethylene oxide gas followed by aeration and lyophilization. Results showed that aeration and lyophilization were effective in reducing residual levels to within acceptable limits. Bone which is not lyophilized should be well aerated before clinical use.[7,22] Soaking of bone in an excess of solution before implantation is also effective in reducing residue levels.[20]

FREEZE-DRYING

Freeze-drying, or lyophilization, is a process in which frozen bone is dehydrated by sublimation. Tissue moisture passes directly from the solid phase to the vapor phase to be converted to ice on the condenser of the machine. A vacuum is maintained in the freeze-drier during the process, which allows bottles of bone grafts to be sealed under vacuum and stored at room temperature for several years. The cycle takes 14 to 16 days to attain a maximum dryness of 3% to 5% of residual water as determined by gravimetric methods.[16]

A reduced or undetectable immune response in the recipient has been reported with the use of freeze-dried grafts.[10,12] The mechanism of this reduced antigenicity is unclear in view of findings that the normal proteins found in bone have been shown to be stable chemically, antigenically, and electrophoretically after freeze-drying.[4]

Deleterious effects of freeze-drying have been reported, including a lessened torsional and bending strength in grafts. If bone is freeze-dried in addition to sterilization by irradiation, a significant decrease in the breaking strength occurs.[18] Other studies have shown decreased osteogenesis and callus production, delayed revascularization, and the collection of lymphocytes around the graft, in addition to the changes in biomechanical characteristics caused by microfractures and dehydration.[5]

When ordering banked bone, it is important to know the effects of various preservation methods on bone strength and to evaluate the effect of these changes in view of the type and magnitude of the load to which the graft will be subjected.[18] When used in appropriate cases, freeze-dried bone serves well by retaining sufficient biologic potential and providing a nonviable structure on which new bone can be built.

Nonfreeze-Dried Bone

Cloward's 45 years experience using cadaver bone for interbody spinal fusions has led to the development of a simplified bone bank. Unsterile bone removed from fresh cadavers is cut into appropriate sizes and shapes, washed clean, packaged and sterilized with ethylene oxide gas, then aerated and stored at room temperature.[7]

QUALITY CONTROL

The sterility of grafts should be demonstrated by extensive culturing of specimens before any are distributed for clinical use. It is advisable to use at least two different media[20] in aerobic and anaerobic conditions for at least 7 days of incubation.

If ethylene oxide is used to sterilize grafts, periodic testing for residuals should be performed on all types of specimens produced.[20] If freeze-drying is the preservation method used, periodic testing for residual water levels will allow the bone bank to be certain that sufficient dryness is achieved.

ORGANIZATIONAL CONSIDERATIONS

The following guidelines represent suggestions for the banking of musculoskeletal allografts. It is expected that these guidelines will change as knowledge of allotransplantation increases and as applications of allografts continue to evolve.

1. *General.* The nature and purpose of the banking facility should be clearly defined. It should have functional indentity with a professional staff and a commitment to maintain and preserve records and operating procedures for future reference and historical continuity.[1]

2. *Facilities and equipment.* Each facility should be self-contained, having the equipment necessary for the required tasks and its own separate space where its activities can progress and security can be maintained.

3. *Personnel qualifications.* The tissue banking procedures should be under the supervision of a currently licensed medical or osteopathic physician, dentist or oral surgeon, or an individual whose past training clearly indicates competence in the application and evaluation of all procedures involved in the safe banking of effective tissues. Other personnel involved in the banks must be trained and/or judged competent by the tissue bank supervisor for those procedures he or she performs.[1]

4. *Operational procedures.* An *operational manual* should be kept for the bank. This should be the document in which all aspects of donor election, procurement processing, storage, quality control, distribution, and general record keeping should be recorded.

Other important information includes:
1. Records
   a. Donor identification, age, sex, and social security number
   b. A detailed description of the specimen, including radiograph(s) where indicated
   c. Cause of death
   d. Significant past medical history
   e. Blood and tissue types, if known
   f. Identification of methods used for procurement, processing, and storage of the graft, including mention of any antibiotics employed
   g. Summary of laboratory, culture, and autopsy records
   h. Results of quality control
   i. Place where tissue was procured and the individual responsible[1]
2. Recipient information
   a. Recipient identification, age, sex, address, social security number
   b. Transplant surgeon identification and address
   c. Application for which graft used, date, and location of the procedure
   d. Adverse reactions attributed to the graft[1]

(Record any additional information.)
   e. Recipient blood and tissue type
   f. Report of graft culture at time of graft use
   g. Any deviations from recommended directions for reconstitution of grafts or from suggestions for their handling
   h. An estimate of clinical graft success

RECORD KEEPING

Complete and current records should be kept in the bone bank, covering all aspects of donor acquisition, laboratory testing, storage, processing, and distribution. A detailed procedure manual should be made available to all staff members. This manual should be reviewed and updated, if necessary, on an annual basis.[1]

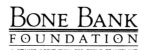

```
              BONE BANK
              FOUNDATION
           A SERVICE INSTITUTION FOR TISSUE TRANSPLANT
           San Antonio, Texas 78229
                 (512) 734-8738


           AIRDRIED BONE ALLOGRAFT INFORMATION

TISSUE NUMBER:_____
DESCRIPTION:_____
EXPIRATION DATE:_____
SIZE: _____
```

This bone allograft has been sterilized with gasseous ethlene oxide following air drying. It has been double packaged and has a shelf life of 2 years. It should be stored at room temperature. The donor was screened for malignancy, neurological disorders, active infectious disease, sepsis and disease of unknown etiology. A blood sample was shown to be negative for hepatitis-B surface antigen by radioimmunoassay. The tissue has passed rigid bacteriological quality control testing. It should be returned to the Bone Bank Foundation on its expiration date.

REHYDRATION OF AIR DRIED ALLOGRAFT BONE

1. Use aseptic precautions throughout.

2. Open the outside peel pack, avoiding touching or otherwise contaminating the inside peel pack.

3. The inside peel pack is received by the scrub nurse and opened in the sterile field for use of the surgeon.

4. Transfer the bone into an antibiotic solution of your choice and allow to soak prior to implantation. This helps reconstitute bone matrix to its original texture and removes unwanted residues from the transplant.

5. The bone should be cut with an air powered saw and/or air powered burr to fashion it in whatever shape is needed for the allograft transplant.

6. If the tissue is not used for the procedure after opening the sealed pack, it must be discarded.

7. Please complete the enclosed transplant record form and return to the above address

NOTE: If you have any questions about this tissue graft, please phone the Bone Bank Foundation.

        4330 Medical Dr. • Suite 200 • San Antonio, TX 78229 • 512/696-4912

Fig. 40-3 Air-dried bone allograft information.

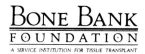

```
              BONE BANK
              FOUNDATION
           A SERVICE INSTITUTION FOR TISSUE TRANSPLANT

              San Antonio, Texas 78229

                   (512) 734-8738


              ALLOGRAFT TRANSPLANT RECORD

    This form has been included with the tissue allograft information
    sheet.  It is a very important part of our transplant record.  It
    must accompany the graft material to surgery and be returned to
    the above address after the graft is used.

    Thank you.

    1.  Date graft used:_____

    2.  Hospital where graft was used:_____

    3.  Tissue type and number:_____

    4.  Name of recipient:_____

    5.  Age and sex of recipient:_____

    6.  Recipient's chart number:_____

    7.  Surgeon using graft:_____

    8.  Procedure requiring graft:_____
        _____

    9.  Any comments about the graft (i.e. malleability, shape, suggested
        improvements, etc.)
        _____
        _____
        _____
        _____
        _____




        4330 Medical Dr. • Suite 200 • San Antonio, TX 78229 • 512/696-4912
```

Fig. 40-4   Allograft transplant record.

With each specimen distributed by the bone bank, a package insert (Fig. 40-3) should be included that indicates the method of processing used for that specimen as well as instructions on proper storage and reconstitution.[1] A form requesting information about the surgical procedure in which the tissue was used may also be included (Fig. 40-4). The surgeon or the assistant should complete this form and return it to the bone bank, where it is placed in the permanent records of the tissue donor.

SUMMARY

The advantages of using allogeneic bone include a reduction of morbidity, an excellent means of physical stabilization and prevention of collapse, a good matrix for new bone growth, and a means of stimulating induction by host tissues.

Bone-banking methods will change as more knowledge is gained about the biomechanical and biologic aspects of bone grafting. Sterilization methods, cleaning of bone, storage, preservation, and packaging are all subject to improvement when better methods are discovered. Bone banks have a responsibility to the surgeons and to the graft recipients to attain new information and to respond to it in a responsible manner.

Editorial comments on p. 470.

REFERENCES

1. American Association of Tissue Banks, Standards for tissue banking, Mowe, J.C., editor, 1984.
2. Bonfiglio, M.: Repair of bone-transplant fractures, J. Bone Joint Surg. **40A:**446, 1958.
3. Brown, K.L., et al.: Bone and cartilage transplantation in orthopaedic surgery, J. Bone Joint Surg. **64A:**270, 1982.
4. Burchardt, H., and Enneking, W.F.: Transplantation of bone, Surg. Clin. North Am. **58:** 403, 1978.
5. Burchardt, H.: The biology of bone graft repair, Clin. Orthop. **174:**28, 1983.
6. Cloward, R.B.: Creation and operation of a bone bank, J. Neurosurg. **33:**682, 1980.
7. Cloward, R.B.: Gas-sterilized cadaver bone grafts for spinal fusion operations: a simplified bone bank, Spine **5:**4, 1980.
8. Friedlaender, G.E.: Current concepts review: bone banking, J. Bone Joint Surg. **64A:**307, 1982.
9. Friedlaender, G.E.: Guidelines for banking osteochondral allografts. In Osteochrondral allografts, biology, banking, and clinical applications, Boston/Toronto, 1983, Little Brown & Co., Inc.
10. Friedlaender, G.E.: Immune responses to preserved bone allografts in humans. In Osteochondral allografts, biology, banking, and clinical applications, Boston/Toronto, 1983, Little Brown & Co., Inc.
11. Friedlaender, G.E., and Mankin, H.J.: Bone banking: current methods and suggested guidelines. In Instructional course lectures, The American Academy of Orthopaedic Surgeons, vol. 30, St. Louis, 1981, The C.V. Mosby Co.
12. Friedlaender, G.E., et al.: Studies on the antigenicity of bone, I. Freeze-dried and deep-frozen bone allografts in rabbits, J. Bone Joint Surg. **58A:**854, 1976.
13. Glowacki, J., et al.: Fate of mineralized and demineralized osseous implants in cranial defects, Calcif. Tissue Int. **33:**71, 1981.
14. Glowacki, J.: Application of the biological principle of induced osteogenesis for craniofacial defects, Lancet **8227:**959, 1981.
15. Inclan, A.: The use of preserved bone grafts in orthopaedic surgery, J. Bone Joint Surg. **24:** 81, 1942.
16. Malinin, T.I., et al.: Freeze-drying of bone for allotransplantation. In Osteochondral allografts, biology, banking, and clinical applications, Boston/Toronto, 1983, Little Brown & Co., Inc.
17. Mulliken, J.B., and Glowacki, J.: Induced osteogenesis for repair and construction in the craniofacial region, Plast. Reconstr. Surg. **65:** 553, 1980.
18. Pelker, R.R., et al.: Biomechanical properties of bone allografts, Clin. Orthop. **174:**54, 1983.
19. Prolo, D.J.: The neurosurgeon in transplantation: provision and use of cadaver tissues and organs, Neurosurgery **6**(3):342, 1980.
20. Prolo, D.J., et al.: Ethylene oxide sterilization of bone, dura mater, and fascia lata for human transplantation, Neurosurgery **6:**529, 1980.
21. Reynolds, F.C., et al.: Clinical evaluation of the merthiolate bone bank and homogenous, bone grafts, J. Bone Joint Surg. **33A:**873, 1951.

22. Tomford, W., et al.: 1983 bone bank procedures, Clin. Orthop. **174:**15, 1983.
23. Tuli, S.M., and Singh, A.D.: The osteoinductive property of decalcified bone matrix: an experimental study, J. Bone Joint Surg. **60B:**116, 1978.
24. Urist, M.R.: Surface-decalcified allogeneic bone (SDAB) implants: a preliminary report of 10 cases and 25 comparable operations with undecalcified lyophilized bone implants, Clin. Orthop. **56:**37, 1968.
25. Urist, M.R.: Practical applications of basic research on bone graft physiology. In Instructional Course Lectures, The American Academy of Orthopaedic Surgeons, St. Louis, 1976, The C.V. Mosby Co.
26. Urist, M.R., and Hernandez, A.: Excitation transfer in bone, Arch. Surg. **109:**486, 1974.
27. Urist, M.R., et al.: A chemosterilized antigen-extracted autodigested alloimplant for bone banks, Arch. Surg. **100:**416, 1975.
28. Urist, M.R., et al.: Human bone morphogenetic protein (BMP), Proc. Soc. Exp. Biol. Med. **173**(2):194, 1983.

EDITORIAL COMMENTARY

One third of our authors do not use bank bone. One third find bank bone of some value and one third find bank bone of great value. Richard Rothman does use bank bone occasionally in the rare fusion that he does. Half of the authors have experienced significant complications with bank bone.

Because of the great theoretical advantage but lack of studies comparing rates of incorporation and fusion several of the authors use a mixture of bank bone with the patient's bone.

We do not have a bone bank at our spine center. We have purchased bone from several bone banks for our interbody fusions. We have had no difficulty obtaining adequate bone for grafting in any of the other types of fusions. In the wide decompressions of multiple levels, especially with internal fixation in the form of pedicle screws and plates, so much of the posterior elements are removed that there is adequate bone simply from the posterior elements. We rarely need to take bone from the iliac crest in such procedures.

The iliac crest is easily accessible through the midline lumbar wound. We take as much bone as is necessary from the posterior third of the iliac crest. We will take one or both of the cortices as necessary. We have had no significant complications from taking bone graft in this fashion.

It is surprising to me how successful solid fusions can be both clinically and in the lack of pseudarthrosis when we use only the ground up posterior elements from the decompressive laminectomy. This may be because of the rigid internal fixation. It may be that partial fusion is as clinically successful as complete fusion. It has been suggested by many in the past that pseudarthrosis in themselves are not painful. At any rate, as our internal fixation has become more and more rigid, we have used less and less ancillary bone graft.

Arthur H. White

CHAPTER

41

SYNTHETIC BONE GRAFT

Vert Mooney   Craig Derian

The purpose of this discussion is to focus at a constant surgical problem—how bone can be built when there was none there before. This problem taxes all skeletal surgeons and touches the field of tumor surgery, trauma surgery, total joint replacement, and certainly spinal fusion surgery. Although living donor bone graft is always available, the concept of donation is a euphemism. Certainly, the patient pays a price of additional morbidity, additional threat for complications, and certainly additional potential for pain at the donor site on every occasion of extraction of bone graft from one skeletal location to another. Yes, alternatives are available. Cadaver allograft, now either fresh frozen or freeze-dried, is available. But will it incorporate as readily as autogenous? This material has been with us for many years, but it still has not received total acceptance. Is there a better material to enhance spinal fusions?

The discussion that follows answers the question proposed with a fuzzy "not yet." It will, however, suggest the potentials for the future and leave the reader with the expectation that ultimately synthetic bone graft will be available.

HISTORICAL BACKGROUND

Until recently the quest for a bone graft substitute has been focused mostly on homograft (cadaver graft). The standard of comparison to autogenous graft was established by the classic paper of Chase and Herndon,[6] which was updated and confirmed by Heiple and coworkers in 1974.[10] In both studies clearly it was autogenous cancellous graft that was superior. The explanation of failure of the processed cadaver bone to be as successful as autogenous bone was thought to be due to minor immunologic aspects, as well as the apparent absence of bone inductive or stimulating qualities of the dead tissue.

In an effort to enhance the potential of the dead scaffold of mineral (hydroxyapatite), additives were suggested in the form of autogenous marrow by Burwell in 1966.[4,5] Boyne[3] also advocated the mixture of autogenous marrow cells as a method of induction to various bone mineral granules. This method is still used frequently in the oral surgical and maxilla facial reconstructive surgery areas.

One of the persistent problems of all clinicians dealing with autogenous graft, however, is the unpredictable nature of its stability. It has been noted frequently that resorption, especially of cancellous graft, occurs for undefined reason. Thus there was a reasonable need to supply a bone graft substitute that would allow new bone formation at least at a rate comparable to autogenous graft but also be predictable for its persistence.

One type of material that seems to have the appropriate physical characteristics of purely a scaffold of mineral with hopefully no reactive protein characteristics about it is xenograft. Coming from an unlimited animal source such as a calf, it is quite easy to provide a material of any dimension, cortical cancellous ratio, and strength. Bassett[1] first reviewed the potential of this material in the early 1960s. At that time the recorded results were somewhat glowing. Depending on the location, origin, manufacturer, and historic background, various products, known as Oswestry bone, Kobe bone, Kiel bone, and Surgibone, became intermittently available. Currently, this processed animal bone is available for implantation in Europe; the recent history of its use has been summarized by Salama[21] in 1983. He reported on the addition of marrow graft. This series seemed to suggest that now not only was the material bone conductive, but also bone induction as well. Clinical experience has failed to confirm its use in general in America.[17]

As always, in the discussion of new bone formation, there is the constant trade-off between strength and speed of incorporation. Cortical bone with its strength (or other materials with cortical bonelike scaffold) potentially has insufficient void space to allow the rapid proliferation of new bone-forming cells, as well as the vascular supply necessary for metabolic support. Thus incorporation occurs by creeping substitution. One material has been advocated that completely avoids the subject of mechanical strength and looks completely to inductive possibilities of the material. The antigen extracted allogenic bone matrix gelatin (AAA) was developed by Urist[22] in the early 1970s.

Clinical application of this material when compared to autogenous graft for an intertransverse process fusion was quite successful.[21] The fusion rate with autogenous graft in a parallel series reported by Dawson[8] was 92%; with the AAA graft it was reported by Urist as 88% in similar patients. This material has never become commercially available and thus a repeat of the series has not been accomplished. The advantage of the material, which is gelatin in characteristic, was that it would rapidly stimulate new bone formation. When applied to tumor void spaces,[15] it was successful in 91% of the patients, that is, the material was metabolized and replaced by new bone formation. Again, this experience was conducted in Japan; the material is not currently out of the experimental stage in America. It offers no structural contribution, but apparently a significant stimulus to new bone formation.

However, there certainly are clinical settings where structural strength is desirable. With the anticipation that bone can form over a scaffolding of mineral and in an environment where bone is already forming, the application of ceramics to bone substitutes seems reasonable. The first clinical application of a ceramic specifically designed as a bone substitute was by Smith.[20] This material was an impure ceramic, but porous, and achieved its structural strength characteristics by the impregnation of epoxy resin in the porous ceramic. Thus by adjusting the porosity of the material one could vary the mechanical characteristics. The material was known and marketed as Cerosium. In the period before the acceptance of methylmethacrylate bonding (bone cement), this material was an early pioneer for bone ingrowth into porous structures. It failed in early clinical applications, however.

Enthusiasm for the potential of the ceramic material to serve as a bone substitute continued into the early 1970s. The materials scientists, especially at Clemson University, took an interest in the characteristics of bone ingrowth. Hulbert and coworkers[14] demonstrated that at least a 50 μm-diameter aperture was necessary in the ceramic to expect bone ingrowth. Predecki and associates[18] demonstrated that bony ingrowth could only be expected for a millimeter or so in a cylindric channel. For greater ingrowth it was necessary to have interconnecting apertures within the channels. Both studies pointed out that probably over 100 μm diameter porosity was necessary to have reliable bony ingrowth. The primary ceramic model for these studies was aluminum oxide. The Predecki study also pointed out that from the standpoint of bone ingrowth one material seemed about as good as another as long as it was biologically inert. Thus polymers such as polyethylene and metals such as titanium—as well as ceramics, if made in a porous structure—could all expect bony ingrowth. In addition, the expectation of bony ingrowth was far greater if interface between living tissue in a bony environment, and the implant, were stable. If a significant degree of motion occurred between the interface of implant and living material, fibrous ingrowth would result, rather than bone.

Alternative bonelike minerals have emerged as ceramic bone substitutes, which are expected to serve as scaffolding for new bone formation. In addition, there is the theoretic potential of developing a mineral so bonelike that its difference from true bone mineral (hydroxyapatite) cannot be defined by the living system; thus the mineral would participate in bone turnover according to physiologic principles. A porous ceramic with controllable biodegradation is thus a theoretic possibility. If the implanted mineral lost is replaced by living bone, this class of ceramics has a distinct advantage over other bone-substitute materials. The class of materials known as tricalcium phosphates has the potential to slowly desolve in physiologic environments, but because of the high concentration of mineral, the structure can be replaced by bone. The foundation for this work was laid by Bhaskar.[2] This material seemed to have superior biocompatible characteristics compared to the aluminum oxide ceramics.[9] Originally marketed as Synthograft, it now appears commercially as Orthograft and currently has its major application in the maxilla facial/oral surgery field for periodontal defect repair.

One of the most interesting materials is one that presents a mineral scaffolding with the appearance of human bone, and with a mineral characteristic extremely similar to human bone. The similarity of sea coral to bone is evident.[24] Webber and White[23] suggested specific types of coral that might be converted to ceramic or polymer materials for biomedical applications. Since coral itself is calcium carbonate, it has been recognized that this is not ideally biocompatible. At the materials laboratory at Pennsylvania State University a method of converting limestone structural coral into pure hydroxyapatite was developed,[25] and the process was called Replanineform.[19] The first animal study of this material was reported by Chiroff.[7] The study noted that a cylinder of 1 cm by 5 mm placed in the cancellous bone of the distal femur and proximal tibia of a dog was uniformly filled with new bone. No other material described had been so fully incorporated by ingrowing bone. Other porous ceramics reported an invasion up to perhaps 2 mm.

The clinical potential for this material was recognized by Holmes[11] and was initially applied to facial reconstruction. He proposed a concept that the hydroxyapatite mineral model on the Porites coral skeleton appeared so similar to osteoevacuated bone with its parallel channels and frequent interconnecting fenestration that it became an ideal material for implantation.[12] It was noted in the dog mandibles, which had a 2-cm defect replaced by the hydroxyapatite model on the coral structure, that the entire length became incorporated with bone. At 2 months 11% of the void was filled with new bone and at 4 months 46%. In fact, it was noted that in this laboratory-fabricated hydroxyapatite material at 12 months 29% of the material was lost because of biodegradation and replacement by bone. Overall, this seemed to offer the most favorable characteristics for a bone-substitute mineral scaffold. In none of the experimental work has the hydroxyapatite mineral modeled on coral demonstrated an allergic or adverse biologic response.

One additional material has been tried as a bone-graft substitute in lumbar fusions. In 1983 Lemons and coworkers[17] reported on an animal study of synthetic materials for lumbar fusions in dogs. In addition to nonporous calcium hydroxyapatite (Durapatite), porous biodegradable tricalcium phosphate ceramic (Synthograft) and invert soda-lime glass (Bioglass) were used as alternatives to autogenous iliac crest bone. A series of dogs was used who were evaluated 6 months after fusion procedure. In this group it became apparent that the hydroxyapatite most often showed continuous bone to biomaterial interfaces. Trabecular bone surrounded the calcium hydroxyapatite particles. The tricalcium phosphate ceramic showed varying amounts of resorption with some adjacent bone and some fibrous tissue. The glass particulate material showed very little bone incorporation and largely incapsulation by fibrous tissue. In all settings the incorporation was enhanced by the application of autogenous bone graft.[16]

Thus, to summarize the historic perspective, we have learned a few things over the past several decades. There are various bonelike minerals available that are well tolerated in the living system and can be expected to supply a framework in which bone will grow. There are certain characteristics of porosity that are more ideal for bone growth than others. The presence of living cells in an environment of bone formation is a positive environment. Finally, no perfect material has been proposed that can supply the potential for rapid new bone induction and also the strength necessary to maintain the structural integrity of the system without auxiliary support.

CURRENT DEVELOPMENTAL WORK

At our institution we decided to pursue the experimental studies and ultimately clinical application of hydroxyapatite made from coral as the best choice of the various possible bone substitute systems. Holmes and coworkers reported an experimental study of 16 foxhounds in which was used the cortical bone replacement Porites. In this diaphyseal defect model the implant was incorporated as rapidly and completely as the control side, which was grafted with iliac crest autogenous graft in the usual manner. There was no rejection. In another study an alternative coral material, which has a microstructure similar in appearance to that of cancellous bone (goniopora), was implanted into the metaphyseal defect of eight foxhounds. This material was well incorporated at 2, 4, 6, and 12 months. Incorporation of the material was actually complete by 2 months and was thus far more rapid than in the case of the cortical-like coral structures from Porites. A third experimental model was used. In this setting 16 foxhounds had lumbar spinal fusions with autogenous graft on one side and Porites implants on the other. No fixation was used in these lumbar spine fusion models. In this setting incorporation of the autogenous and the coral material was equal in settings where there was no motion, but no solid spine fusions occurred. No complete incorporation occurred traversing the joints. Distribution of bony ingrowth was similar in implants and grafts. In all of these studies biodegradation at 12 months was minimal. The material used for implantation was more greatly standardized than the previous studies in the dog mandible.

The mechanical characteristics of the hydroxyapatite made from coral were also studied. Although the material was quite weak when compared either to cancellous or cortical bone, once incorporated it actually became stronger than the native material. For instance, hydroxyapatite from the cancellous-appearing coral (goniopra) was found to have 1.6 times the energy absorption capacity compared to cancellous grafts.[13] The implant therefore presents itself as slightly stronger and more flexible and able to absorb energy better than cancellous graft. In the dog model, which compared Porites graft to the cancellous graft in the radius defect, the ultimate strength of the implant was about three fifths that of the dog radius at 6 months (the cancellous graft was stronger than either the intact radius or the Porites implant).

In another study, which was a comparative study of porous hydroxyapatite to tricalcium phosphate, Shimazaki[21a] attempted to quantitate the bone ingrowth in biodegradability of tricalcium phosphate compared to hydroxyapatite. All the implants had totally interconnecting pores. The pores averaged around 500 for the goniopora vs. 200 for the Porites vs. about 150 for the tricalcium phosphate. In this study cylinder co-implants, 3 mm in diameter by 8 mm, were implanted into the diaphyses of rabbit tibias. The quantity of regenerated bone, remaining implant and nonmineralized space was evaluated. At 24 weeks, although more bony incorporation occurred in the goniopora implant (56% vs. 45% for TCP), a greater degree of biodegradation occurred in the TCP vs. the hydroxyapatite (46% compared to 27%). This study seems to present the evidence that a larger pore size encourages more rapid incorporation. Biodegradation seems to be a factor of exposed surface area, and in settings where surface was "shielded" by bony overlay of implant, less degradation occurred. This study also suggested that biodegradation of TCP could occur without vascularization. New bone formation only occurred in apposition to bony areas not within the intermedullary canal. Thus TCP did not seem to be quite as osteoconductive as the larger-pore hydroxyapatite.

CLINICAL EXPERIENCE WITH BONE GRAFT SUBSTITUTES FOR SPINAL FUSIONS

Based on excellent histologic response to hydroxyapatite made from coral, in 1982 we planned a prospective clinical trial of hydroxyapatite as a bone graft substitute. The model chosen was similar to the one described by Dawson and Urist[9] for an intertransverse process fusion. In addition, it was anticipated that additional stabilization could be achieved by the use of Knodt rods; thus a series was planned to use standard methods of intertransverse process fusion with Knodt-rod stabilization and autogenous bone graft placed on one side with hydroxyapatite bone-graft substitute on the other side. The decision of left or right side was left to be completely random.

Initially, only the morselized posterior elements were used for the donor graft material on the autogenous side. It rapidly became apparent, however, that this provided insufficient bone to achieve an adequate volume. Although it has been hoped that the use of a bone graft substitute would allow the physician to avoid the need to search for donor graft from the traditional posterior iliac crest, in general this was impossible; supplemental bone graft was provided from the iliac crest in addition to the morselized posterior elements. Also, as the series progressed, it became apparent that an adjunct to new bone formation was necessary on the hydroxyapatite side; thus granules of autogenous bone were sprinkled on that side as well.

The necessary physical characteristics of the hydroxyapatite for implantation were not clear. Because the customary bone-grafting technique for this particular fusion location usually required the implantation of long slivers of cortical cancellous and cancellous bone, a similar physical characteristic of the hydroxyapatite from coral was sought. Thus, using the Porites material (200 μm diameter porosity), "matchstick"-size staves of material were applied, which measured 4 mm on a side and were of several centimeters length; these were placed in parallel fashion traversing the facet joints and transverse processes. This material is somewhat brittle; frequently at the time of application the "matchsticks" broke. However, because they were to offer no structural stability—merely a matrix for new bone formation—this event was considered noncontributory to success or failure. Aside from the implantation of the hydroxyapatite, all other characteristics of the surgery were routine and as required by the specific needs of the clinical problem.

Our associate in the study was Dr. David Selby. In the study 53 patients underwent consecutive posterior spinal procedure by Selby or Mooney in a 6-month period, 1982 through 1983; 34 were operated by Dr. Selby and 19 by Dr. Mooney. Cases were reviewed by Dr. Derian. The patients were all private patients followed in routine manner after surgery. X-ray films were taken in standard manner of follow-up. The evaluations were performed independently by Dr. Derian, who participated in none of these specific surgeries. His evaluations were accomplished without the participation of the surgeon, but with a rating system in total agreement with the surgeon's views. The evaluations were accomplished at 1, 3, 6, 9, 12, 18, and 24 months. At this time 81% (43/53) of the patients had been followed for 12 months or more. The majority carried the diagnosis of either primary or postoperative segmental instability (47%) or primary or surgical spinal stenosis (32%). The rest of the patients had variations of degenerative and herniated disc disease. There were 18 women in the group of 53 patients, and 49% of the patients had had at least one previous posterior lumbar procedure. In fact, 20% had had two or more previous procedures. The levels operated on are shown in Table 41-1.

Results: Of the original 53 patients 48 had sufficient data for follow-up. Of these 48 patients, 85% (41/48) had fusion of the autogenous side; 12% had fusion of the hydroxyapatite side (6/48). No patient had fusion of the hydroxyapatite

Table 41-1 *Levels operated on*

Level	No. patients	%
L3-L4	2	3.7
L4-L5	6	11.3
L5-S1	7	13.2
L4 to S1	29	54.7
L3 to S1	7	13.2
L2 to S1	2	3.7

side and not the autogenous side. Fusion appearance was purely on a subjective rating scale by one interpreter without initial correlation to clinical findings or past history. The average time of radiographic solid fusion on the autogenous side was 8.5 months. On the hydroxyapatite side, the numbers were so few that figures are not significant. It is interesting, however, that three fusions seem to be apparent at 4 to 8 months, whereas three fusions were not evident until 24 months. Review of the records fails to identify what different technique was applied on those who fused early.

There were no complications that could be specifically assigned to the use of the hydroxyapatite material. There was one deep infection that required reoperation and removal of Knodt rod. The coral was not disturbed (nor was the autogenous graft), and the wound healed without residual effects and eventually became a solid fusion.

Although the purpose of this study was essentially to evaluate the efficacy of a bone graft substitute to achieve solid fusion, a relationship to clinical outcome is necessary for any clinical study. Of the 48 who were followed long enough to identify clinical outcome 73% returned to work (35/48). Interestingly, 69% of those who returned to work (24/35) had only a unilateral radiographic fusion on the autogenous side.

Obviously, this is a poor application of this material. Its role in stabilized skeletal defects, however, has been excellent. In a series by Bucholz of 35 patients with a metaphyseal fractures and internal fixation the fusion rate has been 100%. However, the significant differences are environment and stability. Experience has pointed out that the Knodt rods cannot truly immobilize the motion segments of the lower lumbar segments. Moreover, the hydroxyapatite from coral grafts are not in an ideal bone-forming environment. Although they are placed in a bony bed, they certainly are not enveloped by bone-forming tissue as is the case in a metaphyseal defect. The historical and clinical experience suggests that the significant environment of bone-forming cells is necessary for this scaffold of mineral to serve adequately for new bone formation, that is, the interbody environment. Certainly, here a more significant environment of cancellous bone could be developed. Unhappily, as was demonstrated in our basic studies, hydroxyapatite material is of insufficient strength to tolerate the mechanical loads at this site. On the other hand, pressed tricalcium phosphate is a far stronger material; it was believed appropriate to try this application in the interbody space. Figs. 41-1 to 41-4 demonstrate its application.

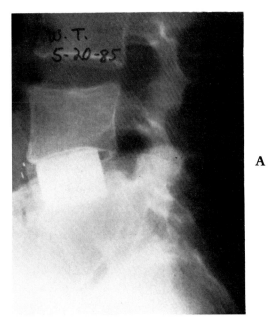

Fig. 41-1 A, L4-L5 anterior interbody fusion (Crock technique) with the implantation of solid tricalcium dowel. Similar autogenous iliac crest graft was placed parallel to this in interspace.

Continued.

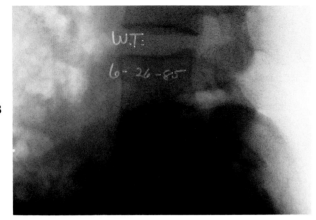

Fig. 41-1, cont'd B, 1 month later the bone substitute dowel has fragmented. Patient went on to fuse. Solid dowel had insufficient strength to tolerate the loads of function.

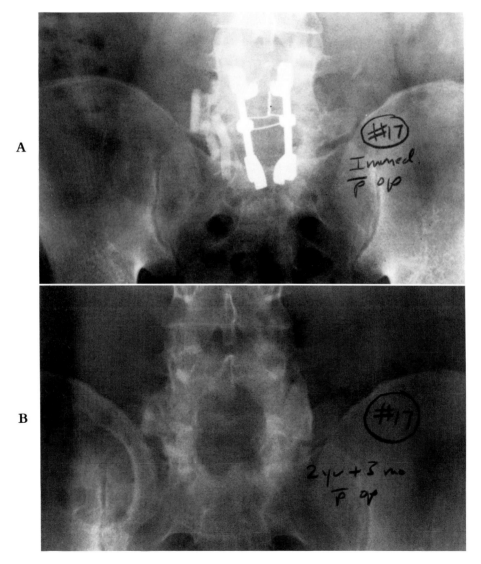

Fig. 41-2 A, Status immediately after intertransverse process fusion with autogenous graft on right and hydroxyapatite on left with Knodt rod fixation. Patient was a 26-year-old manual laborer with spondylolisthesis at L5, S-1 and herniated disc at L4-L5. **B,** Knodt rods had been removed approximately 1 year earlier due to irritation; 6-month films had indicated solid fusion at the autogenous side on the right at that time. At present both sides are defined as radiographically solid, and the patient is back to work as a heavy laborer.

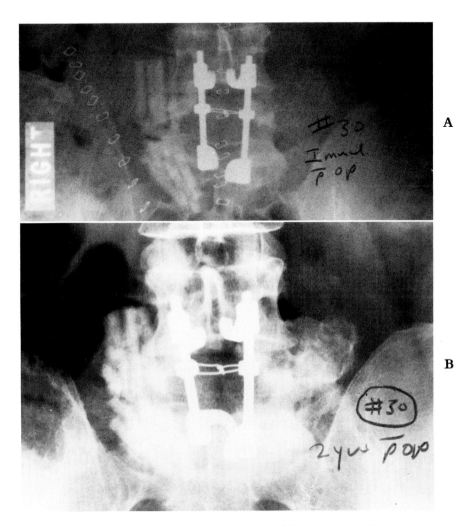

Fig. 41-3 **A,** A 59-year-old businessman with herniated disc at L4-L5 and spinal stenosis at L5-S1 underwent facetectomy at L5 and fusion, L4, S1, with Knodt rod stabilization. **B,** At 2-year follow-up solid fusion noted on autogenous side, as well as on the coral side, L-5, S-1, but not L4-L5. The patient had returned to full activities at 1 year after surgery.

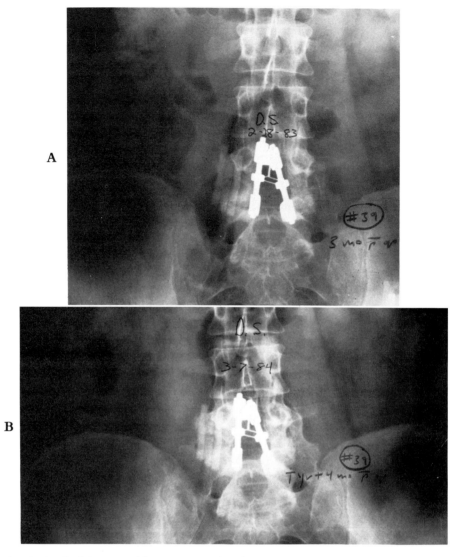

Fig. 41-4 A, A 35-year-old optometrist after chymopapain failure at L4–L5 had a Knodt rod fusion at L4–L5 with autogenous bone on the right and hydroxyapatite on the left. At 3 months after surgery no union is noted. **B,** At 16 months after surgery, autogenous graft appears united, but the hydroxyapatite does not appear incorporated. Patient had returned to work as an optometrist 8 months after surgery with only minor back pain.

SUMMARY

One of the reasons for limited enthusiasm for spinal fusion in lumbar reconstructive surgery is the morbidity associated with the procedure. The group of individuals to whom the procedure is applied in degenerative disc disease or for postsurgical failures is an older age-group than the typical, more successful fusions for scoliosis. Also, seldom are these scoliosis fusions traversing the lower lumbar segments. These segments have the greatest mobility and greatest mechanical stresses, again limiting potential for fusion. The addition of a large amount of donor graft to all of the physiologic-negative factors greatly increases the discrepancy between human cost and potential benefit. This is probably the most demanding site for bone-graft substitute in terms of the need to increase healing rate and the need to offer inherent structural stability. Unhappily, we currently have no real substitute to autogenous graft material. For a while longer we will have to pay the price of a human source of graft material. However, basic studies indicate that ultimately a solution will be found. *Editorial comments on p. 482.*

REFERENCES

1. Bassett, C.A.L., and Creighton, D.K.J.: A comparison of host response cortical autografts and processed calf heterografts, J. Bone Joint Surg. **44A**:842, 1962.
2. Bhaskar, S.N., et al.: Biodegradable ceramic implants in bone, Oral Surg. **32**:336, 1971.
3. Boyne, P.J.: Induction of bone repair by various bone-grafting materials: hard tissue growth, repair and remineralization, Ciba Foundation Symposium 11, Elsevier Excerpta Medica, 1973, Elsevier North Holland.
4. Bucholz, R.B.: Personal communication, 1985.
5. Burwell, R.G.: Studies in the transplantation of bone, J. Bone Joint Surg. **48B**:532, 1966.
6. Burwell, R.G.: Studies in the transplantation of bone. VII. The fresh composite homograft-autograft of cancellous bone: an analysis of factors leading to osteogenesis in marrow transplants and in marrow-containing bone grafts, J. Bone Joint Surg. **46B**:110, 1964.
7. Chase, S.W., and Herndon, C.H.: The fate of autogenous and homogenous bone grafts, J. Bone Joint Surg. **37A**:809, 1955.
8. Chiroff, R.T., et al.: Tissue ingrowth of replamineform implants, J. Biomed. Mat. Res. Symp. **6**:29, 1975.
9. Dawson, E.G., et al.: Intertransverse process lumbar arthrodesis with autogenous bone graft, Clin. Orthop. **154**:90, 1981.
10. Graves, G.A., et al.: Resorbable ceramic implants, J. Biomed. Mater. Res. **2**:92, 1971.
11. Heiple, K.G., et al.: A comparative study of the healing process following different types of bone transplantation, J. Bone Joint Surg. **45A**:1593, 1974.
12. Holmes, R.E., and Salyer, K.E.: Bone regeneration in a coralline hydroxyapatite implant, Surg. Forum, **24**:611, 1978.
13. Holmes, R.E.: Bone regeneration within a coralline hydroxyapatite implant, Plast. Reconstr. Surg. **63**:626, 1979.
14. Holmes, R.E., et al.: A coralline hydroxyapatite bone graft substitute, Clin. Orthop. **88**:252, 1984.
15. Hulbert, S.F., et al.: Tissue reaction to three ceramics of porous and nonporous structures, J. Biomed. Mater. Res. **6**:347, 1972.
16. Iwata, H., et al.: Chemosterilized autolyzed antigen-extracted allogeneic (AAA) bone matrix gelatin for repair of defects from excision of benign bone tumors, Clin. Orthop. **154**:150, 1981.
17. Lemons, J.E., et al.: Synthetic biomaterials for spinal fusion, Orthop. Trans. **7**(2):331, 1983.
18. Pieron, A.P., et al.: Bone grafting with bioplant results in 33 cases, J. Bone Joint Surg. **50B**:364, 1968.
19. Predecki, P., et al.: Kinetics of bone ingrowth into cylindrical channels of aluminum oxide and titanium, J. Biomed. Mater. Res. **6**:375, 1972.
20. Roy, D.M., and Linnehan, S.K.: Hydroxyapatite formed from coral skeletal carbonate by hydrothermal exchange, Nature **247**, 1974.
21. Salama, R.: Xenogeneic bone grafting in humans, Clin. Orthop. **174**:113, 1983.
21a. Shimazaki, K., and Mooney, V.: Comparative study of porous hydroxyapatite and tricalcium phosphate as bone substitute, J. Orthop. Res. **3**:301, 1985.
22. Smith, L.: Ceramic plastic material as a bone substitute, Arch. Surg. **87**:653, 1963.
23. Urist, M.R., and Dawson, M.E.: Intertransverse process fusion with the aid of chemosterilized autolyzed antigen-extracted allogenic (AAA) bone, Clin. Orthop. **154**:97, 1981.
24. Urist, M.R., and Iwata, H.: Preservation in biodegradation of the morphrogenic property of bone matrix, J. Theor. Biol. **38**:155, 1973.
25. Webber, J.N., and White, E.W.: Carbonate materials as precursers to new ceramic and polymer materials for biomedical applications, Minerals Sciences Engineering, **5**:151, 1973.
26. Wells, J.W.: Scleractinia in treatise on invertebrate paleontology. In Moore, R.C., editor, Kansas City, 1967, University of Kansas Press.
27. White, E.W., et al.: Materials useful in prosthetic devices and the like, U.S. Patent no. 3,890,107, June 17, 1975.

EDITORIAL COMMENTARY

The rather recent development of polymeric pins for biodegradable bone strut material by Russian authors may prove to be important for certain fusion techniques in the future. The material is fabricated from a copolymer of polyvinylpyrrolidone and methyl methacrylate reinforced with polyamide fibers and calcium gluconate. Intramedullary rods formed from this material are claimed to be as strong as metal implants but have superior flexibility. These easily cut and trimmed rods have been shown to promote long bone fusions and to become incorporated within the new bone mass; the rods then virtually disappear 1 to 3 years later.* Other porous, fused-sintered synthetic materials (high-density polyethylene, polyprophylene or fluorocarbon) some of which may be bonded to a steel or carbon substrate, are now being tried for the fabrication of prostheses to which bone will attach.†

Of considerably greater interest, however, is the discovery of an embryonic cartilage activation factor. This hormone-like material, whose molecular structure is as yet unclear, has been found to promote rapid healing of fractures of causing osteoblasts to become cartilage cells which then rapidly convert to osteocytes with restitution of the bone, rather like a recapitulation of long bone growth from cartilagenous end plates. This substance is now being manufactured from bovine embryo chromatin implanted into E. Coli organisms which are then cloned in massive numbers. This process of genetic engineering is similar to that which is used in the bacterial production of human insulin, growth hormone, nerve growth factor, interferon and many others. In animal studies so far available, the process of new bone formation and therefore fusion has been reduced from months to only a few weeks. Clearly, if this or some similar substance can be found to materially shorten the fusion process (without the production of massive overgrowth, osteophytes, tumors, etc.) there will follow a dramatic change in nearly all methods of reconstructive bone surgery, as well as the instrumentation used! Perhaps the "orthopaedic Nirvana" lies at hand.

Charles D. Ray

---

*Merendino, J., et al.: Use of biocompatible orthopaedic polymer for fracture treatment and reconstructive orthopaedic procedures, J. Int. Med. Res. **12:**351, 1984.
†Porex, manufactured by Glasrock, Fairburn, Ga.

CHAPTER 42

OSTEOPOROSIS

Jerome Schofferman

Osteoporosis is a skeletal disorder characterized by a decrease in the mass per unit volume of bone. The bone that remains is normal. Clinically it is more appropriate to use the nonspecific term *osteopenia* to indicate the generalized decrease in bone density, until definitive diagnosis is reached.[18,31,34]

Osteopenia is most commonly due to osteoporosis, but 8% to 30% of patients may have osteomalacia.[17,26] Osteoporosis in turn may be primary (involutional, idiopathic, juvenile) or secondary to disorders of the endocrine system, bone marrow, collagen, or gastrointestinal tract, or it may be due to neoplasia or a number of miscellaneous causes.[17,26] Osteopenia may be discovered as an incidental finding on x-ray films, or the patient may have back pain or fracture. Patients who require spinal fusion—with or without instrumentation—should be screened for underlying metabolic bone disease because treatment may dramatically reduce the incidence of pseudoarthrosis.[23]

MAGNITUDE OF THE PROBLEM

Osteoporosis is a major health problem and will become even more important as our population ages. Medical or orthopedic problems related to osteoporosis accounted for 5% of the hospital days in patients over the age 65 and led to cumulative expenses of 3.8 billion dollars in 1984.[17] The incidence of hip fracture doubles every 5 years after age 50 in women, and by age 80 fractures of the hip resulting from osteoporosis have occurred in one woman in three and in one man in six.[26] Over a billion dollars is spent each year to care for these patients.[10] There is a 10% to 15% mortality rate; 40% to 50% of patients require long term extended care.[26] Vertebral compression fractures occur in 25% of women over age 65 and in approximately 50% of women by age 80.[18] Effective prevention of osteoporosis and effective treatment for patients with established disease would result in significant decreases in morbidity, mortality, and expenditures of health care dollars.

BONE

Bone is in a constant state of remodeling. Formation and resorption are normally well balanced, although factors that control the interactions are not fully understood. Osteoporosis can occur if there is either decreased formation of bone, increase in resorption, or a combination of both.

Bone is composed of organic and inorganic components. The organic matrix is produced by osteoblasts and is composed primarily of collagen with small amounts of glycoprotein, phosphoproteins, mucopolysaccharides, and lipids. The mineral phase consists of hydroxyapatite deposited on the matrix first as calcium phosphate salts, which are transformed to apatite crystals. Osteoblasts also play a role in mineralization. Other minerals are also found in bone.[16] As the extracellular matrix forms, the osteoblasts become encased in it. The encased cells are now called *osteocytes,* and gradually lose their ability to synthesize.

Resorption is carried out by osteoclasts, which contain multiple enzymes capable of resorbing mineral and matrix.[34] Control of resorption is multifactoral with parathyroid hormone (PTH), vitamin D, and osteoclast activating factor each playing some role.

Skeletal bone mass increases until about age 40. Bone formation continues at a constant rate in most individuals, but resorption increases to average 0.5% per year.[16] After menopause, women may lose 1% to 2% of cortical bone per year and even greater amounts of axial bone if not treated.[10] By age 80 women may have lost one third to two thirds of their bone mass, compared to 14% to 25% for men.[19,20,28]

RISK FACTORS

Knowledge of risk factors, or traits that predispose to the development of osteoporosis, may allow the clinician to prevent or detect the problem at an earlier stage. Aging is an obvious risk factor and appears to play an equal role in men and women. Richelson and coworkers[25] have suggested that one fourth of postmenopausal bone loss in women is due to aging and three fourths of the bone loss is due to superimposed estrogen lack.

The exact mechanism of age-related osteoporosis is not clear, perhaps because of the heterogeneity of the disorder.[27] There is an age-related decrease in calcium absorbtion that may be due to impaired conversion of 25 hydroxy vitamin D to 1,25 dihydroxy vitamin D. Poor calcium absorbtion may stimulate PTH production. Riggs[27] has noted higher levels of PTH in osteoporosis in patients aged 75 and older (type II osteoporosis) compared to the normal or low levels seen in osteoporosis in patients aged 51 to 65 (type I osteoporosis).

Estrogen lack is the major cause of osteoporosis in postmenopausal women.[25] There is accelerated bone loss that begins at the menopause and continues for up to 6 to 10 years.[10] Bone loss then slows somewhat. There are several proposed mechanisms. Bone lacks estrogen receptors, implying that all mechanisms are indirect. Lack of estrogen may increase the bone responsiveness to PTH. Some investigators have shown that the low levels of 1,25 dihydroxy vitamin D and low calcium absorption found in some postmenopausal women can be reversed by estrogen administration, but others have not been able to confirm this.[10] Calcitonin deficiency has been said to play a role, but recent data do not support this.[35] It is equally confusing that some studies have demonstrated lower levels of estrogens, testosterone, and 25 hydroxy vitamin D in postmenopausal women with osteoporosis compared to age-matched controls without osteoporosis, but other studies have not.[1,27]

Risk factors for osteoporosis in men have been examined and include exogenous or endogenous hypercorticolism, gastrectomy, intestinal resection, nephrolithiasis, liver disease, childhood rickets, anticonvulsants (osteomalacia?), radiation therapy, and hypogonadism.[32] In the same study tobacco and alcohol consumption were significantly higher in osteoporotic men than those men without osteoporosis. Aloia[1] has also identified cigarette smoking as an independent risk factor and showed an inverse relationship between smoking and calcium absorption. Daniell[7] stated that lower body weight of smokers is important in the development of osteoporosis, but there are direct and indirect factors acting on bone resorption as well. Interestingly, Brown has noted a 500% greater incidence of pseudoarthrosis after attempted lumbar spine fusion in smokers compared to nonsmokers.[5]

It is agreed that nutritional factors are important, but details are controversial.[20] Calcium intake and bone mineralization during the growing years and young adulthood determine bone mass at skeletal maturity. The greater the bone mass is, the more bone that can be lost during aging before osteoporosis develops. Children require 400 to 700 mg of calcium per day, adolescents 1300 mg per day, premenstrual women 700 to 1000 mg per day, and postmenopausal women and senior men need 1400 to 1600 mg per day. Unfortunately, the average American woman consumes only about 550 mg per day.

Excess protein intake may be deleterious.[20] Doubling protein intake increases urinary calcium loss by 50%. Vitamin D deficiency resulting from inadequate sun exposure, decreased dietary intake, poor absorption, or abnormalities in metabolism may lead to osteomalacia, but they are not directly linked to osteoporosis. Young adults need 400 IU per day and the elderly may need 800 IU per day.

Blacks rarely develop osteoporosis, whereas Caucasians of northern European extraction have a high incidence. Sedentary individuals lose more bone than people who are active. Prolonged immobilization leads to hypercalciuria and decreased bone density. Osteoporosis is more common in relatives of persons with osteoporosis.

Various endocrine disorders may cause osteoporosis. Postmenopausal estrogen deficiency has been discussed. Hypogonadism in the male also leads to osteoporosis. Hyperparathyroidism receives a good deal of attention and occasionally may present as generalized osteopenia. Hyperthyroidism, acromegaly, and insulin-dependent diabetes mellitus have each been linked to osteoporosis.[18] Exogenous or endogenous glucocorticoid excess causes osteoporosis, and patients on prolonged therapy should be considered for prophylactic treatment.[2]

The decreased bone density and increased fracture rate recently described in elite women runners with secondary amenorrhea may be of particular interest to orthopedists.[21] Prophylactic therapy with estrogens and calcium should be considered.[13]

Multiple myeloma, metastatic carcinoma to bone, or lymphoma can present with diffuse osteopenia. Hyperplastic marrow disorders such as sickle cell anemia or thallassemia may cause bone rarefaction. Other medical disorders with an increased frequency of osteoporosis include rheumatoid arthritis, malabsorption syndromes, systemic mastocytosis, primary biliary cirrhosis, and other forms of obstructive liver disease. Osteoporosis has been associated with anorexia nervosa,[30] alcohol abuse,[4] and may of course appear in an idiopathic form. Long-term use of heparin, methotrexate, phenytoin (osteomalacia?) can cause osteopenia. There are hereditary forms such as osteogenesis imperfecta or homocysteinuria. Blonds, redheads, persons with many freckles, and patients with scoliosis have been identified as being at higher risk.

CLINICAL PRESENTATION

Osteopenia may be an incidental finding on x-ray films or patients may have acute fractures after minimal or no trauma. Complaints of acute or chronic back pain, easy fatiguability, or shortness of breath resulting from kyphosis and loss of lung volumes may bring the patient to the physician.

Back pain may be of sudden onset because of acute vertebral compression fracture or may develop more gradually. If kyphosis develops, there may be pain resulting from mechanical stresses on joints, muscles, or ligaments.[20] Progressive kyphosis may cause pain as the lower ribs come in contact with the anterior iliac crest.

HISTORY AND PHYSICAL EXAMINATION

The extent and specifics of the evaluation of osteopenia will depend on the degree of disease and clinical suspicions. The history should seek predisposing factors and underlying diseases already discussed. Determine menstrual history, especially the date of menopause. General inquiries should include prior surgeries (gastric or intestinal resection), past and present diet with particular attention to milk products, calcium supplements, protein intake, and alcohol use. Determine cigarette use, past and present levels of physical activity, sun exposure, and family history of bone disorders and fractures. Specific inquiries should seek weight loss (cancer, malabsorption, hyperthyroidism), weight gain (corticosteroid excess), loss of height (prior compression fractures), ulcer (antacids), diarrhea (malabsorption, lactase deficiency) or arthritis. Determine medications used.

The physical exam must screen for systemic illness, adenopathy, clubbing, lung disease, skin changes, and changes in fat deposition, thyromegaly or scars from surgeries. Height and weight are measured. The prostate must be felt for cancer.

LABORATORY EVALUATION

Laboratory investigation is designed to screen for underlying disease and to delineate the specific cause of osteopenia. Routine studies include hemoglobin (multiple myeloma, cancer, systemic illness), white blood cell count, sedimentation rate, urinalysis, serum and urine protein electrophoresis, liver function tests, magnesium, creatinine and creatinine clearance, serum calcium, phosphorous, alkaline phosphatase, immunoreactive PTH, thyroid function tests, fasting glucose, and 24-hour urine calcium. Most patients will need a measurement of 25 hydroxy vitamin D to assess total stores and to screen for osteomalacia. Low levels require further investigation. Other testing such as measurement of 1,25 dihydroxy vitamin D, 24-hour urine hydroxyproline or cyclic AMP, serum cortisol and dexamethasone suppression test, or testosterone are indicated if initial testing is not diagnostic.

The laboratory profile in most patients with osteoporosis is normal. Alkaline phosphatase is elevated after a fracture, but persistent elevation will prompt a work-up for osteomalacia, bone metastases, Pagets disease, or liver disease. During immobilization, serum calcium may increase transiently which lowers the PTH level which in turn lowers the level of 1,25 vitamin D. Elevations of calcium lead to a further workup for hyperparathyroidism, malignancy, granulomatous disease, Addison's disease, or thyroid disease. Low serum calcium may suggest osteomalacia, malabsorption, or hypoparathyroidism. Low phosphorous can be seen in humoral hypercalcemia of malignancy, primary hyperparathyroidism, or osteomalacia. High levels can be seen in renal failure.

RADIOLOGIC EVALUATION

Radiologic techniques are used to detect, quantify, and follow the course of osteopenia. Plain radiographs are insensitive. There must be bone loss of 30% or greater before osteopenia can be detected. Although plain films are not useful for screening or following osteopenia, bone loss may first be noticed as an incidental finding and suggest the need for further investigation. Even radiogrammetry, the technique of measuring cortical thickness, is too insensitive to be clinically useful.[31]

Single photon absorptiometry is a quantitative technique to measure bone mineral content in the peripheral skeleton, usually the cortical bone of the nondominant radius. Correlation is high with bone mineral content of the femoral neck but not with bone density of the spine, thereby limiting its usefulness. The test is inexpensive, quite accurate and precise, requires no special preparation, and takes 10 to 15 minutes; radiation exposure is about 10 to 15 millirads.

Dual photon absorptiometry is a quantitative technique that can measure bone mineral content in the spine. The test is more expensive than single photon studies but is much more useful. It is quite precise, requires no special patient preparation, and takes about 30 to 45 minutes. Radiation exposure is about 15 millirads, which is low enough to allow serial measurements. Most researchers believe the accuracy is quite high, but others disagree.[9,13] Vertebral compression fractures or significant osteophyte formation may lead to erroneously high readings, which must be considered when interpreting the data.

Quantitative computed tomography is quite valuable in expert hands, and results are comparable or better than dual photon studies.[9] Cortical and trabecular bone of the spine can be measured and compared to a bone-mineral equivalent phantom. The cost is high, and the test is not readily available. It takes about 15 minutes, and it is sensitive and accurate. However, the radiation dose is 200 to 250 millirads, which limits its usefulness for serial measurements or screening. Scanning compressed vertebrae may also present falsely high readings, and increases in marrow fat may also make results less useful. It is not settled whether dual photon studies or quantitative computed tomography is preferred.[12]

Radionucleotide scanning with technetium-99m is a qualitative technique that is universally available, has a low radiation dose, and is inexpensive. It is useful to date compression fractures. Fractures that have occurred in the previous few months show a high uptake of technetium. Uptake fades with time and is usually gone by 24 months. Uptake may be increased with fracture, infection, malignancies, and degenerative changes. However, the pattern of uptake may help differentiate between these conditions and may suggest alternative diagnoses such as osteomalacia.[31]

Bone biopsy is a very reliable technique to diagnose bone disease. Biopsy of an osteopenic vertebra may be useful to find evidence of malignancy or infection. However, biopsy from the region near the superior anterior iliac crest is gaining favor as an excellent way to diagnose metabolic bone disease. Doubling labeling of the bone with two oral courses of tetracycline helps to evaluate bone dynamics. Special handling of specimens is necessary, and at the present time the procedure is limited to a few centers.[18]

TREATMENT

The treatment of osteoporosis must be individualized and based on the patient's age, menopausal status, sex, degree of disease, diet, underlying medical problems, or medications. Some aspects of treatment remain under investigation and others are controversial; however, some are straightforward although they are too frequently neglected.

Calcium supplementation is indicated in all patients unless there are specific contraindications such as hypercalcemia or hypercalciuria. Calcium supplementation alone in established disease does not increase bone density, although it does seem to slow further deterioration.[24,29] Riggs[29] demonstrated that calcium supplementation alone decreased the incidence of vertebral fractures compared to an untreated control group in women with previous fractures and established osteoporosis. Postmenopausal women should receive calcium supplementation to bring the total daily intake to 1500 to 1600 mg. Urinary calcium should be maintained at 150 to 250 mg per 24 hours.

Calcium is available in many forms. Calcium carbonate is convenient and inexpensive. The 650 mg tablets are 40% calcium (260 mg). Tums contain 500 mg of calcium carbonate. Calcium lactate tablets, 650 mg, are 13% calcium (85 mg). Calcium gluconate tablets, 1.05 gm, are only 9% calcium. Neocalglucon syrup contains 23 mg calcium per ml.

The use of estrogens for the postmenopausal woman is still debated as treatment for established osteoporosis. There is no doubt estrogens are effective for prophylaxis when given at or soon after the menopause. However, fears of causing or exacerbating endometrial carcinoma, breast cancer, hypertension, thromboembolic phenomena, cerebrovascular disease, hyperlipidemia, or gallbladder disease have limited their use.[11,15] Recent studies do not support these fears. In fact, Bush and coworkers[6] demonstrated a significant decrease in the all-cause mortality in women treated with estrogens compared to women not treated. Not only did the estrogen group have a lower mortality, but there was no difference in the use of antihypertensive medication, diuretics, anticoagulants, or medications for angina, implying no significant increase in these problems. There was, however, an increased incidence in cholelithiasis.

Recently, Haber[11] reviewed the association between estrogen use and endometrial cancer. There is a 200% increase in cancer incidence in patients treated with estrogen alone, but the mortality in this group was actually lower than that of the women who developed the same cancer but were not receiving estrogens. In the estrogen-treated group, the cancers were better differentiated and less advanced. More impressive is the fact that women treated with cyclic progestins in addition to estrogens actually had a lower incidence of endometrial cancer compared to patients not treated at all. The risk of breast cancer does not appear to be increased.

Estrogen replacement begun soon after menopause significantly slows bone loss and decreases fracture rate. The effect is sustained.[8] Some data indicate that estrogen therapy begun later in the menopause also slows further bone loss.[10,22,24] Not all agree.[18] Riggs[29] has shown that calcium plus estrogen prevents vertebral fractures better than treatment with a calcium alone in postmenopausal women with established osteoporosis and prior fracture.

Gordon[10] suggests the need for full replacement doses of estrogen, 1.25 mg of conjugated estrogen, 50 μg of ethinyl estradiol, or 1 mg of stilbesterol. Others have suggested that only one half these doses is necessary.[12,14] Contraindications to estrogen therapy include a history of breast cancer, endometrial cancer, bleeding uterine fibroids, migraine, congestive heart failure, unexplained vaginal bleeding, liver disease, or venous thrombosis. In the presence of an intact uterus, cyclical therapy with progestins is desirable. One useful schedule is to give estrogens on days one through twenty-five of the calendar month. A progestin such as medroxyprogesterone, 10 mg or DL-norgestrel, 150 μg, is added for days fifteen through twenty-five of the calendar month. Neither medication is given the last 5 or 6 days of the month. Patients will experience withdrawal bleeding when not receiving hormones. Patients should be informed to seek medical attention for any breakthrough bleeding and will need curettage.

Treatment with vitamin D alone in any form is not useful unless there is superimposed osteomalacia. Lane[19] recommends 400 to 800 IU of vitamin D_2 per day, but only as part of a comprehensive regimen. Larger doses are not helpful and may be potentially toxic.

Fluoride treatment for postmenopausal osteoporosis appears promising.[3] Riggs[29] compared multiple treatment regimens for osteoporosis with an untreated control group. The fluoride treatment group did best. The vertebral fracture rate per thousand person-years was 834 in untreated patients, 419 in patients treated with calcium with or without vitamin D, 304 in patients on fluoride and calcium with or without vitamin D, but only 53 in those given fluoride, estrogen, and calcium with or without vitamin D. The results were most dramatic after 12 months of therapy. Side effects from fluoride were seen in 38% of patients and included joint pain or swelling, plantarfascia pain, nausea, vomiting, dyspepsia with or without blood loss in the stool, and combinations of these. Of patients treated with fluoride 60% had readily distinguishable improvement in bone mass on plain x-ray films of the lumbar spine. These patients did the best with the lowest incidence of repeat fractures.

Lane[19] has reported 10 well-studied patients treated with sodium fluoride, 1 mg/kg/day, calcium 1.6 gm per day, and vitamin D, 400 to 800 IU per day but no estrogen. The pretreatment fracture rate was 1250 fractures per 1000 patient-years. The posttreatment fracture rate was only 110 fractures per 1000 patient-years. Lane believes that fluoride acts by stimulation of osteoblast replication and functions to increase osteoid production and stabilize the hydroxyapatite crystal. He considers the calcium to be a parathyroid gland suppressant, but others feel calcium prevents fluoride induced osteomalacia.

It seems worthwhile to consider fluoride treatment, especially for patients who have already suffered one or more vertebral fractures. Patients should be treated with 1.6 gm of calcium and 400 to 800 IU of vitamin D per day for 1 to 6 months before adding fluoride, depending on the degree of osteoporosis. Cyclic estrogen therapy is optional for established osteoporosis, but it is definitely indicated and beneficial if started early in the postmenopausal years. Some would add estrogens at any time in women who can tolerate them and I tend to favor this position. Fluoride is then added gradually to reach a dose of 1 mg/kg/day of sodium fluoride. The dose is reduced in the presence of renal insufficiency by the same percentage as the decreased renal function. Sodium fluoride is available as 2.2 mg tablets and is usually started at three tablets after each meal, three times per day. The dose is increased each week by three tablets each dose until the desired level is reached. Serum levels may be followed and the dose adjusted to maintain a level of 5 to 10 μmol/L. The dose is adjusted downward for side-effects. Edema resulting from sodium accumulation can be treated with diuretics. Treatment with fluoride should be continued for at least 2 years and until technetium bone scans are normal for 1 year. Calcium should be continued indefinitely.

Calcitonin has been used to treat postmenopausal osteoporosis. Recent interpretation of the available data indicates that calcitonin may slow bone loss but does not replace previously lost bone, nor does it decrease the incidence of vertebral fractures. In addition, it is expensive and must be given by injection. It is not currently recommended.[36]

REFERENCES

1. Aloja, J.F., et al.: Risk factors for postmenopausal osteoporosis, Am. J. Med. **78:**95, 1985.
2. Baylink, D.J.: Glucocorticoid-induced osteoporosis, N. Engl. J. Med. **309:**306, 1983.
3. Bikle, D.D.: Fluoride treatment of osteoporosis: a new look at an old drug, Ann. Int. Med. **98:**1013, 1983.
4. Bikle, D.D., et al.: Bone disease in alcohol abuse, Ann. Int. Med. **103:**42, 1985.
5. Brown, C.W.: The rate of pseudoarthrosis (surgical nonunion) in smoking versus nonsmoking patients (abstract), Orthop. Trans. **7:**453 1983.
6. Bush, T.L., et al.: Estrogen use and all-cause mortality, JAMA **249:**903, 1983.
7. Daniel, H.W.: Osteoporosis of the slender smoker, Arch. Int. Med. **136:**298, 1976.
8. Ettinger, B., et al.: Long-term estrogen replacement therapy prevents bone loss and fractures, Ann. Int. Med. **102:**319, 1985.
9. Genant, H.K., et al.: Osteoporosis. I. Advanced radiologic assessment using quantitative computed tomography, medical staff conference, University of California, San Francisco, West. J. Med. **139:**75, 1983.
10. Genant, H.K., et al.: Osteoporosis. II. Prevention of bone loss and fractures in women and risks of menopausal estrogen therapy, medical staff conference, University of California, San Francisco, West. J. Med. **139:**204, 1983.
11. Haber, R.J.: Should postmenopausal women be given estrogen? Medical staff conference, University of California, San Francisco, West. J. Med. **142:**672, 1985.
12. Heath, H., III: Progress against osteoporosis, Ann. Int. Med. **98:**1011, 1983.
13. Heath, H., III: Athletic women, amenorrhea and skeletal integrity. Ann. Int. Med. **102:**258, 1985.
14. Horsman, A., et al.: The effect of estrogen dose on postmenopausal bone loss, N. Eng. J. Med. **309:**1405, 1983.
15. Judd, H.L., et al.: Estrogen replacement therapy: indications and complications, Ann. Intern. Med. **98:**195, 1983.
16. Kaplan, F.S.: Osteoporosis, Ciba Clinical Symposia, **35**(5), 1983.
17. Lane, J.M.: Introduction, symposium on metabolic bone disease, Orthop. Clin. North Am. **15:**569, 1984.
18. Lane, J.M., et al.: Osteoporosis, Orthop. Clin. North Am. **15:**711, 1984.
19. Lane, J.M., et al.: Treatment of osteoporosis with sodium fluoride and calcium: effects on vertebral fracture incidence and bone histomorphometry, Orthop. Clin. North Am. **15:**729, 1984.
20. Lukert, B.P.: Osteoporosis: a review and update, Arch. Phys. Med. Rehabil. **63:**480, 1982.
21. Marcus, R., et al.: Menstrual function and bone mass in elite women distance runners: endocrine and metabolic features, Ann. Intern. Med. **102:**158, 1985.
22. Nordin, E.C., et al.: Treatment of spinal osteoporosis in postmenopausal women, Brit. Med. J. **1:**451, 1980.
23. Raney, F., and Kolb, F.O.: Metabolic abnormalities in patients with pseudoarthrosis (abstract), Orthop. Trans. **7:**452, 1983.
24. Recker, R.R., et al.: Effect of estrogen and calcium carbonate on bone loss in postmenopausal women, Ann. Intern. Med. **87:**649, 1977.
25. Richelson, L.S., et al.: Relative contribution of aging and estrogen deficiency to postmenopausal bone loss, N. Engl. J. Med. **311:**1273, 1984.
26. Riggs, B.L.: Osteoporosis. In Wnygaarden, J.B., and Smith, L.H., editors: Cecil textbook of medicine, Philadelphia, 1985, W.B. Saunders Co.
27. Riggs, B.L., and Melton, L.J.: Evidence for two distinct syndromes of involutional osteoporosis, Am. J. Med. **75:**899, 1983.
28. Riggs, B.L., et al.: Effects of oral therapy with calcium and vitamin D in primary osteoporosis, J. Clin. Endocrinol. Metab. **42:**1139, 1976.
29. Riggs, B.L., et al.: Effect of the fluoride/calcium regimen on vertebral fracture occurrence in postmenopausal osteoporosis, N. Eng. J. Med. **306:**446, 1982.
30. Rigotti, N.A., et al.: Osteoporosis in women with anorexia nervosa, N. Eng. J. Med. **311:**1601, 1984.
31. Schneider, R.: Radiologic methods of evaluating generalized osteopenia, Orthop. Clin. North Am. **15:**631, 1984.
32. Seeman, E., et al.: Risk factors for spinal osteoporosis in men, Am. J. Med. **75:**977, 1983.
33. Synthetic calcitonin for postmenopausal osteoporosis, Med. Letter **27:**53, 1985.
34. Tannenbaum, H.: Osteopenia in rheumatology: pathogenesis and therapy, Sem. Arth. Rheum. **13:**337, 1984.
35. Tiegs, R.D., et al.: Calcitonin secretion in postmenopausal osteoporosis, N. Engl. J. Med. **312:**1097, 1985.
36. Vigorita, V.J.: The tissue pathologic features of metabolic bone disease, Orthop. Clin. North Am. **15:**613, 1984.

CHAPTER

43

COMPUTER ASSISTANCE IN SPINE SURGERY

James Zucherman   Richard Derby

COMPUTER TECHNOLOGY IN SPINE SURGERY

Along with our increasing depth of understanding of disease processes and the availability of new and very sensitive diagnostic tests, the task of organizing, reporting, and recording pertinent information for medical management and research on the spine is becoming increasingly complex. This complexity has been compounded by the increased demands by the legal, industrial, and social systems for documentation. As is evident from the diversity of opinions in this book innumerable fundamental questions regarding the nature and treatment of back disease are still unanswered. This is in part due to the time and difficulty required for meaningful research. The recent advantages in computer technology and reduced costs of hardware have made it worthwhile to develop the following spine patient medical record system. This system incorporates report generators, a comprehensive data base with a function for research purposes, and a diagnostic program.

In the traditional office system, the physician gathers information from the patient and then dictates that information, which is transcribed by a stenographer into a report form (Fig. 43-1). This system is somewhat redundant, inefficient, and costly. Sorting through patients' past charts for research data is further time-consuming and often inaccurate. It entails another step in organizing data once found in the charts. Computerizing this system greatly streamlines the process, resulting in reduced physician involvement and data recording and processing, which are irrelevant tasks of drudgery not necessarily contributing to optimal patient care. For example, application of the system for a new patient is as follows.

Instead of spending 30 to 45 minutes asking questions of a patient with complex problems for a complete history, the physician asks the patient to complete a comprehensive multiple-choice questionnaire (Fig. 43-2). This can be sent to new patients before the office visit. On seeing the patient, the physician may scan the questionnaire and obtain more information or occasionally clarify ambigu-

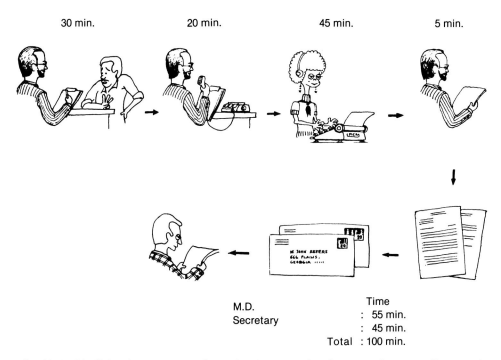

Fig. 43-1 Traditional system. Lengthy patient interview by physician, dictation of historical factors, transcription of dictation, review of transcription.

ities. The complete physical examination form also produces multiple-choice answers and is completed by the physician or assistant. The physician may then dictate a discussion based on the data obtained after reviewing any x-ray films or records (Fig. 43-3). This dictation then is added to the computer-generated narrative history and physical examination. The latter usually comprises 90% of the text in that evaluation. Thus most of the report is produced by rapid entry of multiple-choice responses by a data entry employee into the computer (Fig. 43-4). The resultant text approaches the true narrative report in its flow and in most cases surpasses it in its completeness (Fig. 43-5).

Since the history represents patient's direct written responses, it is the most valid historical document. Complete records can be produced with physician time reduced by 80% and stenography expense reduced by 60%. In addition, the patient data is automatically filed according to the patient's demographic information and is instantaneously retrievable, as is all information relative to the patient's progress (Fig. 43-6).

Follow-up visits and their reports are managed similarly. Diagnostic test results such as EMG, CT scan, myelogram, MMPI, block injections, discograms, and operative reports are likewise reduced to computer-easy forms and entered under each patient's demographic file. Narrative reports for each can be generated instantaneously if desired. Indexing allows one to scan all entrys for a particular patient and review any particular entry in totality instantaneously. This is extremely useful in multidisciplinary centers where network systems can allow complete access to any patient record in various locations. Additionally, patient progress and its relationship to therapeutic interventions can be graphically demonstrated over time.

4. Which of the following activities change the nature of your pain:

		Aggravates Pain	Relieves Pain
1)	Sitting	_____	_____
2)	Standing	_____	_____
3)	Rising from sitting	_____	_____
4)	Leaning forward (brushing teeth)	_____	_____
5)	Walking	_____	_____
6)	Lying on your side	_____	_____
7)	Lying on your back	_____	_____
8)	Lying on your stomach	_____	_____
9)	Driving	_____	_____
10)	Coughing/Sneezing	_____	_____
11)	Bending forward	_____	_____

Now go back and put an asterisk (*) next to the most aggravating activity and the most relieving activity.

5. Please answer the following questions using the following chart:

```
1 = unable to tolerate
2 = several minutes only
3 = about 10 minutes only
4 = about 20 minutes only
5 = about 1/2 hour only
6 = about 1 hour
7 = several hours
8 = indefinite period
```

1) How long can you sit?   _____

2) How long can you stand? _____

3) How long can you walk? _____

Fig. 43-2 One page of comprehensive history questionnaire.

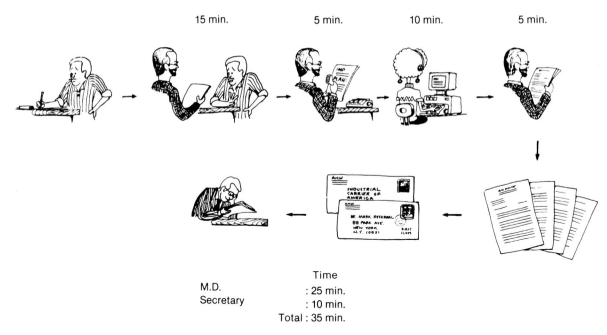

Fig. 43-3 Computer-based system. Patient fills out lengthy 18-page historical questionnaire at home before physician visit, history form is reviewed and clarified by physician with the patient, and physical examination form is completed by physician. Physician dictates additionally, if necessary, secretary enters data, and dictation, if any was done, is reviewed by physician.

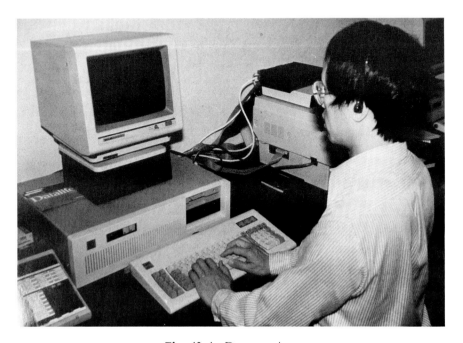

Fig. 43-4 Data entering.

SAN FRANCISCO ORTHOPAEDIC SURGEONS MEDICAL GROUP, INC.
2235 Hayes Street
San Francisco, CA 94117
(415) 750-5556

January 14, 1987

Dr. Donald Benson
555 California Street
San Francisco, CA 94102

                              RE: xxxxx xxxxx

Dear Dr. Benson:

Thank you for referring xxxxx xxxxx to us for consultation. She was seen and examined today, January 14, 1987.

PRESENT COMPLAINTS: On her pain drawing, this 44-year old female indicates pain in the following areas: the midline lower back, the right buttock, the right posterior thigh, the right posterior knee, the right anterior lateral leg, the right posterior leg, the right dorsal lateral foot and the right plantar foot. The ratio of back to leg pain is fifty per cent back and fifty per cent leg. In addition, the patient complains of weakness in the right ankle, the right knee and the right hip.

The patient describes her pain intensity as follows: intense, making normal functions impossible at its worst; severe, limiting all activities most of the time; moderate and can be controlled by analgesics at its best. In the morning, before getting out of bed, the pain is moderate and can be controlled by analgesics. After getting out of bed, it is severe, limiting all activities, and by midday, it is intense, making normal functions impossible. In the evening, the pain is intense, making normal functions impossible, and during the night, it is moderate and can be controlled by analgesics. The pain is made worse by sitting, leaning, walking, driving, coughing and/or sneezing and bending. The pain is decreased by lying in a decubitus position with legs curled up, lying in a supine position with knees bent, lying in a prone position, standing and arising from sitting.

Current medications used for pain control include Acetaminophen, which she feels is helpful in relieving symptoms. Additionally, the patient takes Tylenol #3, which she feels is helpful for symptomatic relief.

Currently, in the waking hours between 7:00 a.m. and 11:00 p.m., the patient spends no time working, less than one-half hour driving, about two to four hours housekeeping, about one-half to one hour sitting, about one-half to one hour walking, no time in bed and about two to four hours reclining on a couch.

McGill Pain Questionnaire: The patient selected the following words to describe her pain: Throbbing; Sharp; Cramping; Burning; Aching; Tender; Troublesome; Radiating; Numb; and Cold.

(c) MKS 1986

Fig. 43-5 Typical first page of computer-generated report.

```
                    PRESCRIPTION FOR TREATMENT
                  Patient:
                  Date of Visit:_____/_____/_____

        TREATMENTS                          ORTHOPAEDIC SUPPORT

    1.  Rest                             1.  Corset
    2.  Body mechanics                   2.  Body jacket
    3.  Back school                      3.  Lumbar cushion
    4.  Chiropractor                     4.  Ergonomic chair
                                         5.  Home traction
Physical Therapy                         6.  Stationary bicycle
5.1   Mobilization                       7.  Home gym
5.2   Flexion                            8.  Neighborhood gym
5.3   Extension                          9.  Home exercise program
5.4   Stabilization                     10.  Swimming
5.5   Soft tissue mobilization          11.  Other:
5.6   Traction
5.7   Pelvic traction
5.8   Gravity traction
5.9   Auto traction                               BLOCKS
5.10  Inpatient spine rehab
5.11  Outpatient spine rehab             1.  Caudal epidural
5.12  Other:                             2.  Lumbar epidural
                                         3.  Thoracic epidural
Modalities                               4.  Selective nerve root
6.1   Ice                                5.  Facet block
6.2   Heat                               6.  Facet rhizotomy
6.3   Ultrasound                         7.  Costovertebral joint
6.4   Diathermy                          8.  Indwelling block
6.5   Spray & stretch                    9.  Hook block
6.6   TENS unit                         10.  Sympathetic block
6.7   Acupuncture

Medications
7.1   Antiinflammatory:_____
7.2   Muscle relaxant :_____
7.3   Antidepressant  :_____
7.4   Analgesic       :_____
7.5   Other           :_____

                          SURGERY (and Level)

Instrumentation                          Decompression
1.1   Luque rods:_____       4.1  Central     :_____
1.2   Harrington:_____       4.2  Subarticular:_____
1.3   Knodt     :_____       4.3  Foraminal   :_____
1.4   Steffe    :_____
1.5   Edwards   :_____       Chemonucleolysis
1.6   Wires     :_____       5.1  Chemonucleolysis:

Fusion                                   Hardware Removal
2.1   Fusion            :_____  6.1  Removal of rods
2.2   Posterior lateral :_____  6.2  Removal of plates
2.3   Anterior interbody:_____  6.3  Removal of bone plug
2.4   Posterior interbody:_____

Discectomy                               Surgical Repair
3.1   Micro           :_____  7.1  Pseudarthrosis
3.2   Standard        :_____  7.2  Repair dural leak
3.3   Fragment removal:_____
```

Fig. 43-6 Disposition form is completed on all patient visits and often obviates the need for any physician dictation.

FURTHER DIAGNOSTIC STUDIES

1. Psychological _____
2. Multidisciplinary _____
3. X-ray _____
4. EMG _____
5. Bone scan _____
6. Myelogram _____
7. MRI _____
8. Discogram _____
9. CT scan _____
10. Thermogram _____
11. Brevital _____
12. Bone densitometry _____
13. Other: _____

CURRENT DIAGNOSIS

	Cervical	Thoracic	Lumbar
1. Annulus tear	___	___	___
2. Segmental instability	___	___	___
3. Facet arthropathy	___	___	___
4. Bulging disc syndrome	___	___	___
5. Sprain	___	___	___
6. Ligament dysfunction	___	___	___
7. Herniated nucleus pulposus	___	___	___
8. Herniated nucleus pulposus w/radiculopathy	___	___	___
9. Spinal stenosis	___	___	___
10. Spinal stenosis w/radiculopathy	___	___	___
11. Spondylolysis—acute	___	___	___
12. Spondylolisthesis—unstable	___	___	___
13. Spondylolisthesis w/radiculopathy	___	___	___
14. Internal disc disruption	___	___	___
15. Fracture	___	___	___
16. Infection	___	___	___
17. Neoplasm	___	___	___
18. Functional	___	___	___
19. Metabolic	___	___	___
20. Systemic arthritis	___	___	___
21. Failed surgery	___	___	___
22. Postoperative—Early	___	___	___
23. Postoperative—Late	___	___	___
24. Osteoporosis	___	___	___
25. Other: _____	___	___	___

EVALUATION

Overall Response
1 = Excellent
2 = Good
3 = Fair
4 = Poor
5 = Worse

Physical Examination
1 = Yes
2 = No
3 = No change

ENVIRONMENTAL FACTORS

Expected RTW date : ____/____/____   RTW: FT   PT   No. of hrs. ____
  Limitations   : 1 = No repetitive bending, stooping, or pushing
                     2 = No lifting more than _____ pounds
                     3 = No sitting more than _____ hours
                     4 = No standing more than _____ hours
                     5 = No driving more than _____ hours
Perm. & stationary: 1 = Yes   2 = No
Disability rating : A   B   C   D   E   F   G   H   Totally disabled
Next appointment : ____/____/____   Ready for voc. rehab.: ____/____/____

COMPUTER INSTRUCTIONS

1. Is this: H & P   Follow-up   2. Dictation? Yes   No   Tape no.: _____
3. Copies : Insurance _____ Referring MD _____ Attorney _____ Chart _____ Pt. _____
4. Special instructions: _____

Fig. 43-6, cont'd

A query program enables any variable or variables to be retrieved and analyzed with ease for clinical research. Study flags may be placed on those entries that are involved in prospective studies, allowing for rapid retrieval and organization. A statistical program that runs all commonly used statistical tests is used to assess the population distribution significance levels.

A diagnostic program runs simultaneously with the history, physical, and diagnostic test report generators off their data base. This program gives a diagnostic profile (Fig. 43-7) by rating each response in terms of its consistency with each diagnosis. The program can substitute as a "spine expert" in some situations, as when used by a general practitioner or physical therapist. Additionally, conservative care algorithms on the data base instruct the user on the specific form of treatment indicated. In cases where urgent diagnostic or therapeutic evaluation by a spine expert is indicated by the history and physical or other data, directions for such are given to the user by the program. Since each diagnostic profile is a result of over 8,000 relative items of in formation from the history and physical alone, the program is as thorough and reliable in many respects as the current level of expertise in the field.

TECHNICAL ASPECTS

The design, production, and implementation of a medical data base system, with the aforementioned features, is not a trivial undertaking; it requires years of effort in both the medical and system programing fields. As evidence, there are many medical office management systems on the market, but there are few, if any, true medical record systems. In order to collect and process this large amount of data, more demanding requirements are made on the data base software (how to collect and process the

---

Diagnosis Based on History and Physical Examination

October 07, 1985

DIAGNOSIS	CONSISTENCY SCORE
Annulus Tear	105%
Segmental Instability	106%
Facet Arthropathy	26%
Bulging Disc Syndrome	32%
Sprain	52%
Ligament Dysfunction	0%
Herniated Nucleus Pulposus	46%
Herniated Nucleus Pulposus + Nerve Damage	35%
Spinal Stenosis	23%
Spinal Stenosis + Nerve Damage	24%
Spondylolysis -- Acute	0%
Spondylolisthesis -- Unstable	117%
Spondylolisthesis + Nerve Damage	36%
Internal Disc Disruption	0%
Fracture	0%
Infection	44%
Neoplasm	108%
Functional	0%
Metabolic	9%
Systemic Arthritis	12%

Fig. 43-7 Diagnostic profile derived from history and physical examination.

date), the loading of the data base (what to collect), and the hardware with which to collect and store this information. In addition, both hardware and software compatability must exist with current accelerating technology so that more complex use and interfaces can be easily accomplished.

All data base systems collect and store information on secondary devices such as hard- and soft-sectored disks and tape backups. More than just a filing system, however, the system has a central program code (driver or core), which interacts with modules of specially formatted information which the driver uses (in the same way a computer language interprets source or pseudocompiled code) to do its various tasks. These modules are defined by the system's data definition, screen, report, and query languages.

Traditionally, data base systems have been either relational, hierarchical, or network in design. Most data bases are currently used for business applications and use a relational type of model with a very limited data definition language. These are unsuitable for the collection of a full medical-records system. Medical information is highly structured and possesses attributes of all three designs. The implementation of a system without this structure (the DBase approach) can and is being done, but it will fall far short of physician expectations.

Before any of the data can be collected, it must be described to the data base via the data definition language. The power of this module, and in particular its ability to structure the data, sets the stage for all the requirements to follow. Medical data have a hierarchical-network structure with multiple levels of repeating groups, thus the data definition must likewise facilitate this organization. Further, in addition to the usual data element attributes, that is, character, number, date, there must be strong support for keyed-type data. The amount of information and the time required to collect it absolutely require that most data collected on any individual patient are only a pointer or key to information described in the data definition file.

Imagine, for example, the problem of how to describe to the data base the location and character of a patient's pain pattern. As seen in Fig. 43-8, the logical structure is a repeating group of hierarchical data elements that includes at the highest level the body location. Related to body location is body symmetry, and related to body symmetry is a repeating group of a pain type associated with that repeat of body location. These data elements, in turn, point to their respective keyed answers, which again can have a hierarchical format with pointers (network structure). All that is stored in the patient's data file are the key locations of the answers.

In addition to structuring the data within the patient record, the data definition module, controlled by the central program core, must incorporate a secondary file storage scheme that allows patients to own many repeating groups of records (most likely in different files) based on several indexes. The most commonly used and reliable is the "Balanced Tree Indexing method" using either a Index Sequential Access Method (ISAM) or Variable Sequential Access Method (VSAM). This relational method ties all records together via common data elements present in each record (the patient name).

The screen design language with which the screens are created and with which the data are primarily collected must be fast. With the volume of data that must be collected it is too much to expect the data entry person to accept a mediocre performance. Key choices must be displayed instantaneously. Windowing, color, and all the amenities of the new

16. Use the body diagrams below to indicate the location of any of the sensations listed. Mark the areas on the drawings with the symbol that best describes the sensation that you feel.

```
= = = =    Numbness
O O O O    Pins and needles
X X X X    Burning pain
/ / / / /  Stabbing pain
∧ ∧ ∧ ∧ ∧  Aching pain
```

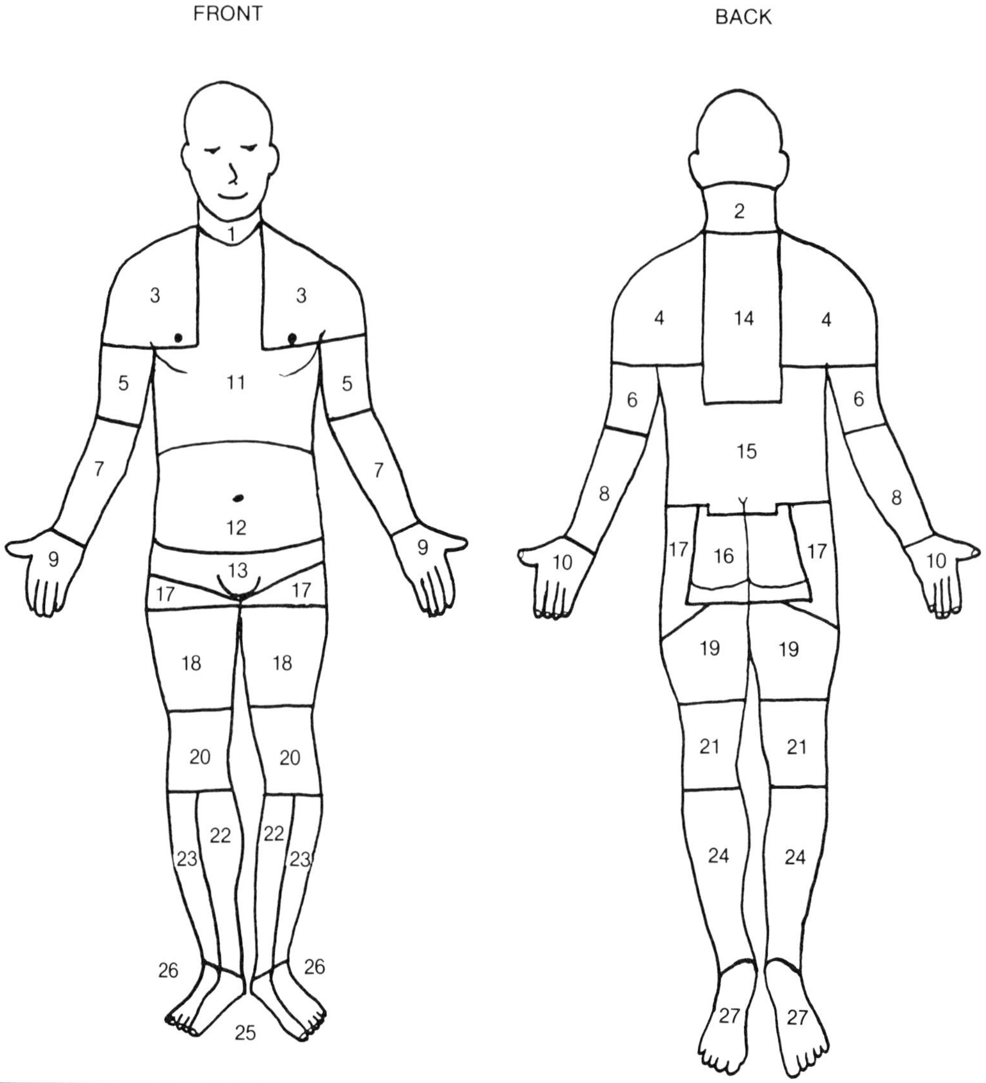

FRONT   BACK

```
PAIN DRAWING - Section Header
  BODY REGION - Keyed answer repeats 15 times
    SYMMETRY  - One keyed answer for each "Body Region" selection
      SENSATION - Three keyed answers for each "Symmetry" selection
```

Fig. 43-8 **A,** Sectored pain diagram. **B,** Repeating hierarchic data elements.

generation of computer technology must be standard. If any of these features are missing, the data base is already outdated and probably of marginal quality.

A data base is only as good as the quality and quantity of reports it is able to produce. In order to produce narrative reports there must be a very extensive and specially designed report language that allows the gathering, testing, transformation, checking, and formating of keyed information into a narrative report that approaches the quality of the physician-dictated report. In addition to usual programing constructs such as multiple levels of if-then-else statements, printer commands, and page formating, there should be special constructs to handle repeating groups, virtual access and testing of any data elements in the data base, and specialized tests to deal with work substitution, to mention only a few.

Finally, the query module must allow on-screen keyed access to any portion of the data definition hierarchy network structure with the ability to define multiple "and/or" conditions for gathering and display of patient information. The module should format outputs that can be used with graphic software.

Just as saws, hammers, and lumber do not equal a house, the data-base software tools and computers do not equal a medical records system. However, given the proper tools, the job can begin. The job entails deciding what to collect, organizing and structuring the data (data domain), and the building (loading) of the data base itself.

Domain is an important key word. The domain must be limited and well defined. Trying to collect all possible occurrences and situations of a patient medical chart is best avoided. This is not to say that a near complete record is not desired or cannot be achieved. A standard, however, must be in the particular medical domain (for example, back care)

such that the information to be collected and the keys to be stored are agreed on and accepted by the majority of physicians in the field. Given the disagreement among most physician experts, this is difficult at best. The more practical approach would be a center devoted to the domain that would set a de facto standard, which could later be changed and improved as the input of other users of the system are accumulated.

The smallest obstacle to overcome is the hardware requirement. The new generation of microcomputer technology has far outpaced the available software. Storage requirements will be large. An active patient with multiple visits and extensive testing and treatment records will require approximately 20 to 30 thousand bytes of secondary storage, with an average patient requirement of 15 to 20 thousand bytes. This translates to a 150-megabyte disk for a practice of 10,000. This storage capacity is already available for a very reasonable price, and costs are rapidly decreasing while storage capacities are increasing. Laser technology, which stores gigabytes of information, will be available in the near future.

Although it is a common buzzword, compatibility in both hardware and software is of vital importance. It does not take much computer knowledge to see the direction development is taking:

1. *Hardware compatibility*. IBM is using the Intel's IAPX family of microprocessors.
2. *Software compatibility*. C or Pascal languages are by far the favorite and most common language currently used for system development.
3. *Operating system*. The MSDOS by Microsoft or possibly a UNIX environment is available (UNIX, however, is not very user friendly).

We are currently using a developmental system by Medical Knowledge Systems of San Francisco, California. The data-base system embodies most of the requirements outlined above. The loading has been a continuous and evolving process; at the time of this writing, we are collecting a full history and physical examination, follow-up visits, and minor procedural data. Over 50% of our physician dictation time is done by the system. Our hardware consists of an IBM AT with a 52-megabyte hard disk and 3.5-million byte memory, an enhanced color display monitor, and an HP laser jet printer.

In conclusion, I believe that the computer will play an important role in the organization of spine surgery programs by allowing spine surgery research to answer the many unsolved problems and controversies presented throughout this book. The gradual acceptance of a standardized method of evaluation and treatment along with the general acceptance of computer-aided dictations may encourage more software companies to develop such systems.

CHAPTER

44

EPIDURAL FAT GRAFTS FOR THE PREVENTION OF POSTOPERATIVE ADHESIONS IN THE LUMBAR SPINE

Charles D. Ray

EPIDURAL AND PERINEURAL FIBROSIS

It has been well established that the primary source of fibrosis after spinal decompression is the outpouring of fibroblasts from the undersurface of injured muscle, stripped away from the bone and rendered hypoxic by the compression from prolonged retraction.* To reduce the likelihood of postoperative massive fibrosis, three elements must be resolved: (1) there must be little or no remaining fluid accumulation (good hemostasis, watertight repair of any dural leaks); (2) there must be little or no unfilled tissue void (dead space); and (3) there must be a mechanical barrier to the ingrowth of fibroblasts. Barbera and associates[1] found experimentally that a solid barrier is necessary to effectively prevent the so-called "laminectomy membrane" from forming. Here solidity is equated with microscopic continuity, that is, without a gross break in the integrity of the barrier. It is clear that there is no way to prevent all fibrosis, nor would this be desirable.

In an editorial comment on a paper about fat grafting by Bryant and co-workers,[2] Watts noted that the ultimate value of routine fat grafting after lumbar spine surgery would have to await clear proof that epidural scarring produces definitive if not chronic postoperative pain. Reasonably, any operation in the epidural space produces scarring, and yet few patients become disabled from pain after surgery. In his opinion, there had been no proof that postoperative scarring in any part of the body, in and of itself, produces pain. Although it is a valid commentary, this appears to go counter to the clinical experience and belief of many surgeons who have reported numerous cases where lysis of adhesions and opening of entrapment have resulted in restoration of function, as well as reduction in pain.

---

*References 2, 6, 7, 10, 12, 28.

Furthermore, the evidence is clear that tethering or constriction of neural elements can cause irritation and interference with normal neuronal function.

Perhaps there might be interference with circulation to the nerve or with its axonal transport, if the entrapment or tethering is severe. Triano and Luttges[24] have shown in mice that chronic, mild mechanical irritation of sciatic nerves by soft silastic plugs (affixed adjacent to the living nerve) significantly altered nerve conduction velocity and refractoriness. In addition, histologic evidence of chronic irritation was documented, and the animals exhibited objective signs of alteration in behavior. What they found was objective evidence of compression neuropathy without gross mechanical entrapment. There is reason to believe that a clump of relatively inflexible scar tissue, or a small, partly calcified mass, may act in a similar way. Clearly, the issue will wax hot for some time, but in the meanwhile prevention of massive epidural and perineural scar tissue formation will continue to be a goal of spinal surgeons and researchers.

Adhesive arachnoiditis is an entirely different matter. The entrapment produced by this disorder can indeed produce severe clinical problems including chronic, intractable pain radiating into the extremities, perhaps by mechanical interference with normal mobility of the rootlets.[3]

FREE FAT GRAFTING

Of all the substances studied to date, autogenous (or autologous) fat grafts are the most useful in preventing fibrosis. Fat is a remarkable tissue, serving mechanical and metabolic functions. Peer[18] discusses the differences between the two types of body fat: white, subcutaneous fat, having cell nuclei located around the periphery (signet ring cells) and brown fat (extensively developed in hibernating animals) having central nuclei. The latter type is not used in grafting, since it is too dense, too scarce, and too difficult to harvest. White fat is ubiquitous and ordinarily rather plentiful. Considerable variation in white fat is seen between patients as to consistency, color (content of lipochrome and exogenous vs. dietary fat contribution), globular size, and friability. Fatty tissues vary in respect to firmness, relative to their supporting or padding function. Mature free fat grafts actually resemble encapsulated lipomas, they forever reflect the metabolism of their originating donor site, for example, changing fat content with diet. Furthermore, Peer stressed that in harvesting a graft one should avoid random cutting through the fat, rough handling, or permitting it to dry before host site implantation. If infection occurs, the entire graft will probably be lost; therefore there is reason to protect the patient with antibiotics before the surgery and afterward. He makes a most interesting point, mentioned by a few other authors, that there may be an advantage to having patients on a fat-reducing diet for some time before surgery. This ensures that specific fats synthesized from the patient's own carbohydrates and protein will be present in the fat cells, unmodified by dietary fats.

With the normal process of degeneration in the graft, fat cells atrophy and release complex oils and grease. Where there is a high content of one's own specific fats, these breakdown products may be less irritating to the host (receiving) site than might be modified food (dietary) fats.[17] A fat-free diet also reduces the fat content of fat cells, allowing them to better withstand trauma and manipulation during harvesting of the graft. Indeed, fat grafts in lean patients lose much less bulk than do those in obese cases. Because they are more easily damaged while being dissected free, one should therefore probably avoid the use of the super-large globular, areolar fat cells found deeply in the buttocks of obese patients.

Burton[3] and I did a limited retrospective study using CT scanning to estimate the viability of fat grafts placed after surgery following simple and extensive lumbar decompressions. After approximately 2 years there was no discernible difference in the extent of epidural fibrosis formation between patients having had small, particulate fat grafts (where the fat was collected from the walls and depths of the decompression and then placed over the exposed dura) and those having had no grafts at all. However, in a group of 183 patients receiving large (20 to 30 cc) fat grafts taken from the superior gluteal region, there was a significant graft still present in about two thirds of the cases (Fig. 44-1). Burton has estimated that approximately one third of the transplanted fat will undergo a shrinkage (necrosis with absorption) over a matter of some months or years. This he has demonstrated with the use of serial CT scanning of selected patients. Although there was a clear positive correlation between the viability of the fat graft and the extent of postoperative epidural fibrosis in these cases, unfortunately there was no comparison drawn among these groups as to clinical outcome. More recently Burton,[4] who continues to use large, full-thickness, free fat grafts, has had three patients in whom the fat graft proved too large. These patients developed a cauda equina syndrome within 48 hours and had to be immediately reoperated on for the removal of a major portion of the graft. It is therefore possible to have grafts of excessive volume. The use of subsequent CT scans to follow the progress of fat graft viability has also been reported by Bryant and coworkers.[2] They found that fat grafts greater than 1 cm in thickness are easily identified. This presents a convenient means to follow the progress of such grafts. My findings are similar.

Jacobs and associates[7] compared a variety of hemostatic agents, antiinflammatory drugs and mechanical barriers as to their relative inhibitory action on postlaminectomy scar formation in animals. Among the results, they showed that as a barrier material, microfibrillar collagen (Avitene) was superior to gelatin foam (Gelfoam). Cortisone injected into the experimental wounds of laminectomized mongrel dogs delayed healing and often resulted in abscess formation with an eventual filling of the wound with scar. On the other hand, Williams[26] reported that oral or parenteral cortisone given from the day of surgery for 9 days had no particular effect on the ultimate outcome of homografts. Jacobs and coworkers[7] found that bone wax was also moderately guilty of both scar formation and protracted inflammation. Free fat grafts proved the superior material in all criteria. They extended this work to 50 human cases and noted that microfibrillar collagen was superior to gelatin foam as a hemostatic agent, as well as a barrier to fibrosis. Once again, however, free fat grafts proved the preferred means for preventing scar formation. Keller and associates[9] likewise found that Gelfoam did not prevent the ingrowth of scar tissue, but autogenous fat grafts clearly did so.

In a related vein, experimental and clinical work with autologous fat sewn directly into the margins of a dural defect has enjoyed excellent results.[9,19,20,21] Mayfield[15] thus reported success with the use of fat as a material not only for protection of the dura but also as a graft for dural repair. Indeed, where the dura cannot be closed (because of inaccessibility or impracticality), a fat graft placed over the defect (sewn in or not) is among the preferred means for dealing with this unfortunate problem.

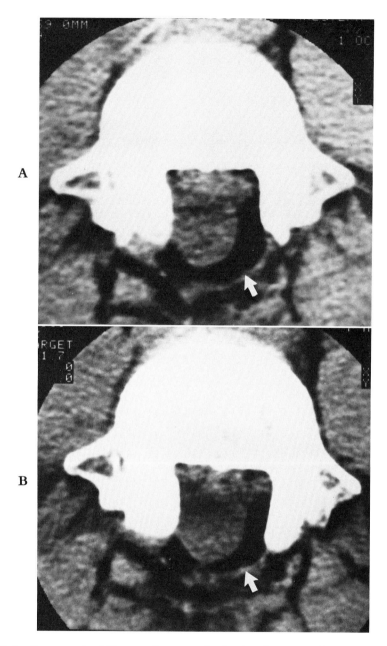

Fig. 44-1 Postoperative CT scans after extensive lumbar decompression. Note surviving fat graft and formation of an outer fibrous tissue capsule *(arrow)*. **A,** 6 months after surgery. **B,** 2½ years after surgery. Note small difference between this scan and **A,** made 2 years earlier.

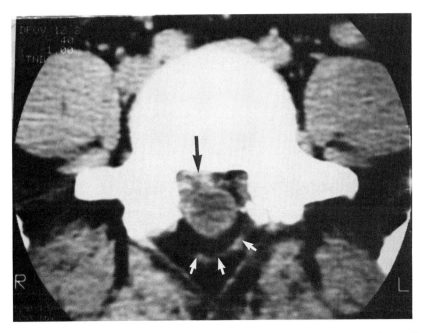

Fig. 44-2 Postoperative CT scan 3 years after removal of HNP showing fat graft with overlying, encapsulating membrane *(short arrows)* and recurrent disc fragment *(long arrow)*. Presence of fat simplified diagnosis by scanning and also in removal of fragment.[14]

If there were no other major reason for the use of fat grafts, Long and many others[3,10,28] have observed the comparative ease of reexploration and repeat decompression where patients have had a previous fat graft. There is no question that a good-sized fat graft that remains intact over the surface of the dura and nerves is of distinct advantage if one has to reoperate the patient at the same level (Fig. 44-2). Furthermore, should there be a change in the mechanical relationship of nerve structures (such as with a disc reherniation or the development of a mechanical stenosis or slippage) then a scar tissue mass or the presence of adhesions will probably complicate the clinical problem. In such cases the nerve or dura is unable to escape the presence of the new compressive situation. The lack of adhesions or the presence of fat may allow the neural structures more space to move aside (remain less tethered), as would be so in the normal condition.

Gill and coworkers[6] report the use of a pedicle fat graft taken from the wound margins and passed downward to the recipient site. In my experience this is technically quite difficult; such a graft can only be obtained in relatively overweight patients since paraincisional fat is sparse in slender patients. Furthermore, one must be careful not to close the deep fascia of the wound too tightly, otherwise the already slender blood supply to the graft will become strangulated and thus lose the advantage of pedunculation. I therefore believe that this technique is not a very practical one. In addition, there is no clear evidence that this method is more effective than a simple free fat graft.

Peer[17] reported, as a result of an extended animal study plus scattered human observations, that isogenous fat grafts completely disappear following transplantation. This would serve to rule out the use of cadaver fat as a graft source. Human autogenous fat grafts, on the other hand, lose about 45% of weight/volume in one or more years after transplantation. A composite (particulate) graft made of multiple small pieces of autogenous fat loses a larger percentage of its weight and volume than does an intact piece of equal size; about 79% of the particulate fat mass over 1 year or more. This is similar to what Burton and Ray[3] had found. In general, areas of fat degeneration are usually scattered within a graft but the margins show more loss, probably due both to injury while dissecting out the grafts and to drying before insertion. Surviving graft cells appear as normal fat, whereas degenerating cells become fibrotic, with mixed types of connective tissue.[8,13,21,26]

OBTAINING A FAT GRAFT

The usual volume required when harvesting a graft is 20 to 30 cc (as measured in a sterile medicine glass) per bilateral lumbar level decompressed. Only 5 to 15 cc are needed for a simple hemilaminotomy or hemilaminectomy. For the larger volume the superior gluteal region is the best donor site (Fig. 44-3, A). One must make the incision approximately a hand's width from the midline to avoid the cluneal nerves in the deeper layers. If this is not done, one may produce an area which is more painful than that of the decompression, since small, painful neuromas might develop from these injured sensory nerves. The more superficial layers of fat around the buttocks, arising in Camper's fascia, have smaller globules than the deeper ones, which come from around the Scarpa's layer[3] (Fig. 44-3, B). Either of these is quite acceptable, although the smaller the globules—in general—the less likely they will be transected or injured while harvesting the graft.

A simple incision, about 5 to 8 cm in length, is placed about 12 to 15 cm from the midline; immediately beneath the skin one angles the cutting (using Metzenbaum scissors and a rat-tooth

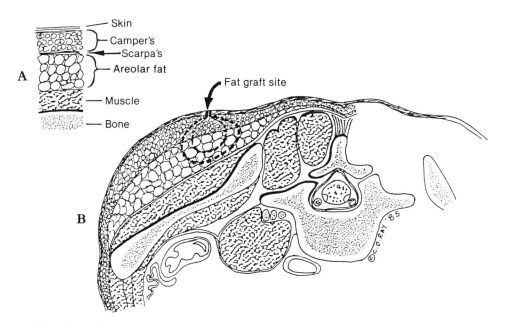

Fig. 44-3 Diagram of cross-section of skin, fat, fascia and muscle layers of gluteal area showing approximate location of fat graft donor site *(dashed line)*. Larger globules from areolar fat layer may be less desirable for grafting in that they are more easily injured while being harvested; damaged fat cells usually undergo atrophy and fibrosis (see text).

forcep) so that the graft resembles a shortened canoe. A few singular globules are also good to take, if they are not injured. One must be careful not to pass so deeply that a muscle biopsy is taken. The donor bed must have good hemostasis, otherwise it will likely accumulate fluid or a hematoma, which may produce a painful lump or possibly act as a pocket for infection. Deep, space-filling sutures of 2-0 absorbable material reapproximate the cavity in at least two layers. A subcuticular skin closure aids in prevention of skin-stretch scarring. In the thin patient, obtaining fat may be quite difficult. Although most of the posterior and lateral fat may be missing, especially in slender males, there is often some to be found in the lumbodorsal triangle, laterally. Other sites for obtaining very suitable grafts of fat-fascia may be found by tunneling under the skin from the wound laterally (in the direction of the iliac crest, much as when striking out for a bone graft) or to progress downward to the retrosacral fat pad. In addition, in relatively obese patients, an excellent graft may be obtained in the paraincisional area during the initial opening of the wound. This graft of some intact volume should be obtained just after the skin incision, before the fat is split in half by a deep midline dissection.

In any case, one should not obtain a large mass of fat from the margins close to and under an incision, because the tissue void that remains may be hard to close and the cosmetic result may be poor (a deep dimple). On the other hand, there is clinical and experimental evidence that fat donor sites will regenerate to some extent with time.[25]

LIGAMENTUM FLAVUM AND OTHER TISSUES AS BARRIERS

It is clear that harvesting relatively intact tissue, fat, fascia, ligament, omentum, dermis, or other tissue having relatively less capability of fibroblastic proliferation than injured muscle may well make that tissue acceptable as a graft for the prevention of adhesions. For example, Yong-Hing and associates[27] showed that the ligamentum flavum (containing about 80% elastin and 20% collagen fibers, much like all elastic ligaments and tendons) makes a good free-graft material to protect exposed nerve tissue from invasion by adhesions. Their work further confirmed that free fat grafting was particularly effective in epidural scar prevention, but Gelfoam was ineffective. I have used ligamentum flavum split or shaved into layers about 2 mm thick to cover exposed dura in several cases. Such barriers, however, must be essentially an unbroken blanket of tissue to be effective; furthermore, they have no mass effect to prevent accumulation of fluids in the void between dura and overlying resected structures.

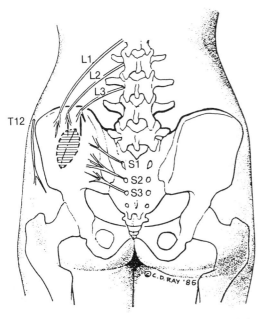

Fig. 44-4 Sketch of relative location of usual fat graft site, gluteal area *(shaded ellipse)*. Note approximate location of the iliohypogastric (T12), cluneal (L1 to L3), and sacral nerves relative to midline and to location of fat graft incision. Generally, fat is obtained from side opposite radiating leg pain so that patient will not confuse postoperative laminotomy pain from that arising from fat donor site.

Stark and associates[23] reported the practical use of paratenon as a graft material to prevent adhesions in hand tendons. Paratenon is the thin, almost transparent layer of loose areolar tissue found covering the deep fascia overlying muscle compartments. I have used this tissue to cover exposed nerve or dura after decompression, especially in thin individuals. It can be dissected, along with substantial fat cells, from its loose attachment to the dorsal fascia overlying the spinal erector muscles during initial exposure for the lumbar decompression. It is a continuous tissue that meets the criteria of a barrier sheet and can also have some volume-filling effect. I refer to this as a fat/fascial graft, and more recently I employ it extensively, even preferentially to larger fat grafts.

O'Neal and Both[16] reported in a 2-year study of 28 human cases, using porcine dermis to wrap lumbar nerve roots at the time of surgery for herniated discs or extradural adhesions, no untoward or foreign-body inflammatory response was found. They suggested, but could not confirm, the potential role of this interesting material in prevention of fibrotic invasion in and around nerve or dura.

SYNTHETICS AS BARRIERS TO FIBROSIS

Unfortunately, it is extremely difficult if not impractical, after dissections in the central canal, to place a significant fat graft on the ventral surface of the dura or nerves. Here, and perhaps on the dorsal surface of exposed dura and nerves, there may be a place for an inert-material shield. Many materials have been tried and reported, for example, gelatin foam, but most of these apparent early results have not held with time.[22] Keller and co-workers[9] studied several materials that might serve as dural substitutes and found that polyester fiber mesh was effective. Silicone-coated Dacron produced connective tissue encapsulation sufficient, in some animals, to produce compression of the underlying spinal cord. Feild and McHenry[5] fabricated a plastic shield made of Dacron polyester–supported silicone rubber that could be placed both ventral and dorsal to the dura and nerve, through a laminotomy window. To date, however, all such synthetic membranes may act to prevent or hinder ingrowth of fibrosis (although this evidence is not well established), but they do not help to fill the void created by the resection and stripping of muscle away from bone. This has also been my experience, where dural substitute material has been tried. It appears that the preferred barrier membrane must also retain some permeability to fluids and therefore to nutrients.[7,9,15,26]

The ideal synthetic material, acting both as barrier and void-filler, has yet to be developed.

REFERENCES

1. Barbera, J., et al.: Prophylaxis of the laminectomy membrane, J. Neurosurg. **49**:419, 1978.
2. Bryant, M.S., et al.: Autogenic fat transplants in the epidural space in routine lumbar spine surgery, Neurosurgery **13**:367, 1983.
3. Burton, C.V.: Diagnosis and treatment of lateral spinal stenosis: implications regarding the "failed back surgery syndrome." In Genant, H.K., editor: Spine update 1984 San Francisco, Radiology Research and Education Foundation, 1983.
4. Burton, C.V.: Personal communication, December 1986.
5. Feild, J.R., and McHenry, H.: The lumbar shield: a progress report, Spine **5**:264, 1980.
6. Gill, G.G., et al.: Pedicle fat grafts for the prevention of scar formation after laminectomy, Spine **4**:176, 1979.
7. Jacobs, R.R., et al.: Control of postlaminectomy scar formation, Spine **5**:223, 1980.
8. Keller, J.T., et al.: The fate of autogenous grafts to the spinal dura, J. Neurosurg. **49**:412, 1978.
9. Keller, J.T., et al.: Repair of spinal dura defects: an experimental study, J. Neurosurg. **60**:1022, 1984.

10. Langenskiold, A., and Kiviluoto, O.: Prevention of epidural scar formation after operations on the lumbar spine by means of free fat transplants, Clin. Orthop. **115**:92, 1976.
11. Langenskiold, A., and Valli, M.: Epidurally placed free fat grafts visualized by CT scanning 15-18 years after discectomy, Spine **10**:97, 1985.
12. LaRocca, H., and Macnab, I.: The laminectomy membrane: studies on its evolution, characteristics, effects and prophylaxis in dogs, J. Bone Joint Surg. **56B**:545, 1974.
13. Lexer, E.: Die freien Transplantation. I. Neue Deutsche Chirurgie 26. Stuttgart, 1919, Ferdinand Enke.
14. Long, D.M.: Free fat graft in laminectomy (letter), J. Neurosurg. **54**:711, 1981.
15. Mayfield, F.H.: Autologous fat transplants for the protection and repair of the spinal dura, Clin. Neurosurg. **27**:349, 1980.
16. O'Neill, P., and Booth, A.E.: Use of porcine dermis as a dural substitute in 72 patients, J. Neurosurg. **61**:351, 1984.
17. Peer, L.A.: Loss of weight and volume in human fat grafts, Plast. Reconstr. Surg. **5**:217, 1950.
18. Peer, L.A.: The neglected free fat graft, Plast. Reconstr. Surg. **18**:233, 1956.
19. Rehn, E.: Die Fetttransplantation, Arch. Klin. Chir. **98**:1, 1912.
20. Rehn, E.: Die Verwendung der autoplastischen Fetttransplantation bei Dura—und Hirndefecten, Arch. Klin. Chir. **101**:962, 1913.
21. Saunders, M.N., et al.: Survival of autologous fat grafts in humans and in mice, Connect. Tissue Res. **8**:85, 1981.
22. Scheuerman, W.G., et al.: The use of Gelfoam film as a dural substitute, J. Neurosurg. **8**:608, 1951.
23. Stark, H.H., et al.: The use of paratenon, polyethylene film or silastic sheeting to prevent restricting adhesions to tendons in the hand, J. Bone Joint Surg. **59**:908, 1977.
24. Triano, J.J., and Luttges, M.W.: Nerve irritation: a possible model of sciatic neuritis, Spine **7**:129, 1982.
25. Van, R.L.R., and Roncari, D.A.K.: Complete differentiation in vivo of implanted cultured adipocyte precursors from adult rats, Cell Tissue Res. **225**:557, 1982.
26. Williams, R.G.: Studies of autoplastic and homoplastic grafts in rabbits, Am. J. Anat. **93**:1, 1853.
27. Yong-Hing, K., et al.: The ligamentum flavum, Spine **1**:226, 1976.
28. Yong-Hing, K., et al.: Prevention of nerve root adhesions after laminectomy, Spine **5**:59, 1980.

EDITORIAL COMMENTARY

Epidural fat grafts are not used by one third of our authors. One third finds them of some value and one third finds them of great value. Richard Rothman finds fat grafts of some value and uses them in most of his laminectomy cases. One half of the authors have experienced significant complications with the use of fat grafts.

I have several times done a series of patients with fat grafts and have not found my success rate to change significantly. Over the long range I agree with Leon Wiltse who finds the fat grafts to attach firmly to the dura and resemble "a beaver hat." The dissection of this firmly adherent fat graft from the dura is frequently as difficult as normal postoperative scar tissue. Since I find no increase in my success rate I am not willing to use a fat graft if it requires significantly increased surgical time, a separate incision, or cosmetic deformity.

Arthur H. White

CHAPTER

45

TOWARD PERCUTANEOUS SPINE FUSION

Noel Goldthwaite   Arthur H. White

The purpose of this chapter is to stimulate investigation into techniques of and indications for spine fusion by minimally invasive techniques. Newer understanding of the biology of osteoinduction, isolation of bone inducing substances, and advances in instrumentation in several areas should put percutaneous lumbar spine fusion within relatively easy reach.

Advantages of such an approach, which in its ideal form would be performed under local anesthesia and not require harvesting of graft from the patient, should include reductions in surgical trauma, scarring, disfigurement, transfusions, burden of medications, post operative confinement, rehabilitation time, operating room time, hospital stay, pain, and suffering. As presently envisioned, this method could be developed to the point of performing many spine fusions on an outpatient basis. The financial implications are enormous. The medical implications have yet to be explored.

BENEFITS OF PERCUTANEOUS LUMBAR FUSION

Which patients might benefit from percutaneous lumbar fusion? In many cases some conditions are already treated by fusion alone. These include symptomatic spondylolisthesis, facet syndrome, and segmental instability.[27] Other conditions are treated with instrumentation and fusion, such as scoliosis and unstable fractures. Some of these cases might be treatable by a percutaneous method without instrumentation—if fusion were rapid and highly reliable—or at least attempted by this method as a minimally invasive initial procedure.

Certain cases of spinal stenosis, such as those with milder degrees of lateral recess or foraminal stenosis who obtain early and dramatic relief from epidural injections or bracing, might obtain long-term or even permanent relief from fusion alone, either interbody or posterolateral. The low-trauma, low-risk nature of percutaneous fusion would allow extensive clinical trials to identify this class of patients. If decompression became necessary, it could be done secondarily with the spine already fused and would thus be far less debilitating in the recovery period, as is already the practice of some surgeons who use anterior interbody fusion or posterolateral fusion through a paramedian approach as primary procedures. Or percutaneous fusion might be carried out in patients with more severe stenosis with full intention of secondary decompression.

More speculatively, some cases of advanced osteoporosis in which any amount of bony resection for the relief of stenosis, mild or severe, would run the risk of destabilization, and in which instrumentation would not hold and conventional interbody fusion could not be relied on, might be well handled by percutaneous combined interbody and posterolateral fusion and secondary decompression. Again speculatively, the quality of local bone may be greatly enhanced by the agents used to induce new bone formation.

Percutaneous fusion may conceivably be combined with percutaneous discectomy or microdiscectomy, gaining the advantages of fusion when relatively indicated and preserving the advantages of minimal surgery for discal decompression.

Finally, there may be a highly select group of patients who would benefit from stabilizing their spines but who cannot tolerate either restrictive appliances or major surgery, and who could tolerate a procedure involving minimal trauma and only local anesthetics. For example, patients with segmental instability, facet syndrome, moderate stenosis, or fractures and also multisystem disease such as COPD and cardiovascular disease that makes them poor surgical risks, patients with paralytic scoliosis in advanced states of weakness, or patients afflicted with neuromuscular diseases who are subjected to malignant hyperthermia under general anesthesia all may eventually be treatable with percutaneous fusion.

The principles on which this hoped-for therapeutic modality are based may have extensive application in arthrodesis elsewhere in the skeleton and also for reconstruction of large and small bone defects.[43,71,72]

Thus the potential indications and potential benefits of percutaneous fusion are vast. How is it to be accomplished? The first requirement is safe mechanical access to the structures to be fused. For many years now spine surgeons, radiologists, and anesthesiologists have been injecting and sampling the component parts of the lumbar spine through small- and large-bore needles, trocars and cannulae, and even arthroscopes to accomplish such procedures as epidural injections, discograms, selective nerve-root blocks, chemical facet rhizotomies, enzymatic discolysis, vertebral and discal biopsies, and most recently, mechanical discectomies.[18,22,23,31,32] In the majority of cases these are done with the patient under local anesthetic and with minimal morbidity.

It is already possible, if not routine, to approach the disc spaces with an access channel up to 6 mm or more in diameter through a stab wound, without undue hazzard. A large variety of existing or easily adapted instruments can be passed through a cannula only 4.5 mm in diameter, including graspers, rongeurs, burs, rotary cutters, and reciprocating cutter-aspirators. Adequate access to the upper four lumbar discs, then, is available for tissue removal and placement of bone forming agents.

The most difficult aspect of preparing the intervertebral spaces for fusion will undoubtedly be decortication of the vertebral end-plates, if indeed this is an absolute requirement for interbody fusion, and it may not be. Another difficulty will be approaching the lumbosacral disc space over, or through, the iliac wing with instruments large enough to accomplish decortication.

Although it does not at this point seem necessary, it may turn out that some advanced technologies may need to be brought to bear on the end-plates, such as ultrasonic osteotomes or laser drills.

The approach to the transverse processes for posterolateral fusion is easier. In our preliminary (unpublished) work with dogs it has proven a relatively simple matter to decorticate the dorsal surface of the transverse process by placing a bone biopsy cannula on the bone through a stab wound. The serrated rim of the cannula gives secure purchase on the bone, thus preventing the decorticating bur or drill from slipping off and injuring a nerve root or otherwise plunging too deeply into soft tissues. By adjusting the length of the decorticating drill, depth of penetration is limited by the driver abutting the hub of the biopsy cannula (Fig. 45-1). Indeed, through a few stab wounds the entire surface of the spinous process, the dorsal surface of the laminae, the medial, lateral, and dorsal aspects of the facets, and the facet joints themselves—in addition to the dorsal surface of the transverse processes—can be decorticated. Safety would dictate the use of fluoroscopic control, but as a practical matter this can be done safely entirely by "feel" where there are no defects in the bony structures and the operator is thoroughly familiar with the anatomy.

The second requirement for the accomplishment of percutaneous fusion is the manipulation of biologic processes to produce a bony bridge that is firmly anchored at both ends. We usually think of spine fusions just as we think of fusions elsewhere in the skeleton: bleeding bone plus corticocancellous graft plus immobilization equals rigid fusion. The work of Urist over the last 30 years and others more recently has provided much new information about the biology of bone grafting and bone induction.* The isolation and purification of bone morphogenetic protein (BMP) has opened the possibility of fusion without grafting, without decortication, and indeed without operation.

CONDUCTION AND INDUCTION

Bone can be encouraged to enter areas where it never previously existed by conduction or by induction. Conduction is the process by which new bone forms by extension from adjacent normal bone on a guiding framework. This is what occurs when inert substrates are implanted, such as bone in which the active bone-

---

*References 19, 33, 34, 37-39, 49, 50, 53-56, 58, 62, 69, 72, 75, 98-101.

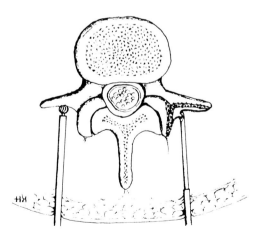

Fig. 45-1 Dorsal surfaces of transverse processes and lateral surfaces of facets can be decorticated with a burr protected within a cannula and passed through a stab wound in skin and muscles. A large-bore needle can then be used to inject a variety of bone-inducing substances.

inductive principle has been destroyed, as in autoclaved or irradiated banked bone, or as in porous inorganic implants such as hydroxyapatite or "ingrowth" inplants. Induction, on the other hand is the process of *de novo* formation of bone in situ, independent of extension from existing bone. This occurs in normal skeletal development, fracture healing, osteosarcomas, and myositis ossificans, for example.[76,79,80]

An active bone-inducing principle was first isolated from osteosarcomas and has since been purified from normal cortical bone of many mammalian species, including man.* Human BMP has a molecular weight of 17,000 to 18,000 daltons. It is associated with other protein fractions of 14,000 and 24,000 daltons that enhance its action. Intensive investigations have demonstrated that BMP stimulates DNA synthesis and mitosis in target cells. It does not directly affect collagen synthesis. When implanted into skeletal muscle in laboratory animals it produces *de novo* osteosynthesis by its action on multipotent mesenchymal cells normally found in the perivascular spaces of soft tissue (pericytes). These cells are influenced to differentiate first into cartilage-forming cells and eventually osteoblasts and osteocytes. Over approximately a 3-week period the process results in the formation of woven bone, and by 4 weeks it results in lamellar bone, which is colonized by circulating marrow elements and develops a marrow cavity.†

In general BMP is not species specific in biologic assays, although the protein (glycoprotein?) has not been sequenced and species differences may exist.[63] It is apparently tightly bound to but distinct from collagen and thus is difficult to solubilize, while still maintaining its biologic activity.[105,106] This accounts for the difficulty in characterizing it. Many properties of clinical significance are known, however. A typical assay method consists of enclosing a preparation of BMP within a membrane envelope, which is then implanted into skeletal muscle of a test animal. The result is that bone forms on the exterior of envelopes with pore sizes of at least 0.25 μm. The effective diffusion distance is about 300 μm.[25,92,93] This and other assay methods have been used to establish the following facts.*

Osteogenic activity is destroyed by:
1. Collection of bone more than 12 hours after death (presumably by autodigestion, especially by BMPase)
2. Prolonged storage above 0° (slow autodigestion)
3. Immediate freeze-drying without pretreatment of bone (preserves BMPase activity)
4. Irradiation sufficient for sterilization (2 rads Cobalt-60)
5. Autoclaving
6. Trypsin and some other proteases, especially BMPase
7. Bacterial infection
8. Benzalkonium chloride (Zephrian), a disinfectant
9. Delayed hypersensitivity (cell-mediated) immune response
10. Zinc and magnesium deficiencies
11. Grinding decalcified bone matrix to a particle size of less than 125 microns

Osteogenic activity is resistant to:
1. DNA-ases
2. RNA-ases
3. Neuraminidase
4. Beta-galactosidase
5. Chondroitinase
6. Phospholipases
7. Lipase
8. Purified collagenase
9. Thimerosol (Merthiolate) and povidone-iodine (Betadine), anti-

---

*References 20, 25, 45, 73, 74, 82, 89, 94, 96.
†References 3, 10, 11, 16, 21, 64, 65, 70.

*References 2, 7, 8, 17, 51, 68, 77, 81, 83, 88, 92.

bacterial/antifungal/antiviral agents
Osteogenic activity is enhanced by:
1. Dispersal of purified bone morphogenetic protein (BMP) on carrier substances such as tricalcium phosphate (TCP) or gamma-carboxyglutamic acid-rich proteins
2. Pelletizing ground decalcified bone matrix of particle size greater than 125 μm into macrostructures of 12 by 3 mm
3. Associated matrix protein fractions of 14,000 and 24,000 daltons

BMP can be purified from cortical bone by complex and costly procedures that are detailed in the references.[96] The yield is meager, a few milligrams from many kilograms of bone. By present methods it would be prohibitively expensive to accumulate sufficient quantities of BMP to be of general clinical utility. However, another substance that is produced early in the purification process by simple methods and that retains osteogenic activity and can be produced in large quantities is decalcified bone matrix (DBM).

DBM has been used sporadically since before the turn of the century for filling large bone defects. It is prepared by soaking cortical bone in 0.6 normal solution of hydrochloric acid (HCl), typically in a ratio of 200 ml of acid for each gram of bone, at 2° C for 24 hours. The result is a gelatinous material that retains BMP activity, can be carved or ground into convenient shapes, and is nearly as good a bone inducer as autogenous cancellous bone in experimental grafts.[12,13,80,90]

Not all bones have the same inductive capacity when decalcified. Urist[87] has shown that DBM from diaphyseal bone of the humerus, femur, tibia, and fibula, and also dentin are good osteoinducers, whereas most soft tissues, most cartilage, bone from the calvarium, scapula, and interestingly, the pelvis are poor osteoinducers. Urinary bladder epithelium is also a good osteoinducer as long as the cells are viable, there is little BMP activity in the interstitial matrix of bladder epithelium.

Urist and others[40,46,78,84] have described the process of incorporation of grafted bone. The host must decalcify and resorb the matrix of the graft. If the graft is inert, that is, its osteogenic activity has been destroyed, incorporation occurs by creeping substitution (conduction)—a slow and incomplete process. Only about 10% of a cortical graft is replaced by new bone. If the graft retains its osteogenic capacity and also has large surface area, as in the case of fresh autogenous cancellous graft, the process is much more rapid and complete. There is an element of osteoinduction, as well as osteoconduction. If the graft is first decalcified, the process of resorption and replacement is much more rapid than in the case of undecalcified graft. Finally, if there is no matrix at all, as in the case of purified bone morphogenetic protein, bone is formed by induction alone. Since this is a surface phenomenon, the effectiveness of a given amount of BMP can be increased manyfold by dispersal on a carrier substance such as tricalcium phosphate (TCP), which itself is absorbed, or on hydroxyapatite, which is not absorbed.[24,26,97]

Farley[14,15,42] isolated a protein of 83,000 daltons from femoral heads called human skeletal growth factor (hSGF), which enhances bone growth significantly but does not cause differentiation of more primitive mesenchymal cells. Other bone growth factors are known, as well.[9,95]

Oikarinen[57] has used 5 mm spicules of DBM in a study of experimental spine fusions in rabbits, comparing DBM to autogenous cancellous bone and allogeneic frozen bone. He found DBM to be nearly as good a bone inducer as autogenous cancellous graft and vastly superior to frozen bone. There was no evidence of immunologic reaction to the decalcified bone matrix. These were interspinous fusions performed by open operation.

Although there are no reports of the use of purified BMP in clinical settings, there is a growing volume of literature on the use of DBM maxillofacial surgery for the reconstruction of alveolar ridges and facial bone loss. Hydroxyapatite is also used in alveolar ridge reconstruction.* Results have been encouraging. Immune rejection is not a prominent feature in these reports, and infection rates run about 5%.

If these products are to be used in humans in large volume three important issues must be addressed: sterility, immunogenicity, and tumorogenicity. As noted earlier, radiation sufficient to sterilize bone or DBM destroys its osteoinductive capacity, as does autoclaving. Collection and processing under sterile conditions, as is done for maxillofacial work, results in a 5% infection rate. Some work has been done mixing large amounts of antibiotic with bone without loss of osteoinductive capacity, but this report does not address large numbers of implants over the long term.[59] Gas sterilization with ethylene oxide is effective, but it must be followed by lyophilization to prevent transfer of toxic material to patient and personnel.[60]

There are no reports on the incidence of infection with implants of purified BMP in animals or of cultures of the preparation before implantation. The extensive chemical extraction process would seem to preclude the survival of any organisms. Furthermore, BMP can be passed through filters with a pore size of 0.25 μm, which would exclude any cellular forms but might not exclude some smaller infectious particles. BMP activity is resistant to Merthiolate and Betadine; other, more elaborate chemical sterilization schemes are under study.[35,61] Is there a need to screen donors for processed bone products as thoroughly as organ donors are screened? Routine bone bank screening and surveillance of stores varies widely from place to place. Since a certain degree of biologic activity is preserved in these products, minimal standards for donor screening and product testing will need to be established.

It has long been known that freezing to very low temperatures, on the order of −70° C, reduces the immunogenicity of bone. Immune reactions to allogeneic DBM prepared with a normal solution of 0.6 HCl have not been a feature in the literature of animal experimentation, except when the issue was addressed specifically. This has certainly not been a problem with human maxillofacial implants.

Experimentally, immunogenicity can be reduced with Cobalt-60 irradiation up to 0.4 rad without seriously affecting osteogenic capacity. This will not sterilize the specimen. Serial extractions with organic and inorganic solvents during the process of purification of BMP also reduce immunogenicity. Although xenografts are quite immunogenic, the immunologic response to purified BMP has not been reported on. In general, immunologic reactions to DBM do not seem to present a problem and can be reduced further.[104] Urist has presented a processing technique to produce autodigested, antigen-extracted, allograft (AAA) which he feels is a very acceptable osteoinductive graft material for general use.[84,90,93]

Urist[85,91] has reviewed the known relationships between bone morphogenesis and tumorogenesis. Osteosarcomas produce what appears to be normal BMP. Osteosarcoma cells confined within a diffusion membrane release BMP, which

---

*References 1, 5, 28-30, 41, 46-48, 107.

causes normal bone to form outside the membrane. No tumor-associated virus particles appear outside the membrane or within its pores. No tumor appears beyond the envelope. Osteosarcomatous tissue killed by lyophylization and implanted into animals also induces normal bone morphogenesis without tumor formation.

These studies are encouraging that BMP is not, by itself, tumorgenic. But they do not address the issue of the long-term effect of higher-than-physiologic concentrations of BMP that has been treated with a variety of chemical agents. There are no reports on long-term follow-up of implanted purified BMP.

DBM would seem to be less hazardous, since the concentration of BMP is comparable to that in natural bone. Similar concerns apply, however, when DBM has been partially digested with collagenase to increase the concentration of BMP and treated with several agents to reduce autodigestion and immunogenicity. DBM has been implanted in humans; these patients should be followed closely and reported on.

PROBLEMS OF PRACTICAL APPLICATION

How can all this information help us to bring percutaneous spine fusion to clinical practice? The ultimate goal as we conceive it is to inject BMP, or some other bone inducing agent, into the connective tissue between mobile segments, inducing ossification there and thus producing fusion without any other treatment except external immobilization. In the case of posterior or posterolateral fusion it may not be necessary to decorticate if the osteogenic agent can incorporate Sharpie's fibers into the induced fusion mass. In the case of interbody fusion it may not be necessary to decorticate end plates. What might be the effect of injecting and osteogenic agent into the annulus fibrosis?

Technically more complicated procedures will no doubt precede this ideal situation, partly because of the shortage of human BMP. In fact, Hoppenfeld has done several percutaneous interbody fusions, decorticating the end-plates with manual instruments and packing the evacuated disc space with chips of banked bone. There is a broad range of osteoinductive substances available: (1) fresh autogenous cancellous bone, (2) decalcified bone matrix, (3) collagenase-treated enriched DBM in spicules, granules, and powders, (4) purified BMP with or without carriers, which are or are not resorbable and supplemented with enhancers such as (hSGF), and (5) somatomedin; thus a great variety of experiments will be in order.[101] To all the conceivable combinations of these can be added electrical stimulation[44,52,66,67,103] and pretreatment of the nucleus pulposus with collagenase or chymopapain before injection.

Progress in research is hampered by the difficulty of obtaining large quantities of hBMP. Several remedies are possible. Xenogeneic BMP may be tolerated by human hosts if sufficiently free of immunogenic contaminants. Lesser purified precursers such as enriched DBM may serve, as well as purified BMP if it can be delivered to fusion sites in the proper physical form. More efficient purification processes may become available. Finally, hBMP may be synthesizable by genetic engineering techniques. Although osteosarcomas are a rich source of BMP and could be maintained in culture, it would seem imprudent to use tumor-derived products clinically.

No doubt new instrumentation will be needed. We have found it tedious to implant ground cancellous bone or hydroxyapatite granules through biopsy needles using the obturator as a plunger.

A power-driven injector would be helpful. Approach to the lumbosacral disc space with instruments large enough to perform end-plate decortication may require a straight path through a hole in the iliac wing or instruments that can work at an angle through an approach from above.

Finally, theoretic and real complications must be anticipated and investigated. For example, what would be the effect of an intrathecal injection of BMP or BMP plus tricalcium phosphate (TCP). How can the effect of implanted BMP be restricted to the area of interest? What are the consequences of errant BMP in the perispinal soft tissues? How permanent is the bone induced by BMP? Will it resorb over time? What are the long-term immunologic and tumorologic implications? Will infection require open management?

SUMMARY

Advances in our understanding of bone induction, isolation of bone-inducing agents, and the development of percutaneous discectomy, taken together, suggest the possibility of percutaneous spine fusion, both interbody and intertransverse. Beginning with traditional principles of decortication and grafting (this has been done percutaneously in humans) and leading to the ultimate goal of injection techniques alone, a large array of intervening experiments is suggested using DBM, purified BMP, TCP, hydroxyapatite, hSGF, somatomedin, and electrical stimulation. Problems of mechanical access are already largely solved. Problems of supply of the various agents are discussed, as are questions of sterility, immunogenicity, tumorogenicity, and complications.

It is hoped that the information and speculations presented here will kindle enthusiasm in many investigators so that percutaneous spine fusion may be brought to safe and reliable clinical practice and a long list of potential benefits and indications evaluated and possibly extended.

Editorial comments on p. 523.

REFERENCES

1. Alling, C.C.: Hydroxyapatite augmentation of edentulous ridges, J. Prosth. Dent. **52**:828, 1984.
2. Bab, I., et al.: Assessment of an in vivo diffusion chamber method as a quantitative assay for osteogenesis, Calc. Tiss. Intl. **36**:77, 1984.
3. Bab, I., et al.: Ultrastructure of bone and cartilage formed in vivo in diffusion chambers, Clin. Orthop. **187**:243, 1984.
4. Bauer, F.C.H., et al.: Formation and resorption of bone induced by demineralized bone matrix implants in rats, Clin. Orthop. **181**:139, 1984.
5. Block, M.S., and Kent, J.N.: Healing of mandibular ridge augmentations using hydroxyapatite with and without autogenous bone in dogs, J. Oral Maxillofac. Surg. **43**:3, 1985.
6. Bombi, J.A., Ribas-Mujal, D., and Trueta, J.: An electron microscopic study of the origin of osteoblasts in implants of demineralized bone matrix, Clin. Orthop. **130**:273, 1978.
7. Burning, K., and Urist, M.R.: Effects of ionizing radiation on the bone induction principle in the matrix of bone implants, Clin. Orthop. **55**:225, 1967.
8. Burning, K., and Urist, M.R.: Transfilter bone induction, Clin. Orthop. **54**:235, 1967.
9. Canalis, E.: Effect of growth factors on bone cell replication and differentiation, Clin. Orthop. **193**:246, 1985.
10. Canalis, E., et al.: Effect of partially purified bone morphogenetic protein on DNA synthesis and cell replication in calvarial and fibroblast cultures, Clin. Orthop. **198**:289, 1985.
11. Craven, P.L., and Urist, M.R.: Osteogenesis by radioisotope labelled cell populations in implants of bone matrix under the influence of ionizing radiation, Clin. Orthop. **76**:231, 1971.
12. Dawson, E.G., et al.: Intertransverse lumbar arthrodesis with autogenous bone graft, Clin. Orthop. **1**(54):90, 1981.
13. Dubuc, F.L., and Urist, M.R.: The accessibility of the bone induction principle in surface-decalcified bone implants, Clin. Orthop. **55**:217, 1967.

14. Farley, J.R., and Baylink, D.J.: Purification of a skeletal growth factor from human bone, Biochemistry **21**:3502, 1982.
15. Farley, J.R., et al.: Human skeletal growth factor: characterization of the mitogenic effect on bone cells in vitro, Biochemistry **21**:350B, 1982.
16. Firschein, H.E., and Urist, M.R.: Enzyme induction, accumulation of collagen, and calcification in implants of bone matrix, Clin. Orthop. **84**:263, 1972.
17. Friedman, B., et al.: Ultrastructural investigation of bone induction by an osteosarcoma, using diffusion chambers, Clin. Orthop. **59**:39, 1968.
18. Friedman, W.C.: Percutaneous discectomy: an alternative to chemonucleolysis? Neurosurgery **13**:542, 1983.
19. Gray, J.C., and Elves, M.W.: Donor cells' contribution to organogenesis in experimental cancellous bone grafts, Clin. Orthop. **163**:162, 1982.
20. Hanamura, H., et al.: Solubilized bone morphogenetic protein (BMP) from mouse osteosarcoma and rat demineralized bone matrix, Clin. Orthop. **148**:281, 1980.
21. Harakas, N.K.: Demineralized bone matrix-induced osteogenesis, Clin. Orthop. **188**:239, 1984.
22. Hausmann, B., and Forst, R.: Nucleoscope: instrumentation for endoscopy of the intervertebral disc space, Arch. Orthop. Trauma. Surg. **102**:57, 1983.
23. Hausmann, B., and Forst, R.: Shaving the lumbar disc space—a new technique in lumbar nucleotomy, Arch. Orthop. Trauma. Surg. **103**:284, 1984.
24. Hoogendoorn, H.A., et al.: Long-term study of large ceramic implants (hydroxyapatite) in dog femora, Clin. Orthop. **187**:281, 1984.
25. Iwata, H., and Urist, M.R.: Protein polysaccharide of bone morphogenetic matrix, Clin. Orthop. **87**:257, 1972.
26. Jarcho, M.: Calcium phosphate ceramics as hard tissue prosthetics, Clin. Orthop. **157**:260, 1981.
27. Johnson, J.R., and Kirwan, K.O'G.: The long term results of fusion in situ for severe spondylolisthesis, J. Bone Joint Surg. **65**(B):43, 1983.
28. Jones, J.C., et al.: Mandibular bone grafts with surface decalcified bone, Oral Surg. **30**:269, 1972.
29. Kaban, L.B., and Glowacki, J.: Augmentation of rat mandibular ridge with demineralized bone implants, J. Dent. Res. **63**:998, 1984.
30. Kaban, L.B., et al.: Treatment of jaw defects with demineralized bone implants, J. Oral Maxillofac. Surg. **40**:623, 1982.
31. Kanter, S.L., and Friedman, W.A.: Percutaneous discectomy: an anatomical study, Neurosurgery **16**:141, 1985.
32. Kambin, P., and Gellman, H.: Percutaneous lateral discectomy of the lumbar spine. Clin. Orthop. **174**:127, 1983.
33. Katthagen, B.D., and Mittelmeier, H.: experimental animal investigation of bone regeneration with collagen-appatite, Arch. Orthop. Trauma. Surg. **103**:291, 1984.
34. Kline, S.N., and Rimer, S.R.: Reconstruction of osseous defects with freeze-dried allogenic and autogenous bone, Am. J. Surg. **146**:471, 1983.
35. Kramer, S.J., et al.: Antibacterial and osteoinductive properties of demineralized bone matrix treated with silver, Clin. Orthop. **181**:154, 1981.
36. Ksiazek, T.: Bone induction by calcified cartilage transplants, Clin. Orthop. **172**:243, 1983.
37. Ksiazek, T., and Moskalewski, S.: Studies on bone formation by cartilage reconstructed by isolated epiphyseal chondrocytes, transplanted syngeneically or across known histocompatibility barriers in mice, Clin. Orthop. **172**:233, 1983.
38. Lindholm, T.S., et al.: Extraskeletal and intraskeletal new bone formation induced by demineralized bone matrix combined with bone marrow cells, Clin. Orthop. **171**:251, 1982.
39. Macewen, W.: The growth of bone, Clin. Orthop. **174**:5, 1983.
40. Malinin, T., et al.: Healing of fractures with freeze-dried cortical bone plates, Clin. Orthop. **190**:281, 1984.
41. Marx, R.E., et al.: A comparison of particulate allogeneic and particulate autogenous bone grafts into maxillary alveolar clefts in dogs, J. Oral Maxillofac. Surg. **42**:3, 1984.
42. Maugh, T.H.: Human skeletal growth factor isolated, Science **217**:819, 1982.
43. McLaughlin, R.E., et al.: Enhancement of bone ingrowth by the use of bone matrix as a biological cement, Clin. Orthop. **183**:255, 1984.
44. Miller, F., et al.: The use of bone allograft: a survey of current practice, J. Ped. Orthop. **4**:353, 1984.
45. Mizutani, H., and Urist, M.R.: The nature of bone morphogenetic protein (BMP) fractions derived from bovine matrix gelatin, Clin. Orthop. **171**:213, 1982.

46. Mulliken, J.B., and Glowacki, J.: Induced osteogenesis for repair and construction in the craniofacial region, Plast. Reconstruct. Surg. **65**:553, 1980.
47. Mulliken, J.B., et al.: Use of demineralized allogenic bone implants for the correction of maxillocraniofacial deformities, Ann. Surg. **194**:366, 1981.
48. Mulliken, J.B., et al.: Current research review: induced osteogenesis—the biological principle and clinical application, J. Surg. Res. **37**:487, 1984.
49. Nade, S.: Osteogenesis after bone and bone marrow transplantation, Acta Orthop. Scand. **48**:572, 1977.
50. Nade, S., et al.: Osteogenesis after bone and bone marrow transplantation, Clin. Orthop. **181**:255, 1984.
51. Nilsson, O.S., et al.: Microdissection specimens of connective, chondrous, or bone tissue of human osteosarcomas and chondrosarcomas transplanted to athymic nude mice, Clin. Orthop. **171**:232, 1982.
52. Noda, M., and Sato, A.: Calcification of cartilaginous matrix by constant direct-current stimulation, Clin. Orthop. **193**:281, 1985.
53. Nogami, H., and Urist, M.R.: Explants, transplants and implants of a cartilage and bone morphogenetic matrix, Clin. Orthop. **103**:235, 1974.
54. Nogami, H., et al.: Radioactive isotope labeled diffusible components of a bone morphogenetic substratum, Clin. Orthop. **122**:307, 1977.
55. Nogami, H., et al.: Ultrastructure of chondrogenetic interactions between bone matrix gelatin and mesenchymal cells, Clin. Orthop. **133**:238, 1978.
56. Oikarinen, J., and Korhonen, K.: The bone inductive capacity of various bone transplanting materials used for treatment of experimental bone defects, Clin. Orthop. **140**:208, 1979.
57. Oikarinen, J.: Experimental spinal fusion with decalcified bone matrix and deep-frozen allogeneic bone in rabbits, Clin. Orthop. **162**:210, 1982.
58. Oni, O.O.A.: Osteogenetic activity of the bone marrow (letter to the editor), Clin. Orthop. **184**:309, 1984.
59. Petri, W.H.: Osteogenic activity of antibiotic-supplemented bone allografts in the guinea pig, J. Oral Maxillofac. Surg. **42**:631, 1984.
60. Prolo, D.J., et al.: Ethylene oxide sterilization of bone, dura mater, and fascia lata for human transplantation, Neurosurgery **6**:529, 1980.
61. Prolo, D.J., et al.: Superior osteogenesis in transplanted allogeneic canine skull following chemical sterilization, Clin. Orthop. **168**:230, 1982.
62. Reddi, A.H., and Huggins, C.B.: Influence of geometry of transplanted tooth and bone on transformation of fibroblasts, Proc. Soc. Exp. Biol. Med. **143**:634, 1973.
63. Sampath, T.K., and Reddi, A.H.: Homology of bone-inductive proteins from human, monkey, bovine, and rat extracellular matrix, Proc. Natl. Acad. Sci. **80**:6591, 1983.
64. Sato, K., and Urist, M.R.: Bone morphogenetic protein-induced cartilage development in tissue culture, Clin. Orthop. **183**:180, 1984.
65. Sato, K., and Urist, M.R.: Induced regeneration of calvaria by bone morphogenetic protein (BMP) in dogs, Clin. Orthop. **197**:301, 1985.
66. Simmons, J.W.: Posterior lumbar interbody fusion with posterior elements as chip grafts, Clin. Orthop. **193**:85, 1985.
67. Simmons, J.W.: Treatment of failed posterior lumbar interbody fusion (PLIF) of the spine with pulsing electromagnetic fields, Clin. Orthop. **193**:127, 1985.
68. Syftestad, G., and Urist, M.R.: Degradation of bone matrix morphogenetic activity by pulverization, Clin. Orthop. **141**:281, 1979.
69. Syftestad, G.T., and Urist, M.R.: Bone aging, Clin. Orthop. **162**:288, 1982.
70. Syftestad, G.T., et al.: An osteo-inductive bone matrix extract stimulates the in vitro conversion of mesenchyme into chondrocytes, Calcif. Tiss. Int. **36**:625, 1984.
71. Takagi, K., and Urist, M.R.: The reaction of the dura to bone morphogenetic protein (BMP) in repair of skull defects, Ann. Surg. **196**:100, 1982.
72. Takagi, K., and Urist, M.R.: The role of bone marrow in bone morphogenetic protein-induced repair of femoral massive diaphyseal defects, Clin. Orthop. **171**:224, 1982.
73. Takaoka, K., et al.: Solubilization and concentration of a bone-inducing substance from a murine osteosarcoma, Clin. Orthop. **148**:274, 1980.
74. Takaoka, K., et al.: Partial purification of bone-inducing substances from a murine osteosarcoma, Clin. Orthop. **164**:265, 1982.
75. Terashima, Y., and Urist, M.R.: Chondrogenesis in outgrowths of muscle tissue onto modified bone matrix in tissue culture, Clin. Orthop. **127**:248, 1977.
76. Thielemann, F.W., et al.: Osteoinduction, Arch. Orthop. Trauma. Surg. **100**:73, 1082.

77. Tornkvist, H., et al.: Influence of indomethacin on experimental bone metabolism in rats, Clin. Orthop. **193**:264, 1985.
78. Tsuyama, K., et al.: Origin of the marrow cells in bones induced by implantation of osteosarcoma-derived bone-inducing factor in mice, Clin. Orthop. **172**:251, 1983.
79. Tuli, S.M., and Singh, A.D.: The osteoinductive property of decalcified bone matrix, J. Bone Joint Surg. **60**(B):116, 1978.
80. Urist, M.R.: Surface-decalcified allogenic bone (SDAB) implants, Clin. Orthop. **56**:37, 1968.
81. Urist, M.R.: Osteoinduction in undemineralized bone implants modified by chemical inhibitors of endogenous matrix enzymes, Clin. Orthop. **87**:132, 1972.
82. Urist, M.R.: A bone morphogenetic system in residues of bone matrix in the mouse, Clin. Orthop. **91**:210, 1973.
83. Urist, M.R., and Iwata, H.: Preservation and biodegredation of the morphogenetic property of bone matrix, J. Theor. Biol. **38**:153, 1973.
84. Urist, M.R.: Practical applications of basic research on bone graft physiology, Instructional course lectures: The American Academy of Orthopaedic Surgeons, St. Louis, 1976, The C.V. Mosby Co.
85. Urist, M.R.: Bone morphodifferentiation and tumorogenesis: perspectives in biology and medicine **22**:589, 1979.
86. Urist, M.R., and Dawson, E.: Intertransverse process fusion with the aid of chemosterilized autolyzed antigen-extracted allogeneic (AAA) bone, Clin. Orthop. **154**:97, 1981.
87. Urist, M.R., et al.: Osteogenic competence, Clin. Orthop. **64**:194, 1969.
88. Urist, M.R., et al.: Quantitation of new bone formation in intramuscular implants of bone matrix in rabbits, Clin. Orthop. **68**:279, 1970.
89. Urist, M.R., et al.: Bone morphogenetic protein and proteinase in the guinea pig. CORR **85**:275, 1972.
90. Urist, M.R., et al.: A chemosterilized antigen-extracted autodigested alloimplant for bone banks, Arch. Surg. **110**:416, 1975.
91. Urist, M.R., et al.: An osteosarcoma cell and matrix retained morphogen for normal bone formation, Clin. Orthop. **124**:251, 1977.
92. Urist, M.R., et al.: Transmembrane bone morphogenesis across multiple-walled diffusion chambers, Arch. Surg. **112**:612, 1977.
93. Urist, M.R., et al.: Solubilized and insolubilized bone morphogenetic protein, Proc. Natl. Acad. Sci. **76**:1828, 1979.
94. Urist, M.R., et al.: A bovine low molecular weight bone morphogenetic protein (BMP) fraction, Clin. Orthop. **162**:219, 1982.
95. Urist, M.R., et al.: Bone cell differentiation and growth factors, Science **220**:680, 1983.
96. Urist, M.R., et al.: Human bone morphogenetic protein (hBMP), Proc. Soc. Exp. Biol. Med. **173**:194, 1983.
97. Urist, M.R., et al.: Beta-tricalcium phosphate delivery system for bone morphogenetic protein, Clin. Orthop. **187**:277, 1984.
98. Vandersteenhoven, J.J., and Spector, M.: Histological investigation of bone induction by demineralized allogeneic bone matrix: a natural biomaterial for osseous reconstruction, J. Biomed. Mater. Res. **17**:1003, 1983.
99. Vukicevic, S., et al.: 1a,25-Dihydroxy vitamin D_3 stimulates alkaline phosphatase activity and inhibits soft-tissue proliferation in implants of bone matrix, Clin. Orthop. **196**:285, 1985.
100. Weiss, R.E., and Reddi, A.H.: Synthesis and localization of fibronectin during collagenous matrix-mesenchymal cell interaction and differentiation of cartilage and bone in vivo, Proc. Natl. Acad. Sci. **77**:2074, 1980.
101. Wittbjer, J., et al.: Bone formation in demineralized bone transplants treated with biosynthetic human growth hormone, Scand. J. Plast. Reconstr. Surg. **17**:109, 1983.
102. Wittbjer, J., et al.: Osteogenetic activity in composite grafts of demineralized compact bone and marrow, Clin. Orthop. **173**:229, 1983.
103. Wittbjer, J., et al.: On direct currents and bone formation in demineralized bone transplants, Acta. Odont. Scand. **42**:141, 1984.
104. Yablon, I.G., et al.: Matrix antigens in allografts, Clin. Orthop. **172**:277, 1983.
105. Yoshikawa, H., et al.: Biochemical stability of a bone-inducing substance from murine osteosarcoma, Clin. Orthop. **163**:248, 1982.
106. Yoshikawa, H., et al.: Soluability of a bone-inducing substance from a murine osteosarcoma, Clin. Orthop. **182**:231, 1984.
107. Zaner, D.J., and Yukna, R.A.: Particle size of periodontal bone grafting materials, J. Periodontol. **55**:406, 1984.

EDITORIAL COMMENTARY

Percutaneous fusion has been a long-sought concept. At levels above the iliac crest the method (although clearly not without potential hazard to nerve and vascular structures lying in the path of access) may become relatively simple; below the iliac crest (the L5-S1 space) there is another story entirely. Direct linear (or nearly linear) lateral access to the L5-S1 space is a far greater challenge. Not only the gluteal musculature, iliac bone, and iliacus muscle must be penetrated, but several structures must be avoided, for example, the upper trunks of the sacral plexus, lying in the sacro-alar gutter, and their accompanying vessels and laterally placed bowel. (See editorial commentary on Chapter 15.) The present methods of C-arm fluoroscopy are already difficult enough for intraoperative use, but for percutaneous fusions (or discectomy) one may have to resort to intraoperative CT scanning, a method (and machine) that is rather rare at this time. Of course, fusions performed at L5 to S1 by any approach other than posterolateral (or PLIF) may for some time to come best be achieved via a formal anterior approach. (See Chapter 38.) J.A.N. Shepperd (Royal East Essex Hospital, Hastings, England TN341ER) has reported on the percutaneous fusion technique in a few cases (Alternatives in Spinal Surgery, International Symposium, Paris, June 1985, poster session). He uses nested sets of tubing, each being slightly larger than the previous one, to dilate the path to the disc space until a 16 mm diameter is reached. The boring out of the disc space, the emptying of the nucleus, and the driving the bone plug are all accomplished through the 16 mm internal bore. The final instrument roughly resembles an operating proctoscope. Biopsy forceps are used to pull out the nucleus; this can be achieved through an additional cannula tube placed on the side opposite to that into which the fusion plug will be driven. Thus removal of the nucleus may be performed under direct observation from the opposite side.

Charles D. Ray

CHAPTER

46

MOTION STUDIES OF THE LUMBAR SPINE

Neil Chafetz   Sheldon Baumrind   James Morris

It has been estimated that between 8000 and 12,000 lumbar fusions are performed annually in the United States. These fusions are performed for the correction of mechanical or segmental instability resulting from extensive or multiple decompression procedures and for patients with advanced spondylosis and extensive facet joint arthropathy. Approximately one third of those patients who have undergone lumbar fusion are beset with persistent or recurrent pain. Failure of bony fusion (pseudarthrosis) has been implicated as a causal or contributing factor in a significant number of these cases. Appropriate treatment of the failed back fusion patient is dependent on correct diagnosis. Routine techniques for demonstrating pseudarthrosis are less effective than would be desired. Current methodologies for the diagnosis of post-lumbar fusion pseudarthrosis may be divided conceptually into two groups: evaluations of structural integrity and evaluations of functional integrity.

STRUCTURAL AND FUNCTIONAL INTEGRITY

Assessments of structural integrity rely on radiographic methods demonstrating the bone fusion and the vertebral segments that were intended to be fused. Routine radiographs on both AP and lateral projections have been employed for this purpose. In order to demonstrate the bony structures better, conventional tomography has also been used. Improved spatial resolution for bony structures became available with the advent of computed tomography (CT) (Fig. 46-1, *A*). Routine axial scans obtained in the course of a spinal CT examination may, for technical reasons, fail to demonstrate a break in the bony fusion that has occurred in the axial plane. Consequently, the information generated from the axial images frequently has been reformatted in a perpendicular plane (coronal or parasagittal reformations) (Fig. 46-1, *B*). Preliminary reports of a new method for direct coronal CT scanning of lumbar

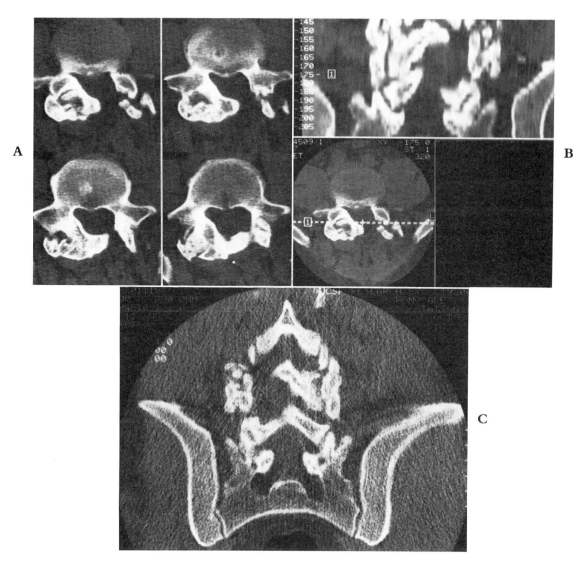

Fig. 46-1 **A,** Sequence of four CT axial images demonstrates posterior fusion with apparently solid fusion on right side. **B,** Coronal reformations from axial CT scan of same patient reveal no definite solid fusion. Bone fusion appears not to be firmly attached to vertebral segments. **C,** Direct coronal image reveals apparent pseudarthrosis. Note superior delineation of bony structures when compared to reformations demonstrated in **B.**

fusions suggest that higher resolution, lower radiation dose, reduced time, and lower cost are all associated with this new technique[1] (Fig. 46-1, C). The fundamental assumption underlying interpretation is that if bone fusion material appears to be adherent to the vertebral segments at which fusion was intended and the bony fusion appears unbroken, then successful fusion has taken place.

Tests of functional integrity are designed to detect the presence of motion at the levels at which fusion was intended. A routine radiograph of the lumbar spine in the lateral projection with the patient in flexion can be compared to one in extension. An attempt is made to determine if motion has occurred. This method, as well as those designed to determine structural integrity, is of limited precision and

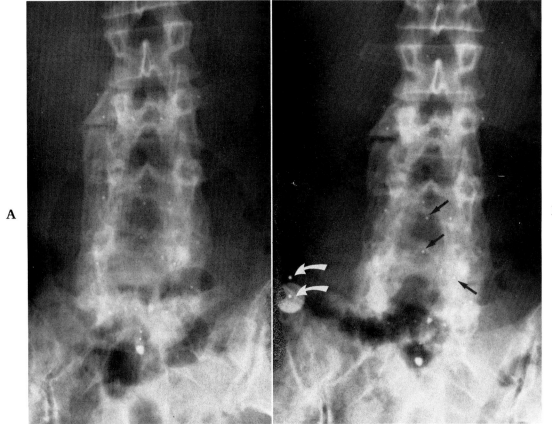

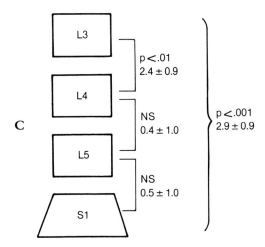

Fig. 46-2 AP radiographs with bending to patient's right, **A,** and to patient's left, **B,** demonstrate posterolateral fusion from L3 to S1. This patient with postfusion pain was suspected of having pseudarthrosis. Representative implanted metallic spheres are visible at each vertebral level *(black arrows)*. Additionally seen are two anterior markers, which are located on calibration cage, external to patient *(white arrows)*.

Although little difference between distribution of vertebral markers may be seen in these two films with the unaided eye, SPG analysis (summarized in Fig. 46-2, **C**) indicate that there is an overall probability of movement ($p < .001$) somewhere in the segment of the four vertebrae. Best estimate of magnitude of movement between these particular left-bending and right-bending stereopairs is 2.9 degrees with a standard error of .9 degrees.

Remaining values in **C** aim at defining where in vertebral segments movement actually occurred. Probability of movement between L4-L5 or between L5-S1 is not significant. However, probability of movement between L3-L4 is very high ($p < .01$ with a best estimate of 2.4 degrees and a standard error of .9 degrees).

may fail to detect subtle but clinically important motion between vertebrae within the fusion area.

STEREOPHOTOGRAMMETRY

What appears to be the most sensitive method for the detection of functional integrity of the fusion is a method called stereophotogrammetry (SPG).[2-5] This method uses geometric techniques originally developed for surveying land and making maps from aerial and satellite photographs. The SPG procedure may be sumarrized as follows. At surgery, after the facet joints have been excised and curetted as much as is safely allowable and bone has been harvested from the ilium and spinous processes, four cobalt-chromium spheres (0.5 mm in diameter) are inserted through a stylet into each vertebra to be included in the fusion. One sphere is inserted into the base of each transverse process and one into each lamina near the base of the spinous process. The procedure of placing four such spheres in each of the vertebra adds approximately 5 minutes to a surgical procedure that on the average requires 3 to 4 hours to perform.

At the time of radiologic evaluation a stereo radiographic pair of conventional films is obtained in the anteroposterior projection, with the patient bending to one side. Then a second stereo pair is obtained with the patient bending to the other side (Fig. 46-2, A and B). At the time these stereo pairs are obtained, the patient stands within a specially designed calibration device. Markers on the calibration device are projected onto the film surface. These markers aid in defining precisely the geometry of the x-ray image. At the present stage of development of the system, the two radiographs of each stereo pair are generated sequentially using a single, nondedicated x-ray machine, which is moved mechanically by the radiologic technician between the two exposures.

The data acquisition and data processing operations demand no expenditure of physician time. In the present version of the system the metallic implants are located on the radiographs by a semiskilled technician, and their coordinates are obtained by a computer-linked digitizer. All further processing and statistical analysis are then conducted automatically by a specially designed set of computer programs. Operating in this mode rotational movements as small as 1 degree between vertebrae can be detected. With dedicated stereo x-ray machines and fully automated scanner digitation it should be possible to improve this performance by a factor of at least 5. Sample output from the analysis of stereo radiographs taken for a single patient whose axial spinal CT scans with coronal reformations were equivocal is summarized in Fig. 46-2, C.

REFERENCES

1. Chafetz, N., et al.: Pseudarthrosis following lumbar fusion: Detection by direct coronal CT scanning, Radiology **162**:803, 1987.
2. Kratky, V.: Analytical x-ray photogrammetry in scoliosis. In Karara, H.M., editor: Close range photogrammetric systems, Falls Church, Va., 1975, American Society of Photogrammetry.
3. Moffitt, F., et al.: A stereoroentgenographic with portable calibration cage for use in clinical medicine, Proc. Soc. PhotoOptical Instrument. Eng. **361**(39):210, 1982.
4. Morris, J., et al.: Stereophotogrammetry of the lumbar spine—a technique for the detection of pseudarthrosis, Spine **10**:368, 1985.
5. Olsson T.H., et al.: Mobility in the lumbosacral spine after fusion studied with the aid of roentgen stereophotogrammetry, Clin. Orthop. **129**:181, 1977.

CHAPTER

47

ELECTROPHYSIOLOGIC EVALUATION OF LUMBAR PAIN: ESTABLISHING THE RATIONALE FOR THERAPEUTIC MANAGEMENT

Jeffrey A. Saal   Joel S. Saal

The treatment of low back pain is a formidable challenge. Lumbar pain is a common problem that has tremendous economic and social impact. It is second only to the common cold as a cause for days lost from work in the United States. Acute low back pain frequently represents a self-limiting condition that 80% of the population will sometime suffer. However, among patients with complaints lasting longer than 6 weeks, only a small percentage (10% to 15%) will undergo resolution without intervention.

The treatment of lumbar pain tests the mettle of the clinician's anatomic, physiologic, and social skills. A successful outcome requires an accurate anatomic, physiologic, and biomechanic diagnosis with an appropriately tailored treatment program. The electrophysiologic evaluation supplies key information in this regard. Patient selection, method of evaluation, and interpretation of data must be considered in a discussion of the electrophysiologic evaluation of lumbar pain syndromes. It is composed of a group of confusing clinical syndromes with multiple possible pain generators. Electromyography (EMG) is a valuable tool to aid in sorting out these different subsets. A successful outcome depends on accurate diagnosis of pain generators and clinical subtypes.

REFERRAL PAIN AND POTENTIAL PAIN GENERATORS

Essential to the proper application of electrophysiologic studies is an under-

---

Portions of this chapter are excerpted from (or originally appeared in) Saal, J.A.: Electrophysiologic evaluation of lumbar pain: establishing the rationale for therapeutic management, Spine, State of the art reviews, vol. 1, no. 1, September 1986, and White, A.H., editor: Failed back surgery syndrome, pp. 21-46, Philadelphia, Hanley & Belfus, Inc.

standing of the multiplicity of sites for pain generation in the lumbar spine. A major use of the EMG is to document nerve injury as the primary or the associated source of pain.

The annulus fibrosis and lumbar zygoapophyseal joints can by themselves cause back pain with radiation to the lower extremity, or secondarily inflame nerve fibers to cause referral pain. Anatomic studies demonstrate nociceptive nerve endings in the annulus fibrosis,[6] and tears of this structure can cause pain referral into the low back, buttock, sacroiliac region, and lower extremity in the absence of nerve compression. An annular tear that progresses to protrusion with frank compression of the nerve is an obvious source of pain. Even in the absence of direct nerve compression, disc protrusion can trigger an inflammatory response, causing secondary radiculitis with subsequent neurogenic pain referral.[40]

Facet arthropathy (zygoapophyseal joint synovitis) can cause spinal nerve compression or irritation in the intervertebral foramen with the buttock and lower extremity pain referral. Back pain combined with paresthesias in a nonspecific distribution in the lower extremity may result from irritation of those sensory fibers in closest proximity to the facet capsule and the inflammatory process. Additionally, low back pain with referral to the buttocks and lower extremity can result from irritation of the medial branch of the dorsal primary ramus. This nerve, which supplies sensory innervation to the facet capsule and motor supply to the multifidus, can theoretically become entrapped in the fibroosseus tunnel created as it courses around the superior articular process at the root of the transverse process.[17]

Reliance on the physical examination to demonstrate neurologic deficit as the sole indicator of significant injury is too insensitive an approach. Observable neurologic deficit (for example, reflex, motor loss, dermatomal sensory loss) usually appear only in the presence of high degree neural element compression (although this is not uniformly the case).[47] Electrophysiologic studies can be a far more sensitive indicator of nerve injury in the context of the low back pain patient. The differentiation of neural and non-neural pain generators is a crucial factor in determining the appropriate therapeutic plan. The demonstration of the relevant neural and non-neural pain generators in a given clinical situation must be specific before surgical decision-making can be considered complete.

Fundamental to the assessment of the pain generator is the judicious combination of diagnostic studies to adequately examine both structure and function. Unsuccessful attempts have been made to correlate structural changes alone (lumbar x-ray, myelography, CT scan) to the patient's pain complaints.[3,12,13,41] The combined use of EMG and CT scan (with and without selective nerve root blocks) can be highly specific.[32,51] The finding of structural injury or disease must be correlated to the clinical context with physiologic studies such as the EMG. Overreliance on structural changes alone too often results in the failed back syndrome, not infrequently with multiple surgeries.

Numerous studies have demonstrated efficacy in the use of electrodiagnostics in the diagnosis of lumbar spine root lesions.[15,28,32,60] Additionally, Wilborne[70] has discussed its limitations. A high rate of reproducibility and accuracy has been demonstrated in the correlation of clinical EMG findings and selective nerve root block, in both "virgin" and previously operated spines.[51] Clearly, electrodiagnostics can be extremely useful in sorting out the site of pain, and it is essential for assessment of location and degree of nerve injury. In the following sections, we will attempt to establish a rationale for the use of electrodiagnosis for treatment of the spine patient based on the type of electrodiagnostic findings.

BASIC ANATOMY AND PATHOPHYSIOLOGY OF LUMBAR NERVE INJURY

Certain structural relationships and anatomic differences may reflect in disproportionate injury to the lumbar roots. Similarly, the structure of spinal nerves differs from the rest of peripheral nerves with a predictable result. The dorsal and ventral roots course toward the intervertebral foramen within the confines of the dural sheath. The dorsal root merges to the (bulbous swelling) dorsal root ganglion (DRG) at the center of the intervertebral foramen. The DRG may be an important source of pain, and cases of pain syndromes due to compression/entrapment of more medially placed DRGs have been reported.[62] Distal to the DRG, the dorsal (sensory) and ventral (motor) root merge to form the mixed spinal nerve. They pass dorsally and laterally to the intervertebral disc. The dorsal nerve roots have a greater diameter than the ventral roots, and some authors have described an increased susceptibility of the sensory axons to a compressive force on this basis.[59] The greater length (L1, 60 mm length; S1 170 mm length) of the lower lumbar and sacral roots may explain their increased predisposition to injury. Each lower extremity peripheral nerve is composed of axons distributed from the various lumbosacral roots in an established pattern. The axon's health, and the health of its cell body (in the substance of spinal cord for motor axons and DRG for sensory) are interconnected, dependent on the maintenance of normal axoplasmic flow, in both antero- and retrograde directions.[20,63] Nerve injuries severe enough to cause cell body disruption or completely sever axoplasmic flow result in pain syndromes that can be refractory to treatment.

Similarly, the structure of spinal nerves differs from peripheral nerves with a resultant increased susceptibility to injury. Spinal nerve roots (SNR) lack the connective tissue protection that sheaths the peripheral nerves.[54] This sheathing has a considerable mechanical strength and possesses properties to form a barrier to diffusion of certain molecules. Therefore the SNRs are at a biochemical, as well as mechanical, disadvantage. However, the nerve roots are surrounded by cerebrospinal fluid (CSF), which in combination with the dura affords some mechanical protection.

The dura of the SNRs appears to be continuous with the epineurium of the peripheral nerve. This complex as a whole must be extraordinarily mobile. The nerve root complex should be considered mechanically as other soft tissue structures, with requisite adaptation to the dynamic change of spinal position. Nerve roots must change length dependent on the degree of flexion, extension, lateral bending, or rotation of the lumbar spine. Lumbar nerve roots limited in motion by fibrosis of either intraspinal or extraspinal cause will create traction on the nerve root complex, causing ischemia and secondary neural dysfunction. This fact must also be kept in mind during the rehabilitation process. Flexibility exercises must be designed to maintain nerve root mobility. The use of corticosteroids placed into the foramen or in the epidural space followed by a vigorous stretching program may sometimes be necessary to restore the normal and neural movement pattern in the patient where dural adhesions or fibrosis plays a role in pain generation.

Intraneural blood flow is another critical factor in the pathogenesis of nerve injury with a structural dependence. It is markedly affected when the nerve is stretched more than 8% over the original length. Complete cessation of all intraneural blood flow is noted at 15% elongation.[37] The spinal nerve root is not entirely free to move within its own environment. Suspensory ligaments have been demonstrated within the dura and the level of the intervertebral foramen that limit spinal nerve root excursion.[56] Instability with or without epidural fibrosis or stenosis may cause significant traction on the spinal nerve root, potentially causing dysfunction. Direct neural compression significantly compromises intraneural blood flow with resultant nerve injury as well.[59] Elevated compartment pressures demonstrated in the carpal tunnel syndrome provide another example of neuropathy associated with ischemic changes secondary to compressive forces.[38]

Instability in the presence of stenosis will cause a combination of compression and traction, limiting intraneural blood flow even further. The interruption of intraneural blood flow will cause a secondary increase in capillary permeability with subsequent development of intraneural edema. If intraneural edema is allowed to remain, fibroblasts will enter the interstitium and begin to lay down collagen, causing intraneural fibrosis. Intraneural fibrosis will secondarily limit axoplasmic flow and generally disrupt the milieu of the axonal fibers, causing neural dysfunction and a sick nerve.[59] This situation is not infrequently the case in the presence of severe spinal stenosis. Mechanical forces can interrupt axoplasmic flow directly and cause neuropathy. Because of the presence of its fibrous capsule and its rich vascular supply, the DRG may be more susceptible to interruptions and/or alteration in intraneural blood flow and the subsequent development of secondary intraneural edema and fibrotic change.[49] This may explain sensory symptoms even in the absence of sensory loss on gross neurologic exam.

Sunderland[59] has commented on the promotion of friction fibrosis in spinal nerve roots and secondary inflammatory response, terminating in the formation of adhesions. He describes this phenomenon secondary to the continuous "piston movement of the nerve in the foramen." He has also stated that spinal nerves will tolerate remarkable degrees of deformation, providing that it occurs slowly and does not alter the blood supply. Normal spinal nerves appear to demonstrate high degrees of tolerance to mechanical deformation, whereas damaged nerve fibers are less tolerant, resulting in ischemia disproportionately large to force applied. Therefore a patient with a long-standing radiculopathy will tolerate less instability and mechanical stress than the patient with healthier nerve root. Extraneural fibrosis can cause fixation and secondary ischemia of the spinal nerve root within the intervertebral foramen. The relationship of fiber size and its susceptibility to ischemia is open to question.[54,59] It cannot be categorically stated that sensory nerve fibers that are of larger diameter than the motor nerve fibers would be more susceptible to traction- and/or compression-induced ischemia. We have found that in the presence of solely sensory symptoms, the EMG often demonstrates denervation in the motor axons, as noted by the presence of fibrillation potentials and positive sharp waves on needle EMG examination.

Sunderland[59] has described five types of nerve injuries. Lumbar radiculopathy is best explained by the neurophysiologic principle of conduction block. In this situation the conduction of an action potential down the spinal nerve is slowed or completely interrupted. This would be considered a grade one through three lesion, using the Sunderland classification. Most radiculopathies are a grade one lesion, best explained by neurapraxia. These types of injuries are not associated with structural changes in the axon and consequently are immediately reversible when the intraneural circulation is returned to normal. As long as the myelin tube remains intact, the axons have the potential of regenerating and reconstituting the normal neural pathway.

Sunderland[59] describes three categories of conduction blocks. Category one is transient and is corrected in seconds or minutes when the affected nerve is no longer being stretched or compressed. An example of this would be a position-induced paresthesia in the lower extremity that is relieved by change of position, such as going from sitting to standing in the presence of a discogenic radiculitis. A category two conduction block is divided into two types. A mild lesion where conduction is blocked for 3 to 4 weeks and a severe lesion where it is blocked for up to 3 months. In a category three lesion there is gradual compression of a slowly progressive lesion. In this situation progressive neurologic deterioration will occur. If this compression is not dealt with rapidly, it can progress to a higher degree nerve injury, which will lead to a residual neurologic loss, despite efforts at late surgical decompression. The second type of category three (gradual compression) lesion is described as a persistent stationary lesion where the nerve is essentially placed in "suspended animation." If a constriction is relieved rapidly, dramatic relief can ensue. This has been demonstrated in removal of a herniated disc, which is compressing the spinal nerve root, with return of normal SSEP.[9] The same has been noted with removal of a constricting scar from a peripheral nerve.[46] The third type of category three lesion is intermittent conduction block, which is most likely of vascular origin. This intermittent type of conduction block will therefore cause intermittent neural dysfunction and only intermittent symptomatology. The intermittent variety leads to the most confusion and to the most difficulty in diagnosis (see discussion under instability). The recognition and differentiation of these types of conduction block have great diagnostic and prognostic value in the treatment of the lumbar pain patient.

Compression of a normal nerve root usually induces a sensation of numbness but not pain. However, mechanical deformation of a previously compressed nerve does cause pain. Within the nerve root complex the dorsal root ganglion appears to be the structure most sensitive to mechanical deformation. Compression of the normal dorsal root ganglion has been found to induce prolonged repetitive firing of the sensory axons, which might induce pain.[24] The lowering of pH, which has been associated with epidural fibrotic change, may act as a chemical irritant to the spinal nerve and secondarily cause pain.[45] One must also keep in mind that pain is a perceptual phenomenon with great individual variability.

THE NEUROPHYSIOLOGY OF ELECTRODIAGNOSIS
Definition of Terms

Nerve conduction studies are routinely used in the electrodiagnostic evaluation of neural function. Nerve conduction velocity can be determined by stimulating the peripheral nerve at two locations and using the simple formula of distance divided by time. The distance (meters) the nerve potentials traveled along the nerve pathway is divided by the time (milliseconds) it took the impulses to traverse that segment. Nerve conduction velocities can be computed for both motor and sensory peripheral nerves. In general, velocity is a myelin-dependent factor. The evoked response or compound action potential is recorded over the motor point of the associated muscle after motor nerve stimulation, and the sensory evoked response is measured either by surface or needle electrodes adjacent to the sensory nerve fibers. The evoked response is an axon-dependent phenomenon. The analysis of the evoked response for rise time, duration, amplitude, and configuration yield important information to the skilled electromyographer.

In the case of lumbar radiculopathies, nerve conduction velocities are normal. The lesion in lumbar radiculopathy affects the proximal segment axons and therefore does not affect the conduction velocity along the distal nerve segment.[70] However, alteration of the motor-evoked response does occur in the presence of lumbar radiculopathy. This is due to conduction block as described previously. The sensory evoked response does not change in lumbar radiculopathy because the lesion is proximal to the dorsal root ganglion. Therefore the sensory synapse from the periphery will occur at the dorsal root ganglion in an uninterrupted fashion. With a proximal lesion (root), even in the face of a totally anesthetic limb, the sensory conduction responses are obtained normally.[57] If changes occur in sensory conduction or evoked response, a peripheral neuropathy or peripheral nerve lesion must therefore be the cause. Changes in the motor evoked response can help differentiate degrees and types of conduction block[35] and will be discussed in a later section of this chapter.

One of the greatest values of nerve conduction studies in evaluation of lumbar radiculopathy is to search for the possibility of a peripheral neuropathy and peripheral nerve entrapment. The most common peripheral neuropathies are induced by diabetes mellitus or alcohol abuse. This will lead to nerve dysfunction that can confuse the clinical picture. It has been postulated that sick nerves are more easily injured when mechanically manipulated[59] and should therefore be taken into consideration in these individuals. Lower extremity nerve entrapments may mimic radicular syndromes and must therefore be sorted out by thorough electrophysiologic studies. A double-crush syndrome with both a proximal and distal lesion along the same axon pathway must also be considered.[50,61] An S1 radiculopathy and a tarsal tunnel entrapment of the tibial nerve is an example of this double-crush phenomenon. On the other hand, distal symptomatology of foot and calf pain that the patient with peripheral neuropathy reports can often be confused with lumbar radiculopathy. The burning feet of a patient suspected of having spinal stenosis may, indeed, be on the basis of a peripheral neuropathy. Moreover, the patient with peripheral neuropathy may not respond well to spine surgery even in the presence of a well-documented radiculopathy. In addition to the motor and sensory nerve conduction studies, there are three other types of nerve conduction studies commonly employed; H-reflex, F-waves, and somatosensory evoked potentials.

The H-reflex is essentially the electrophysiologic correlate of the Achilles deep tendon reflex. It has been shown to be a monosynaptic reflex with motor and sensory pathways traveling primarily through the S1 nerve root and it has been demonstrated to be useful in the diagnosis of S1 nerve root lesions.[5,8,52] In our experience, when the latency is prolonged, there is a high correlation with S1 nerve root pain reproduction as noted by selective nerve root blocks.[51] The converse, however, may not apply. Normal H-reflex latencies or H-reflex changes do not absolutely exclude the presence of an S1 lesion. Therefore an asymmetrically prolonged H-reflex (greater than 1.2 msec side-to-side differential) is diagnostic of an S1 nerve root lesion in the absence of sciatic mononeuropathy. Symmetric and normal H-reflex latencies can still be consistent with the presence of an S1 nerve root lesion. Potentiation of the H-reflex on the involved side has been reported to occur early after the onset of the radicular syndrome. Therefore, this paradoxic reaction must also be taken into consideration when attempting to interpret asymmetric H-reflex latencies.[34] Absolute reliance on the H-reflex to determine the presence or absence of an S1 nerve root lesion can therefore be misleading. The H-reflex is obtained with submaximal stimulation of the tibial nerve in an antidromic fashion at the popliteal space with surface recording electrodes over the medial head of the gastrocnemius (soleus). The latencies obtained from both lower extremities are compared, looking for asymmetry as described. The values obtained from both lower extremities are then compared to the normative data available based on age, leg length, and temperature. Improper technique and poor relaxation of the patient will often lead to incorrect assumption that the H-reflex is absent. Proper technique along with proper positioning of the patient to obtain maximal relaxation of the gastrocnemius musculature is imperative.

Attempts to correlate H-reflex amplitude with intraresponse latency variability have been disappointing.[33] H-reflex accuracy may be improved with the use of a subtraction technique, using S1 nerve root stimulation.[38] The H-reflex latency will also be prolonged in the presence of a proximal sciatic nerve lesion (pyriformis syndrome) and in the presence of segmental demyelination associated with a peripheral neuropathy. H-reflex abnormalities become evident within the first day of onset of radicular symptoms.

Motor conduction along with the most proximal segment of the nerve can be assessed by measurement of the F-wave. The F-wave is a late muscle potential that results from the backfiring of antidromically and supramaximally activated anterior horn cells.[39] In the assessment of lumbar radiculopathy, F-wave studies can be carried out on the tibial nerve to assess L5-S1 and potentially S2 lesions and on the peroneal nerve to assess L5 and S1 nerve root lesions. F-waves have been found to be useful in the diagnosis of lumbar nerve root lesions.[16] Side-to-side latency difference is considered abnormal if greater than 2.0 msec and can be diagnostic in a setting where peripheral nerve injury has been excluded by sensory and motor conduction studies.

Some authors have commented on the number of F-waves present after a series of 10 stimulations as an indicator of nerve root lesions.[29] F-wave latency abnormalities are useful adjunctive information and only rarely occur as the only abnormality.[16] There are many pitfalls in the interpretation of F-wave responses that make reliance on F-waves in the diagnosis of lumbar radiculopathy tenuous.[72] We have found F-wave responses measured from the extensor digitorum brevis after stimulation of the peroneal nerve, either at the ankle or at the fibular head, to be helpful in the diagnosis of L5 radiculopathy. Tibial nerve F-wave studies do not appear to add information regarding S1 nerve root lesions above and beyond the data supplied by the H-reflex studies and needle examination. F-wave studies are most appropriate as an adjunctive test and by no means should be used as the sole finding for determining the absence or presence of a radiculopathic process. We have never found F-wave latency abnormalities or changes in persistence of stimulated F-waves to be the sole finding in a radiculopathy. Theoretically, F-wave latency changes should occur at the same time as H-reflex changes on the day of radicular symptom onset.

Somatosensory evoked potentials (SSEPs), although theoretically attractive, have to this date only found a limited place in the diagnosis of lumbar radiculopathy.[31] Recent reports using dermatomal somatosensory evoked potentials to diagnose lumbar radicular lesions demonstrated an accuracy of 85.7% in a group of 70 patients when using myelography as the standard and 87.5% accuracy in a group of 38 patients when surgery was used as a standard.[14] The analysis of preoperative and postoperative SSEPs in patients who have undergone spinal stenosis decompressive surgery has shown improvement in latency and amplitude, correlating with postoperative clinical improvement.[18] SSEP evaluation may become most useful for the serial evaluation of nerve root lesions. The preoperative, intraoperative, and postoperative SSEP evaluations can be compared and potentially correlated with the persistence and/or resolution of the painful neural lesion. We are currently working on a project analyzing this type of data. We are attempting to analyze electrophysiologic data and determine the prognostic factors. The clinical situation where SSEP function appears to have its greatest value is in the workup of the individual with a purely sensory radiculopathy.[21] In this particular situation the clinical EMG studies may indeed be entirely normal, and only SSEP evaluation can electrophysiologically determine the injury of the sensory pathway.

Considering the sensitivity of the dorsal root ganglion to mechanical stresses, SSEP sensory evaluation of patients suspected of having radicular injury should become a more valuable and routine portion of the diagnostic workup in the future. SSEP evaluation of spinal pain patients who are experiencing bowel and bladder dysfunction can also be of extraordinary value. Clinical EMG studies have great limitation in their ability to evaluate the sacral plexus. In this clinical situation, SSEP evaluation of the sacral plexus is therefore an integral part of the electrodiagnostic evaluation.

The needle portion of the EMG examination is an integral part of the electrodiagnostic evaluation. It can be performed with either a monopolar electrode or a concentric needle electrode. The monopolar needle is an electrode with a bare tip and requires the use of a separate reference electrode. The concentric needle electrode has a reference and active electrode within a single cannula. We routinely use the concentric needle electrode. It allows for a more sensitive exam than the monopolar, allowing insertional activity analysis to be performed at a 50 μv sensitivity without baseline interference. This allows for careful scrutiny for the presence of extremely small spontaneous activity (that is, 20 μv fibrillation potential). These findings in the distal musculature may be the only abnormalities noted in a chronic radiculopathy. Our patients have not found concentric needle electrodes to be any more uncomfortable than monopolar electrodes. We have performed the needle examination comparing the two types of electrodes in the same individual and have found the patient unable to detect any significant difference in discomfort between the two. In the initial phase of the needle examination the muscles are evaluated at rest. After an initial electrical burst of insertional activity there should be electrical silence, a flat baseline. It is in this postinsertional period that spontaneous activity is sought. Spontaneous activity includes fibrillation potentials, positive sharp waves, fasiculations, and complex repetitive discharges. Fibrillation potentials have a duration of one to five msec and are 20 to 200 μv when recorded with concentric electrode. Fibrillation potentials typically fire on a regular pattern at a rate of 1 to 30 pulses per second. When heard over the EMG loudspeaker, the fibrillation potentials produce a crisp clicking type noise that is quite distinct.

The finding of fibrillation potentials is an unequivocal sign of abnormality. They should not be confused with miniature end-plate potentials recorded in the end-plate zone, nor should they be confused with small voluntary motor unit action potentials. This differentiation can be made by analyzing the potentials for regularity and noting the initial positive deflection that is invariably present in the fibrillation potential wave form. Voluntary motor unit potentials will tend to be irregular and change firing frequency with muscle contraction.

Usually, miniature end-plate potentials (MEPPs) will have an initial negative deflection, an irregular firing pattern, and be found only in the end-plate zone. The end-plate zone is easily recognizable by its distinctive seashell background noise. Fibrillation potentials are usually seen in denervated muscle but may also occur in certain primary muscle diseases and in certain lesions of the upper motor neuron. Fibrillation potentials arise from a single muscle fiber secondary to a combination of denervation hypersensitivity and changes in the resting membrane potential.[33] The quantity of fibrillation potentials noted appears to have no bearing on the degree of muscle denervation present.[11,43] The only fact to consider is the absolute presence or absence of these wave forms in at least two separate locations in the same muscle. Therefore, grading of spontaneous activity from 1 to 4+, as is customarily done, is of limited value. Severely denervated muscle, as in the case of a peripheral nerve severance, will have greater amounts of fibrillation potentials, but the precise correlation of the amount of fibrillations to the degree of denervation remains quite poor. Severely atrophic muscle, due to either denervation or disuse, will actually have a decrease in the amount of spontaneous activity present.[11] Moderate cooling of the muscle and hypoxia will suppress fibrillation potential generation. Rewarming of the musculature will therefore be necessary to note the abnormalities present.[33]

Positive sharp waves are encountered in denervated muscle and are postulated to have the same origin as fibrillation potentials.[66] Positive sharp waves appear in the paraspinal musculature 7 to 10 days after the onset of lumbar radiculopathy. After approximately 14 days, positive sharp waves begin to appear in the proximal muscles of the extremity. At 14 days the paraspinals begin to demonstrate fibrillation potentials where there previously had been positive sharp waves. By 21 days after onset of radicular symptomatology, the proximal and distal musculature innervated by the involved nerve root will demonstrate the findings of positive sharp wave and fibrillation potentials. Positive sharp waves appear to be the most acute finding and start out as large amplitude waves of approximately 200 μv that slowly drop in amplitude with the evolution of fibrillation potentials to approximately 100 to 150 μv in amplitude.[29] This process continues to evolve over time. The postive sharp waves become smaller, as do the fibrillation potentials. Eventually the positive sharp waves will almost entirely disappear and the fibrillation potential's amplitude falls to values between 20 and 50 μvs. These chronic fibrillation potentials can often only be found in the distal musculature. Just as the paraspinal musculature is the first to demonstrate the findings of radiculopathy, they are also the first to become "normal" with the evolution of chronicity. Lumbar myelography has been shown to cause the propagation of fibrillation potentials that last for up to 3 days after the procedure in the paraspinal musculature.[64]

No studies have specifically mentioned

the finding of fibrillation potentials in the paraspinal musculature after lumbar epidural injections, but it has been our experience that translumbar epidural injections will induce similar changes in the paraspinal musculature that must be taken into account. Sacral epidurals do not appear to elicit the propagation of spontaneous activity in the paraspinal musculature (unpublished data). Likewise, lumbar selective nerve root blocks or intraarticular facet injections, as well as trigger point injections, traumatize the paraspinal musculature and will induce fibrillation potentials, which should not be misinterpreted as evidence of true neural involvement. Lumbar selective nerve root blocks will cause the propagation of spontaneous activity secondary to mechanical and possibly chemical irritation of the nerve directly as well. These abnormalities have been noted to persist for as long as 4 weeks following the procedure.[51] Previous sites of intramuscular injection of pain medications into the extremity musculature can also cause the propagation of spontaneous activity, which will usually recede in 7 to 21 days. It is therefore preferable that EMG studies be carried out before injection procedures.

Obviously, in the clinical circumstance of the failed back pain patient, a surgical scar through the lumbar paraspinal musculature is present. This will induce changes in the paraspinal musculature that may go on for many years following the procedure. Some authors feel that paraspinal musculature can still be evaluated but at a distance of at least 3 cm lateral to the scar.[27] In a study reviewing 77 electromyograms on 60 patients, Johnson concluded that electromyographic abnormalities present at one level at least 3 cm lateral to the scar are probably diagnostic. See[53] found widely distributed abnormalities in the paraspinal musculature and concluded that recurrences could not be reliably established on the basis of paraspinal findings.

I reviewed 50 consecutive EMG studies carried out on previously operated on spinal pain patients and found paraspinal findings did not add information of clinical utility. This may be due not only to the denervation secondary to the surgical disruption of the musculature, but also to the repetitive insults the paraspinal musculature had undergone by needle techniques such as trigger point injections, acupuncture, previous EMG studies, injections, epidural injections, and myelographic examinations (unpublished data). In the failed back pain patient, I prefer to use a careful needle examination of the extremity musculature of both lower extremities to localize and establish the possibility of persistent or recurrent nerve root pathology or combinations of both. In the "virgin" spine, paraspinal musculature spontaneous activity may be the sole abnormality in the presence of radiculopathy in 5% to 15% of the cases.[26,29,67,70] The findings of fasiculation potentials and complex repetitive discharges are not uncommon in chronic radiculopathies.[33] When fasiculation potentials occur in the depth of a muscle, they may not necessarily be accompanied by a visible twitch. In a chronic radiculopathy without any acute denervation, fasiculations and/or complex repetitive discharges may be the only findings noted.

The needle examination is the most error-prone portion of the electrodiagnostic examination. An absolute minimum of two muscles from each myotome in each lower extremity must be sampled, and each muscle must be sampled with a minimum of 20 insertions over three separate locations for the test to be considered complete.[29,33] Simply placing the needle electrode into a single muscle without doing the necessary amount of insertions and declaring it either normal or abnormal is inappropriate and will yield misleading information. It is not uncommon for only one out of a total of two or three muscles that receive innervation from a spinal nerve root segment to show abnormalities in the presence of a nerve root lesion. Therefore meticulous technique and study is imperative for useful information to be obtained. A careful bilateral electromyographic examination is imperative, and a unilateral study can be considered an incomplete examination.

A motor unit potential represents the sum of a number of single muscle fiber potentials belonging to the same motor unit. A motor unit potential may be characterized by its amplitude, rise time, duration, phases, stability, and territory. The motor unit potential is examined initially with low-level voluntary contraction of the muscle with needle electrode in place. With increased voluntary contraction force, a greater number of motor unit potentials are recruited and the speed of firing of motor unit potentials increases.[10] Changes in recruitment of motor unit potentials occur very early in the onset of a radiculopathic process.[29,67]

Another early finding is the presence of polyphasic motor units in the appropriate musculature. Polyphasia indicates increased temporal dispersion of the muscle fiber potentials within a motor unit. This probably relates to the difference in conduction time along the terminal branches of the nerve or over the muscle fiber membrane.[7] Axonal sprouting secondary to a radiculopathy will give rise initially to small polyphasic motor units. These units will evolve to become large polyphasic motor units, which will in turn evolve to become large-amplitude, prolonged-duration motor units that are nonpolyphasic (polyphasic motor units have four phases and can be considered abnormal when they exceed 5% to 15% of the total population of motor units recorded).

The finding of early polyphasic motor units appears to be on the basis of synchronous but not simultaneous activation of two motor units firing together to give the appearance of polyphasic motor units, but in the true sense these are not indeed polyphasics.[29,48] This differentiation becomes important in sorting out acute vs. chronic lesions. The reinnervation process as noted by the changes of motor unit phases and amplitude may begin to occur as early as 5 to 6 weeks. The finding of large-amplitude, prolonged-duration (mature-type reinnervated motor unit potentials) occur only rarely as early as 6 weeks, usually taking 8 to 12 weeks to develop. Single-fiber EMG studies may be useful to evaluate the progress of reinnervation[58] but would only be clinically worthwhile if carried out serially during the entire course of reinnervation process.

Motor unit recruitment is classically evaluated with a maximal voluntary contraction while the needle electrode is within the substance of the muscle.[33,67] Because of the painful stimulus the needle electrode creates, patients are usually unable to maximally contract the muscle, leading to misleading results. Most electromyographers are trained to look for "whiting out" of the baseline at the time of maximal contraction to determine if there is "full" recruitment. Because of the inaccuracy of the measurement, as well as the variability of patient contraction, the determination of "full interference pattern" has limited clinical utility. The electrophysiologic evaluation of muscle strength and the onset of muscle fatigue may have great value in the diagnosis and rehablitation of patients with lumbar radiculopathy and chronic nerve dysfunction.[4]

We are currently working on computer programs to assess muscle fatigue correlated with muscle force applied. Clinically, one of the earliest signs of radiculopathy may be muscle fatigue and poor work capacity endurance. Using electrophysiologic parameters to determine fatigue would assist in rehabilitation decision-making and prognostication. The electrophysiologic diagnosis is based on finding signs of denervation and/or reinnervation in the distribution of one or more nerve root levels. Denervation is determined by the presence of spontaneous activity in the musculature. The use of H-reflex and F-wave studies is adjunctive. Motor evoked response adds information regarding the number of functioning nerve fibers. SSEP diagnosis of lumbar radicular injury is based on latency and amplitude changes after dermatomal or sensory nerve stimulation and scalp recording.

The paraspinal musculature can only be used to determine nerve root level if the needle examination includes the multifidus muscle. This appears to be the only segment of the dorsal primary ramus that does not overlap innervation with other segments.[19,30] Therefore the examiner must depend on the extremity musculature to determine segmental involvement.

Electrophysiologic findings can be divided into acute findings and chronic findings. The acute findings, as described previously, would include large positive sharp waves, large fibrillation potentials recorded in both proximal as well as distal musculature but often only in the proximal musculature. The motor units would initially be small and polyphasic with a shortened recruitment interval and early signs of fatigue. Motor unit changes would be noted initially in the proximal musculature and later be present in the remainder of the lower extremity.[67] F-wave and H-reflex findings are usually early findings and are not helpful in differentiating acute from chronic lesions. We have observed the reappearance of an H-reflex in a patient with an L5-S1 disc herniation and S1 radiculopathy after an epidural injection of corticosteroids.

The examination of compound motor unit action potentials (the evoked response obtained from the muscle on motor nerve stimulation) can be analyzed to differentiate between acute and chronic abnormalities, but it is most helpful when used serially in the same individual. When it is used serially, an initial loss in evoked response size and area under the curve would stabilize at the same level in the presence of a purely neuropractic lesion, that is, a lesion where there is a condition block, without structural loss of axons of any great degree. If there was progressive loss of axons, there would be concomitant progressive loss in evoked response amplitude and in the area measured under the evoked response curve.[65,69]

Comparing side-to-side differences of evoked response amplitude, an area under the curve can likewise yield important information regarding the integrity of the motor axons. In developing the prognostic factors for the return of function in a patient with a footdrop associated with L5 radiculopathy, the neuropractic subset described has an excellent prognosis, whereas the patient described with a progressive loss of axonal function would have a poorer prognosis for return of function if intervention is delayed (see the discussion of conduction block types). Small polyphasic motor units with recruitment abnormalities represent the earliest motor unit potential changes. Early fatigue, as noted by a frequency shift of recruited motor units with prolonged maximal contraction would also be noted.[4]

Chronic changes would include the finding of small fibrillation potentials in distal musculature, the relative absence of positive sharp waves, and the possible finding of fasiculation potentials and complex repetitive discharges in the appropriate muscles. Motor unit potentials that are large and polyphasic and/or large amplitude nonpolyphasic prolonged duration motor units can be found in the distal musculature.[67] Poor recruitment of motor units with changes in recruitment interval, along with early onset of fatigue, can also be noted. Small amplitude polyphasic motor unit potentials may persist in chronic radiculopathies, especially in the distal musculature.[70] Many times, the presence of acute findings combined with chronic changes are noted. These findings are especially helpful in the evaluation of failed back pain patients.

Responsibilities of the Electrodiagnostician
The values
1. *Assess the presence or absence of nerve injury.* A test with positive findings correctly administered and interpreted can yield unequivocal evidence of nerve injury.
2. *Differentiate root level injury or disease from a peripheral nerve lesion.* The pattern of insertional examination findings coupled with the presence or absence of abnormalities in the nerve conduction studies will accurately differentiate these two entities.
3. *Determine the segmental level of root injury or disease.* The pattern of spontaneous activity in a myotomal distribution will determine the nerve root level involved. (See discussion of nerve root anomalies and variations in innervation pattern.)
4. *Localize sites of peripheral nerve entrapment that may mimic radicular pain.* Abnormalities on nerve conduction studies coupled with peripheral nerve distribution spontaneous activity findings rather than a myotomal distribution will determine the presence of peripheral nerve injury.
5. *Differentiate acute vs. chronic findings.* Changes in motor unit action potentials configuration and recruitment, coupled with the more distal distribution of spontaneous findings, will determine the presence and degree of chronicity.
6. *Determine the degree of motor axon loss and the degree of reinnervation.* Noted by the amount and timing of changes in the compound motor action potential coupled with the changes in the configuration and recruitment of motor unit action potentials.
7. *Provide objective neurophysiologic data to correlate with physical examination findings.* Gross neurologic exam findings of weakness and reflex loss can be objectified by the test findings. For example, an absent Achilles deep tendon reflex by definition should correlate with an abnormal H-reflex study. In the same vein, a weak muscle should correlate with recruitment abnormalities.
8. *Provide objective neurophysiologic data to correlate with anatomic studies.* The presence or absence of nerve injury will assist in the differentiation between neural and non-neural causes of pain.
9. *Assist in sorting out the subsets of the failed back surgery syndrome* (FBSS).

The limitations
1. *The EMG exam may be devoid of findings in the case of a pure sensory radiculopathy.* in this situation, SSEP evaluation can be used to assess the sensory portion of the neuraxis.
2. *In the FBSS, examination of paraspinals muscles* can give false positive results, and in some cases the segmental level of involvement cannot be made with certainty using EMG

alone. See the earlier discussion.
3. *The results of the study depend most heavily on the experience and expertise of the electrodiagnostician.*
4. *Limitations of older equipment* with poor sensitivity and improper electrode selection and handling can significantly affect the test results.
5. *Variations in segmental innervation and nerve root anomalies occur.*

In 1983 Young and coworkers[70] found the tibialis anterior received dominant L5 nerve root innervation in 90% of cases, the extensor digitorum brevis in 74% of cases, the lateral gastrocnemius in 60% of cases, and the medial gastrocnemius in only 8% cases. The medial gastrocnemius received dominant S1 nerve root innervation in 82% of cases, whereas the lateral head of the gastrocnemius received dominant S1 nerve root innervation in only 20% of cases. Additionally, 20% of the lateral heads of the gastrocnemius received equal innervation from L5-S1 segment. The abductor hallucis longus received dominant innervation 80% of the time from the S1 nerve root and only 10% of the time from the L5 nerve root.

Variations in lumbosacral myotomes occur frequently in patients with bony segmental anomalies.[42] Studies using selective nerve root blocks to correlate clinical EMG findings[51] are in agreement with the myotomal map of Young and associates. In Young's report of 100 consecutive patients, there were no false positive EMG results but incorrect EMG diagnosis was present in 16 patients. Of these 16, the wrong level was predicted in seven patients, and in nine patients only one abnormal root was detected when two were involved. This again points out the necessity for clinical correlation of electrophysiologic findings and lumbar selective nerve root blocks before surgical intervention. The L5 and/or S1 nerve roots are involved in 90% of patients who had lumbar radiculopathy.[36] Because of the multisegmental innervation pattern of the lower extremity musculature, it can often be difficult to differentiate an L5 from an S1 lesion, as well as to determine whether the L5 and S1 nerve roots are both involved. This presents one of the greatest pitfalls in EMG localization.

Nerve root anomalies can present a significant problem for the operating surgeon. Correlating the electrophysiologic findings with lumbar selective nerve root blocks, selective nerve root stimulation studies can help to avoid difficulties.

6. *The "true" false negative.* One could eliminate the possibility of nerve root injury with a high level of confidence in the presence of a normal electrophysiologic testing coupled with normal anatomic studies; however a very small percentage of false negative studies can occur. The actual incidence of the "true" false negatives is not clear. (In our laboratory it is less than 3%, but in others it has been reported as high as 30%.)
7. *The degree of nerve injury does not necessarily correlate with the patient's reported amount of pain.* The electrophysiologic evaluation of the spinal pain patient cannot be done in isolation. It cannot be viewed as a purely technical endeavor done by a technician. Nor should it be performed by a physician operating in a void. To offer worthwhile information in the workup of the spinal pain patient, the electrodiagnostician must have a full grasp of the clinical situation. The closer the working relationship between the electrodiagnostician, spine surgeon, and the rest of spinal pain team, the better will be the quality of care.

In a multidisciplinary setting the (electro) diagnostician–physiatric team member's role is in three arenas. The first is diagnostic to assist the surgical team member in finding the causes of pain, not only by well-designed electrodiagnostic studies, but with thoughtful and careful physical examination and history skills. The appropriately skilled physiatrist should be able to carry out the selective block procedures and correlate their findings with findings of structural and electrophysiologic studies. Utilizing this information, the physiatrist faces the second chore, assisting the surgeon in surgical decision making, not only to help decide if a surgery should be performed, but on the type, level, and timing of that procedure. The third portion of this role is the designing of rehabilitation programs based on the diagnostic subsets. This multidisciplinary team approach allows all of the members to contribute their strengths and allows other team members to concentrate on areas in which they are better trained, more interested, and more capable of performing.

The major determinants of the true value of electrophysiologic data obtained from the studies is based on the ability to correlate the electrophysiologic data with the clinical situation. Electrophysiologic data that is evaluated and used in isolation has extremely limited, if any, use in the evaluation of the pain patient.

Reporting of test results

The semantics used in reporting electrophysiologic findings are extremely important.[28] A single examination can only evaluate a single moment in time; it has been compared to an isolated frame in a movie. Caution must therefore be exercised to avoid overreading or underreading of abnormalities. Remember, an electrophysiologic examination without findings does not necessarily mean the patient has no pain, nor does it mean there is no neural injury. It simply means there has been no electrophysiologic evidence of nerve injury on the evaluation at that moment. There are situations in a chronic radiculopathy in which potentially no electrophysiologic findings of lumbar radiculopathy will be noted. Isolated painful lesions of the dorsal ramus can also be missed because of the confusing status of the paraspinal evaluation in the failed back pain patient. The examiner can only comment on the presence or absence of electrophysiologic findings on that particular examination, based on the muscles and nerves they examined. Interpretation of the examinations using terminology indicating the presence or absence of electrophysiologic evidence of lumbar radicular injury is therefore most appropriate. For example, "no electrophysiologic evidence of lumbar radiculopathy on this examination," would indicate that no signs of denervation were found on electrophysiologic examination. This would not include an impression based on history and physical examination that, when combined with the electrophysiologic data, will yield the overall clinical impression of the case. When only soft findings of denervation are present, such as isolatated H-reflex changes, F-wave abnormalities, or motor unit changes, the impression would state, "electrophysiologic evidence suggestive of lumbar radiculopathy." Comments regarding the severity of the lesion can be based on decrements in motor evoked response and recruitment abnormalities but not on the quantity of spontaneous activity, as previously discussed.

Using older EMG methods without the use of SSEPs as tertiary evaluation, the rate of normal examinations in the presence of a high suspicion patient could approximate 10% to 35%.[70] Combining all electrophysiologic evaluations using state of the art electronic equipment, this number falls to 2% to 5%. One could eliminate the possibility of nerve root injury with a high level of confidence in the presence of an electrophysiologic evaluation that demonstrates no physiologic

Table 47-1 *Timing of appearance of electrophysiologic findings (in days)*

	1	7	14	21	30	60	90	120	>180
H-reflex asymmetry	+	+	+	+	+	+	+	+	+
F-wave asymmetry	+	+	+	+	+	+	+	+	+
SSEP abnormalities	+	+	+	+	+	+	+	+	+
CMAP changes*	+	+	+	+	+	+	+	+	+
Positive sharp waves: paraspinals	−	−	+	+	+	−	−	−	−
Proximal extremity	−	−	+/−	+	+	+	+	−	−
Distal extremity	−	−	−	+	+	+	+	+	−
Fibrillation potentials: paraspinals	−	−	+/−	+	+	+	+	+	−
Proximal extremity	−	−	−	+	+	+	+	+	−
Distal extremity	−	−	−	+	+	+	+	+	+
MUAPs: recruitment changes	+	+	+	+	+	+	+	+	+
Small polyphasics	−	+/−	+	+	+	+	+/−	+/−	+/−
Large polyphasics	−	−	−	−	−	−	+	+	+
Large, prolonged duration	−	−	−	−	−	−	+	+	+

*CMAP changes may persist or revert to normal dependent upon persistence and severity of the lesion.
+/−, Possibility these findings may be present. Timing is counted from the onset of radicular symptomatology.

evidence of nerve injury, coupled with normal anatomic studies (CT examination, magnetic resonance imaging [MRI], and discography). In this clinical situation, the search for non-neurol causes of pain should be sought, such as soft tissue origins, facet origin, and/or functional.

ELECTROPHYSIOLOGIC FINDINGS BASED ON CLINICAL SUBSETS

See Tables 47-1 and 47-2.

Previously Unoperated on "Virgin" Spine

Disc subsets

1. *Annular tear.* Findings are scant, and consistent with denervation.
2. *Disc protrusion.* Denervation findings in the distribution of the nerve root adjacent to the protrusion. There may also be findings on the contralateral side involving the same nerve root secondary to the inflammatory response created by the disc protrusion.
3. *Disc herniation.* Denervation findings similar to those noted with disc protrusion, but there may also be findings of two nerve roots involved on the side of the major portion of the herniation. The most severe findings of denervation are noted with foraminal disc fragments. Far lateral disc herniations can also envelop the mixed spinal nerve distal to the foramen and cause severe findings of a single unilateral root.
4. *Large radial annular tear without protrusion or herniation.* Definite signs of denervation of a mild degree may be noted with signs of reinnervation and chronicity in the distribution of the nerve root adjacent to the tear. There may also be findings of denervation of the contralateral nerve root secondary to the inflammatory response caused by the annular tear.
5. *Degenerative disc with recurrent tears with bulge pattern only, without signs of focal protrusion.* Inflammatory radiculitis may be noted, with signs of minimal ongoing low grade de-

Table 47-2 *Appearance and disappearance of electrophysiologic findings*

	Appearance	Disappearance*	Disappearance*
		Nonpersisting lesion	Persisting lesion
H-reflex asymmetry	Day 1	Remain	Remain
F-wave asymmetry	Day 1	Remain	Remain
SSEP	Day 1	Immediate	Remain
CMAP (amplitude, area changes)	Day 1	Revert to normal after lesion corrected	Further decrement or unchanged
Positive sharp waves: paraspinals	Day 7-10	>2 mos. (Persist postsurgery)	>2-3 mos.
Proximal lower extremity	Day 10-14	>2 mos.	>2-3 mos.
Distal lower extremity	Day 14-21	>4-6 mos.	>4-6 mos.
Fibrillation potentials: paraspinals	Day 10-14	>2-3 mos. (Persist postsurgery)	>6-10 mos.
Proximal lower extremity	Day 14-21	>3-4 mos.	May persist
Distal lower extremity	Day 21-28	4-6 mos.	Persist as small amplitude potentials
MUAPs (motor unit action potentials)			
Recruitment abnormalities	Day 1	1-3 mos.	Persist
Small polyphasic potentials	Day 14	5-6 wks.	5-6 wks.
Large polyphasic potentials	5-6 wks.	May persist	Persist
Large, prolonged duration potentials	>12 wks.	Persist	Persist

*Timing is counted from the onset of radicular symptomatology. Disappearance/nonpersisting lesion; pertains to lesions that have been corrected and are asymptomatic. Disappearance/persisting lesion; pertains to unresolved lesions that continue to be symptomatic.

nervation with findings of chronicity and reinnervation. The distribution may encompass the exiting and traversing nerve root at that motion segment.
6. *Internal disc disruption.* Signs of inflammatory radiculitis may be noted as described earlier.

Stenosis subsets

1. *Foraminal stenosis.* Denervation in the distribution of the nerve root(s) compressed in the foramen.
2. *Lateral recess stenosis.* Denervation in the distribution of the traversing nerve root(s) compromised in the recess.
3. *Central canal stenosis.* Denervation in a multisegmental and bilateral pattern. The findings are most amplified in the distribution of the nerve root(s) that are compromised in both their traversing and exiting segments. (See discussion in FBSS section.)

Posterior element subsets

1. *Facet pain (with or without leg pain referral).* Usually no findings of denervation exist, but in the case of dorsal ramus entrapment or significant inflammatory involvement of the dorsal complex, findings of denervation in the paraspinal musculature may be noted. As mentioned earlier, interpretation of isolated

findings in the paraspinal musculature must be done with caution.
2. *Spondylolysis without listhesis.* May show findings of denervation of a mild degree in the distribution of the exiting nerve secondary to fibrocartilage build-up on the inferior portion of the pars intraarticularis.
3. *Spondylolisthesis.* In the case of lytic variety of listhesis nerve root denervation can occur in the case of the exiting nerve root entrapped or tethered in the foramen or extraforaminal zone. In the case of a degenerative spondylolisthesis, this most often represents a variety of central canal stenosis with mild to moderate degrees of foraminal stenosis at that level.

Combined subsets

When any of the entities of disc injury or disease, stenosis, and posterior element abnormalities occur in variable combinations, more complex electrophysiologic findings will be observed.

FAILED BACK SURGERY SYNDROME SUBSETS
Stenosis

The first clinical subset of the failed back pain patient is stenosis. Stenosis can be divided into previously unappreciated stenosis, usually of a lateral variety, as has been pointed out by Burton,[12] or may be the postoperative type, which is of delayed onset and may be combined central and lateral variety. In the patient with previously unappreciated stenosis, the stenotic lesion was not decompressed in the original surgical procedures. In this clinical situation, the pain was never changed by surgery and, because of the possibility of iatrogenically induced instability, the pain may have become worsened and have gone from unilateral to bilateral. The electrophysiologic evaluation in these circumstances would demonstrate the presence of a chronic nerve root lesion on the side of the initial symptomatology. These findings would include polyphasic motor units combined with large-amplitude, prolonged-duration motor units in the distal musculature. The distal musculature would also demonstrate small fibrillation potentials. Quite often there will be signs of ongoing persistent deinnervation with scant findings of small- to medium-size (50 to 100 μv) positive sharp waves in the proximal musculature. Changes in recruitment interval in the involved musculature will be noted, possibly of early fatigueability with frequency phase shift and decrease in total recruitment of motor units in the involved musculature.

If this individual has developed symptomatology in the contralateral lower extremity since surgery, the findings in that extremity would be more of acute to subacute, with fibrillations and positive waves of small to moderate size in the proximal musculature, and some polyphasic motor unit action potentials without the finding of enlarged motor units of prolonged duration. Obviously, the longer the delay in diagnosis, the greater the chronicity of the electrophysiologic findings will be in the contralateral lower extremity. If the pain is truly from intraspinal nerve entrapment of the particular root or roots found in EMG study, there should be perfect correlation with selective nerve root blocks and at least short-term beneficial results from epidural local anesthetic and corticosteroid instillation.

Postoperative stenosis is of a delayed onset. Therefore there will be a period of time after the initial surgery where the nerve compromise and secondary radicular pain has been relieved. The pain will then return either in the same extremity or in the opposite extremity, either in the same radicular distribution or other radicular distributions, or any combination of these. In this particular situation the finding of a previously uninvolved spinal nerve root segment would be a hallmark. In my experience the findings usually are of a chronic reinnervated picture combined with acute changes in the extremity involved before the first surgery. This is usually combined with findings in the contralateral lower extremity, quite often involving two spinal nerve root segments. The findings in the contralateral lower extremity are of an acute nature, which would include findings in the proximal musculature of large positive waves and fibrillations and the finding of polyphasic motor units without signs of increased amplitude or prolonged duration.

Serial EMG studies in this clinical situation can be invaluable, especially in the analysis of compound motor action potentials (CMAPs) of the tribal and/or peroneal nerves. A continued decrement in evoked response size would be consistent with the continued loss of axons in the involved nerve roots and would go along with continued compressive change of the nerve root with secondary ischemia, interneural edema, and the development of interneural fibrotic change. We have observed a number of cases where small evoked responses of the CMAP preoperatively return to normal size postoperatively and then, with the return of symptoms, drop out of evoked response to the preoperative lower amplitude level. Instability will often complicate postoperative stenosis, which will help lead to the multiradicular pattern. In this situation, the already narrowed lateral recess and foramina will be narrowed further by changes in spinal position, causing traction on the nerve roots, which have become fixed in position by fibrotic change, secondarily causing a compromise in neural function. Instability may also be the reason for the contralateral abnormality findings, even in the presence of only intermittent and fleeting symptoms in that extremity.

In 1976 Jacobsen[25] discussed the electromyographic evaluation of lumbar stenosis and found multiradicular and bilateral radicular findings to be the most frequently observed abnormalities. He went on to state, as noted earlier in this chapter, that a unilateral study is an incomplete examination.

The nerve lesion in stenosis appears to be secondary to ischemia. This will then lead secondarily to intraneural edema and fibrotic change. Therefore nerve roots compromised in the stenotic spinal canal will often become "sick nerves," which may continue to cause pain despite adequate decompressive surgical procedures.

Intraneural Fibrosis: Sick Nerve Syndrome

Chronic nerve root lesions can lead to intraneural fibrosis and a sick nerve syndrome. Electrophysiologically, this is demonstrated by chronic motor unit action potential changes, as well as a poor recruitment of motor unit potentials on voluntary contraction and early fatigueability, noted by early frequency phase shifts on low level muscle contraction. There will also be small evoked responses noted on motor nerve stimulation with temporal dispersion of the wave form. The sensory evoked response should remain unchanged unless the DRG is affected.

Fibrillation potentials usually can be found only in the most distal musculature. They will be of the very small variety, 20 μv in amplitude, and will be scant in number. It is imperative in this situation to differentiate the sick spinal nerve root from a distal peripheral neuropathy. In peripheral neuropathy, conduction velocities will often be altered along with changes in sensory nerve action potentials, both of which are not noted in the presence of chronic lumbar radicular syndromes.

As is sometimes the case with a patient who has diabetes and long-standing degenerative spinal stenosis, the differentiation between neuropathy and radiculopathy can be almost impossible. In this particular situation, paraspinal muscle findings and findings in the proximal musculature can help differentiate the distal peripheral neuropathy from the chronic radicular syndrome. But as pointed out earlier, there are significant limitations in using the paraspinal abnormalities. The use of selective blocks, such as epidural nerve root blocks, will often become necessary to sort out this difficult clinical picture.

Unless stenosis is present, one can expect only a single nerve to be involved in the sick nerve syndrome. When multiple nerve roots are involved, a stenotic lesion should be sought.

SPINAL ADHESIVE ARACHNOIDITIS

Spinal adhesive arachnoiditis as a cause for continued radicular pain in the failed back pain patient has been discussed in numerous reports.[2,23] The only study on the electromyographic changes associated with chronic spinal arachnoiditis demonstrated no specific localizable abnormalities.[27] The only findings they noted were findings in the paraspinal musculature. These findings in the paraspinal musculature of the failed back pain patient can often lead to interpretation difficulties. If no findings are noted in the extremity musculature, the sole findings in the paraspinal muscles are insufficient evidence of neural involvement. The nerve root condition in adhesive arachnoiditis is best explained by a combination of ischemia and mechanical distortion of the nerve root. Chronic changes of a multiple nerve root distribution, as noted in the extremity musculature, without signs of acute degeneration, has been our clinical experience in these patients.

EPIDURAL FIBROSIS

Epidural fibrosis will often occur along with instability and stenosis, thereby creating a multisegmental radicular distribution in both lower extremities. In our experience, epidural fibrosis is usually associated with normal electrophysiologic studies unless there is associated bony stenosis. In the presence of normal stability and no demonstrable stenosis, it is difficult to prove that epidural fibrosis by itself is the cause for persistent lumbar radicular pain. Chronic electrophysiologic changes with small fibrillation potentials in the distal musculature, along with large polyphasic motor units, are the hallmark findings when a radicular syndrome is present. The distribution tends to be multisegmental, but in rare situations single nerve root involvement by the fibrosis can be demonstrated as the sole lesion.

If EMG testing demonstrates abnormalities in a single or multiple nerve root distribution in the presence of suspected epidural fibrosis, the surgeon should make an exhaustive effort to determine if there is, indeed, instability or stenotic lesion present.

INSTABILITY

The neural manifestations of instability are usually delayed, compared to the onset and severity of mechanical lumbar pain. Radicular involvement as a pain source in the presence of instability is not always consistent. Chronic nerve traction through narrowed lateral recesses and narrowed neural foramina combined with dynamic and static stenotic lesions may cause intermittent symptomatology consistent with the intermittent-type category three conduction block previously described.

Electrophysiologic abnormalities may only be noted after a period of 2 to 3 weeks of provoked symptomatology. If the patient has had no symptomatology in the 3 weeks before the examination, then no neural abnormalities may be found on EMG exam, leading to a false impression. In the intermittent variety of conduction block that has gone through a period of exacerbation, signs of acute denervation with findings of positive waves and fibrillations of a moderate to large size in the proximal musculature will be combined with a pattern of chronic denervation changes in the same nerve root distribution in the distal musculature.

If instability has caused chronic radicular pain of a static rather than intermittent variety, then purely chronic changes will be noted without signs of acute change in the proximal musculature. Therefore a carefully administered and interpreted EMG exam can help decipher a complicated clinical situation. Nerve root changes should be confined to the unstable movement segments only, unless adjacent levels have other conditions. An example of this would be a spondylolisthesis at L5-S1 that was previously fused but still remains unstable and a herniated nucleus pulposus and foraminal stenosis at the level above.

The use of facet blocks will also help sort out the picture of neural versus mechanical pain in the instability subset.

RECURRENT DISC PROTRUSION

Recurrent disc protrusion as a cause for failed back pain syndrome is unusual.[12] It most often occurs secondary to delayed instability with resultant shear stress across the previously operated on disc space, thereby causing continued disc pathology at that level. If there is indeed a recurrent disc protrusion at the same level, the pain syndrome will be unilateral in origin and in the same anatomic distribution as preoperatively. The EMG findings will demonstrate acute findings in a single nerve root segment, possibly in the presence of a previously fully reinnervated nerve root lesion. Indeed, if more than one nerve root is found to be involved by EMG testing, then a careful investigation for associated lesions such as instability and stenosis, as well as pathology, at adjacent levels should be sought.

INFECTION

Chronic denervation patterns of a multisegmental nature are the notable findings in the presence of chronic epidural abscess. There are no electrophysiologic abnormalities associated with discitis or chronic osteomyelitis unless there is direct neural compression as a consequence of the infective process.

Serial SSEP evaluations preoperatively and postoperatively could have tremendous potential utility in sorting out all the lesions described. Serial EMG studies combined with serial SSEP studies should be able to fully elucidate and follow the circumstances of recurrent and/or persistent lumbar radicular pain syndromes. This could lead one to argue for the routine use of preoperative and postoperative studies. The probability theory as it applied to the use of diagnostic tests would need to be applied to determine if this path of action is appropriate. Sox[55] has discussed the use of probability theory in evaluating the use of diagnostic tests in a recent report. He points out that diagnostic tests should only be obtained when they can alter management in a case. We have demonstrated in this report that the electrophysiologic data obtained can indeed alter the therapeutic management of the low back pain patient, specifically the failed back pain patient. This is accomplished not only by making a diagnostic localization of a nerve root injury but grading the lesion and eliminating the involvement of adjacent segments and peripheral neuropathies. Difficult to interpret manual muscle testing in a patient suspected of malingering can also be sorted out by carefully planned and executed EMG studies.

The cost effectiveness of electrophysiologic examinations need to be established. Considering the economic impact of the failed back pain patient, the diagnostic yield of electrophysiologic studies appears to demonstrate a significant cost-benefit ratio. The information obtained from electrodiagnostic studies should be used to streamline care and establish a rational management program. Careful preoperative electrophysiologic evaluation is mandatory in all patients. Denying the patient the benefit of this decision-making data tempts disaster. If we are to avoid iatrogenically producing the failed back pain patient, we must endeavor to establish a precise diagnosis before any surgical intervention. This will necessitate the correlation of the electrodiagnostic studies with selective block procedures and anatomic studies. If success is to be achieved, we must be certain that the clinical picture exactly fits the findings of diagnostic studies. In this day of technologic advances, guessing the level of nerve root involvement is inappropriate and potentially injurious.

SUMMARY

The physiatrist/electrodiagnostician is an important team member involved in the management of the spinal pain patient. Electrodiagnostic studies yield important information and clues that are extremely helpful in sorting out the dilemma of low back pain. When this input is combined with the resources of the other team members, solutions for the patient with persistent lumbar pain can be found. The skill of the electrodiagnostician combined with his or her level of involvement in the team effort are the most important factors in determining the utility of the electrophysiologic findings.

REFERENCES

1. Arvidson, B.: A study of the perineural diffusion barrier of a peripheral ganglion, Acta Neuropath. (Berlin) **46**:137, 1979.
2. Auld, A.W.: Chronic spinal arachnoiditis: a postoperative syndrome that may signal its onset, Spine **3**:55, 1975.
3. Barton, P.N.: The significance of anatomical defects of the lower spine, Ind. Med., **17**:37, 1948.
4. Basmajian, J.V.: Muscles alive: their function revealed by electromyography, ed. 5, Baltimore, 1985.
5. Baylan, S.P., et al.: H-reflex latency in relation to ankle jerk electromyographic, myelographic and surgical findings in back pain patients, Electromyogr. Clin. Neurophysiol. **21**:201, 1981.
6. Bogduk, N., et al: The innervation of the human lumbar intervertebral disc, J. Anat. **132**:39, 1981.
7. Borenstein, S., and Desmedt, J.E.: Range of variations in motor unit potentials during reinnervation after traumatic nerve lesions in humans, Ann. Neurol. **8**:460, 1980.
8. Braddom, R.I., and Johnson, E.W.: Standardization of H-reflex and diagnostic use in S1 radiculopathy, Arch. Phys. Med. Rehabil. **55**:161.
9. Brown, M.D.: Intraoperative SSEP in compressive lumbar root lesion, Int. Soc. Study Lumbar Spine, Cambridge, England, April 1983.
10. Buchtal, F.: The general concept of the motor unit. In Abanor, R.D., Eaton, L.M.M., and Sheg, G.M., editors: Neuromuscular disorders, Baltimore, 1960, Williams & Wilkins.
11. Buchtal, F.: Fibrillations: clinical electrophysiology. In Culp, W.J., and Ochoa, J., editors: Abnormal nerve end muscles as impulse generators, Oxford, England, Oxford University Press.
12. Burton, C.V., et al.: Causes of failure of surgery on the lumbar spine, Clin. Orthop. **157**:191, 1981.
13. Diveley, R.L., and Oglevie, L.L.: Preemployment examination of the low back, JAMA **160**:556, 1956.
14. Dvonch, V., et al: Dermatomal SSEP: their use in lumbar radiculopathy, Spine, **9**:291, 1984.

15. Fischer, M.A., et al.: Clinical and electrophysiological appraisal of the significance of radicular injury in back pain, J. Neurol. Neurosurg. Psychiatry **41**:303, 1978.
16. Fischer, M.A., et al: the F-response: a clinically useful physiological parameter for the evaluation of radicular injury, Electromyogr. Clin. Neurophysiol. **19**:65, 1979.
17. Fischer, M.A., et al.: Electrodiagnostic exam, back pain, and entrapment post rami, Electromyogr. Clin. Neurophysiol. **25**:183, 1985.
18. Gonzalez, E.G., et al.: Lumbar spinal stenosis: analysis of pre and postoperative somatosensory evoked potentials, Arch. Phys. Med. Rehabil. **66**:11, 1985.
19. Gough, J.G., and Koepke, G.M.: Electrophygraphic determination of motor root levels in erector spinae muscles, Arch Phys. Med. Rehabil. 9, Jan. 1966.
20. Hahnenberer, R.W.: Effects of pressure on fast axoplasmic flow: an in vitro study in the vagus nerve in rabbits, Acta Physiol. Scand. **104**:229, 1978.
21. Haldeman, S.: The electrodiagnostic evaluation of nerve root function, Spine **9**:42, 1984.
22. Hoffman, G.S.: Spinal arachnoiditis: what is the clinical spectrum? Spine **8**:538, 1983.
23. Hoppenstein, R.: A new approach to the failed, failed back syndrome, Spine **5**:371, 1980.
24. Howe, J.F., et al.: Mechanosensitivity of dorsal root ganglion and chronically injured axons: a physiological basis for radicular pain of nerve root compression, Pain **3**:25, 1977.
25. Jacobsen, R.E.: Lumbar stenosis: an electromyographic evaluation, Clin. Orthop. **115**:68, 1970.
26. Johnson, E.W., and Melvin, J.L.: Value of electromyography in lumbar radiculopathy, Ach. Phys. Med. Rehabil. **52**:239, 1971.
27. Johnson, E.W., et al.: Electromyography in post-laminectomy patients, Arch, Phys. Med. Rehabil. **53**:239, 1972.
28. Johnson, E.W., and Parker, W.D.: Interpretation and reporting. In practical electromyography, Baltimore, 1980, Williams & Wilkins.
29. Johnson, E.W.: Electrodiagnosis of radiculopathy: advanced concepts in evaluation focal neuropathy, Am. Assoc. Electromyog. Electrodiagnosis, Las Vegas, 1985.
30. Jonnson, B.: Morphology, innervation and electromyographic study of the erector spinae, Arch, Phys. Med. Rehabil. **30**:638, 1969.
31. Jones, S.J.: Clinical applications of somatosensory evoked potentials: peripheral nervous system, international symposium on SSEP, Kansas City, Missouri, 1984.
32. Khartri, B.O., et al.: Correlation of electromyography with CT in evaluation of low back pain, Arch. Neurol. **41**:594, 1984.
33. Kimura, J.: Electrodiagnosis in diseases of nerve and muscle: principles and practice, Philadelphia, 1983, F.A. Davis Co.
34. Koehler, F.K., and Burger, A.A.: Facilitation of H-reflex in low back pain, Electromyogr. Clin. Neurophys. **21**:207, 1981.
35. Lambert, E.: Diagnostic value of electrical stimulation of motor nerves. Electroncephalgr. Clin. Neurophysiol. Suppl. **22**:9.
36. Leyshon, A., et al.: Electrical studies in the diagnosis of compression of the lumbar root, J. Bone Joint Surg. **63B**:71, 1981.
37. Lundborg, G., and Rydevik, B.: Effects of stretching the tibial nerve of the rabbit: a preliminary study on the intraneural microcirculation and the barrier function of the perineum, J. Bone Joint Surg. **55B**:390, 1973.
38. Lundborg, G., et al.: Median nerve compression in carpal tunnel syndrome: the functional response to experimentally induced controlled pressure, J. Hand Surg. **7**:252, 1982.
39. Marshall, L.L., et al.: Chemical radiculitis, Clin. Orthop. **129**:61, 1977.
40. McCrae, D.L.: Asymptomatic intervertebral disc protrusion, Acta Radiol. **46**:9, 1956.
41. McCullogh, J.A., and Waddel, G.: Variation of the L5 myotomes with bony segmental abnormalities, J. Bone Joint Surg. **62B**:475, 1950.
42. Miller, R.G.: Nerve injury, advanced concepts in evaluating focal neuropathies, Am. Assoc. Electromyog. Electrodiagnosis, Las Vegas, 1985.
43. Mooney, J., and Robertson, J.: The facet syndrome, Clin. Orthop. **115**:149, 1976.
44. Nachemson, A.: Intradiscal measurements of pH in patients with lumbar rhizopathies, Acta. Orthop. Scand. **40**:23, 1962.
45. Ochoa, J. et al.: Anatomical changes in peripheral nerves compressed by a pneumatic tourniquet, J. Anat. **113**:433, 1972.
46. Porter, R.W., et al.: The natural history of root entrapment syndrome, Spine **9**:418, 1984.
47. Roth, G., and Magistris, M.: Ephase Between Two Motor Units in Chronically Denervated Muscle, Electromyog. Clin. Neurophysiol. **25**:331, 1955.

48. Rydevik, B., et al.: Pathoanatomy and pathophysiology of nerve root compression, Spine **9**:7, 1984.
49. Saal, J.A.: The multiple crush lesion of the median nerve in the presence of clinical root compression, Phys. Med. Rehabil., Los Angeles, 1983.
50. Saal, J.A.: The correlation of clinical EMG findings and lumbar selective nerve root blocks, paper presented at North American Spine Society, Laguna Niguel, California, 1985.
51. Schuchmann, J.A.: H-reflex latency in radiculopathy, Arch. Phys. Med. Rehabil. **59L**:185, 1978.
52. See, J.H., and Kraft, G.H.: Electromyography in paraspinal muscles following surgery for root compression, Arch. Phys. Med. Rehabil. **56**:50, 1975.
53. Sedden, H.: Surgical disorders of peripheral nerves, London, 1972, Churchill Livingstone.
54. Sox, H.C.: Probability theory in the use of diagnostic tests: an introduction to initial study of the literature, Ann. Int. Med. **104**:60, 1956.
55. Spencer, I.L., Anatomy and fixation of the lumbosacral nerve roots in sciatica, Spine **8**:672, 1983.
56. Stanwood, J., and Kraft, G.: Diagnosis and management of brachial plexus injury, Arch. Phys. Med. Rehabil. **52**:52, 1971.
57. Stalberg, E., and Ekstedt, J.: Single fiber EMG and microphysiology of the motor unit in normal and disease muscle. In Desmedt, J.E., editor: New developments in electromyography and clinical neurophysiology, vol. 1, Basel, Switzerland, 1973, Karger.
58. Sunderland, S.: Nerve and nerve injuries, ed. 2., New York, 1978, Churchill Livingstone.
59. Tonzola, R.R., et al.: Usefulness of electrophysiological studies in the diagnosis of lumbrosacral root disease, Ann. Neurol. **9**:305, 1980.
60. Upton, R.M., and McComas, A.J.: The double crush syndrome in nerve entrapment syndromes, Lancet **2L**:359, 1973.
61. Vanderlinden, G.R.: Subarticular entrapment of the dorsal root ganglion as a cause of sciatic pain, Spine, 9:19, 1984.
62. Varons, A.R.: Nerve growth factors and control of nerve growth: current topics in developmental biology. vol. 16, Moscana, A.A., et al., editors: New York, 1980, Academic Press, Inc.
63. Weber, R.J., and Weingarden, S.I.: EMG abnormalities following myelography, Arch. Neurol. **36**:588, 1979.
64. Weber, R.J., and Piero, D.: Entrapment syndromes. In Practical electromyography, Baltimore, 1981, Williams & Wilkins.
65. Weicher, D.O.: Mechanically provoked insertional activity before and after nerve section in rats, Arch. Phys. Med. Rehabil. **58**:402, 1977.
66. Weingarden, H.P., et al.: Radiculopathies. In Practical electromyography. Baltimore, 1980, Williams & Wilkins.
67. Wexler, I.: Nerve action potential changes associated with proved lumbrosacral root compression, Electromyogr. Clin. Neurophysiol. **19**:453, 1979.
68. Wilbourn, A.: The value and limitation of EMG in examination in the diagnosis of lumbrosacral radiculopathy. In Hardy, R.W., editor: Lumbar disc disease, New York, 1982, Raven Press.
69. Young, A., et al.: Variation in the pattern of muscle innervation by the L5 and S1 nerve roots, Spine **8**:616, 1983.
70. Young, R.R., and Shahani, B.T.: Clinical value and limitation of F-wave determination, Muscle Nerve, **13**:248, 1978.

INDEX

A

AAA; see Autolysed antigen-extracted allogeneic bone
AATB; see American Association of Tissue Banks
Abdominal aorta, 369, 373
Abdominal approach to Raney fusion, 405
Abdominal decompression, 87, 96
Abdominal retraction in anterior fusion, 374-376
Abdominal wound closure, 379-381
Abdullah, A., 18
Aberrant structures, percutaneous discectomy and, 118
Abradil, 10
Absorptiometry, 487
Acetaminophen, 319
Action potentials, 539
Activity level, 165
  Knodt rods and, 319
Adamkiewecz, A.A., 9
Adhesions, perineural, 117, 292, 503-504
Adhesive arachnoiditis, 504
Adkins approach to posterolateral fusion, 268
Adson, 17
Age
  fusion and, 411-412
  lateral extraforaminal herniations and, 198
  lumbar decompression and, 165
  osteoporosis and, 484
  spinal stenosis and, 277
  type II spondylolisthesis and, 282
Air-dried bone allograft, information sheet for, 467
Aitken, A.P., 115
Ala, fusion and, 277
  distraction rods and, 311-312
  spondylolisthesis, 280-281
Alajouanine, T.H., 7, 8
Alar hook, 310, 311
Albee, F.H., 11, 76, 237, 286
Albee bone graft method of spinal fusion, 238
Alcohol, excessive, 247
ALIF; see Anterior lumbar interbody fusion
Alkaline phosphatase, 486
Allen-Ferguson pelvic fixation, 84-85
Allergy to bone wax, 259
Allograft, 448-451; see also Bone graft
  information sheet for air-dried, 467
  in posterior lumbar interbody fusion, 293
  in posterolateral fusion, 270
  rehydration of, 467
  transplant record of, 468
Alpha-2-macroglobulins, 106
Alumina, 453
Ambulation after spine plating with pedicle screws, 330
American Association of Tissue Banks, 460
Analgesic pump, patient controlled, 401
Anaphylaxis, 105, 107
Anatomy, 65-71
  facet joint, 66-71
  intervertebral foramen, 196
  ligamentum flavum, 65-66
Ancef, 369, 381
Anderson, G.B.J., 10
André hook, 78
Andrews frame, 91-94, 281, 324
  lateral thigh supports of, 94
  microdiscectomy and, 125
  moving patient from, 94
  positioning in, 93-94
Anesthesia, 149-150
  epidural
    laminectomy and, 149
    microcatheter for, 161-162
    paralateral approach and, 178
  local; see Local anesthesia
  positioning for low back surgery and, 87-88
Angulation of spine, 266
Animal bone, 472
Ankle, valgus deformity of, 448
Annulus fibrosus, 37, 289
  anterior lumbar interbody fusion and, 376
    Raney, 405, 406, 407
  chymopapain and, 106, 107
  delamination of, 38
  electrophysiology and tear in, 543
  functions of, 38
  lateral extraforaminal herniations and bulge in, 207

Annulus fibrosus—cont'd
  pain and, 36, 529
  posterior, window in, 159
  posterior lumbar interbody fusion and, 289, 301
  structure of, 38, 48
  tensile properties of, 50
Antacids, 247
Anterior column pain, 383-384
Anterior cortex, pedicle screws and, 342
Anterior displacement, isthmic spondylolisthesis and, 280
Anterior iliac crest graft, 435-438
  anterior fusion and, 400
Anterior lumbar interbody fusion, 368-432
  abdominal retraction and, 374-376
  abdominal wound closure and, 379-381
  advantages of, 368-369, 419
  approach for, 384-392
  bone grafts in, 400
  complications in, 401
    rate of, 414, 415
  contraindications to, 384
  disadvantages of, 369
  dowel cutters and, 400
  failure rate in, 432
  graft harvesting and, 377-378
  graft site closure and, 381
  history of, 14-15, 368
  inability to obtain solid union in, 411
  indications for, 383-384, 415-419, 432
  kidney rest and, 400
  morbidity and, 414-419
    preoperative, 408-409
  occupation and, 417-419
  orthopedic technique for, 393-399
  postoperative care and, 381, 400-401
  postoperative clinical improvement in, 418, 419
  preoperative and postoperative morbidity and, 417-419
  published reports of, 415-417
  Raney technique for, 403-407
  results of, 408-432
    diagnostic studies and, 409-410
    editorial commentary on, 432
    indications and, 410-412
    morbidity criteria and, 414-419
    preoperative evaluation and, 412-414
    review of, 408-409
  team and equipment and, 384
  technique of, 369-373

Anterior lumbar interbody fusion—cont'd
  term of, 70
  transperitoneal exposure and, 373-374
  union rate in, 418
Anterior segment, 289
Anterior spinal flexion, 54, 55, 56
Anterior superior iliac spine
  avulsion or fracture of, 436, 438
  inguinal ligament attachment to, 438
Antibiotics
  bone for grafts and, 450, 451
  fat graft and, 504
  Raney anterior interbody fusion and, 403
Antibody, human thyrotropic lymphocytic virus-III, 463
Antidepressants, 116
Antigen
  chymopapain and, 107
  hepatitis B surface, 463
  transplantation, 451
Antigen extracted allogeneic bone, 451, 464, 472, 517
Antiinflammatories, 319
Anulus fibrosus; see Annulus fibrosus
A-O plate bender, 329
A-O screw, 344
Approach
  for anterior interbody fusion, 409
  for decompression in spinal stenosis, 171-174
  for laminotomy, 161
  for lateral extraforaminal herniations, 203
  for percutaneous lumbar fusion, 513-514
  for posterior lumbar intertransverse process fusion, 277
Arachnoiditis, adhesive, 150, 153, 504
  electrophysiology and, 547
Arch autografting, 219-220, 224
Arcuate line, 369, 370, 371
Arnell, S., 10
Arterial pressure, prone-sitting frame and, 101
Arteriosclerosis, 384, 401
Arteriovenous fistula, superior gluteal, 444
Arthropathy, facet, 529
Articular facet joint dysfunction, 58, 529
Articular process resection, 283
Articulating clamp, short-segment internal fixation and, 345-346, 349, 355, 360
Ascani, C., 16
Ascending transverse myelitis, 105
Asher, M., 13

Aspiration probe, automated nucleus, 143-145
Aspirin
  anterior lumbar interbody fusion and, 381
  hemostasis and, 135
  Knodt rod and, 319
  preoperative reduction of, 165
Autoclaving of bone, 450
Autodigested antigen-extracted allograft, 451, 464, 472, 517
Autodonation; see Autograft
Autogenous cancellous bone harvesting, 435; see also Autograft
Autogenous fat graft; see Fat graft
Autogenous marrow cells as additive, 471
Autograft, 434-442; see also Bone graft
  anterior lumbar interbody fusion and, 377, 400
  bilateral-lateral lumbar spine fusion and, 255-259
  extensive lumbar decompression and, 219-220, 224-226
  fat graft and; see Fat graft
  harvesting of cancellous, 435
  marrow cells and, 471
  microdiscectomy and, 124
  neural arch, 172, 219-220
  pars, 172
  unilateral arch, 224
Autolysed antigen-extracted allogeneic bone, 451, 464, 472, 517
Autostabilization in extensive lumbar decompression, 217-229; see also Lumbar decompression, extensive
Avitene, 505
Avulsion of anterior superior iliac spine, 436, 438
Axial compressive load, 38-39, 49-50
Axial pain, anterior fusion and, 411, 420, 421-422
Axial rotation of lumbosacral spine, 55
Axilla, protection of, 88
Axis of rotation
  helical, 57-58
  instantaneous, 55-57
    center of, 75
  internal fixation and, 75
Axon, 530

B
Babinski, 6
Bacitracin, 407

Back pain
  causes of, 266-267
  after disc excision, 272
  isthmic spondylolisthesis and, 280
  lateral extraforaminal herniations and, 200
  low, 53
    clinical biomechanics of, 40-43
  lumbar interbody fusion and
    anterior, 411, 420, 421-422, 429-430
    posterior, 287
Baer, W.S., 241
Bailey, P., 17
Balanced Tree Indexing method, 499
Balls, A.K., 103
Bank bone; see Bone banking
BAPNA; see DL-Benzoyl arginine-p-nitroanilide
Barr, J., 8, 103
Basildon frame, 90
Battson, O.V., 9
Beaver blade, microdiscectomy and, 130-131
Beckman retractor, 136
Beebe, S.P., 238
Bell and Lavyne modification of Taylor retractor, 137
Bennett retractor, force-fulcrum and, 137
Benzalkonium chloride, 451
DL-Benzoyl arginine-p-nitroanilide, 106
Benzyl alcohol, 150
Bertolotti, 7
Beta-propiolactone, 450, 451, 464
Bilateral laminectomy, 69, 70, 172
Bilateral-lateral lumbar spine fusion, 250-264
  in older patients, 271
  success rates for, 263-264
Bioactive material, 453
Biocompatible orthopaedic polymer, 482
Biodegradable ceramic, porous, 454
Bioglass, 474
Bioinert material, 453
Biomechanics, 35-64
  disc and, 37-40
    degeneration of, 40-43
  historical review of, 35-36
  internal fixation of spine and, 44-45
  kinematics of, 53-55
  pain and, 36-37, 40-43
  of pedicle screws, 323
  range of motion and, 55-59
    stability and, 59-61
  spinal fusion and, 43-44, 414

Biomechanics—cont'd
  stability and, 40-43
  surgical procedures and, 40-43
Biopsy
  bone, 248, 249, 487
  Craig needle, percutaneous discectomy and, 118
Biotolerant material, 453
Bipolar coagulation, 87
  forceps for, 208
  microdiscectomy and, 126
Bleeding; *see also* Hemostasis
  in anterior lumbar interbody fusion, 373
  chymopapain and, 106
  paralateral approach to decompression and, 182
  positioning for low back surgery and, 87
Block, facet nerve, 153
Block, F., 11
Blood flow, intraneural, 530-531
Blood tests, metabolic bone workup and, 248
Blood transfusion, 124
Blume dowel technique for posterior lumbar interbody fusion, 298
BMP; *see* Bone morphogenetic protein
Bohr, N., 11
Boiling of bone, 450
Bonding osteogenesis, 453
Bone
  allograft; *see* Allograft
  animal, 472
  banked; *see* Bone banking
  biopsy of, 248, 249, 487
  cancellous
    harvesting of, 435
    histology of, 459
  composition of, 484
  cortical
    histology of, 459
    iliac, 436, 437
  cutting of, lumbar surgery and, 213-214
  donor, 276, 460-463
  grain of, 214
  homologous, 278
  Kiel, 472
  Kobe, 472
  microdiscectomy and removal of, 120-121, 123, 130
  morphogenesis of
    percutaneous fusion and, 514-518
    synthetic grafts and, 472

Bone—cont'd
  Oswestry, 472
  resorption of, 484
  synthetic grafts and ingrowth of, 473
Bone banking, 459-470
  demand for, 460
  demineralization and, 464
  donor for, 276, 460-463
  editorial commentary and, 470
  facility for, 466
  freeze-drying and, 465
  operational manual for, 466
  organizational considerations and, 466
  posterior lumbar interbody fusion and, 304
  processing for, 463
  quality control and, 465-466
  record keeping and, 466-469
  secondary sterilization and, 464-465
  use of, 449, 470
Bone biopsy, 248, 249, 487
Bone cement, 446; *see also* Methylmethacrylate
  biodynamics and, 453
Bone densitometry, 248, 249
Bone disease, metabolic, 246-249
Bone flap from sacral ala, 325
Bone graft
  Albee spinal fusion method and, 238
  allograft; *see* Allograft
  anterior lumbar fusion and, 376-377, 400
    Raney technique for, 403, 404-405, 406-407
  autograft; *see* Autograft
  bilateral-lateral lumbar spine fusion and, 255-259
  complications of, 442-448
  failure of
    lumbosacral spine and, 434
    posterior lumbar interbody fusion and, 297, 298
  fibular, 403, 404-405, 406-407
  histology of, 459
  history of, 238-239, 241
  lumbar fusion with distraction rods and, 312
  methylmethacrylate cement and, 454; *see also* Methylmethacrylate
  muscle-pedicle, 448
  pedicle screw and, 329-330
  posterior, 343
  posterior interbody fusion

Bone graft—cont'd
  posterior interbody fusion—cont'd
    insertion of, 301, 303
    retropulsion of, 299
    slipping of, 295
  posterior migration of, 296
  posterolateral, preparation for, 325
  synthetic, 452-454, 471-482; see also Synthetic bone graft
    ingrowth of bone and, 473
    temperature and, 449
    uses of, 434
    xenografts and, 451-452
Bone graft substitute, 471-482
Bone impactor instruments, 231-233
Bone matrix, percutaneous lumbar fusion and, 516-518
Bone mineral content, 487
Bone morphogenetic protein, 451, 459, 464
  percutaneous lumbar fusion and, 514-518
Bone plug, 83
Bone spurs, 230-236
Bone transplant, history of, 459; see also Bone graft
Bone wax
  bilateral-lateral spine fusion and, 259
  microdiscectomy and, 130
  posterior iliac crest graft and, 439
  scar formation and, 505
Bone-cutting instruments, 181
Bone-forming cells
  percutaneous lumbar fusion and, 515
  synthetic grafts and, 472
Bone-screw interface strength, 344-345
Bony bridge, percutaneous lumbar fusion and, 514
Bony encroachment, lumbar decompression of, 230-236; see also Lumbar decompression
Bony ingrowth, synthetic bone grafts and, 473
Bony obstruction, chemonucleolysis and, 109-110
Booth, R., 12
Boplant, 452
Bosworth, 12
Bosworth technique for donor site hernia, 447
Boucher, H.H., 13, 84
Boucher method of screw fixation, 322
Bovine bone, 452

Bowel defect and bone abnormalities, 247
Bracewell, R.N., 10
Brachial plexus protection, 88
Brackett, E.G., 241
Bradford, C.H., 115
Bradford, D., 16
Breakage
  of Knodt rod, 320
  of screw, 331, 338, 343-344
Briggs, H., 15
Brissaud, 6
Broad decompressive laminectomy, 69
Brodsky, A.E., 17
Broken pedicle or screw, 331, 338
Brown, J., 104
B-tricalcium phosphate and bone morphogenetic protein, 454
Buck, R.E., 16
Bulging disc, 38-39; see also Herniated disc
  computed tomography scans of, 347
  loading and, 38, 49
Bupivacaine
  discography and, 414
  laminectomy and, 149, 158
    epidural, 162
  microdiscectomy and, 126, 129, 131
  paralateral approach and, 186
Burnout, sciatic, 148
Burns, B.H., 14
Burr
  high-speed, 214, 231
  for plate and pedicle screw system, 325
Buttocks
  cushions for, 98
  neuritis of, bone grafts and, 443
Buttress thread, 359-360

C

Cable, Dwyer, 80
Cadaver graft, history of, 471
CADUCEUS; see Committee Advocating the Development and Use of Chymopapain to Eliminate Unnecessary Surgery
Calciferol, 247
Calcitonin, 484, 489
Calcium, 248, 249
  bone abnormalities and, 247
  oral supplements of, 248, 249
  osteoporosis and, 485, 487-488
  serum, 486

Calcium aluminate, 453
Calcium carbonate, 488
Calcium gluconate, 482, 488
Calcium hydroxyapatite, 453, 454, 474
Calcium lactate, 488
Calcium loading, 248, 249
Calcium phosphate ceramic, 453
Calcium phosphate–coated metallic implant, 454
Calderol, 247
Campbell, W.C., 12, 15, 25
Campbell exposure in posterolateral fusion, 268
Cancellous bone
  harvesting of, 435
  histology of, 459
Cancer, endometrial, 488
Cannula tube in percutaneous fusion, 523
Carbon, biodynamics of, 453
Carbon dioxide laser, 210, 211
  cutting mode of, 215
Carbonizing of tissue, 209, 211
C-arm fluoroscopy, 88, 413
Cartilage, excision of facet, 277
Cartilage activation factor, embryonic, 482
Casamajor, C., 17
Catheter
  Fogarty, 444
  Foley, 87-88
    anesthesia access during surgery and, 87-88
    anterior lumbar interbody fusion and, 369
Cauchoix, J., 7
Cauda equina, damage to nerve roots of, 369
Cautery
  bilateral-lateral lumbar spine fusion and, 251-252
  lateral extraforaminal herniations and, 203
  laminotomy and, 228
Cell membrane lipoprotein, 451
Cellulose, 203
Center of instant axis of rotation, 75
Central canal
  electrophysiology and stenosis of, 544
  herniations in, 197, 198
Central laminectomy, results of, 173
Central recess stenosis, bilateral-lateral fusion and, 260, 261
Ceramics, 454, 472
  calcium phosphate, 453
  glass, 453

Ceramics—cont'd
  hydroxyapatite, 453
  porous biodegradable, 454
Cerebrospinal fluid, 530
Cerosium, 473
Chemical treatment of grafts, 450-451
Chemolase, 105, 106
Chemonucleolysis, 68, 103-114
  bony obstruction and, 109-110
  complications of, 31, 105
  criteria for, 108-109
  danger of intravenous injection in, 113-114
  first, 9
  injection technique in, 109-112
  lateral extraforaminal herniations and, 203
  patient selection in, 107-108
  pharmacology in, 105-107
  preoperative evaluation and preparation in, 109
  toxicology in, 105-107
Chest cushions, 97, 98-99
Chiba needle, 413
Chisel, 214
  anterior iliac crest bone grafts and, 436
  circular, anterior fusion and, 393-398
  Cloward Puka, 378
Chord length, 347, 351, 352, 357-358
Chymodiactin, 105
Chymopapain, 68, 103-114; see also Chemonucleolysis
Cimetidine, 162
Circular chisel, 393-398
Circumflex iliac artery, deep, 443-444, 446
Clamps, articulating, 345-346, 349, 355, 360
Cleveland, M., 12
Clinical biomechanics; see Biomechanics
Clinical instability, 42; see also Instability
Clinical stability, 40; see also Stability
Closure; see also Suture
  abdominal, 379-381
  microdiscectomy and, 131
  of rectus sheath, 391, 392
Clothespin graft, 76
Cloward, R.B., 15, 25, 286
Cloward's indications for lumbar spine fusions, 288
Cloward chisel, 378
Cloward impactor, 378
Cloward osteotome, 220, 222
Cloward posterior lumbar interbody fusion, 15, 286
  results of, 298

Cloward retractor, microdiscectomy and, 126, 127, 130
Cloward spinous process spreader, 220, 222
Cluneal nerves
  injuries to, 442
  posterior iliac crest graft and, 439, 443, 445
Coagulation, bipolar, 87, 126
  forceps for, 208
Cobalt radiation, 450, 464
  immune reaction to, 517
Cobb dissector, 135, 136
Cobb elevators, bilateral-lateral lumbar fusion and, 252, 257
Coccygeal pain, Knodt rods and, 320
Cold, bone grafts and, 449
Collagen, 38, 48, 160
Collagenase, 68
Collis indications for posterior lumbar interbody fusion, 287
Collis posterior lumbar interbody fusion, results of, 299
Committee Advocating the Development and Use of Chymopapain to Eliminate Unnecessary Surgery, 104
Common iliac vessel, left, 390
Common peroneal nerve protection, 88
Compartment syndrome, postoperative, 96
Compatibility of hardware and software, 501
Compere, E., 8
Complex nerve sheath, 67-68
Complex repetitive discharges, 537
Composite graft of autogenous fat, 508
Compound action potential, 532-533, 539
  postoperative stenosis and, 546
Compression neuropathy, 503-504, 532
Compression strength of vertebral bodies, 51
Computed tomography
  anterior interbody fusion and, 412
  cutting scar tissue with hot wire and, 213
  fat grafts and, 505, 506, 507
  laminectomy and, 150, 151, 152
  lateral extraforaminal herniations and, 201, 202
  of lumbar spine, 524-527
  before microdiscectomy, 124
  of neural arch autograft, 222, 223
  osteoporosis and, 487
  paralateral approach to decompression and, 182, 183, 184, 185
  pars autograft and, 226, 227
  pedicle measurements and, 347-348, 350-353, 357-358

Computed tomography—cont'd
  percutaneous nuclectomy and, 141, 142, 143, 146
  subarticular stenosis and, 159
  whole-body, 177-178
Computer assistance, 491-502
  technical aspects of, 498-502
Computer-generated report, 495
Concentric needle electrode, 535
Conduction, percutaneous spine fusion and, 514-518
Conduction blocks, 531-532
Conjugated estrogens, 488
Conray, history of, 10
Consent, informed, 109, 460-461, 462
Conservative measures, trends in, 3-4
Contact osteogenesis, 453
Contact pressure of plates and screws, 341
Continuous-wave laser mode, 215
Contrast media
  computed tomography scan and, 412; see also Computed tomography
  discography and, 413
  laminectomy and, 150
Contraves microscope stand, 126
Coordinate system in kinematics of spine, 53-54
Coral, 473
  hydroxyapatite modeled on, 474-480
    disadvantages of, 477-480
    mechanical characteristics of, 475
Cord lesion, scans of, 347
Core evacuation gouge, 398, 399
Cormak, A.M., 10
Cortical bone, histology of, 459
Cortical engagement of pedicle screws, 342
Cortical window, iliac crest, 436, 437, 440
Corticosteroids
  after laminectomy, 162
  microdiscectomy and, 126, 129
  neural movement and, 530
  scar formation and, 505
Cortisone, 505
Cosmetic results
  in fusion for high-grade spondylolisthesis, 281
  incision and, 135
Cotrel, 13
Cotugno, D., 5
Coupling, 57-58, 266
Coventry, 8
Craig needle biopsy, 118

Cramer, F., 17
Creep of fixator, 341
Creeping substitution, 459, 472
Crock, H., 9, 14
Crock curette, 393, 396
Crock indications for lumbar spine fusions, 288
CSF; *see* Cerebrospinal fluid
Culture, banked bone, 465
Curette
    Crock, 393, 396
    down-cutting, reoperation and, 191, 192
    Epstein, 131
    for iliac gutters, 255, 257
    O'Brien, 393, 396
    posterior iliac crest graft and, 440
    scraping ligament or osteophyte from bony margin, 231
    sharpening of, 252-254
    sonic, 214-215
Cushing dissector, 136
Cushions
    attaching and adjusting, 98-100
    face rest, 100-101
    kneeling frame, 96-98
    positioning patient and, 95-96
    prone-sitting frame, 96-98
Cutaneous nerve, lateral femoral
    injuries to, 436, 442
    protection of, 88
Cutting tools
    lumbar surgery and, 213-215
    osteophyte spurs and bony encroachments and, 231
    sharpness of, 214, 215
CW laser mode; *see* Continuous-wave laser mode

D

Dacron, 510
Damadian, R., 11
Dandy, W.E., 7, 10
Danforth, M., 7
Data base systems, 499-501
Data recording and processing, 491-502
Dawson floating fusions, 270
De novo osteosynthesis, 515
Decompression
    abdominal, in surgery, 87
    by driving spur or bar into vertebral body with impactors, 235-236
    extent of, in laminectomy, 159, 163

Decompression—cont'd
    far lateral, 175-186; *see also* Far lateral decompression
    indications and selection of approach to, 171-174
    lumbar, 230-236; *see also* Lumbar decompression
        exposures for, 134-140; *see also* Exposure
        extensive, 69, 164-174, 217-229; *see also* Lumbar decompression, extensive
        positioning patient for, 95-102; *see also* Positioning
        results of, 173
    midline
        dysplastic spondylolisthesis and, 279
        intertransverse process fusion and, 172
    paralateral, 175-186; *see also* Far lateral decompression
        results of, 173
    percutaneous lumbar fusion and, 512
    posterior
        Knodt rods and, 316
        spinal instability and, 42-43
    posterior lumbar interbody fusion and, 292-293; *see also* Posterior lumbar interbody fusion
        indications for, 415
    posterolateral fusion using spine plates and pedicle screws and, 324
    reoperation after failed spine surgery and, 189
    spondylolisthesis and, 284, 285
    subarticular, results of, 173
Decompressive laminectomy
    broad or wide, 69; *see also* Lumbar decompression, extensive
    in reoperation after failed spine surgery, 189
Decortication
    lumbar fusion and
        bilateral-lateral, 254-255, 256
        percutaneous, 513-514
    transverse process, Knodt rod and, 318
Deep circumflex iliac artery, 443-444, 446
Deep paraspinal procaine anesthesia, 149-150
Degeneration, disc
    biomechanics of, 40-43
    computed tomography of, 347
    posterior intertransverse process fusion and, 270
    posterior lumbar interbody fusion and, 292

Degeneration, disc—cont'd
  in recurrent tears with bulge pattern and without signs of focal protrusion, 543-544
  spinal implant for, 339-367; *see also* Internal fixation; Short-segment internal fixation
Degenerative spondylolisthesis, 283
  biomechanics of, 41
  posterior intertransverse process fusion and, 272
Demineralization, bone banking and, 464
Demirleau, J., 12
Densitometry, bone, 248, 249
DePalma, A., 12
Depo-Medrol, 126, 129
Depression, low back pain and, 116
Dermis, porcine, 510
Destabilization; *see* Instability
Device removal, short-segment internal fixation and, 342
Dexamethasone, 162
Diagnostic techniques
  computer reports and, 498
  failed surgical patient and, 188
  history of, 10-11
  trends in, 2-3
Diagnostician-physiatric team member, 541-542
Diazepam, 149, 178
Diet, fat-free, 504
1,25 Dihydroxy vitamin D, 484
Dimeray, history of, 10
Dimerex, history of, 10
Diphenhydramine, 162
Disc, intervertebral, 37
  bilateral excision of, 70
  biomechanics of, 37-40, 48-50
  bulging, 38-39; *see also* Herniated disc
    loading and, 38, 49
  degeneration of; *see* Degeneration, disc
  geometry and material properties of, 52
  herniation of; *see* Herniated disc
  history of disease of, 5-10
  loads on, 49
  microdiscectomy and, 130-131
  ruptured, first diagnosis of, 8
  standup, 150, 159
  structural specifications of, 36-37
Disc bars, 230-236
  impaction along posterior ridge of, 235
Disc center depth determination, 110, 111

Disc degeneration; *see* Degeneration, disc
Disc disruption syndrome, 384
Disc material, anterior fusion and removal of, 393, 395
Disc osteophyte
  lumbar decompression of, 230-236; *see also* Lumbar decompression
  posterolateral, 67
Disc protrusion; *see* Herniated disc
Disc space
  determining depth of, 393, 397
  infection of, anterior interbody fusion and, 427-428
  internal fixation and, 83-84
  lamina relationship to, 65, 66
Disc stability, biomechanics of, 40-43; *see also* Stability
Disc surgery, history of, 5-10
Discase; *see* Chymopapain
Discectomy, 70, 141, 149, 158-159; *see also* Laminectomy
  facet joint removal and, 153
  microdiscectomy and, 130-131
  percutaneous, 115-122; *see also* Percutaneous discectomy
  results of midline, 173
Discogenic pain; *see* Pain
Discography
  anterior interbody fusion and, 412, 413-414
  disc disruption syndrome and, 384
  integrity of anterior joint of three-joint complex and, 383
  lateral extraforaminal herniations and, 200-201, 202
  multilevel, 412
  needle for, 413
Disc-oriented scanning, 151
Dislocation, internal fixation for unstable, 336; *see also* Internal fixation
  Knodt rods in, 320
Displastic spondylolisthesis, 279
Disposition form, 496-497
Dissection, laminectomy and laminotomy and, 130, 136, 153-158
Dissector
  Cobb, 136
  Cushing, 136
  Hoehn, 135, 136
  Penfield, 130
Distance osteogenesis, 453
Distraction rod, 306-314; *see also* specific rod

Dommisse, G.F., 9
Donor bone, 276
   information form for, 460, 461
   length of time between death and tissue procurement of, 460
   selection of, 460-463
Donor site
   posterior iliac crest graft and, 439
   Raney anterior interbody fusion and, 404
Dorsal primary ramus, 529
Dorsal root ganglion, 530
Double-crush phenomenon, 533
Double-needle technique, 110
Dowel, precut, 304
Dowel cutter
   anterior fusion and, 398, 400
   anterior iliac crest bone grafts and, 437
Down-cutting curettes, reoperation and, 191, 192
DRG; *see* Dorsal root ganglion
Drills, 214
Drummond and Keene spinous process fixation, 76-77
Dual photon absorptiometry, 487
Dubausset, 13
Dunn device for anterior instrumentation, 82-83
Dura
   chymopapain and, 106
   fat graft for defect in, 505-507
   Knodt rods and, 320
   posterolateral fusion using spine plates and pedicle screws and, 325
   of spinal nerve root, 530
   tear of, in redo surgery, 193
Dural sac, transversing, 66
Dural sheath, microdiscectomy and, 130
Durapatite, 474
Dutaillis, D.P., 8
Dwyer cable fixation of pedicles, 80
Dwyer screw fixation of pedicles, 78, 79
Dwyer vertebral body instrumentation and fusion, 82
Dyck, W., 13

E

Edema
   entrapment and, 169
   intraneural, 531
Edward sleeve in laminar fixation, 78
Edwards, C., 308
Edwards system for internal fixation, 194, 313
   history of, 13
Ehni, G., 17
Ejaculation, retrograde, 373, 401
Elastic stockings, 88
Elasticity of disc and vertebral body, 50
Electric knife in, laminotomy, 228
Electrodiagnostician-physiatric team member, 541-542
Electrocautery
   bilateral-lateral lumbar spine fusion and, 251-252
   posterior iliac crest graft and, 439
Electrodiagnostics, 540-543; *see also* Electrophysiology in lumbar pain
   efficacy of, 529
Electromyography, 528-551; *see also* Electrophysiology in lumbar pain
   limitations of, 540-542
   values of, 540
Electrophysiology in lumbar pain, 528-551; *see also* Electromyography
   clinical subsets and, 543-545
      failed back surgery, 545-547
   epidural fibrosis and, 547
   findings in
      acute and chronic, 539-540
      appearance and disappearance of, 544
   infection and, 548-549
   instability and, 547-548
   nerve injury and, 530-532
   neurophysiology in, 532-543
      electrodiagnostician responsibilities and, 540-543
      terms in, 532-540
   potential pain generators and, 528-530
   recurrent disc protrusion and, 548
   referral pain and, 528-530
   spinal adhesive arachnoiditis and, 547
Electrosurgery, 135, 209-210
   laser resection of tissues vs., 211
   reopening and resecting with hot wire loop in, 211-213
Elevator
   Cobb, 252, 257
   Fraser, 122
Elsberg, C., 17
Emboli to femoral artery, 384, 401
Embolization, bone grafts and, 444
Embryonic cartilage activation factor, 482

Emotional status, 165
Endocrine disorders, 485
Endometrial cancer, 488
Endorphins, 319
End-plate, 37
    biomechanics and, 50, 51
    separation of, 393, 395
    subperiosteal exposure of, 393, 394
Entrance zone, 196
Entrapment, 230-236, 503-504; see also Lumbar decompression
    edema and, 169
    estimating degree of freedom from, 160
    hypoxia and, 169
    between moving elements, 169
    between nonmoving elements, 169
    peripheral nerve, nerve conduction studies in, 533
Epidermal migration of reparative cells, 211
Epidural anesthesia
    fibrillation potential of paraspinal muscles and, 537
    laminectomy and, 149
    microcatheter for, 161-162
    paralateral approach and, 178
    after redo surgery for failed spine surgery, 194
Epidural fat graft, 503-511; see also Fat graft
    complications of, 31
    editorial commentary on, 511
    epidural fibrosis and, 503-504
    free, 504-508
    ligamentum flavum and, 509-510
    microdiscectomy and, 130
    obtaining, 508-509
    perineural fibrosis and, 503-504
    synthetics as barriers to fibrosis and, 510
Epidural fibrosis, 503-504
    electrophysiology of lumbar pain and, 547
    posterior lumbar interbody fusion and, 304
Epidural morphine, 161-162
Epinephrine
    bilateral-lateral lumbar spine fusion and, 251
    lumbar surgery and, 135
    microdiscectomy and, 129
Epineurium, 530
Epstein curette, 131
Erratic motion patterns, 41-42
Estrogen, 484, 488
Ethinyl estradiol, 488

Ethylene chlorohydrin, 465
Ethylene dioxide, 450, 451
Ethylene glycol, 465
Ethylene oxide gas, 464, 465
Euler equation, 50
Evoked response, 532-533, 539
Ewing, J., 238
Excision, disc; see Discectomy
Exercises, therapeutic, 124
Exit zone, 196
Exposure
    anterior fusion, 369-374, 386
    laminectomy and laminotomy, 153-158
    lumbar decompression and fusion, 134-140
        force-fulcrum retractors in, 136-137
        muscle stripping and, 136
        retraction in, 136
        skin marking and incision in, 134-136
        stability at tip in, 137-140
    retroperitoneal, 369-373
    subperiosteal end-plate, 393, 394
    of thecal sac, 260
    transperitoneal, 373-374
Extension of lumbar spine, 54, 55, 56
    positioning patient and, 96
Extensive lumbar decompression, 164-174, 217-229; see also Lumbar decompression, extensive
External fixator, disadvantages of, 342-343
Extradural morphine, 182
Extraforaminal disc, 195
    herniation of lateral, 197, 198; see also Herniated disc lateral to intervertebral foramen
    level of, 198, 199
Extreme lateral disc, 195; see also Herniated disc lateral to intervertebral foramen
Eyes, protection of, 88

F

Face rest cushion, 100-101
Facet; see also Facet joint; Facetectomy
    decompressing ganglion and nerve through, 229
    decompressing stenosing uncinate spur through, 174
    destruction of, 171
    drilling through, 174
    orientation of, 58
    rods or plates and damage to, 278
    vertical loading and, 51, 52

Facet block, 153
  after redo surgery for failed spine surgery, 194
Facet capsule
  microdiscectomy and, 130
  pain mechanism and, 36
Facet cartilage excision, 277
Facet joint, 66-67; *see also* Facet; Facetectomy
  anatomy of, 66-71
  capsules of
    microdiscectomy and, 130
    pain mechanism and, 36
  discectomy and removal of, 153
  dysfunction of articular, 58
  fixation of
    internal, 84
    Mangerl, 84
  function of, 39-40
  fusion of, 70
    oblique screw in, 343
  pain in
    arthropathy, 529
    electrophysiology and, 544-545
    percutaneous lumbar fusion and, 512, 513
  spreading of, 229
Facet nerve block, 153
  after redo surgery for failed spine surgery, 194
Facet screw, 70
Facet syndrome, percutaneous lumbar fusion and, 512, 513
Facetectomy, 69
  anterior interbody fusion and, 427-428
  failed spine surgery and, 189, 191
  laminotomy with partial, 69
Failed back surgery syndrome, 117; *see also* Failed posterior lumbar interbody fusion; Failed posterior spine surgery
  decision on reoperating in, 188
  electromyography and, 540-541, 545-547
Failed posterior lumbar interbody fusion, 187-194, 296-305; *see also* Failed back surgery syndrome
  clinical series of, 298-300
  technical aspects of, 301-305
Failed posterior spine surgery, 187-194; *see also* Failed back surgery syndrome; Failed posterior lumbar interbody fusion
  discussion of, 187-189
  technique in, 189-194

Far lateral decompression, 175-186
  additional considerations and, 181-182
  choice between midline approach and, 175
  clean-out of disc space and, 181-182
  drainage and, 182
  exposure in, 179
  fascia and, 179
  procedure in, 178-181
  results of, 173
  using midline incision, 203, 204
Far lateral disc, 195
Far lateral zone, 196
Far out syndrome, 67
Farfan, H.F., 9
Far out entrapment, 169, 170
Fascial planes, dissection through, 179, 208
Fasciculation potentials, 537
Fat graft
  bilateral-lateral spine fusion and, 261
  epidural; *see* Epidural fat graft
  free, 504-508
    microdiscectomy and, 131
  harvesting of, 504
  incision and, 135
  isogenous, 507
  laminectomy and, 160, 161-162
  neural arch autograft and, 222
  paralateral approach and, 179
  pedicle, 507
  posterior intertransverse fusion and, 276
  scar formation and, 213, 505
  too large, 505
Fat pad preservation, 67
Fat-fascia graft, 135, 510
  laminectomy and, 160
Fat-free diet, 504
Fatigue fracture, tibial, 448
FBSS; *see* Failed back surgery syndrome
Feeding tube, 160
Femoral nerve
  injuries to, 436, 442
  protection of, 88
Femoral vessels
  plaque emboli to, 384, 401
  protection of, 88
Fentanyl, 149, 178
Fiber geometry, 52
Fiberoptic lighting, 126
Fibrillation potentials, 535-536
  postoperative stenosis and, 545
  sick nerve syndrome and, 546

Fibrosis
  epidural, 503–504
    electrophysiology and, 547
    posterior lumbar interbody fusion and, 304
  intraneural, electrophysiology and, 546–547
  perineural, 117, 292, 503–504
Fibular bone graft, 448
  Raney anterior fusion and, 403, 404–405, 406–407
Finite element analysis, 52–53
Fistula, superior gluteal arteriovenous, 444
Fixation; *see also* Fixator
  cement and implant, 454; *see also* Methylmethacrylate
  internal; *see* Internal fixation
  pedicle, 79–81
  sacral, 84–85, 308–310
Fixator; *see also* Fixation
  creep of, 341
  external, disadvantages of, 342–343
  as load transducer, 343
Flap
  from annulus fibrosus, 405, 406, 407
  from sacral ala, 325
Flexion of spine, 54, 55, 56, 291–292
  positioning of patient and, 96
Flexion/extension film, abnormal motion and, 410
Floating fusion, Dawson, 270
Fluoride, 247, 489
Fluorocarbon, high-density, 482
Fluoroscopy
  anterior interbody fusion and, 413
  chemonucleolysis and, 109
  nerve location and, 179
  percutaneous discectomy and, 118
  percutaneous nuclectomy and, 143, 145
  root or ganglion injections and, 179
Fogarty catheter, 444
Foley catheter
  anesthesia access during surgery and, 87–88
  anterior lumbar interbody fusion and, 369
Food and Drug Administration, 104
Footed impactor, 232, 233
Foraminal stenosis
  electrophysiology and, 544
  after spine plating with pedicle screws, 333
Foraminal zone, 196

Foraminotomy, 69
  degenerative spondylolisthesis and, 283
  lumbar fusion with distraction rods and, 311
  pantaloon and spica cast and, 271
  in reoperation after failed spine surgery, 189
Force-fulcrum retractor, 136–137
Forceps, bipolar coagulator, 208
Forestier, 10
Fourth lumbar artery, 443–444, 446
Fracture
  anterior fusion and, 383
  of anterior superior iliac spine, 436, 438
  fatigue, tibial donor site and, 448
  spinal implant for, 339–367; *see also* Internal fixation; Short-segment internal fixation
  stability of, 59–60
  surgical management of, 356
  of transverse processes, 254, 255
  unstable
    internal fixation for, 336
    percutaneous lumbar fusion and, 512, 513
Fraenkel, J., 16
Frame
  Andrews; *see* Andrews frame
  Basildon, 90
  cushioning and; *see* Cushions
  Gardner, 90
  Hall, 90
  Hastings, 91, 251, 281
  Hicks, 91
  Norfolk, 90
  positioning patient and, 95–96
  Relton, 90
  Taylor, 91
    modified, 101
Fraser, R., 10
Fraser elevator, 122
Free fat graft, 504–508; *see also* Fat graft
  microdiscectomy and, 131
Freebody, D., 14
Freeze-dried bone
  allografts and, 449
  biomechanical properties of, 450
  bone banking and, 465
Freezing, allografts and, 449
Friction fibrosis in spinal nerve roots, 531
Friedman, W., 141

Friedman technique for percutaneous discectomy, 118
Front-back stenosis, 168, 169
Frymoyer, J.W., 12
Frymoyer-Vermont internal fixation device, 313
Function
  anterior interbody fusion and, 417-419
  motion studies of lumbar spine and, 524-527
Functional spinal unit, 266
Fusion
  abnormal biomechanics and, 414
  anterior interbody; see Anterior lumbar interbody fusion
  autograft, extensive lumbar decompression and, 224-226
  bilateral-lateral lumbar spine, 250-264
    success rates for, 263-264
  bilateral-lateral lumbosacral, in older patients, 271
  biomechanics of, 43-44, 267-268
  complications of, 44
  distraction rods and, 306-314
  exposures for, 134-140; see also Exposure
  facet joint, 70
    oblique screws and, 70
  failed spine surgery and; see Failed back surgery syndrome; Failed posterior lumbar interbody fusion
  history of, 15, 237-245
  indications for, 43-44
  intertransverse process
    bone graft substitute and, 475-480
    midline approach for, 172
  isthmic spondylolisthesis and level of, 280
  of knee, first description of, 241
  metabolic bone disease and, 246-249
  percutaneous spine, 512-523; see also Percutaneous spine fusion
  positioning patient for, 95-102; see also Positioning
  posterior; see Posterior fusion
  posterior intertransverse; see Posterior intertransverse fusion
  posterior lumbar interbody; see Posterior lumbar interbody fusion
  primary, relative indications for, 411
  results of
    one- and two-level fusion in, 416
    poor, 44
F-wave, 534

G

Gamma radiation, cobalt, 450, 464, 517
Ganglion knife, 325, 327, 328
Gardner frame, 90
Garvin, P.J., 104
Gastrografin, 118
Gelatin foam, 510
Gelfoam
  bilateral-lateral spine fusion and, 259, 261, 262
  microdiscectomy and, 126, 130
  posterior iliac crest graft and, 439
  scar formation and, 505
  in thrombin
    and anterior fusion, 378, 379, 381
    and hemostasis, 87
    and microdiscectomy, 126, 130
Gellman, H., 141
Gelpi retractor, 136
Gerster, A., 17
Ghormley, R.K., 12
Gibson, 76
Gill procedure in spondylolisthesis, 271
Glass ceramic, 453
Glucocorticoids, 67
Glycoprotein, 451
Goald microdiscectomy, 119
Goldner, J.L., 14
Goldthwait, J., 7
Goniopora, 474, 475
Gouge, posterior iliac crest graft and, 440
Graft
  anterior fusion
    closure of site of, 381
    harvesting of, 377-378
    insertion of, 399, 400
    review of technique for, 409
    site preparation for, 398, 399
    slot, 376-377
  bone; see Bone graft
  extrusion of, after posterior lumbar interbody fusion, 301, 302
  fat; see Fat graft
    epidural; see Epidural fat graft
  fat/fascial, 510
    laminectomy and, 160
  maintaining viability of, 222-224
  neural arch, results of, 173
  sterility of, 465
  synthetic; see Synthetic bone graft
Graham, C.E., 10
Grain of bone, 214

H

Hadra, B., 11, 76
Hall frame, 90
HAM; *see* Helical axis of motion
Hamstring tightness, spondylolisthesis and, 279, 280, 282
Hardware, computer, 501
Harman, P.D., 14
Harmon, P., 14
Harrington, P.R., 13, 16
Harrington hook, 308, 341
Harrington rod, 3
  with alar hooks and intersegmental wires, 310
  attached to pedicle screw, 308-309
  contouring of, 78, 79
  in failed surgery patient, 193
  history of, 13
  internal fixation with fusion and, 70-71
  laminar fixation and, 77-78
  length of, 340, 341
  lumbar spine and, 277-278, 307, 311
  lumbosacral spinal fusion and, 45
  motion limitation and, 341
  pedicular fixation and, 80
  procedure for, 311
Harvesting
  of autogenous cancellous bone, 435
  of fat graft, 504
Hastings frame, 91, 251, 281
Healing, wound
  electrosurgery and, 209, 211, 212
  laser surgery and, 211
Heat, grafts and, 450-451
Helical axis of motion, 57-58
Helium-neon pilot-light beam, 210
Hemifacetectomy, 69
Hemorrhage; *see* Bleeding; Hemostasis
Hemostasis, 87, 160
  anterior lumbar interbody fusion and, 378-379
  bone grafts and, 444
  microdiscectomy and, 121
  Raney anterior interbody fusion and, 407
Hemostatic agent, 160
Hemovac drain, 263
He-Ne pilot-light beam; *see* Helium-neon pilot-light beam
Heparin, 485
Hepatitis B surface antigen, 463
Hernia through iliac bone graft donor site, 444-447

Herniated disc, 40
  in central canal, 197, 198
  choice of procedure for, 116-117
  classification of, 197, 198, 199
  computed tomography scans of, 347
  electrophysiology and, 543, 548
  finding exact location of, 158
  laminectomy for; *see* Laminectomy
  lateral to intervertebral foramen, 195-207
    anatomy in, 196-197
    classification of, 197
    clinical appearance of, 198-200
    editorial commentary and, 207
    incidence of, 197-198
    level of, 198, 199
    radiographic findings and, 200-202
    treatment options and, 203-206
  lumbar laminotomy and, 148
  recurrent
    electrophysiology in, 548
    failed spine surgery and, 189
  results of procedures for, 117
  unilateral, stenosis with, 172
Hibbs, R.A., 11, 238-239, 240-241, 242, 244, 286
Hibbs retractor, 135
Hicks frame, 91
Hidden zone, 169, 170, 218
High-speed burr, 214, 231
Hip, protection of, 88
Hirsch, C., 8, 103
Histology
  of bone graft, 459
History
  of bone transplant, 459
  lumbar spine surgery, 5-23
    anterior interbody fusion in, 14-15, 368
    clinical biomechanics in, 35-36
    diagnostic techniques in, 10-11
    disc surgery in, 5-10
    internal fixation in, 13-14
    intervertebral disc disease in, 5-10
    lumbar spine fusion in, 11-12, 237-245
    metallic implants in, 12-13
    neurosurgeon and, 24-26
    posterior lumbar interbody fusion in, 15
    spondylolisthesis reduction in, 15-16
    sacroiliac joint fusion in, 15
    spinal stenosis in, 16-18
History questionnaire, comprehensive, 493
Hitjikata, S., 141
Hittoff-Crookes tube, 6

Hodgson, A.R., 14
Hoe retractor, 372, 375
Hoehn dissector, 135, 136
Hofmann apparatus, history of, 13
Homogenous bone, 400
Homologous bone, 278
Hook
 Andre design for, 78
 complications of, 342
 Harrington, 308, 341
 Knodt, 308, 316, 317
Hoop stress in annulus fibrosus, 37
Hormone replacement, 247
Houndsfield, G.N., 10
H-reflex, 533-534
hSGF; *see* Human skeletal growth factor
Hudgins microdiscectomy, 123
Hudgins modification of Williams microsurgical discectomy, 119-120
Hult, L., 10
Human skeletal growth factor, 516
Human thyrotropic lymphocytic virus III antibody, 463
Humphries, A.W., 14
Hurd retractor, 260
Hutter posterior lumbar interbody fusion, results of, 299
Hydrochloric acid, 464
Hydrogen peroxide, 451, 464
25 Hydroxy vitamin D, 247, 484
Hydroxyapatite, 453, 471
 synthetic bone grafts and, 473
 modeled from coral, 474-480
  disadvantages of, 477-480
  mechanical characteristics of, 475
Hyperextension, 96
Hyperlordosis, 96
Hyperostoses, 230-236
Hypogastric plexus, 369
Hypoxia, entrapment and, 169

I

IAR; *see* Instantaneous axis of rotation
Iatrogenic instability, 217, 272-273, 275
IEU; *see* International Enzyme Units
Iliac artery, 443-444, 446
 laceration of, 369
Iliac contour preservation, 436, 438
Iliac crest; *see also* Iliac crest bone graft
 as bone graft reserve, 435
 paralateral approach to decompression and, 179

Iliac crest—cont'd
 Raney anterior interbody fusion and, 403-404, 406
 superior, anterior fusion and, 384
Iliac crest bone graft; *see also* Iliac crest
 anterior, 435-438
 bilateral-lateral lumbar spine fusion and, 255-259
 posterior, 439-442
Iliac gutters, curette for, 255, 257
Iliac spine
 anterior superior
  avulsion or fracture of, 436, 438
  inguinal ligament attachment to, 438
Iliac vessels, 369, 373, 390
Iliac wing defect, 446
Iliohypogastric nerve injuries, 442, 443
Ilio-inguinal nerve injuries, 442, 443
Iliolumbar ligament, 181
Iliolumbar vessels, 373, 443
Iliotransverse ligament stabilization, 219
Iliovertebral ligament stabilization, 219
Illumination, microdiscectomy and, 121, 126
Image intensifier, 109
Immune reaction, 448, 517
Impact osteotomy, 252, 254
Impaction, 231-236
Impactor
 Cloward, 378
 for decompression of bony excrescences, 231-233
 for inferior pedicle, 233-235
 pedicle screw internal fixation and, 335
Implant
 bone; *see* Bone graft
 cement and fixation of, 454; *see also* Methylmethacrylate
 metallic
  calcium phosphate–coated, 454
  history of, 12-13
 spinal
  anterior vs. posterior, 357
  loads on, 360
  titanium mesh, 452-453
In situ transverse process fusion, 279-283
In vivo load, short-segment internal fixation and, 343-344
Inaccessible zone, 169, 170
 extensive lumbar decompression and, 169-171, 218-219
 laminotomy approaches for, 226-229

Incision
  for anterior fusion, 369, 384, 385, 386, 388
  for anterior iliac crest bone grafts, 435-436
  for bilateral-lateral lumbar spine fusion, 251
  for fat graft harvesting, 508
  for laminectomy and laminotomy, 65, 134-136, 153-158
  for lumbar fusion with distraction rods, 311
  midline, 311, 324, 369
  for paralateral approach, 179, 203, 204
  for percutaneous discectomy, 118
  posterior iliac crest graft and, 439
  for posterolateral fusion with spine plates and pedicle screws, 324
  for Raney anterior interbody fusion, 403, 405
Index Sequential Access Method, 499
Indigo carmine, 128
Induction, percutaneous spine fusion and, 514-518
Infection
  disc space, 427-428
  electrophysiology in lumbar pain and, 548-549
  pin track, 342
  spine plating with pedicle screws and, 331
Inferior laminotomy, 161
Inferior vena cava, 373
  laceration of, 369
Inflammatory response, pain and, 529
Informed consent, 109, 460-461, 462
Inguinal ligament, 436, 438
Injection technique for chemonucleolysis, 109-112
Inman, V.T., 10
Instability, 40; *see also* Stability
  checklist for assessing clinical, 60-61
  electrophysiology and, 547-548
  extensive lumbar decompression and, 217
  of first degree, 59
  iatrogenic, 217, 272-273, 275
  low back pain and, 40-42
  mechanical, 40-42
    laminectomy and laminotomy and, 153
    spondylolysis and, 275
  pathomechanics of, 266-268
  posterior decompression and, 42-43
  after posterior lumbar interbody fusion, 270-271, 297, 298
  of second degree, 59-60

Instability—cont'd
  segmental, 42, 266, 356
    anterior interbody fusion and, 417
    percutaneous lumbar fusion and, 512, 513
    posterior intertransverse process fusion and, 270-271
    surgical principles and, 356
  after simple disc excision, 273
  single motion-segment, 356
  of third degree, 60
Instantaneous axis of rotation, 55-57
Instruments
  microdiscectomy and, 125-127
  percutaneous fusion and, 513, 523
Interbody fusion
  anterior; *see* Anterior lumbar interbody fusion
  compared to other techniques, 267-268
  Lin, 83
  pedicle screw internal fixation and, 335
  posterior lumbar; *see* Posterior lumbar interbody fusion
    failed; *see* Failed posterior lumbar interbody fusion
  in redo surgery on failed spine surgery, 193-194
Interlaminar wire, 193
Intermittent conduction block, 532
Internal disc disruption, electrophysiology and, 544
Internal fixation, 276, 277-278, 306-314
  anatomy and, 74-85
    disc space in, 83-84
    facet joints in, 84
    lamina in, 77-79
    pedicle fixation in, 79-81
    sacral fixation in, 84-85
    spinous process in, 76-77
    vertebral bodies in, 82-83
  biomechanics of, 44-45
  complications of, 306
  history of, 13-14
  ideal, 75
  indications for, 45
    posterolateral fusion and, 415
  pedicle screws and, 322-338; *see also* Pedicle screw
  posterior interbody fusions and, 295
  posterolateral fusion and, 415
  problems with current methods of, 75

Internal fixation—cont'd
  in redo surgery on failed spine surgery, 193, 194
  rotational stresses on, 76
  short-segment spinal defects and, 339-367; see also Short-segment internal fixation
International Enzyme Units, 106
Intersegmental wires
  Harrington rod with alar hooks and, 310
  in lumbar fusion, 307-314
  results of, 312
Intertransverse fusion
  bone graft substitute and, 475-480
  midline approach for, 172
  posterior, 265-278; see also Posterior intertransverse fusion
  pseudoarthosis after, 268, 269
Intertransverse ligament, 67
Intertransverse membrane, 252, 253
Intervertebral disc; see Disc, intervertebral
Intervertebral foramen
  disc herniations lateral to, 195-207; see also Herniated disc lateral to intervertebral foramen
Intraabdominal pressures, 49
Intradiscal pressure, 38, 39, 49, 291
Intraneural blood flow, 530-531
Intraneural fibrosis, 546-547
Intraoperative nerve location, 178
Intraoperative x-ray film in microdiscectomy, 128-129
Intravenous medications, 319
Invert soda-lime glass, 474
Iohexol, history of, 10
Iopamidol, history of, 10
Iophendylate, hazard of, 150, 153
Irradiated bone
  biomechanical properties of, 450
  cobalt-60, 450, 464, 517
ISAM; see Index Sequential Access Method
Ischemia
  secondary to compressive forces, 531
  susceptibility to, 531
Isogenous fat graft, 507
Isosulfan blue dye, 154, 179
Isthmic spondylolisthesis, 280-283
  posterior intertransverse process fusion and, 271-272
Ito, H., 14

J

Jaccoud, S., 16
Jansen, E.F., 103
Jaslow, I., 15
Jaslow posterior lumbar interbody fusion, 15
Jenkins, J.A., 14, 15
Joint, facet; see Facet joint
Joint reaction force, 39
Judet, R., 13
Judet system of plates and pedicle screws, 323
Jumping, leg, 154-158
Junghanns, H., 8, 287

K

Kaiwa technique, 219
Kamin, P., 141
Kaneda, K., 13
Keim indications for lumbar spine fusions, 288
Kelly modification of Watkins posterolateral fusion, 268-269
Kennedy, F., 17
Kerrison rongeur, 130
Keyes, D., 8
Kidney, anterior fusion and, 400
Kidney rest, 398, 403, 406
Kiel bone, 452, 472
Kinematics, lumbar spine, 53-55
Kinesiology, 36
King, D., 13
Kirkaldy-Willis, W.H., 17
Kittners in anterior interbody fusion, 371, 373
Knapp, W., 27
Knee, protection of, 88
Knee-chest position, 96
  without frame, 90-91
Knee cushions, 97
Knee fusion, first description of, 241
Kneeling position
  Andrews frame and, 91-94
  cushioning and, 96-98
Knodt, H., 306
Knodt rod, 3, 70, 315-321
  advantage of, 321
  complications of, 319-320, 321
  contraindications for, 316
  distraction force via, 78
  editorial commentary on, 321
  in failed surgery patient, 193, 194
  history of, 13

Knodt rod—cont'd
  indications for, 316
  intertransverse process fusion with autogenous graft and hydroxyapatite with, 475-480
  laminar fixation and, 77-78
  lumbar fusion and, 306-307, 311
  lumbosacral spinal fusion and, 45
  pedicular fixation and, 80
  postoperative management of, 318-319
  results of, 312, 320-321
  technique for, 316-317
Knodt rod hook, 308, 316, 317
Kobe bone, 472
Kocher, T., 6
Kraag, M.H., 13

L

L1-L5 level
  diagnosis of clinical instability in, 60
  microdiscectomy and, 128, 129
L3-L4 level, percutaneous nuclectomy and, 147
L4-L5 level
  degenerative spondylolisthesis and, 283
  lateral herniations above, 198, 199
  percutaneous nuclectomy and, 147
L5-S1 level, 280
  lateral extraforaminal herniations and, 207
  percentage of displacement of, 280
  percutaneous fusion hazard and, 523
  percutaneous nuclectomy and, 147
  scar formation and, 213
  self-stabilizing details of, 218-219
  ventrolateral stenosis and, 169, 170
Lactated Ringer's, 369
Lamina
  disc space relationship to, 65, 66
  internal fixation and, 77-79
    spinous process in, 76-77
  overhang of, 159, 160
  screws through, 219
Laminar wire, complications of, 342
Laminectomy, 68, 69; see also Lumbar decompression
  bilateral, 69, 70, 172
  central, results of, 173
  decompressive
    broad or wide, 69; see also Lumbar decompression, extensive reoperation after failed spine surgery and, 189

Laminectomy—cont'd
  laminotomy vs., 148-163
    diagnosis and approach in, 151-152
    discectomy and, 158-159
    dissection and, 153-158
    editorial commentary on, 163
    epidural morphine and, 161-162
    exposure and, 153-158
    fat grafting and, 161-162
    history of, 149
    incision and, 153-158
    lateral lesions and, 161
    mechanical instability and, 153
    nerve freedom and, 160
    stand-up disc and, 159
    subarticular stenosis and, 159
  lateral extraforaminal herniations and, 203
  lumbar fusion with distraction rods and, 311
  posterolateral fusion using spine plates and pedicle screws and, 324
  with preservation and restoration of removed segments, 219
  spondylolisthesis and, 283
    hazard of, 271
  total, Knodt rods and, 316
Laminectomy frame, Hastings, 91, 251, 281; see also Frame
Laminotomy, 69
  approaches to, 161, 173
    inaccessible zone and, 226-229
    limited exposure in, 154, 155-157
  extensive lumbar decompression and, 226-229
  laminectomy vs., 148-163; see also Laminectomy, laminotomy vs.
  with partial facetectomy, 69
Lane, A., 16
Lange, F., 11
LaRocca, H., 10
Laser, 210-215
Lateral approach to pedicle and disc bar or spur impaction, 235
Lateral decompression, far, 175-186; see also Far lateral decompression
Lateral disc, 195
Lateral extraforaminal herniation, 195-207; see also Herniated disc lateral to intervertebral foramen
Lateral femoral cutaneous nerve
  injury to, 436, 442
  protection of, 88

Lateral fusion, nonhealing, 429-430
Lateral instability after posterior interbody fusion, 297, 298
Lateral laminotomy, 161, 173
Lateral lesion, laminectomy and, 161
Lateral localizing roentgenogram, 128
Lateral position, 89
Lateral spine flexion, 54, 55, 56
Lateral stenosis, 167-169
   bilateral-lateral fusion and, 260, 261
   electrophysiology and, 544
   impactors in, 233
   laminectomy and, 151
   laminotomy for, 161
   popular misconception of, 167
   posterior interbody fusion and, 292
Lateral subluxation after posterior interbody fusion, 297, 298, 300
Lateral-bilateral fusion to sacrum in older patients, 271
Leg
   jumping of, 154-158
   pain in
      isthmic spondylolisthesis and, 280
      lateral extraforaminal herniations and, 200
      spine plating with pedicle screws and, 332
Leg cushions, lower, 97-98
Lidocaine
   discography and, 413
   lumbar surgery and, 135, 150
Lidstrom, F., 10
Ligaments, vertebral, 289-291
   pain mechanism and, 36
   spondylolisthesis and, 284, 285
   sprain and, 36
Ligamentum flavum, 65-66
   epidural fat grafting and, 509-510
   microdiscectomy and, 130
Lin indications for lumbar spine fusions, 288
Lin modification of Cloward posterior interbody fusion, 83, 287
   results of, 298
Lindbloom, K., 9
Link rongeur, 130
Lipids, allograft and, 451
Lipidol, history of, 10
Lipoprotein, allograft and, 451
Litigation, 116
Load sharing, 51-52
Load transducer, fixator as, 343

Loads on disc, 49
Local anesthesia
   discography and, 413
   laminectomy and, 149
   paralateral approach and, 178
   percutaneous nuclectomy and, 143
Localizing roentgenogram, microdiscectomy and, 128
Longitudinal intraspinal veins, 121
Loosening of Knodt rod, 319
Lordosis
   Edwards modular system in, 194
   Harrington rod system in, 341
   in lumbar fusion, 307, 309
   Steffee plate in, 194
   Wiltse pedicle screw fixation in, 194
Louis, R., 13, 15
Louis plate, 80
Love, J.G., 8
Low back pain, 53
   clinical biomechanics of, 40-43
Lower leg cushions, 97-98
Lumbar adhesive arachnoiditis, 150, 153
Lumbar artery, fourth, 443-444, 446
Lumbar decompression, 230-236; see also Laminectomy
   bony entrapment and, 230
   exposures for, 134-140; see also Exposure
   extensive, 164-174, 217-229
      approaches in, 171-174
      autograft fusion and, 224-226
      background of, 219
      editorial commentary on, 174
      graft viability and, 222-224
      inaccessible zone and, 169-171, 218-219
      indications for, 171-174
      laminotomy and, 226-229
      lateral stenosis types and, 167-169
      neural arch autograft and, 219-220
      patient criteria in, 164-165
      procedure for, 220-222
      site selection criteria in, 167
      stability and, 171
      unilateral arch autografting and, 224
   impaction and, 231-236
   positioning patient for, 95-102; see also Positioning
   results of, 173
   surgical methodology and, 230-231
Lumbar fusion; see Fusion
Lumbar nerve
   discography and, 413

Lumbar nerve—cont'd
  electrophysiology of, 528-551; see also Electrophysiology in lumbar pain
  injury to, 530-532
Lumbar radiculopathy; see also Radicular symptoms
  degenerative spondylolisthesis, 272
  motor-evoked response in, 533
Lumbar sagittal mobility, 54-55
Lumbar spinal jacket, Raney fusion and, 407
Lumbar spine
  anterior fusion approach to, 384-392
    Raney, 405
  articulations of, 76
  bilateral-lateral fusion of, 250-264
  biomechanics of, 35-64; see also Biomechanics
  history of surgery of, 5-23; see also History
  internal fixation of; see Internal fixation
    short segment; see Short-segment internal fixation
  kinematics of, 53-55
  motion studies of, 524-527
  paralateral approach to, 175-186; see also Far lateral decompression
  positioning for decompression or fusion of, 96; see also Positioning
  stability of, 59-61
  stenosis of, incidence of, 166, 167
  tissue dissection and resection in, 208-216; see also Tissue dissection and resection
  x-ray series of, before chemonucleolysis, 109
Lumbar zygoapophyseal joint pain, 529
Lumbosacral corset, 330
  anterior lumbar interbody fusion and, 381
  bilateral-lateral fusion and, 263
Lumbosacral flexion, hazards of, 86-87
Lumbosacral myotome variations, 541
Lumbosacral spine
  axial rotation of, 55
  diagnosis of clinical instability in, 60
  fusion comparison and, 267
  biomechanics of fixation of, 44-45
  internal fixator for short segments of, 339-367; see also Short-segment internal fixation
Luque rectangular rod system, 45, 70-71
  history of, 3, 13
  laminar fixation and, 77
  lumbar spine and, 278, 310
  lumbosacral spine and, 45

Luque rectangular rod system—cont'd
  pedicular fixation and, 80
  sacral fixation and, 85
  span of, 341
Lymphazurin, 134, 154
Lyophilization, 465

M

Ma, G., 15
Ma technique for posterior lumbar interbody fusion, 298-299
MacElroy retractor, 136
MacNab, I., 9, 104
α-2-Macroglobulins, 106
Magerl, F., 13, 79
Magerl external fixator, 84, 341
  penetration depth of, 347
Magnetic resonance imaging scan, 153
Malabsorption syndrome, 247
Marcaine; see Bupivacaine
Marking needle in microdiscectomy, 128, 129
Marlex mesh, 447
Marrow, grafts and, 449, 471
Mathematic modeling, 52-53
Mathias plate, 16
Mathieu, P., 12
Matrix, decalcified bone, 516-518
Mayfield, F., 25
McElroy, K.B., 244-245, 250
McElvenny, R.T., 250
McPhee, I.P., 16
Mechanical instability; see Instability
Mechanical low back pain, 40-42, 150; see also Pain
Medial branch of dorsal primary ramus, 529
Median sacral artery and vein, 373
Medical data base system, 491-502
Medical status, 165
Medroxyprogesterone, 488
Menard, V., 242
Mendeleev, 10
Menopause, 247
MEPP; see also Miniature end-plate potentials
Mercer, W., 14, 286
Merthiolate, 450, 451, 464
Metabolic bone disease, 246-249
Metal, synthetic grafts and, 452, 473
  history of, 12-13
Methotrexate, 485
Methylmethacrylate, 454, 482; see also Bone cement

Methylmethacrylate—cont'd
  anterior fusion and, 380, 381
  donor site hernia and, 447
  pedicle screws and, 324, 325
Methylprednisolone acetate suspension, 126
Metrizamide
  discography and, 413
  history of, 10
Meurig-Williams plate, 322
Meyerding retractor, 135
Microcatheter for epidural anesthesia, 161-162
Microdiscectomy, 115-133
  average stay for, 119
  definition of, 68, 123
  disadvantages of, 132-133
  first, 9
  incision in, 135, 154
  instrumentation for, 125-127
  intraoperative x-ray films and, 128-129
  medications for, 125-127
  positioning for, 125-127
  postoperative management in, 131
  preoperative evaluation and preparation for, 124-125
  techniques for, 115-118, 129-131
  term of, 123
Microfibrillar collagen, 160, 505
Microlumbar discectomy, 123
Microscope, operating; *see* Operating microscope
Microscope stand, Contraves, 126
Microsurgery
  techniques for, 117-118
Microsurgical discectomy; *see* Microdiscectomy
Middleton, G., 6
Midline approach; *see also* Midline incision
  for intertransverse process fusion, 172, 277
  in microdiscectomy, 124
  paralateral or, 175
  results of, 173
  spondylolisthesis and,
    degenerative, 283
    dysplastic, 279
Midline incision; *see also* Midline approach
  lateral extraforaminal herniations and, 203, 204
  lumbar fusion and
    distraction rods in, 311
    spine plates and pedicle screws in, 324
Midline paramedial laminotomy, 161

Migration of bone graft, 296, 300
Milipore filter, 162
Milligan, P., 15
Mineral, scaffolding of, 472
Miniature end-plate potentials, 536
Mixed spinal nerve, 530
Mixter, J., 8
MLBS; *see* Mechanical low back pain
MMC; *see* Methylmethacrylate
Models, mathematical, 52-53
Moderately stable segment, 171
Monopolar needle, 535
Monticelli, M., 16
Mooney, V., 11
Morphine
  epidural, 161-162
  extradural, 182
Morphogenesis, percutaneous fusion and, 514-518
Morphometry, vertebral, 344, 347-348, 350-353, 357-358
Morscher, E., 16
Motion, 53
  erratic pattern of, 41-42
  helical axis of, 57-58
Motion segment of spine, 266, 287
Motion studies, 524-527
  after anterior interbody fusion, 409-410
Motor axon loss, 540
Motor unit action potentials, 538
  compound, 539
  sick nerve syndrome and, 546
Motor-evoked response, 532-533, 539
Motor unit recruitment, 538
Multidisciplinary team approach, 2, 541-542
  failed surgical patient and, 188
Multifidus muscle, 539
Multilevel discography, 412
Murphey, F., 25, 149, 150
Murphey blunt nerve probe, 159
Muscle fatigue, electrophysiology of, 538-539
Muscle jump, 154-158, 210
Muscle strengthening exercise, 263
Muscle stripping, 136
Muscle-pedicle bone grafting, 448
Myelography, 149, 150
  disc herniation and, 116
    lateral extraforaminal, 200
  fusion and
    anterior interbody, 412
    posterolateral, 271

N

Nachemson, A., 10
Naloxone, 162
Narcotics, 401
   for epidural laminectomy, 161-162
   paralateral approach and, 182
   preoperative reduction of, 165
Nasogastric tube, 369
Naylor, A., 8
Needle
   chemonucleolysis and, 109
   Craig biopsy, percutaneous discectomy and, 118
   discography and, 413
   electromyography and, 535-538
   microdiscectomy and, 128, 129
Neocalglucon syrup, 488
Neodymium-YAG laser, 210, 211
Nerve; *see also* Nerve root
   injury to
      anatomy and pathophysiology of, 530-532
      bone grafts and implants and, 442-443
      electromyography and, 540
      positioning for surgery and, 88; *see also* Positioning
      posterior lumbar interbody fusion and, 301
      types of injuries to, 531
   interference with circulation to, 503-504
   intraoperative location of, 178
   laminectomy and laminotomy and freeing of, 160
   protection of peripheral, 88
   spinal; *see* Spinal nerve
Nerve block, facet, 153
Nerve conduction velocity, 532
Nerve probe, Murphey blunt, 159
Nerve root, 67-68; *see also* Nerve
   anatomy of, 66
   anomalies of, 541
   chronic lesion of, 546-547
   injury to, after posterior lumbar interbody fusion, 301
   in posterolateral fusion with spine plates and pedicle screws, 325
   microdiscectomy and, 122, 130
   mobility of, 530
   retraction of, 158-159
   traction on, 530
Nerve sheath, 67-68; *see also* Nerve root

Neural and non-neural pain generator differentiation, 529
Neural arch autograft, 172, 219-220
   results of, 173
Neural arch defect, 272
Neural arch en bloc removal, 172, 173
Neural foramen, 180
Neurapraxia, 532
Neuritis of buttocks, 443
Neurologic deficit, 116
Neuromotion segment, 410; *see also* Motion
Neuropathy
   compression, 503-504, 532
   peripheral, 533
Neuro-Trace System, 178
Neurovascular bundle, 67
NG tube; *see* Nasogastric tube
Nitrogen gas envelope, 212, 215
NMR; *see* Nuclear magnetic resonance imaging
Nociceptive irritation, 36
Nomenclature, 65-71
   facet joint and, 66-71
   ligamentum flavum and, 65-66
Non-freeze-dried bone, 465
Nonmetallic synthetic bone implant, 453-454
Non-neural and neural pain generator differentiation, 529
Nonsteroidal antiinflammatory drugs, 135, 165
Nonsurgical treatment failure, 414
Nonunion, posterior, 383
Norfolk frame, 90
Nuclear magnetic resonance imaging, 412
Nuclectomy, percutaneous, 68, 141-147; *see also* Percutaneous discectomy
Nucleotome probe, 143-145
Nucleus aspiration probe, automated, 143-145
Nucleus pulposus, 37, 48, 291; *see also* Disc, intervertebral
   pressure in, 49

O

Obesity
   anterior fusion and, 384
   fat graft and, 504
   spinal surgery criteria and, 165
O'Brien, J., 16
O'Brien curette, 393, 396
Ogilby, C., 237
Oldendorf, W., 10
Older patient; *see* Age

Onlay graft, anterior fusion and, 378, 379
Operating microscope
　discectomy and, 119
　microdiscectomy and, 125-126
　paralateral approach and, 179
　position of patient and, 86
Operating system, computer, 501-502
Operating table, 88
Operative field access, positioning and, 86-87
Opiates, 319
Orthograft, 473
Orthopedist, 27-34
　anterior lumbar fusion and, 393-399
Oscillating saw, neural arch and, 221
Osteoconduction, 464
Osteocyte, 484
Osteogenesis, 453, 464
　percutaneous lumbar fusion and, 514-518
Osteoinduction, 464; *see also* Osteogenesis
Osteomalacia, 247, 483
Osteopenia, 247, 483
Osteophyte, 67, 230-236; *see also* Lumbar decompression
Osteoporosis, 483-490
　bone and, 247, 484
　clinical presentation of, 486
　cost of, 483
　history and physical examination in, 486
　laboratory evaluation in, 486
　magnitude of problem of, 483
　percutaneous lumbar fusion in, 513
　posterior lumbar interbody fusion in, 304
　radiology in, 486-487
　risk factors in, 484-485
　segmental wiring in, 310
　spinal surgery criteria in, 165
　treatment of, 487-489
Osteosarcoma, 517
Osteosynthesis, *de novo; see also* Osteogenesis
Osteotome, 214
　anterior iliac crest bone grafts and, 436
　Cloward, 220, 222
Osteotomy, impact, 252, 254
Oswestry bone, 472
Overdistraction, 321, 341

P

Package insert, bone banking and, 467, 469
Packed red cells, 124
Padding, 95-96; *see also* Positioning
Pain
　anterior column, 383-384

Pain—cont'd
　anterior interbody fusion and, 411, 417-422, 429-430
　chronic severe, 429-430
　data base description of, 499
　disc excision and, 272
　discogenic, 150
　　anterior interbody fusion and, 411
　electrophysiology in lumbar, 528-551; *see also* Electrophysiology in lumbar pain
　facet joint, 150
　generators of lumbar, 528-530
　isthmic spondylolisthesis and, 280
　lateral extraforaminal herniations and, 200
　posterior lumbar interbody fusion and, 287
　Knodt rods and, 319, 320
　leg; *see* Leg, pain in
　low back, 40-43, 53
　mechanical, 40-42
　radicular; *see* Radicular symptoms
　after redo surgery for failed spine surgery, 194
　sectored diagram for, 499, 500
　in segment adjacent to multilevel fusion, 194
Pantaloon, foraminotomy and, 271
Pantopaque; *see* Iophendylate
Papain, 103-114; *see also* Chemonucleolysis
　first injection of, 9
Papaya fruit, 105
Paralateral approach, 175-186
　choice between midline and, 175
　clean-out of disc space and, 181-182
　considerations in, 181-182
　drainage and, 182
　exposure in, 179
　fascia and, 179
　procedure in, 178-181
　results of, 173, 182, 186
Paramedial laminotomy, midline, 161
Paramedian muscle-splitting approach in microdiscectomy, 124
Paraparesis or paraplegia, posttraumatic, 60
Parasagittal reformatted images, 176-177
Paraspinal approach
　to lateral extraforaminal herniations, 203, 204-205
　to posterior lumbar intertransverse process fusion, 277
　to spondylolisthesis, 279, 281, 282
　by Watkins, 244

Paraspinal muscles, 210
  fibrillation potentials and, 537
  postoperative compartment syndrome and, 96
Paratenon graft, 135, 510
Parathyroid hormone, 484
Parker, 17
Pars, transected
  extensive lumbar decompression and, 224-226
  screws through lamina and, 219
Pars autograft, 172, 224-226, 227
Particulate graft of autogenous fat, 508
Patient
  analgesic pump controlled by, 319, 401
  age of; *see* Age
  chemonucleolysis and, 107-108
  extensive lumbar decompression criteria and, 164-165
  positioning of; *see* Positioning
Paulson, 15
Pedicle; *see also* Pedicle screw
  broken, 331, 338
  fixation of, 79-81
  fracture of, after spine plating, 332
  identification of, 66, 325, 326
  impactor for inferior, 233-235
  measurements of, 347-348, 350-353
  structures adjacent and lateral to, 67
Pedicle axis angles, 347, 350, 357
Pedicle fat graft, 507
Pedicle guides, 325, 326, 327
Pedicle plate in failed surgery patient, 193, 194
Pedicle screw, 45, 71, 322-338; *see also* Internal fixation
  alignment of, 332
  breakage of, 331, 338, 343-344
  buttress thread and, 359-360
  complications of, 331-333, 338
  contact pressure and, 341
  diameter of, 278, 347, 348-349, 350-351, 357, 358
  editorial commentary on, 338
  in failed surgery patient, 193, 194
  Harrington rod attached to, 308-309
  insertion of, 325-331
  length of, 340
  load testing and, 343
  mechanical characteristics of, 344
  operative time for, 330
  path length of, 347, 351, 352, 357-358

Pedicle screw—cont'd
  pitch of, 349, 353, 358-359
  placement angle of, 332, 344, 345
  posterolateral graft bed preparation and, 325
  posterolateral fusion and, 324-325
  prototype of, 354, 355-356
  pull-out strength of, 344-345, 358
    experimental types and, 354
    screw design and, 353
  safety of, 342, 356-357
  short-segment internal fixation and, 344-345, 348-349, 353-355, 358-360
  penetration depth in, 347, 349-350, 355
  results of, 312
  sacral, 308, 312
  size of, 278, 357
    limiting factor to, 344
  spine plates and, 322-324
  stress transfer and, 333-334
  through lamina and transected pars, 219
  toe-nailing effect of, 355, 357
  tooth profile of, 353, 359
  variable spine plate/pedicle screw system and, 324
  wound infection and, 331
Pedicle sounder probe, 325, 327, 328
Pedicle zone, 196
Pelvic instability
  Allen-Ferguson fixation and, 84-85
  bone grafts and implants and, 447
  dysplastic spondylolisthesis and, 279
Penfield dissector, 130
Percutaneous discectomy, 115-122; *see also* Percutaneous nuclectomy
  microsurgical discectomy and, 119-122
  technique for, 118-119
Percutaneous nuclectomy, 68, 141-147; *see also* Percutaneous discectomy
  discussion of, 145-147
  procedure for, 143-145
Percutaneous spine fusion, 512-523
  benefits of, 512-514
  conduction and induction and, 514-518
  decalcified bone matrix and, 516-518
  editorial commentary on, 523
  practical application of, 518-519
Perineural fibrosis, 117, 292, 503-504
Perineural ligament, 67
Periosteal elevator, Cobb, 252, 257
Periosteum of vertebra, cuff of, 393, 394

Peripheral nerve
  entrapment of, electromyography in, 533, 540
  protection of, 88
  structure of, 530
Peritoneal sac, ureter mobilized with, 387, 389
Peritoneum, visceral, 369-371, 372
Permission
  for chemonucleolysis, 109
  for donation, 460-461, 462
Peroneal nerve injury, 88, 448
pH, pain and, 532
Phenomenon, double-crush, 533
Phenytoin, 485
Phosphate depletion, 247, 486
Piezoelectric crystals, 214
Pilot-light beam, helium-neon, 210
Pin-hole stenosis, 168, 169
Pin track infection, 342
Plaque emboli to femoral artery, 384, 401
Plate, spine, 322-338; *see also* Pedicle screw
  contact pressure and, 341
  contouring of, 332
  length of, 340
  load testing and, 343
  Louis, 16, 80
  pedicle, in failed surgery patient, 193, 194
  Steffee; *see* Steffee variable spine plate/pedicle screw system
Platform, attaching and adjusting, 98-100
PLIF; *see* Posterior lumbar interbody fusion
Polyamide fiber, 482
Polyethylene, 473, 482
Polymeric pins, 482
Polymers, 473, 482
Polyphasic motor unit, 538, 545
Polypropylene, high-density, 482
Polyvinylpyrrolidone, 482
Porcine dermis for nerve root, 510
Porex, 482
Porites coral implant, 474-480
Porosity, 454, 472
Portal, A., 16
Positioning, 86-102
  access to operative field and, 86-87
  anesthesia access and, 87-88
  attaching and adjusting platform and cushions and, 98-100
  cushioned face rest and, 100-101
  cushions, rolls, frames and, 95-96
  decreased blood loss and, 87

Positioning—cont'd
  extension vs. flexion of lumbar spine in, 96
  kneeling frame, 96-98
  microdiscectomy and, 125-127
  peripheral nerve protection and, 88
  pressure point protection and, 88-89
  prone-sitting frame, 96-98
  techniques for, 89-94
  x-ray access and, 88
Positive sharp waves, 536
  postoperative stenosis and, 545
Postdecompression spinal instability or spondylolisthesis, 42-43
Posterior annulus, window in, 159
Posterior bone graft, 343, 439-442
Posterior decompression, 42-43; *see also* Decompression
  Knodt rods and, 316
Posterior fusion, 70; *see also* Posterior intertransverse fusion; Posterior lumbar interbody fusion
  anterior interbody fusion and, 425-426
  compared to other techniques, 267-268
  computed tomography axial images of, 525
  indications for, 414-415
Posterior iliac crest graft, 343, 439-442
Posterior intertransverse fusion, 70, 265-278; *see also* Posterior fusion; Transverse process fusion
  approaches to, 277
  compared to other techniques, 267-268
  editorial commentary on, 274-278
  indications for, 270-273
  pathomechanics of instability and, 266-268
  results of, 268-270
Posterior lateral disc, 195
Posterior lumbar interbody fusion, 70, 84, 286-295; *see also* Posterior fusion
  advantages of, 275-276, 296
    biomechanical, 288-292
    clinical, 292-293
  anatomic alignment in, 292
  choice of, 275
  complications of, 294-295
  disadvantages of, 276, 296
  editorial commentary on, 294-295
  failed, 296-305; *see also* Failed posterior lumbar interbody fusion
  history of, 15
  indications for, 287-288, 295, 415

Posterior migration of bone graft, 296, 301, 302
Posterior nonunion, anterior fusion and, 383
Posterior plates and screws, disadvantages of, 341
Posterior segment, 289, 290
Posterior spinal decompression, instability and, 42-43
Posterior spine surgery; *see also* Posterior fusion
  failed, 187-194; *see also* Failed posterior spine surgery
  Knodt rods and, 316
  Vermont Spinal Fixator in, 340
Posterior unroofing of nerve structure, 235
Posterior wedge approach, 172, 173
Posterolateral bone graft bed preparation, 325
Posterolateral disc osteophyte, 67
Posterolateral fusion
  anterior interbody fusion and, 425-426
  indications for, 414-415
  pedicle screw internal fixation and, 335
  radiographs of, 526
  surgical exposure in, 268, 269
  type and placement of bone grafts in, 268, 269
Postfacetectomy patient, anterior fusion and, 427-428
Postforaminal stenosis, 169
Postlaminectomy patient
  anterior interbody fusion and, 418, 423-424, 427-428
  posterior lumbar interbody fusion and, 415
Postoperative care; *see also* Postlaminectomy patient
  bilateral-lateral spine fusion and, 263
  electrophysiology and, 548-549
  microdiscectomy and, 131
Posture, 51
Pott, P., 242
Preload, 57-58
Preoperative evaluation and preparation
  chemonucleolysis, 109
  electrophysiology and, 548-549
  microdiscectomy, 124-125
Preoperative morbidity, anterior interbody fusion and, 408-409
Pressure points, 88-89, 95-96
Previously operated cases, 136; *see also* Failed back surgery syndrome

Primary fusion, indications for, 411
Probe, nucleus aspiration, 143-145
Procaine, 149-150
Progestins, cyclic, 488
Progressive lumbar degenerative scoliosis, 277
Progressive neurologic deterioration, 532
Prone position, 96
  bolsters and, 89-90
  frame for, 96-98, 178, 179
    Hall, 90
Propiolactone, 450, 451, 464
Protein
  bone morphogenetic, 451, 459, 464
    percutaneous lumbar fusion and, 514-518
  osteoporosis and, 485
Proteoglycan, 38
Protrusion, disc; *see also* Herniated disc
Pseudarthrosis, 44
  intertransverse fusion and, 268, 269, 277
  metabolic abnormalities and, 247
  Raney anterior interbody fusion and, 403
Pseudomeningocele, 320
Psychosocial problems, 116
PTH; *see* Parathyroid hormone
Puka chisel, Cloward, 378

Q

Quadriceps weakness, 200
Quality control in bone banking, 465-466
Questionnaire
  comprehensive history, 493
  for spinal surgery, 28-29, 32-34

R

Radial annular tear without herniation, 543
Radiation
  allografts and, 450-451
  cobalt gamma, 450, 464, 517
  xenografts and, 450-451
Radicular symptoms, 529
  anterior interbody fusion and, 401, 411
  degenerative spondylolisthesis and, 272
  lateral extraforaminal herniations and, 200
  motor-evoked response in, 533
Radiculitis, secondary, 529
Radiculopathy
  degenerative spondylolisthesis, 272
  motor evoked response in, 533
Radiofrequency current, 209

Radiography
  after anterior interbody fusion, 410
  herniations lateral to intervertebral foramen and, 200-202
  osteoporosis and, 486-487
  range of motion and, 55
Radionucleotide scanning with technetium-99m, 487
Radon, 10
Raney, F., 14
Raney anterior interbody fusion, 403-407
Raney modification of Kerrison rongeur, 444
Raney retractor, 374-375
Range of motion, 54-59
Rapid plasma reagin, 463
Rasps, 214
Ray neural arch autograft, modified, 219-220
Raylor retractor, 137, 138
  laminectomy and, 154
  skin incision and, 135
  stability at tip and, 139
Reciprocating saw, 214
Reconstitution of freeze-dried bone, 449
Record keeping
  bone banking and, 466-469
  computerized, 492-502
Recruitment, motor unit, 538
Rectus abdominis muscle, 369, 370, 371
Rectus sheath
  closure of, 391, 392
  exposure of, 386-387, 388
Recurrent disc protrusion; see also Failed back surgery syndrome
  clean-out of disc cavity and, 159
  electrophysiology and, 548
  failed spine surgery and, 189, 273
  indications for fusion and, 411
Referral pain, lumbar, 528-530
Rehabilitation, failed surgical patient and, 188
Reherniation, see Recurrent disc protrusion
Rehydration of bone, 449, 467
Reichert, F.L., 17
Reid, A., 11
Reimers plate, 322
Reinnervation, electromyography and, 540
Rejection, immunologic, 448
Relton frame, 90
Rene Louis plate, 16, 80
Reoperation, scar tissue removal in, 189, 190; see also Failed back surgery syndrome; Recurrent disc protrusion

Repetitive discharges, complex, 537
Replam Hydroxyapatite-Porites, 453
Resection, tissue, 208-216; see also Tissue dissection and resection
Residual neurologic loss, 532
Resorption, bone graft, 464
Retraction; see also Retractor
  fusion and, 136-137
    anterior lumbar interbody, 374-376
    bilateral-lateral, 252, 253
  lumbar decompressions and, 136-137
Retractor
  Beckman, 136
  Bennett, 137
  Cloward, 126, 127, 130
  force-fulcrum, 136-137
    neural arch autograft and, 221
  Gelpi, 136
  Hibbs, 135
  Hoe, 375
  Hurd, 260
  MacElroy, 136
  malleability of, 137, 139
  Meyerding, 135
  paralateral approach and, 180
  Raney, 374-375, 405
  Raylor, 137, 138
    laminectomy and, 154
    skin incision and, 135
    stability at tip and, 139
  Scoville, 136, 180
  Scoville-Haverfield, 126, 127
  stability of, 137-140
  Stake, 374-375, 379
  Taylor, 136, 137-138
    microdiscectomy and, 126, 127
    posterior iliac crest graft and, 439
    vessel injury by, 443, 444
  Thompson, 375
  Tower, 136
  T-Weinberg, 375
  Waugh, 257-259
  Williams, 126
  Wiltse, 135
Retrograde ejaculation, 373, 401
Retroperitoneal structures
  anterior lumbar interbody fusion and, 369-373
  percutaneous discectomy and, 118
RF; see Radiofrequency current
RHAP; see Replam Hydroxyapatite-Porites
Rigidity, type of fusion and, 267

Ringer's lactate, 369
Risser, J., 241, 244
Robin McKenzie protocol of therapeutic exercises, 124
Rod, distraction, 306-314
  breakage or dislocation of, 320
  Harrington; see Harrington rod
  Knodt; see Knodt rod
  Luque; see Luque rectangular rod system
Rod long, fuse short technique, 340, 342
Rodegerdts sacral plate with pedicle screws, 323
Roentgen, C., 6
Rolls in patient positioning, 95-96
Rongeur, 214
  Kerrison, 130
  Link, 130
Roofe, P.G., 10
Root, nerve; see Nerve root
Rotation, 53, 291-292
  instantaneous axis of, 55-57
Rotational stress on internal fixation, 76
Roy-Camille, R., 13
Roy-Camille plate and screws, 323
  length of, 340
  load testing and, 343
  penetration depth of, 347
Ruby-argon laser, 210, 211
Rugh, J.T., 241
Ruptured intervertebral disc, first diagnosis of, 8; see also Herniated disc
Rutherford, 11

S

S1
  H-reflex and, 533-534
  ventrolateral stenosis and, 169, 170
Sachs, B., 16
Sacral ala
  bone flap and, 277
  ventrolateral stenosis and, 169, 170
Sacral artery and vein, 373
Sacral buttress clamp, 329
Sacral hooks for Harrington or Knodt rods, 45
Sacral laminar thickness, 76
Sacral screw, 308, 312
Sacroiliac joint
  bone grafts and stability of, 447
  history of fusion of, 15
Sacrum
  bilateral-lateral fusion to, 271

Sacrum—cont'd
  fixation of, 84-85, 308-310
  internal fixator attachment to, 356
Sagittal rotation, 280
Saillant, G., 13
Saline injection, 150, 153
Scaffold
  metal, 452
  synthetic bone, 472
Scalpel, 135
Scan, technetium, 248, 249
Scar tissue removal, 189, 190, 213
Scarpa's sheath closure, 391, 393
Schanz pin, 341, 343
  history of, 13
Schöllner spine plate and pedicle screws, 322-323
Schmorl, G., 8, 287
Sciatic burnout, 148
Sciatic nerve
  injuries to, 442, 443
  posterior iliac crest graft and, 439, 444
  protection of, 88
Sciatic notch
  posterior iliac crest graft and, 439, 445
  removal of upper margin of, 444
Sciatica
  after anterior fusion, 429-430
  after Knodt rod fixation, 319
Scoliosis
  percutaneous lumbar fusion and, 512, 513
  progressive lumbar degenerative, 277
Scott, J., 16
Scoville retractor, 136, 180
Scoville-Haverfield retractor, 126, 127
Screw, pedicle; see Pedicle screw
Sea coral, 473
Secondary sterilization, bone banking and, 464-465
Sectored pain diagram, 500
Segmental innervation variations, 541
Segmental instability; see Instability, segmental
Segmental wiring, 307-314
  Knodt rods and, 321
  to sacrum, 310
Selby, D., 15
Semilateral position, 89
Semmes, R.E., 25, 149, 150
Sequestrectomy, 70
Serial somatosensory evoked potentials, 548-549

Seroma, 319
Serum calcium, 486
Shaffer, N.M., 239
Sharpness
    of curette, 252-254
    of cutting edges, 214, 215
Shaw hemostatic scalpel, 135
Shea, J., Sr., 25
Sheath, complex nerve, 67-68; *see also* Nerve; Nerve root
Sherman screw, 344
Shim, anterior fusion and, 379
Shordania, J.F., 9
Short-segment internal fixation, 339-367; *see also* Internal fixation
    design approach in, 343-347
    discussion of, 356-360
    methods of, 347-350
    results of, 350-356
    Vermont Spinal Fixator and, 340-343
Shoulder protection, 89, 100
Sicard, J.A., 10
Sicard plate, 322
Sick nerve syndrome, 546-547
Silicone-coated Dacron, 510
Single photon absorptiometry, 487
Single motion-segment instability, 356
Skin incision, 65
    lumbar decompressions and fusions and, 134-136
    percutaneous discectomy and, 118
Skin marking, 134-136
Skiodan, history of, 10
Sleeve, Edward, 78
Slot graft, 376-377
Smith, L., 9, 103, 104
Smith-Peterson, M.N., 15
Smoking
    bone abnormalities and, 247
    osteoporosis and, 485
Sodium fluoride, 489
Software, 498-501
Somatosensory evoked potentials, 535
Sonic curette, 214-215
Sore disc syndrome, 150
Sottac, 17
SP laser mode; *see* Superpulsed laser mode
Spatial resolution, 524
Specimen, bone bank, 463, 464; *see also* Bone banking
Spengler, D.M., 10

SPG; *see* Stereophotogrammetry
Spica cast, 271
Spiked retractor, 139-140
Spina bifida, 281, 316
Spinal adhesive arachnoiditis, 547
Spinal canal, short-segment internal fixation and, 341-342
Spinal cord injuries, 60
Spinal decompression; *see* Decompression
Spinal flexion, anterior, 54, 55, 56
Spinal fracture, scans of, 347
Spinal fusion; *see* Fusion
Spinal hypermobility from degeneration, 41
Spinal implant; *see also* Implant
    anterior vs. posterior, 357
    loads on, 360
Spinal instability; *see* Instability
Spinal jacket, lumbar, 407
Spinal motion segment, 36-37
    instability of, 42, 43
    pain mechanism and, 36
Spinal nerve, 530
    chymopapain and, 106
    friction fibrosis in, 531
    removal of adherent, 191-192
Spinal retractor, bilateral-lateral fusion and, 252, 253
Spinal stability; *see* Stability
Spinal stenosis; *see* Stenosis
Spinal surgery, questionnaire for, 28-29, 32-34
Spine; *see also* specific approach
    angulation of, 266
    coupling behavior of, 266
    extension of, 54, 55, 56
    functional unit of, 289
    lateral flexion of, 54, 55, 56
    loads on, 49
    translatory movements in, 53, 266
Spine plate; *see* Pedicle screw; Plate, spine
Spine surgery
    failed posterior, 187-194; *see also* Failed posterior spine surgery
    trends in, 3
Spinous process, internal fixation and, 76-77, 308
Spinous process spreader, Cloward, 220, 222
Spiralock, 346
Spondylolisthesis, 279-285
    adult with type II, 282
    clinical success of surgery in, 272
    congenital, 279

Spondylolisthesis—cont'd
  degenerative, 41, 283
    posterior intertransverse process fusion and, 272
  dysplastic, 279
  editorial commentary on, 284-285
  electrophysiology and, 545
  flexion/extension films and, 410
  fusion and
    bilateral-lateral, 260
    indications for, 411
    percutaneous lumbar, 512, 513
    posterior intertransverse process, 271-272
  history of reduction of, 15-16
  isthmic, 280-283
    posterior intertransverse process fusion and, 271-272
  Knodt rods and, 316
  of long duration, 172
  pedicle screw and, 334
  postdecompression, 42
  of recent onset, 172
  risk factors for progression of, 271
  spinal implant for, 339-367; *see also* Short-segment internal fixation
  surgical principles for, 356
Spondylolysis
  electrophysiology and, 545
  indications for fusion and, 411
  painful mechanical instability in, 275
  vertebral movement and, 343
Spondylolysis acquisita, postfusion, 44
Sprain, 36
Spring, Weiss, 78, 84
Spur, lumbar decompression of, 230-236; *see also* Lumbar decompression
Spurling, G., 25
SSEP; *see* Somatosensory evoked potentials
Stability, 59-61; *see also* Instability
  bone graft substitutes and, 477; *see also* Synthetic bone graft
  classification of, 59-60
  clinical, 40
  disc, biomechanics of, 40-43; *see also* Biomechanics
  evaluation of, 60-61
  extensive lumbar decompression and, 171, 217
  fracture and, 59-60
  microdiscectomy and, 120
  retractor, 137-140

Stability—cont'd
  sacroiliac, bone grafts and, 447
  upper limit of procedure for, 153
  Vermont Spinal Fixator and, 340
Stabilizer legs, 98, 99
Stainless steel wire, 453
  neural arch autograft and, 222
  pars autograft and, 226
Stake retractor, 374-375, 379
Standup disc, 150, 159
Statistical program, 498
Stauffer and Coventry posterolateral fusion, 269
Steffee, A., 13, 79, 322
Steffee variable spine plate/pedicle screw system, 313, 324
  advantages and disadvantages of, 312-313
  anatomy and, 79, 80, 81
  biomechanics and, 45
  history of, 16
  as ideal method for maintaining lordosis, 194
Stenosis, spinal
  approach in, 171-174
  decompression of, indications for, 171-174
  electrophysiology and, 544, 545-546
  failed spine surgery and, 189, 287
  far lateral decompression for, 175-186; *see also* Far lateral decompression
  foraminal
    electrophysiology and, 544
    spine plating with pedicle screws and, 333
  front-back, 168, 169
  herniated disc with, 172
  history of treatment of, 16-18
  incidence of, 163, 166, 167
  lateral, 167-169
    electrophysiology and, 544
    impactors in, 233
    incidence of, 163
    laminectomy and, 151
    laminotomy for, 161
    popular misconception of, 167
    posterior lumbar interbody fusion and, 292
  in older patients, 277
  percutaneous lumbar fusion and, 512
  pin-hole, 168, 169
  postforaminal, 169
  postfusion, 44
  subarticular, 159, 160

Stenosis, spinal—cont'd
　ventrolateral
　　herniated disc impingement and, 169, 170
　　lateral extraforaminal herniations and, 207
Stereophotogrammetry, 527
Stereotaxic system for chemonucleolysis, 110-112
Sterilization
　bone for grafts and, 450, 465
　secondary, bone banking and, 464-465
Stilbesterol, 488
Stinchfield, F.E., 250, 255
Straen, W.H., 10
Strain, 36
Stress, 36, 52
　anterior interbody fusion and, 381
Stress transfer, pedicle screws and, 333-334
Stress x-ray film, 381
Structural integrity, 524-527
Stuck, W.G., 12
Subarachnoid hemorrhage, 106
Subarticular stenosis, 159, 160
　results in, 173
Subarticular zone, 196
Subchondral bone, separation of end-plate, 393, 395
Sublaminar wiring, 76
Subluxation after posterior lumbar interbody fusion, 297, 298
Subperiosteal exposure of end-plate, 393, 394
Subperiosteal muscle stripping, 136
Sumita, M., 17
Superior gluteal nerve, 439, 442-443
Superior gluteal vessels
　arteriovenous fistula of, 444
　posterior iliac crest graft and, 439, 443-444, 445, 446
Superior hypogastric plexus damage, 369, 373
Superior laminotomy, 161
Superpressure water jet in cutting technique, 215
Superpulsed laser mode, 215
Surgibone, 472
Surgical approach; see Approach
Surgical procedure
　clinical biomechanics of, 40-43; see also Biomechanics
　frequency of use of, 31
　trends in, 3

Surgicel
　lateral extraforaminal herniations and, 203
　posterior iliac crest graft and, 439
　Raney anterior fusion and, 407
Sussman, B., 9
Suture; see also Closure
　anterior lumbar fusion and, 369, 371, 373, 379-380
　fat graft harvesting and, 509
　laminectomy and, 162
　microdiscectomy and, 131
　neural arch autograft and, 222
　Wolfe and Kawamoto technique and, 442
Sympathetic nerve plexus, 390
　anterior fusion complications and, 401
Synovial joint function, 37
Synovitis, zygoapophyseal joint, 529
Synthetic bone graft, 452-454, 471-482
　clinical experience in, 475-480
　current developmental work in, 474-475
　editorial commentary on, 482
　epidural fat grafting and, 510
　history of, 471-474
　structural strength of, 472
Synthograft, 473, 474
Syphilis, 463

T

Tanaka and associates neural arch autograft, 219
Tangential stress in annulus fibrosus, 37
Tantalum, 447
Tarlov frame, 91
　modified, 101
Taylor, C.F., 239
Taylor, H.L., 237
Taylor blade, 130
Taylor retractor, 136, 137-138
　laminotomy and, 228
　microdiscectomy and, 126, 127
　posterior iliac crest graft and, 439
　vessel injury by, 443, 444
^{99m}TC methylene diphosphate scan; see Technetium scan
TCP; see Tricalcium phosphate
TCP/BMP; see Tricalcium phosphate and bone morphogenetic protein
Teacher, J., 6
Team, multidisciplinary, 2, 541-542
　failed surgical patient and, 188
Technetium scan, 248, 249
Template, pedicle screw and, 329

Tension band fixation, 76, 82
Tension sign, 116
Thecal sac exposure, 260
Therapeutic exercises, 124
Thermal damage, 211, 212-213
Thigh cushions, 98, 99
Thimerosol, 450, 451, 464
Thomas, L., 103
Thompson retractor, 375
Thoracic spine, internal fixator for short segments of, 339-367; see also Short-segment internal fixation
Thorotrast, history of, 10
Three-dimensional imagery, 151
Thrombin, Gelfoam in; see Gelfoam in thrombin
Tibia, grafts from, 447-448
Tissue dissection and resection, 208-216
 cutting of bone in, 213-214
 electrosurgical cutting and, 209-210, 211
 injury in, 211
 laser and, 210-211, 214-215
 laser substitute in, 211-213
 sonic curette and, 214-215
 water jet and, 214-215
Tissue procurement, time between death and, 460
Tissue resection; see Tissue dissection and resection
Titanium implant, 452-453, 473
Tobacco
 bone abnormalities and, 247
 osteoporosis and, 485
Toe-nailing effect of pedicle screws, 354, 355-356
Toothed pedicle screw, 353, 359
Toothed retractor, 139-140
Tower retractor, 136
Towne, E.B., 17
Traction on nerve root complex, 530
Transaxial scan, percutaneous discectomy and, 118
Transected pars, 219, 224-226
Translation, 53, 266
Transperitoneal exposure, 373-374
Transplant; see also Bone graft
 history of bone, 459
 record of allograft, 468
Transplantation antigens, 451
Transverse myelitis, ascending, 105
Transverse process
 decortication of, Knodt rod and, 318

Transverse process—cont'd
 fracture of, 254, 255
 fusion of; see Transverse process fusion
Transverse process fusion; see also Posterior intertransverse fusion
 advantages of, 275-276
 choice of, 275
 degenerative spondylolisthesis and, 283
 Knodt rods and, 316
Transverse wedge, 173
Transversing dural sac, 66
Transversing nerve root, 66
Trap door, iliac crest, 436, 437, 440
Tricalcium phosphate, 453
 bone morphogenetic protein and, 516, 519
 porous biodegradable ceramic, 474
 porous hydroxyapatite compared to, 475
 synthetic bone grafts and, 473
Tricalcium phosphate and bone morphogenetic protein, 454
Tropism, 292
Truchly and Thompson modification of Watkins posterolateral fusion, 268
Tsuji technique of neural arch autograft, 219
Tuberculosis, 383
Tuck position, 96
Tumorogenesis, 517
T-Weinberg retractor, 372, 375

U

Ulnar nerve protection, 88
Uniform Anatomical Gift Act, 460
Unilateral arch autografting, 224
Unilateral herniated disc, stenosis with, 172
Unstable fracture, percutaneous lumbar fusion and, 512, 513
Unstable space, 171
Up-down compression of nerve, 167, 168
Ureter
 injury to, 444
 mobilized with peritoneal sac, 387, 389
 transperitoneal approach and, 374
Urine tests, 248-249, 486
Urist and Dawson posterolateral fusion, 270

V

Valgus deformity of ankle, 448
Valleix points, 6
Variable Sequential Access Method, 499
Variable Spine Plate System, 322, 324
Vascular injury
 bone grafts and implants and, 443-447
 percutaneous discectomy and, 118

Vascular supply, pedicle, 66
Vascular surgeon, 384
Venable, C.S., 12
Ventrolateral stenosis
  with herniated disc impingement, 169, 170
  lateral extraforaminal herniations and, 207
Verbiest, H., 17
Vermont Spinal Fixator, 340-343, 360-361
  history of, 13
Vertebral body
  compression strength of, 51
  internal fixation and, 82-83
Vertebral canal size, 316, 321
Vertebral depth, 393, 397
Vertebral end-plate; see End-plate
Vertebral fracture internal fixation, 335, 336
Vertebral ligaments, 289-291
Vertebral morphometry, 344, 347-348, 350-353, 357-358
Vertebral subluxation after posterior lumbar interbody fusion, 299
Viability of graft, 222-224
Virchow, R., 6
Visceral peritoneum, 369-371, 372
Vitamin D
  bone abnormalities and, 247
  osteomalacia and, 484, 489
Voluntary motor unit action potentials, 536
Von Bechterew, W., 16
Von Luschka, H., 6
Von Luschka nerve, 67
VSAM; see Variable Sequential Access Method
VSF; see Vermont Spinal Fixator
VSP System; see Variable Spine Plate System

W

Wadell, G., 11
Water jet, bone cutting and, 214-215
Watkins, M.B., 12, 244, 250, 251
Watkins paraspinal approach, Wiltse modification of, 175
Watkins posterolateral fusion, 268
Waugh, T.R., 250, 257
Waugh retractor, 257-259
Wax, bone; see Bone wax
Weber, H., 10
Weiss spring, 78, 84
White fat, 504
Whole-body computed tomography, 177-178

Wide decompressive laminectomy, 59; see also Lumbar decompression, extensive
Wilkins, W., 11
Williams, R., 9
Williams microsurgical discectomy, 119, 120-121
Williams plate and screws, 340
Williams retractor, 126
Wilson, P., Sr., 7, 13
Wilson and Harbaugh microdiscectomy, 120, 123
Wilson plate and screw technique, 76, 322
  screw length and, 340
Wiltberger, B.R., 15
Wiltberger posterior lumbar interbody fusion, 287
  results of, 298
Wiltse, L., 251
Wiltse internal fixation pedicle screw device, 45, 194, 313
Wiltse modification of Watkins paraspinal approach, 175
Wiltse posterolateral fusion, 269-270
Wiltse retractor, 135
Window of annulus, microdiscectomy and, 121
Wolfe and Kawamoto technique for iliac crest graft, 440-442
Wound healing, 136
  electrosurgery and, 209, 211, 212
  Knodt rods and, 319
  laser surgery and, 211
  spine plating with pedicle screws and, 331

X

Xenograft, 451-452, 472
X-ray films
  chemonucleolysis and, 109
  fusion and
    anterior, 381
    bilateral-lateral, 262, 263, 264
  metabolic bone workup and, 248, 249
  microdiscectomy and intraoperative, 128-129
  positioning for low back surgery and, 88
Xylocaine; see Lidocaine

Y

Yamamoto and Yamashita spondylolisthesis reduction and stabilization, 323

Yau, A., 79
Young, H., 12
Ytyrium, aluminum, garnet laser, 210, 211

Z

Zeiss operating microscope, 125-126
Zeilke, K., 13
Zielke system for internal fixation, 45, 82
Zindrick, M., 13, 18
Zucherman, Selby, and DeLong posterior lumbar interbody fusion, results of, 299
Zygoapophyseal joints, 529

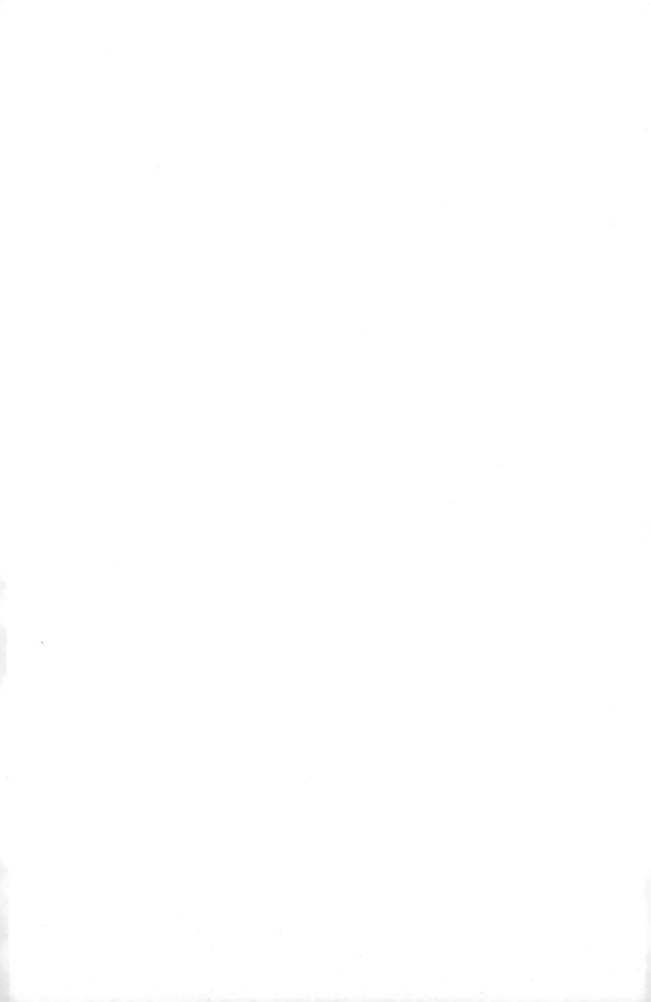